Community
PAEDIATRICS

Commissioning Editor: Ellen Green
Project Development Manager: Jim Killgore
Project Manager: Nancy Arnott
Designer: Sarah Russell

THIRD EDITION

Community
PAEDIATRICS

Edited by

Leon Polnay MB BS BSc FRCPCH FRCP DCH DObst RCOG

Professor of Community Paediatrics
University of Nottingham,
Nottingham, UK

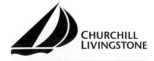

CHURCHILL
LIVINGSTONE

EDINBURGH LONDON NEW YORK PHILADELPHIA ST LOUIS SYDNEY TORONTO 2002

CHURCHILL LIVINGSTONE
An imprint of Harcourt Publishers Limited

© Longman Group Limited 1985
© Longman Group Limited 1993
© Harcourt Publishers Limited 2002

 is a registered trademark of Harcourt Publishers Limited

The right of L Polnay to be identified as editor of this work has
been asserted by him in accordance with the Copyright, Designs
and Patents Act 1988

First Edition 1985
Second Edition 1993
Third Edition 2002

ISBN 0443-06348-6

British Library Cataloguing in Publication Data
A catalogue record for this book is available from the British
Library

Library of Congress Cataloging in Publication Data
A catalog record for this book is available from the Library of
Congress

Note
Medical knowledge is constantly changing. As new information
becomes available, changes in treatment, procedures, equipment
and the use of drugs become necessary. The editors, contributors
and the publishers have taken care to ensure that the information
given in this text is accurate and up to date. However, readers are
strongly advised to confirm that the information, especially with
regard to drug usage, complies with the latest legislation and
standards of practice.

The
publisher's
policy is to use
**paper manufactured
from sustainable forests**

Printed in China
by RDC Group Limited

Preface

Community Paediatrics is now into its third edition. It has grown as the subject has grown and has needed more frequent updating as the pace of change has increased. The number of contributors has increased reflecting the increasing diversity and specialism within the subject. Recruiting contributors from the same District is intended to provide consistency and to provide a snapshot of the service as delivered in our local service.

Community Paediatrics is changing. The time spent in different roles have changed dramatically over the last twenty years, for example, a very large decrease in the primary care role and a parallel increase in secondary and tertiary work. The changes have meant that individual practitioners have found themselves doing a very different job at the beginning, middle and end of their careers. This is reflected in the quite different content and tone of the first, second and third editions of this book.

The age range covered by community paediatrics in generally widening and is now considered to be 0–19, with the greatest expansion being in services to teenagers.

The second edition was rewritten to provide a core text for our newly established MSc in Community Paediatrics. This course will soon be recruiting its tenth intake of students. It is hoped that our experience of running this course as well as in the development of clinical services in the community will add to the educational value of the text. I hope that the new edition will be useful to all paediatric trainees rather than just the group who intend a career in community paediatrics. Some new chapters have been added for example on Child Health in General Practice and Community Nursing. I hope, that these additions will provide a more balanced view of children's health care and expand the range of readers who will find the text useful.

The number of contributors has increased again from the second to the third edition, though I have kept to the principle of local contributors to enable discussion and exchange of material. There is, inevitably, a degree of repetition and overlap between chapters, but hopefully, this serves to link related areas and emphasise important points.

The scientific basis of community paediatrics is given more prominence and important gaps, for example in Social Science, Health Economics and Psychology filled. The service descriptions have been brought up to date. Whilst these largely describe the services in the UK, we hope they will reflect the important principal components of services for all readers. The largest section on clinical services has been written following a Programme of Care framework, reflecting the importance of multidisciplinary teams, in which the paediatrician is only one member and the work co-ordinated between agencies. By adopting this approach, the intention is to capture the essence of Community Paediatrics whilst avoiding duplication of accounts of paediatric clinical diagnosis and management to be found in other books.

During the process of writing, the contributors have discussed the content and presentation of their sections with one another and have asked our trainees for critical comment.

Textbooks, unlike literature, are seldom read for pleasure. The aim is to educate and to help develop an enquiring mind and a critical approach. This is essential so that the reader realises there is a 'sell by' date on the information and that advances are made by challenging current views rather than learning the contents of a book by rote. We cannot include in a book this size, all the evidence that has led us to the words in the text, but the references are intended to fulfil this function rather than simply to impress the reader with the number of sources quoted. The references are not intended for decoration and I hope you will dip into them at least to the knees if not to the neck as the contributors have had to do.

A textbook, at the end of its day, when much in it is obsolete, is still a historical statement of beliefs at that time. I hope we have taken pride in writing well in addition to writing correctly.

For the editor, the process of producing a new edition ensures that he revises his knowledge every five years. The extent to which the subject has changed between editions is astonishing, as the task of revision has, for most chapters, changed to rewriting. It is certainly the most thorough form of continuing medical education imaginable.

The real world of paediatrics does not as easily divide itself into chapters as a textbook. The reader needs to mentally reassemble the pigeon holes, called chapters, into a holistic view of child health. This is not an easy task.

Even in a growing textbook such as this, the contents still have to be selective. However, more extensive referencing, recommended further reading and liberal signposts to relevant websites should facilitate access to the wider literature.

This third edition has required some courage, optimism about the future of the subject and what my great uncle Max called, 'a good backside' to get the task done. The contributors have added the task of writing to very busy working weeks. I am grateful for their patience and persistence and guilty about the loss of sleep that I have caused. My thanks are due to them, to those who have influenced us, those who have encouraged us and those who have put up with our absence from the family life which is the subject of much of this book.

Nottingham   L.P.
2002

Contributors

Jo Aldridge
BA
Senior Research Associate
Young Carers Research Group
Department of Social Science
Loughborough University
Loughborough, UK

Martin Allaby
BA BM BCh DCH DRCOG MFPHM
Consultant in Public Health Medicine
United Mission to Nepal
Kathmandu, Nepal

Saul Becker
BA MA CQSW PhD
Professor of Social Policy and Social Care
Director of the Young Carers Research Group
Department of Social Sciences
Loughborough University
Loughborough, UK

Beryl Bennett
MA
Locum Educational Psychologist
Nottingham City Local Education Authority
 (LEA)
And Nottinghamshire LEA
Nottingham, UK

Giles O. M. Blower
BA (Hons)
Specialist Welfare Rights Adviser for People with
 Severe Learning Disabilities
Nottinghamshire Welfare Rights Service
Nottingham County Council Social Services
 Department
Nottingham, UK

Paul Brennan
BMedSci MBBS MRCP
Specialist Registrar in Clinical Genetics
Clinical Genetics Service
City Hospital
Nottingham, UK

Sandra Buck
MB ChB (Liverpool) DCH (London) MRCPCH
Senior Clinical Medical Officer
Queens Medical Centre University Hospital NHS
 Trust
Teenage Clinic, Victoria Health Centre
Nottingham, UK

Shirley Crosby
RGN RHV
Associate Director Children's Community Services
South Staffordshire Healthcare NHS Trust
Staffordshire, UK

Chris Dearden
BSc MA
Research Fellow
Young Carers Research Group
Department of Social Science
Loughborough University
Loughborough, UK

June Dickens
MA RGN RM RHV
Nurse Consultant in Child Protection
Broxtowe and Hucknall Primary Care Trust
Designated Nurse for Child Protection,
 Nottingham Health Authority
Children's Centre
City Hospital
Nottingham, UK

Elizabeth Didcock
BMBS MRCP DTMH FRCPCH
Consultant Paediatrician, Community Child
    Health
Queens Medical Centre University Hospital NHS
    Trust
Nottingham, UK

Keith Dodd
BSc MBBS FRCP FRCPCH DCH
Consultant Paediatrician
Derbyshire Children's Hospital
Derby, UK

Julia Faulconbridge
BSc (Hons) MSc C Clin Psychol
Consultant Clinical Psychologist
Head of Service
Community Child and Adolescent Clinical
    Psychology Service
Broxtowe and Hucknall Primary Care Trust
Children's Centre
City Hospital Campus
Nottingham, UK

Amanda Hampshire
B Med Sci BM BS MRCGP M Ed
General Practitioner and Lecturer in General
    Practice
Division of General Practice
Community School
University of Nottingham
Nottingham, UK

Pauline Harris
BA MPhil
Research Training Programme Manager
Graduate School
University of Nottingham
Nottingham, UK
Associate Lecturer, Social Science
The Open University

Kim Holt
MB ChB BSc DCH MRCP
Consultant Paediatrician
Child Development Centre
Saltergate
Chesterfield, Derbyshire, UK

Ann Howard
MBBS FRCPCH MFFP Dobst RCOG
Retired Consultant Community Paediatrician
Formerly Nottingham Community Health NHS
    Trust
Nottingham, UK

Helen Heussler
MB BS FRACP
Lecturer in Community Paediatrics
Division of Child Health
School of Human Development
Nottingham University
Queens Medical Centre
Nottingham, UK

Chris Jarvis
BSc SRD Dip ADP
Chief Paediatric Dietician
Nottingham City Hospital NHS Trust
Nottingham, UK

Derek Johnston
MD FRCP FRCPCH DCH
Consultant Paediatrician
Queens Medical Centre University Hospital NHS
    Trust
Nottingham, UK

Joyce Judson
ALA
Information Officer
Broxtowe and Hucknall Primary Care Trust
Children's Centre, City Hospital Campus
Nottingham, UK

Denise Kendrick
DM MRCGP MFPHM DRCOG DCH
Senior Lecturer
Division of General Practice
Community School
University of Nottingham
Nottingham, UK

James Lang
BSc (Hons) MA MSc PhD C Psychol
Consultant Clinical Psychologist
Community Child and Adolescent Clinical
    Psychology Services
Broxtowe and Hucknall Primary Care Trust
Children's Centre
City Hospital
Nottingham, UK

Liz Marder
B Med Sci BM BS MRCP FRCPCH
Consultant Paediatrician, Community Child
    Health
Queens Medical Centre University Hospital NHS
    Trust
Nottingham, UK

Elaine Marlow
BA (Oxon) MB BS MSc
Associate Specialist in Community
    Paediatrics/Paediatric Audiology
Pilgrim NHS Trust
Boston Health Clinic
Boston, UK

Barry McCormick
OBE PhD BSc CertTeach Deaf Dip Audiol
Special Professor in Paediatric Audiology,
    University of Nottingham
Director, Children's Hearing Assessment Centre
Director of Audiology, Nottingham Paediatric
    Cochlear Implant Programme
Nottingham, UK

Paul Miller
BA (Hons) MSc
Trent Institute for Health Services Research
Medical School
University of Nottingham
Queens Medical Centre
Nottingham, UK

Yin Ng
BSc MBBS MD MRCP (UK) FRCPCH DCH DRCOG
Consultant Paediatrician, Community Child
    Health
Queen's Medical Centre University Hospital NHS
    Trust
Nottingham, UK

Lyn Nixon
BA (Lib) ALA
Information Officer
Broxtowe and Hucknall Primary Care Trust
Children's Centre, City Hospital Campus
Nottingham, UK

Jon North
BSc MA
Co-ordinator
Networking Action with Voluntary Organisations
Mansfield, UK

John Pearce
FRCPsych, FRCP, FRCPCH
Professor Emeritus, Child and Adolescent
    Psychiatry
Nottingham University
Nottingham, UK

Catherine Rands
MB BCh MRCPCH
Associate Specialist in Community Paediatrics
Queens Medical Centre University Hospital NHS
    Trust
St Ann's Health Centre
Nottingham, UK

Heather Roberts
PhD MPhil Dip Ad Ed MFPHM
Academic Administrator
Division of Public Health Sciences
University of Nottingham
Nottingham, UK

Richard Slack
MA MB BChir MRCPath FFPHM DRCOG
Consultant and Senior Lecturer, Communicable
    Disease Control
Nottingham Health Authority
Nottingham, UK

Sue Spanswick
RGN BA MSc School Nurse Cert Health Ed Cert FETC
School Nurse Advisor
Broxtowe and Hucknall Primary Care Trust
Calverton Clinic
Nottingham, UK

David Spicer
LLB, Barrister
Head of Personal Legal Services
Nottinghamshire County Council
Nottingham, UK

Andrea Swarbrick
Paediatric Respiratory Nurse
Queen's Medical Centre University Hospital NHS
   Trust
Nottingham, UK

Helen Venning
B Med Sci BM BS FRCP FRCPCH
Consultant Paediatrician
Queens Medical Centre University Hospital NHS
   Trust
Nottingham, UK

Harrish Vyas
DM (Notts) FRCPCH
Consultant in Paediatric Intensive Care and
   Respiratory Medicine
Queens Medical Centre University Hospital NHS
   Trust
Nottingham, UK

Jane Williams
MB BS DCH MRCP FRCPCH
Consultant Paediatrician, Community Child
   Health
Queens Medical Centre University Hospital NHS
   Trust
Nottingham, UK

Contents

1. Origins of Community Paediatrics   1
Leon Polnay

2. Child Public health   7
Martin Allaby

3. Psychological needs of the community paediatrician   29
James Lang

4. Social science   39
Pauline Harris

5. Development   49
Leon Polnay and Liz Marder

6. Clinical genetics and genetic services: principles and practice   67
Paul Brennan

7. Nutrition   95
Chris Jarvis

8. Health Promotion   123
Honey Heussler and Heather Roberts

9. Growth   135
Derek Johnston and Elizabeth Didcock

10. Health Economics   155
Paul Miller

11. A simpleton's guide to management   167
Leon Polnay

12. Health services for children   177
Keith Dodd

13. Child health in primary care   189
Amanda Hampshire

14. Community nursing   205
Shirley Crosby and Sue Spanswick

15. Education services   217
Beryl Bennett

16. Social services   229
Saul Becker

17. Benefits   241
Giles Blower

18. Legal framework   253
David Spicer

19. Voluntary organisations   263
Jon North

20. Child health surveillance and promotion programme   269
Honey Heussler, Leon Polnay and Catherine Rands

21. Avoiding infection   289
Richard Slack

22. Unintentional injuries   309
Denise Kendrick

23. Health inequalities   323
Leon Polnay, Saul Becker, Jo Aldridge, Chris Dearden and James Lang

24. Avoiding harm: child protection   349
June Dickens, Elizabeth Didcock and Yin Ng

25. Young adults   381
Sandra Buck and Ann Howard

26. General paediatrics in the community setting   401
Honey Heussler, Leon Polnay, Catherine Rands, Andrea Swarbrick and Harish Vyas

27. Psychiatric disorder and emotional development   423
John Pearce

28. Emotional and behavioural problems   437
John Pearce

29. Counselling   469
Julia Falconbridge

30. Children with special needs   479
Jane Williams

31. Physical disability   493
Jane Williams and Helen Venning

32. Learning and health   509
Honey Heussler and Leon Polnay

33. Vision   527
Kim Holt

34. Hearing   543
Barry McCormick and Elaine Marlow

35. Speech and language   557
   Elaine Marlow

36. Learning disability   567
   Liz Marder

Appendix 1: Support groups   591
   Joyce Judson and Lynn Nixon

Appendix 2: Sources of information   595
   Joyce Judson and Lynn Nixon

Index   597

1 | Origins of community paediatrics

WHAT IS COMMUNITY PAEDIATRICS?

This area of paediatrics has been given different names over the years — community paediatrics, social paediatrics, ambulatory paediatrics. Some have denied the existence of it altogether and stress the holistic nature of paediatrics. Community-based paediatrics divides into several discrete areas: disability, social paediatrics, community-based general paediatrics (ambulatory paediatrics) and public health paediatrics. It is distinguished by the following hallmarks:

- The promotion of 'Health — Health for all Children' rather than the illness of a few.
- Very close working on a day-to-day basis with other community-based children's services, mainly education and social services and those delivered by primary healthcare teams.
- A population overview of child health as well as the individual perspective.

Community paediatricians do, of course, work closely with colleagues in hospital services and many have both hospital and community components of their post.

The early chapters of this book reflect the wide range of disciplines and services that impact upon the training of a community paediatrician: epidemiology, psychology, sociology, health economics, law. However well trained in these basic sciences and in paediatric medicine, the community paediatrician is not really 'up to speed' until he has detailed knowledge of the population, the environment and the services. In addition, there is the longitudinal element in terms of individual children and families and their histories and the changes

that are taking place within that community and the forces that are driving them.

ROLES OF THE COMMUNITY PAEDIATRICIAN

Not all paediatricians will contribute in every area and the proportion of time spent in any one activity will vary widely from post to post.

- Clinical diagnosis and management:
  — general paediatrics
  — disability
  — emotional and behavioural difficulties.
- Advice and support to:
  — children and young people
  — parents
  — teachers, schools and education authorities
  — social workers and social work departments
  — courts and other legally constituted bodies such as adoption panels.
- Social paediatrics, including:
  — child protection
  — adoption, fostering and children in residential care
  — young carers
  — targeted work with disadvantaged groups:
    family centres
    Health Action Zone programmes
    early intervention programmes, such as Surestart
    local initiatives.
- Health promotion:
  — district child health promotion co-ordinator: content of local programme, including referral pathways
  — local accident prevention programmes

— school-based health promotion programmes
— individual health promotion.
- Service management:
  — medical teams, finance, appointments
  — contributions at health authority, trust, primary care trust, locality and clinic levels
  — risk management
  — clinical governance.
- Service frameworks:
  — clinical guidelines and their audit (based upon clinical effectiveness)
  — service frameworks for each programme of care.
- Teaching and assessment:
  — medical students, postgraduate students, continuing medical education
  — paediatric trainees
  — other professional groups.
- Planning and information:
  — collection of routine and ad hoc enquiry service data
  — analysis of information and trends together with colleagues in the trust, primary care trust and health authority: levels of analysis include school populations, geographical populations, primary health-care team and primary care trust populations
  — Participating in local and district service planning.
- Child advocacy.
- Staff support.
- Research and development.
- Personal continuing medical education.
- Activities related to national and international bodies:
  — government
  — colleges
  — parent organisations
  — professional organisations.

MULTIDISCIPLINARY WORK

Team work is important for all paediatricians and an essential skill for all those who wish to work in the community. It would be very rare for the community paediatrician to be the only person involved with a particular child. The community paediatrician needs to know not only who are the others seeing a particular child (the 'professional-gram'), but also to have an understanding of their role, their training and the organisation to which they belong. This understanding needs to be reciprocated by the other professions, but we need to facilitate this process through excellent communication. We need consent to share information and to be sure that we have communicated as well with the parent and child as we have with our colleagues. This involves both verbal and written communication (letters to parents and children and writing in the Red Book — the personal child health record). The Red Book also serves as a source of information that parents can use to share information with others.

Community paediatricians usually have a geographical area over which they work and the functional multidisciplinary team is the other people in health, education, social services and the voluntary sector who share that same 'patch'. The process of becoming established as a new community paediatrician in a patch can be lengthy in view of the large number of contacts that need to be established. Paediatric training provides the 'driver's license', but the effective community paediatrician also requires a detailed 'map' of which he is a part.

A patch directory for a community paediatrician would include:

- All GPs and primary health-care team members.
- Primary care trust boards and their chief executives.
- Locality management for health services.
- School nurses.
- All schools, head teachers and special educational needs co-ordinators.
- Educational psychologists.
- Pre-school support teachers.
- Education welfare officers.
- Specialist advisory teachers.
- Local social service team members.
- Welfare rights advisers.
- Police child protection unit.
- Local voluntary groups.
- Local counsellors.
- Secondary sources of referral to hospital paediatrics, paediatric surgery, ophthalmology, ENT,

orthopaedics, dermatology, genetics, genitourinary medicine.
- Child and adolescent psychiatry, clinical psychology.
- Public health services.

Effective team work rests upon:

- Mutual respect.
- Ability to reach and keep to joint decisions.
- Knowledge of others expertise.

Places of work

Community paediatricians may work in many sites. 'The patch' minimises travelling times and increases local knowledge. The pattern will, however, be different for those who work in urban and those who work in rural areas. There is usually a central base with an office and secretarial and administrative support. 'Outreach clinics', which are often the largest part of the workload, take place at home visits, schools, nurseries, family centres, residential care homes, primary healthcare teams, hospital and child development centres.

TRAINING

Training posts at senior house officer (SHO) and specialist registrar level for aspiring community paediatricians have been developed from the mid-1980s. It is now a requirement that all paediatric trainees whether planning a career in hospital, community or in a combined service must include 6 months of community paediatrics at both SHO and specialist registrar levels. GP trainees may also include community paediatric posts as part of vocational training.

FUTURE AMBITIONS

The pattern of development of community paediatrics in the UK has been mixed with wide variation in the strength and staffing of the service. In the most developed areas it is becoming the mainstream of general paediatrics delivered at a local community level and a districtwide network of specialty services in each of the workstreams listed above.

HISTORY

Child health services in the community began to develop in Britain 200 years ago. This development was brought about by an interest in the interrelationship between environment and health, 'public health', and also by a change in attitude in which it was not possible to ignore or simply accept the ill health of the poor. The industrial revolution led to an increasing density of population in poor housing and this provided an ideal substrate for devastating epidemics of infectious disease. A combination of social conscience (sometimes tempered with self-interest in terms of fitness to work increasing productivity and reducing the need for charity), with scientific investigation and innovative ideas, led to a wide range of services whose aim was the *prevention* of disease. The main tools for prevention were regulation of the environment at home and at work and education particularly with regard to hygiene and nutrition.

Early landmarks in the development of preventative child health services

1769
George Armstrong established a dispensary for the infant poor and home visiting in London.

1833 Factory Act
This act prohibited the employment of children under 9 and restricted the working day of 9 to 11 year olds to 9 hours a day. It established an inspectorate to judge the fitness of children to work.

1842 Edwin Chadwick: general report on the sanitary conditions of the labouring population of Great Britain
Chadwick recommended that expenditure on sanitation would increase longevity and reduce demand on Poor Law Relief.

1847
The first medical officer of health was appointed in Liverpool.

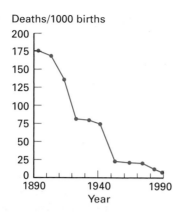

Fig. 1.1 Infant mortality

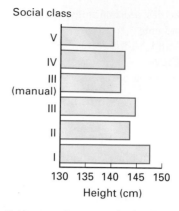

Fig. 1.2 Children aged 11 years, by height and social class

1867

First successful health visiting service established by the Manchester and Salford Ladies Sanitary Reform Association to employ 'a respectable working woman to go from door to door offering physical help and health advice'.

1888 Local Government Act

This act established elected county councils and empowered them to appoint medical officers of health who were required to possess a qualification in public health.

1890

The first school medical officer was appointed by the London School Board.

1891

The first certified course for health visitors was established in Buckinghamshire.

1893 and 1899 Education Acts

These acts gave local authorities discretionary powers to provide special schooling for blind, deaf, defective and epileptic children.

1899

First centre opened in St Helens to supply free sterilised milk to infants and mothers and advice and consultation.

1904 report of the Interdepartmental Enquiry on Physical Deterioration and the 1907 Education (Administrative Provisions) Act

This report was commissioned because of the very high (40–60%) rejection of army recruits for the Boer War. Their 53 recommendations covered an anthropometric survey, air pollution, housing and open spaces, diet and adulteration of food, physical exercise, alcoholism, juvenile smoking, sexually transmitted disease, medical inspection of school children. This important and far-sighted report — most of its recommendations would still apply today — laid the foundations for the school health service.

1908

The first school clinic was opened in Bradford.

1916 Report on Maternity and Child Welfare and 1918 Maternity and Child Welfare Act

This act provided free antenatal and post-natal clinics, medical cover for births and child health services for children under five. It led to the development of child welfare centres.

These developments in the nineteenth and the first part of the twentieth century laid the foundations for community paediatrics in the UK. Impressive and timely annual reports were produced on the health of children in each local authority. They pre-date the National Health Service (NHS) and the widespread development of the specialty of paediatrics practised in a hospital setting. The child health services remained part of the local authority.

1942 Beveridge Report

This report laid down the foundations of the NHS, to provide a social security system which provided access for everyone to comprehensive health services.

1944 Education Act

This Education Act required local authorities to provide free medical treatment for all school children and for parents to allow medical examination in school. School meals and milk were provided, school clinics were to provide services including the treatment of minor ailments, child guidance, orthopaedics, ENT, audiology, speech therapy, orthoptics, remedial exercises and chiropody, and special investigation for rheumatism, asthma and enuresis. The act also expanded the responsibility of the local authority to provide education for children with handicaps and 11 categories were established: delicate, diabetes, educationally subnormal, epileptic, maladjusted, blind, partially sighted, deaf, partially hearing, physically handicapped and speech defective.

1946 National Health Service Act

This act was established to provide 'a comprehensive health service designed to secure improvements in the physical and mental health of the people of England and Wales and the *prevention*, diagnosis and treatment of ill health'. It established a tripartite system of general practitioner, hospital and local authority services with the community child health services in the latter.

1967 Sheldon Report

This report recommended that child health services in the community should be provided by general practitioners.

1973 NHS Reorganisation Act

This 1973 act brought together the tripartite system into area health authorities, removing the child health services from local authority control.

1976 Court Report

This Committee made a comprehensive review of all health services for children with important recommendations for change. Not all these have been implemented, but the report became a powerful catalyst for change, particularly towards an Integrated Child Health Service.

We want to see a child and family centred service; in which skilled help is readily available and accessible; which is integrated in as much as it sees the child as a whole, and as a continuously developing person. We want to see a service which ensures that this paediatric skill and knowledge are applied in the care of every child whatever his age or disability, and wherever he lives, and we want a service that is increasingly orientated to prevention.

Among the committee's recommendations were:

- A multiprofessional team in each health district for the diagnosis, assessment and treatment of handicapped children — the district handicap team.
- At least one consultant community paediatrician per district with special skills in developmental, educational and social paediatrics.
- A general practitioner paediatrician (GPP), with special interest and appropriate accreditation.
- A child health visitor (CHV) who can combine preventive and curative responsibility for children.

Only the first two of these recommendations have been implemented.

Since the Court Report

The first consultant community paediatricians were appointed in Newcastle and Nottingham shortly after the Court Report. The service has changed from one which was responsible to community physicians to one of consultant-led teams. The grading of community health doctors as clinical medical officer (CMO) and senior clinical medical officer (SCMO) has been broadened to include training grades at SHO, registrar and senior registrar levels to prepare them for consultant appointments. New career grade doctors are appointed at

Origins of community paediatrics

staff grade or associate specialist levels, instead of CMO and SCMO, bringing the staffing structure into line with the rest of medicine.

Many roles have or are changing. The central role of health visitors and school nurses in child health surveillance is recognised. Family doctors are taking many of the roles of the child health doctor, mainly in pre-school surveillance. The work in community child health is increasingly demanding higher levels of specialist training operating a referral service for family doctors and a much closer working arrangement with other paediatricians as part of a district service.

At the interface between public health and community paediatrics is the need to establish a district-wide system to ensure that there is information about the health and health needs of the whole population as well as a clinical service for individuals. Community paediatricians need to re-discover, if indeed they have lost them, their roots in public health. The role of community paediatrics as a service that is 'health driven' needs to be recognised, as is the role of the community paediatrician as an advocate for the needs of children.

The interfaces between community paediatrics and education and social services have been of major importance throughout the history of the service. They are being drawn closer together by the consistent emphasis on interdisciplinary working arising in major reports, policy documents and legislation. Important examples are the Court Report, the 1981 Education Act and the 1989 Children Act. Working together at local, district, regional and national levels has always been the key to successful services.

The importance of prevention, highlighted by the first innovations 200 years ago, is reasserting itself.

Successive policies such as 'Health of the Nation' and 'Our Healthier Nation' have set national targets for improving health. Local Health Improvement Plans (HImP) contain national and local targets. Health Action Zones sponsor a wide range of innovative programmes in partnership with local authorities and local communities. These programmes work alongside other national initiatives based on similar philosophies: the New Deal for Communities aims at regeneration of deprived areas; Surestart provides better opportunities for under fours in deprived areas and Education Action Zones seek to raise standards of school achievement. Quality Protects and The Children's Safeguard Review aim to improve the standards of care of children for whom social services carry responsibility. Commissioned NHS research is increasingly directed at areas such as teenage pregnancy, drug and alcohol misuse, nutrition and systematic reviews of topics such as vision screening or the school entrant medical examination. These research programmes will enhance the evidence base of the practice of community paediatrics.

This is an exciting time for the practice of community paediatrics with so much of present UK policy initiatives being directed at promoting health and reducing inequalities. It is hoped that the early pioneers of community paediatrics would be well pleased by what they see today.

REFERENCES AND FURTHER READING

Court SDM (Chairman) 1976 Report of the Committee on Child Health Services. Cmnd 6684. HMSO, London
Harris B 1995 The health of the schoolchild. A history of the school medical service in England and Wales, Open University Press, Milton Keynes

2 | Child public health

Broad vs. narrow approaches to public health

Public Health has been defined as 'the art and science of preventing disease, promoting health, and prolonging life through organised efforts of society' (Acheson 1988). Those who practise public health tend to incline towards one of two approaches: either a broad view that emphasises the social, economic and environmental influences on health, or a narrower view that emphasises the influence of individual behaviour and health services on health (Table 2.1).

Historically, the major improvements in child health as measured by mortality rates occurred before the advent of the National Health Service (NHS) in 1948. The reductions in child mortality up to that point cannot be due to medical care, and are probably the result of improved nutrition, hygiene and housing (Figs 2.1, 2.2).

The relative importance of health services and other determinants of health is a political as well as an academic issue. In 1992 a Conservative Government published the first national strategy for health 'The Health of the Nation'. Although this was welcomed as the first attempt to set targets for improving health, it paid very little attention to the social and economic causes of ill health. In 1999 it was replaced by a new strategy produced by a Labour Government 'Saving Lives: Our Healthier Nation'. Within this strategy are National Contracts for Health which identify what individuals, local communities and government can do to address the social, economic, environmental, behavioural and service provision determinants of cancer, cardiovascular disease, accidents and mental health (Table 2.2).

Long time-scales

As well as recognising the wide range of determinants of health it is important to consider the long time-scales, often decades, over which these factors may operate. For example, there is growing evidence that social and economic circumstances and growth in early life are important determinants of chronic disease such as stroke, stomach cancer and diabetes in adult life (Barker 1994, Davey Smith et al 1998).

Since 1979 there has been a substantial increase in child poverty in Britain, due to two main factors. Firstly, the proportion of children living in one-parent families increased from 12% in 1981 to 23% in 1998 (Office for National Statistics 1999). Secondly, the proportion of children living without a working parent increased from 9% in 1979 to 23% in 1995/96 (Department of Social Security 1998). Given the evidence linking childhood poverty with ill health in later life, these increases may herald unfavourable future trends in adult health.

Individual lifestyle choices regarding smoking, diet and exercise, for example, may not reveal their full effects on health for many years. Although most life-long smokers start their habit as teenagers, its effects on death rates are not apparent until at least 20 years later. Ultimately it becomes a very powerful cause of ill health, shortening life by an average of 7 years (Doll et al 1994).

An example of the potential long-term impact of services is provided by the American Highscope controlled trial of intensive pre-school education for deprived children. This trial demonstrated impressive benefits after three decades of follow up in terms of educational attainment, employment

Table 2.1
Two directions for public health

Characteristics	Broad	Narrow
Definition of health	Foundations for health	Absence of disease
Underlying theory	Socio-structural	'Lifestyle'
Motivating concerns	Inequalities in health; poverty; global environmental issues	Individual risks of disease
Major public health activities	Linkage of public health sciences with policy making	Cost-containment; disease prevention, especially in high-risk groups
Place of epidemiology	Balanced by other methods; participatory research	Emphasis on technique and clinical and molecular epidemiology
Advantages	Potential long-term global benefit	Short-term benefits
Disadvantages	Risk of failure because of breadth of concerns	Failure to address fundamental threats to global health

Reproduced with permission from Beaglehole R, Bonita R, Public Health at the Crossroads: Achievements and Prospects. Cambridge: Cambridge University Press; 1997 (Table 10.1, p. 212)

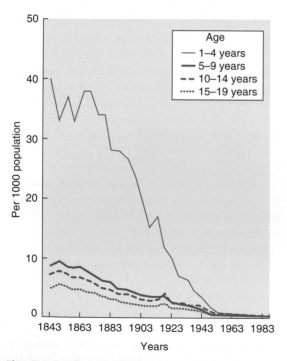

Fig. 2.1 Trend in mortality (5-year averages) under 20 years: 1841–45 to 1986–90. England and Wales. Source data: OPCS DHI/19 and DH2/17 (From Woodroffe 1993)

opportunities and criminality (Schweinhart & Weikart 1993) (Box 2.1).

In view of the long time-scales over which influences on health operate, and the tendency of disadvantages to be passed from one generation to the next, it is entirely appropriate that an Independent Inquiry Into Inequalities In Health (Acheson 1998) recommended that a high priority should be given to policies aimed at improving health and reducing health inequalities in women of child-bearing age, expectant mothers and young children.

Who does public health?

The public health function is fulfilled by anyone whose efforts are designed to improve population health. This includes not just people who would describe themselves as specialists in public health, but a very wide range of individuals and organisations, from health visitors working with individual families at a local level to national policy-makers who determine the priority to be given to improving health and reducing inequalities. At present the vast majority of public health specialists in the UK

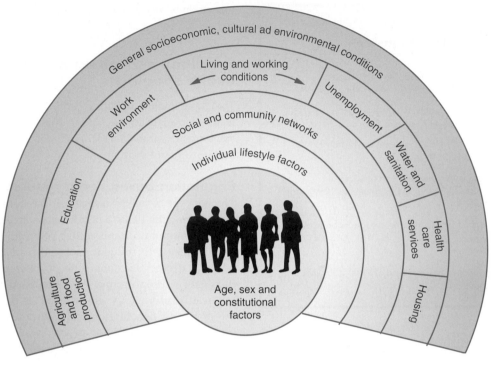

Fig. 2.2 The main determinants of health. (Whitehead & Dahlgren 1991).

Table 2.2
The government's 'Contract for Health' approach to improving health, using prevention of childhood accidents as an example

	People can	Local players and communities can	Government and national players can
Social and economic	Participate in local accident prevention initiatives	Identify and focus efforts on groups with the highest rates of accidents	Target resources to regenerate deprived communities
Environmental	Install, check and maintain smoke alarms	Develop safe play areas	Implement EC regulations on accident prevention
Personal behaviour	Wear cycle helmets	Ensure effective provision/ loans of safety equipment to target groups	Provide education/publicity on drink-driving
Services	Attend cycle proficiency courses	Make accident prevention a priority for health visitors	Make accident prevention part of the national curriculum

Child public health

Box 2.1
Later effects of Highscope

At age 27, graduates of the Highscope programme, a preschool intervention, had:

- Significantly higher monthly earnings (29% vs. 7% earned $2000 or more per month)

- Significantly higher percentage of home ownership (36% vs. 13%)

- A significantly higher level of schooling completed (71% vs. 54% completed 12th grade or higher)

- A significantly lower percentage receiving social services at some time in the last 10 years (59% vs. 80%)

- Significantly fewer arrests (7% vs. 35% with five or more arrests)

---

are medically qualified, but this is changing with the creation of new consultant-equivalent posts of public health specialists which will be open to non-medically qualified staff.

Before 1974 local authorities employed public health doctors as medical officers of health, where it was natural for them to address the social and environmental determinants of health. Since 1974 they have been employed within the NHS, where they were less immediately involved with such issues. The NHS reforms of the 1990s introduced a separation of the purchasing and providing roles within the health service: health authorities (and fund-holding GPs) became responsible for purchasing health services for their residents (or registered patients) from hospital or community trusts (the providers). In this arrangement public health doctors became increasingly preoccupied with advising health authorities about the effectiveness and cost-effectiveness of the health services they were purchasing, at the expense of considering other influences on health. The 1997 White Paper 'The New NHS' has changed the primary role of health authorities from one of purchasing services to taking a strategic lead in improving population health. This should help the public health staff employed by health authorities to broaden their

role again to address the full range of determinants of health.

Functions performed by public health specialists

The three major activities carried out by public health specialists are population-based needs assessment, strategic planning for health, and monitoring and evaluation.

Population-based needs assessment

The concept of needs assessment has been developed during the 1990s, a period when attention was directed more to commissioning of health services than to trying to influence other determinants of health. Current ideas about needs assessment are therefore focused around the assessment of need for health services, in which 'need' is defined as the ability to benefit from a healthcare intervention. A useful model for describing the role of healthcare needs assessment is a Venn diagram with three circles representing need, demand and supply of health services. Within this model the role of needs assessment can be described as the art of maximising the overlap of the three circles (Fig. 2.3).

The overall goal of needs assessment is to limit demand for, and supply of, ineffective or low-priority services in order to make resources available to implement high-priority, effective services. The essential components of any specific needs assessment are:

- The descriptive epidemiology of the problem. (Who does it affect? Where do they live? Is the problem getting better or worse?)
- A review of the effectiveness and cost-effectiveness of potential interventions. (What is known about the potential of different interventions to improve the situation?)
- The corporate view. (What services are currently in place? What is the potential for new ones? What are the views of parents, professionals, other agencies and national policy documents about the way forward?)

Having considered these elements, a good needs assessment should result in a consensus about the

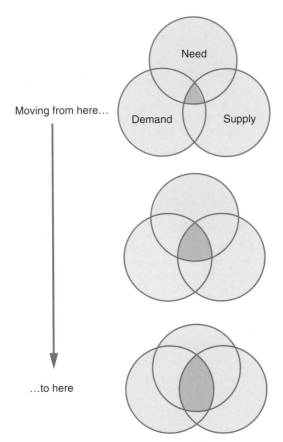

Moving from here...

Need

Demand   Supply

...to here

Fig. 2.3 The aim of needs assessment

best way to improve local services. In the context of child health, needs assessment includes:

- Discouraging the supply of services that are probably ineffective, for example by dissuading ophthalmologists from promoting vision screening before 4 years of age.
- Managing parental demand for services that are not strictly necessary, such as GP home visits for minor self-limiting illnesses.
- Identifying the unmet need for effective services such as screening for deafness in neonates.

Strategic planning for health

Having conducted a needs assessment the next step is to develop a strategic plan for change. Plans that have a primary aim of improving health can be difficult to implement because this is not one of the primary aims of the NHS. The government's over-

riding requirements of the NHS are that it should minimise the number of people on waiting lists, always be able to receive emergency admissions, and manage within its allocated budget.

Although these requirements do not readily lend themselves to improving child health, in the late 1990s substantial amounts of funding have been made available for specific policy initiatives that may benefit children. Examples of such initiatives include the Sure Start Programme, which aims to improve the support available to 0–3 year olds and their families in deprived areas, and Health Action Zones, which in some areas are focusing attention on the health needs of children. Although political demands often require that plans for these initiatives be drawn up at very short notice, they nonetheless provide important opportunities for local action.

Monitoring and evaluation of plans to improve health

This can be a relatively straightforward function of public health if the necessary data is collected in a reasonably complete, accurate and timely way through routine information systems. In practice this ideal is often not met and a judgement must be made whether to use routinely collected data, interpreted with caution, or whether to institute new collection of data specifically for the task in hand. The main sources of routinely collected data are summarised in appendix 2.

Some observations about child public health

- Material prosperity is probably the most important determinant of child health, and obviously it lies outside the control of health services.
- A growing proportion of children in the UK is growing up in relative poverty. Unless this trend is reversed there will be growing inequalities in health between rich and poor.
- There is growing evidence that deprivation in childhood predisposes to common diseases in later life. Therefore investment in improving the circumstances of children now is likely to have substantial benefits in the long term.
- The mental health needs of children and adolescence have been relatively neglected until

recently. Improving emotional health in childhood is probably a major area for improvement in the future (Stewart-Brown 1998).

- The importance of influencing teenagers' decisions about smoking is easily neglected by those who work with them, because its harmful effects are not seen until decades later.
- Because health services make at best a modest contribution to child health, it is important that community paediatricians develop their role as advocates who can champion the cause of children with other local agencies and nationally.

EPIDEMIOLOGY: TYPES OF STUDY, THEIR USES AND INTERPRETATION

Epidemiology is the study of how often diseases occur in different groups of people and why. Epidemiologists usually measure things in terms of rates rather than raw numbers.

Rates

A rate is a measure of the frequency of a phenomenon. In epidemiology, a rate is an expression of the frequency with which an event occurs in a defined population; the use of rates rather than raw numbers is essential for comparison of experience between populations at different times, different places or among different classes of people (Fig. 2.4).

The components of a rate are the numerator, the denominator, the specified time in which the events occur, and usually a multiplier, a power of 10, which converts the rate from an awkward fraction or decimal number to a whole number:

$$Rate = \frac{Number\ of\ events\ in\ specified\ period}{Average\ population\ during\ the\ period} \times 10^n$$

Different sorts of rates

Incidence is: the number of '*new*' cases occurring during a specified time (usually a year) as a proportion of the total population *at risk* of developing the condition.

Prevalence is the number of *existing* cases at a specific point in time as a proportion of the total number of persons in the population at that time.

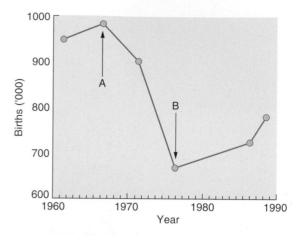

Fig. 2.4 The differences in rates at two different times when the number of cases or events is identical but the denominator changes. If there were 2000 new cases of condition x noted at points A&B, the incidence rates of x in the population would be approximately 2 per 1000 and 3 per 1000 respectively.

Prevalence may be measured at a point in time (point prevalence) or over a period of time (period prevalence). Prevalence measures a combination of new and 'old' cases.

Types of epidemiological study
(Table 2.3)

Descriptive or analytical?

Studies of prevalence or incidence are purely descriptive: they do not, in themselves, involve comparing different rates and drawing conclusions from any differences observed. Studies that compare rates and draw conclusions from any differences are 'analytical'. Prevalence or incidence studies can be combined in an analytical way to draw inferences about causation. For example, in international comparisons across European countries current adult mortality rates from stroke can be shown to be highly correlated with infant mortality rates in the same countries 60 years ago; this may indicate that deprivation in childhood predisposes to stroke in adulthood. Such studies are termed 'ecological'. Because they often use published data they can be relatively quick and cheap to perform. Their main disadvantage is that they compare rates derived from populations, not data obtained from individuals, and correlations that

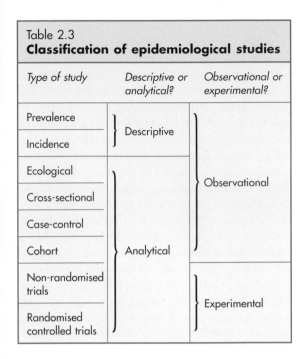

Table 2.3
Classification of epidemiological studies

Type of study	Descriptive or analytical?	Observational or experimental?
Prevalence	} Descriptive	
Incidence		
Ecological		} Observational
Cross-sectional		
Case-control	} Analytical	
Cohort		
Non-randomised trials		} Experimental
Randomised controlled trials		

hold true at population level may not always apply to individuals within them.

Analytical studies of individuals include *case-control* and *cohort* studies. They are generally more expensive and time-consuming to perform than ecological studies, but their results tend to be more dependable (Fig. 2.5).

The British Paediatric Surveillance Unit's findings on Reye's syndrome (a rare and serious childhood encephalopathy) is an example of a case-control study. The parents of 106 children who had had Reye's syndrome and those of 185 children who had febrile illnesses were interviewed in order to compare antipyretic drug exposure prior to admission. The results of interviews showed that 59% of the cases compared with only 26% of the controls had taken aspirin. Significantly more control children had taken paracetamol compared to the cases. The authors concluded that there was a strong association between Reye's syndrome and

Case-control study

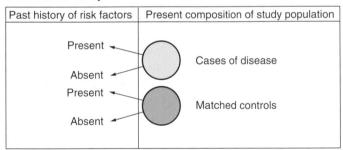

Cohort study

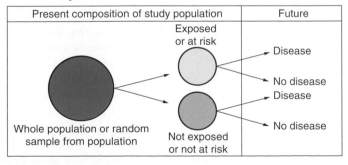

Fig. 2.5 The essential differences between case-control and cohort studies

pre-admission aspirin (Hall et al 1988). The routine use of aspirin in children under 12 years has been discouraged since 1986.

David Barker's studies of the relationship between birth weight, growth in infancy and risk of chronic disease in adulthood are examples of *cohort* studies. One of the largest cohorts he has studied is a group of over 10 000 men born in Hertfordshire between 1911 and 1930. The original midwife and health visitor records of birth weight, feeding method and weight at 1 year provide information about nutrition in early life. The risks of hypertension, stroke, coronary heart disease and diabetes were all greater among those who had lower weights at birth and 1 year, suggesting that good nutrition in early life, perhaps even before birth, may protect against these common diseases in adulthood (Barker 1994).

Observational or experimental?

Many epidemiological studies are observational, in that the study measures the consequences of exposure to risk factors of interest, but does not actually control exposure to those risk factors. Experimental studies are those in which the researcher does control who is exposed to the risk factor or intervention of interest. This degree of control allows the researcher to ensure that any apparent effect is due to the intervention of interest, rather than to baseline differences between the groups being studied or to other unexpected influences. The most rigorous form of intervention study is a randomised controlled trial. Broadly, the robustness of the analytical studies listed increases towards the bottom of Table 2.3.

Uses of epidemiology

There are essentially four things that epidemiology can do:

- Describe the distribution of disease.
- Explain why disease occurs.
- Predict the future.
- Measure the effectiveness of interventions.

Describing the distribution of disease

This is usually expressed in terms of time, place and person. This has traditionally been done for *individual diseases* or problems, such as the distribution of asthma or accidents. Prevalence studies can be used to determine the service needs for chronic conditions like cerebral palsy, diabetes, asthma, rheumatoid arthritis, etc. Surveillance systems can identify areas with a particularly high incidence of childhood accidents and target interventions such as health visitor advice about home safety and subsidised smoke alarms and stair-gates in such areas.

More recently the World Bank and the World Health Organization have taken this approach to describing the *overall burden of disease*, using Disability Adjusted Life Years (DALYs) as units of measurement. This allows one to quantify the relative contribution of different diseases to death and disability by age, sex and area of the world and thereby to identify priorities for action. For example it was estimated that in 1990, taking the world's population as a whole, half of all DALYs lost were due to death and disability among children under 15 years. However, this proportion varied from 66% in sub-Saharan Africa to just 9% in established market economies such as the UK (World Bank 1993).

Explaining why disease occurs

Detailed cross-sectional studies describing environmental and nutritional variables have enabled hypotheses to be postulated about the causes of several diseases, for example, spina bifida and vitamin deficiency, leukaemia and the clustering of cases around nuclear power stations. Case-control studies have enabled the most influential of risk factors to be determined, for example, the link between sleeping position and cot death, maternal rubella and multiple congenital abnormalities, damp housing and asthma, and smoking and glue ear.

Predicting the future

This can be done at the level of the individual, i.e. to establish a clinical *prognosis*, or at population level to *plan services* for the future. In terms of prognosis, for example, it is known from the 1970 National Child Development Study that the majority of asthmatic children under the age of 7 years do not require treatment for this condition by the time they reach 16 years (Butler & Golding 1986). When considering febrile convulsions, a knowledge of the family history and natural history of this condition helps determine treatment options and reassure parents. Children are unlikely to suffer from this condition after the age of 5 years and only 3% of those affected will go on to have true epilepsy.

In the area of service planning a knowledge of trends in the prevalence of, for example, deafness, learning disabilities and physical handicap in a population enables the planning of services for these groups of clients, such as the provision of specialist support teachers in school or the adaptation of public premises to enable access by the disabled. As sickle cell disease became more prevalent in certain communities there arose a need to provide specialist services such as screening mothers at risk antenatally, the provision of a specialist counsellor and the education of hospital and community health staff about the implications for treatment and follow up. The difficulties of non-English-speaking families in accessing health services provided by the NHS has led to the development of interpreter and link worker services in some districts.

Measuring the effectiveness of interventions

The term *efficacy* is used to describe the impact of an intervention under ideal circumstances, often in the context of a randomised controlled trial. One example is a randomised controlled trial which showed that giving women periconceptional folate supplements reduced the risk of neural tube defects in their babies. The term *effectiveness* refers to the impact of an intervention when introduced into routine service use. This can be monitored through surveillance systems that measure whether the incidence or prevalence of a disease is falling. Using the example above, there is concern that despite public information campaigns and professional education programmes about folate supplements, the population incidence of neural tube defects has not yet fallen in the way that would be expected. A more successful example concerns the incidence of cot death, which has fallen substantially following the high profile 'back to sleep' campaign.

For obvious practical reasons, some preventative measures can only be delivered to whole populations, and are therefore not amenable to evaluation through a randomised controlled trial. Provided the impact of such interventions is large it can be reliably assessed through a non-randomised trial. A classic example is the Michigan study of the reduction in dental caries following water fluoridation. One town (Grand Rapids) introduced water fluoridation in 1945 and the prevalence of caries halved. Since there was no change in the caries prevalence in a neighbouring town (Muskegon) which did not introduce fluoridation, the change in Grand Rapids could be confidently attributed to fluoridation.

There is a major international effort to collect in a systematic way the best available knowledge about what is efficacious. This is described further in the section on literature reviews on p 20.

Interpreting epidemiological studies

When interpreting any epidemiological study it is important to consider the roles that chance, bias and confounding may have played in producing the results obtained.

Chance

The role of chance is assessed by considering the statistical significance of results. This has traditionally been indicated by a P value. This indicates the probability that the result obtained could have occurred by chance, simply because the study samples happened to be unrepresentative of the populations from which they were drawn. By convention, if the P value is less than 0.05 (i.e. the probability is less than 1 in 20 that the result could have arisen solely by chance) the result is said to be statistically significant. Increasingly the statistical significance of results is being expressed through *confidence intervals*. These are mathematically related to P values, but convey more information because they provide an estimate of the range of values within which the true result probably lies. Most often, 95% confidence intervals are calculated: in 19 cases out of 20 the true result will lie somewhere between the upper and lower values of the 95% confidence interval.

Bias

Bias results from systematic errors. The data in any study will never be entirely accurate and the errors may be either random or systematic. Random errors may matter to the individuals involved but they do not concern epidemiologists very much because they do not bias the overall results of a study. Systematic errors are of much greater concern because they introduce bias and are therefore likely to produce erroneous overall results. There are no simple rules for assessing the role of bias, but the possible extent of both selection bias and information bias should always be considered. A useful starting point is to determine what study design has been used (case-control, cohort, etc.); in general, designs that appear nearest the bottom as in Table 2.3 are least likely to suffer from serious biases.

Selection bias arises when the subjects studied are not representative of the population about which conclusions are to be drawn. It occurs most commonly when a study achieves a low participation rate. Non-participants are always different from those who do participate, so results obtained from the participants may not be generalisable to the whole group. One example of selection bias concerns the ascertainment of congenital malformations. A change in the way that the Office of National Statistics (ONS) collected data about these in the Trent region in 1999 increased the completeness of coverage three-fold, thereby producing a large, but spurious, increase in the reported incidence of malformations.

A common error is the belief that the problems caused by a low participation rate can be overcome simply by recruiting more individuals to boost the numbers studied. Additional recruitment will increase the study's sample size and statistical power, but will do nothing to reduce bias.

Selection bias can also occur with the denominator populations from which incidence and prevalence rates are calculated. For example, when interpreting the widening gap in mortality rates between social classes V (unskilled) and I (professional) between 1971 and 1991, it has to be remembered that the size of social class V has shrunk substantially over time. Those who remained in class V in 1991 probably had a greater concentration of problems than the larger group who were in class V in 1971. As a result, the class V populations from the different time periods are not directly comparable.

Information bias arises from systematic errors in measuring disease or exposure to risk factors. Criteria for diagnosis may change over time; for example 'asthma' may have become a more fashionable diagnosis than 'wheezy bronchitis'. Meticulous epidemiology studies, using standardised diagnostic criteria for asthma, have been needed to establish that there has been a true increase in the prevalence of asthma in children.

Retrospective ascertainment of exposure to risk factors, for example in case-control studies, is prone to bias. In a study to estimate the risk of congenital malformations associated with maternal exposure to organic solvents such as white spirit, mothers of malformed babies were asked about their contact with such substances during pregnancy. Their answers were compared with those from control mothers with normal babies. With this design there is a risk that 'case' mothers, who were more highly motivated to find out why their babies had been born with an abnormality, might recall past exposure more completely than controls. If so, a bias would result with a tendency to exaggerate any risk.

Confounding

Confounding occurs when a variable other than the possible causal factor being studied is both unevenly distributed between different groups in the study and also related to the outcome of interest. For example, death rates from accidental injury in childhood could not be used to assess the quality of health services in different areas without taking account of the effect of differences in social class between those areas. The death rate from accidental injury is five times higher in class V than in class I, so deprived areas are bound to have higher death rates than affluent areas, regardless of the quality of health services. In this instance social class would be a confounding variable.

The effects of confounding variables can be controlled for either by matching the groups being studied at the design stage or by adjusting for them statistically during the analysis. With the increasing availability of PC-based software that can perform multivariate analysis, confounders are increasingly being dealt with at this stage rather than through matching at the design stage. The question that the reader should ask of any study is whether obvious confounders such as age, sex and social class have been accounted for, either by matching or by statistical adjustment.

Assessing causality

Confounding determines the extent to which observed associations are causal. Although recognised confounders can be dealt with as described above, it is always possible that there are other, unknown confounders that account for a supposedly causal relationship, for example between smoking and lung cancer. In assessing whether a relationship is indeed causal, the following additional criteria are helpful:

- How strong is the association?
- Is the association found consistently in different studies?
- Is there a plausible biological mechanism?
- Is there a dose–response relationship?
- Is there the expected time sequence, with the disease following the suspected cause?

INFORMATION: MAJOR SOURCES OF NUMERICAL DATA

Numerical data about child health comes from a wide variety of sources and is held in a variety of forms of varying accessibility. To build up a comprehensive picture one has to combine information from these various sources, which can be considered in the groups described below.

Populations, births and deaths

Census

This is a regular survey of the population, carried out every 10 years. The Doomsday Book is often considered to be the first national survey of this kind in the UK. Completion of the census form has been a statutory requirement since the Census Act of 1920. The answers given are treated in the strictest confidence and the results are published in an anonymous form. It is designed to count the population and its various attributes including data on the household, the numbers living in that household, amenities (bathroom, central heating, etc.), marital status, occupation, country of birth,

patterns of personal and public transport. The 1991 Census was the first to collect data on long-term illness and self-perceived ethnicity. Analysis is available at levels down to individual electoral wards. Between censuses the Office for National Statistics (ONS) calculates annual population estimates from the numbers identified on census day by adding births, subtracting deaths and adjusting for migration.

Births records

Records are kept of all births within the UK. The midwife or doctor attending the delivery of an infant has to make a notification to the Director of Public Health and the parents have to obtain a birth certificate, within 6 weeks, from the Registrar of Births, Marriages and Deaths. Originally these records were kept by local parishes but now ONS collates the data from around the country and publishes detailed analyses in quarterly and annual reports. The birth rate has been in decline since 1990. All abortions carried out legally are statutorily notifiable. Notification of congenital malformations was instituted in 1964 following the thalidomide epidemic; it is voluntary and coverage is far from complete.

Deaths

All stillbirths and other deaths have to be registered. Statistics derived from these registrations are published by ONS and are analysed by age, sex, cause and social class. It is essential to be aware of the definitions of the various death rates used (Fig. 2.6, Box 2.2).

Why distinguish between the different time-based mortality rates? The causes of perinatal mortality and postneonatal mortality differ, with the former reflecting antenatal, intrapartum and early postnatal care and the latter reflecting more social and environmental factors. In 1986 new stillbirth and neonatal death certificates were introduced which allow the certifier to include both maternal and fetal conditions which contributed to the death. Since 1975 infant death records have been linked to their corresponding birth records to obtain information about the baby's social and biological background.

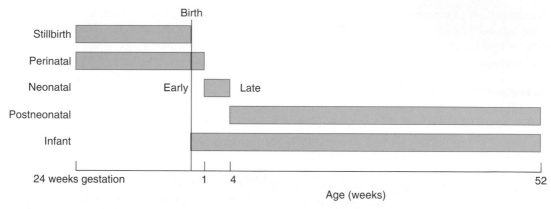

Fig. 2.6 Time period of mortality rates. Source: OPCS monitor DH3 91/2

> **Box 2.2**
> **Commonly used death rates in child health**
>
> **Stillbirth rate:** babies born dead with a gestational age of at least 24 weeks per 1000 *total* births. There are international variations in the definitions used for stillbirths. Sweden uses fetal length (35 cm) and Denmark uses weight (under 1000 g) in addition to gestation to define stillbirths
>
> **Perinatal mortality rate:** stillbirths and babies dying in the first 7 days of life per 1000 *total* births
>
> **Neonatal mortality rate:** babies dying in the first 28 days of life per 1000 *live* births
>
> **Infant mortality rate:** infants dying in the first 12 months of life per 1000 *live* births
>
> **Postneonatal mortality rate:** infants dying between the ages of 1 month and 1 year per 1000 *live* births

ONS longitudinal study

This was set up using a 1% random sample of the 1971 Census in England and Wales. Since 1971, members of the sample have been followed by linking data from birth and death registrations, cancer registrations and data from subsequent censuses. This study is a rich source of data on patterns of family formation, birth intervals, ethnic populations, parity, infant death and stillbirth.

Health-related behaviour (Figs 2.7, 2.8)

Infant feeding

There are 5-yearly surveys of infant feeding practice up to the age of 9 months giving data on the proportions of babies breast and/or bottle fed at different ages by age of the mother, social class based on parents' occupation, education and region.

Health behaviour in school-aged children

This WHO survey is administered at least every 4 years to a nationally representative sample of over 10 000 school children in England aged 11–15 years. Topics covered include smoking, drinking, physical activity and nutrition, psychosocial aspects of health, the school as a work environment, injury and social inequality. The 15 year olds are also asked questions on the use of illegal substances and on sexual health.

Morbidity and use of health services

Health survey for England

This annual survey of the health of people living in private households began in 1991. Children were first included in 1995. It combines questionnaire-based interviews with physical measurements. The 1997 survey was specially designed to yield a large sample (over 14 000) of children aged 2–15 years. In addition to information about smoking, drinking,

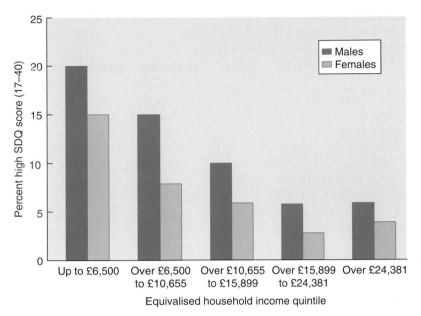

Fig. 2.7 Emotional and behavioural difficulties among children aged 4–15 (high SDQ total deviance score) by household income and sex. Reproduced with permission from: Joint Health Surverys Unit. The health of young people 95–97: Summary of Key Findings. HMSO, London

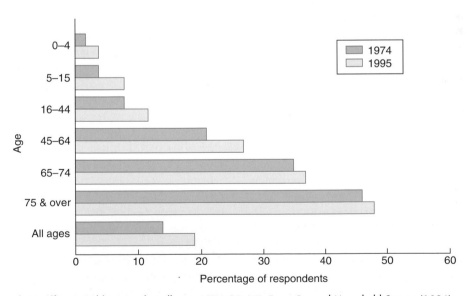

Fig. 2.8 Trends in self-reported longstanding illness: 1974–95, UK. From General Household Survey (1996)

eating and exercise, it provides data on mental health, respiratory problems, accidents, blood pressure and lung function. All of these can be related to social class and household income.

General household survey

This is an annual survey of a sample of over 10 000 households nationally and gives useful data about acute and chronic illnesses, domestic amenities and social and economic circumstances. Respondents who are responsible for children under 16 provide information on their behalf. The proportion of children who are reported as having a longstanding illness has roughly doubled between 1974 and 1995.

GP consultations

There have been three national studies of morbidity statistics in general practice: 1971/2, 1981/2 and 1991/2. These studies involve around 50 volunteer practices, which are therefore not representative of general practice as a whole, but nonetheless they provide valuable information about the pattern of less serious illnesses. The consultation rate in the most recent survey varied with the age of the patient — the highest rate was for the under fives. The commonest reasons for GP consultation in this age group were respiratory tract and infectious disease. The next most frequent reason for attendance was for preventative measures like immunisation and child health surveillance.

Hospital episodes

Hospitals collect data about day-case treatments and inpatient admissions through their patient administration systems. The most widely used measure is the finished consultant episode (FCE), which covers the period during which a patient is in hospital under the care of a specific consultant. If the patient is referred from one consultant to another during a single hospital stay they will be recorded as having two FCEs. The events are coded by clerical staff using the International Classification of Diseases (ICD-10) codes for diagnosis and the OPCS-4 (Office of Population Censuses & Surveys-4) procedure codes for any operations. The data are forwarded to district and regional level and then to ONS. This type of data is useful in examin-

ing trends of hospital usage by children and variations between districts (Fig. 2.9).

Infectious disease

Certain infectious diseases are notifiable (see Chapter 21) and the data is published on a weekly and quarterly basis by ONS. In addition, data is collected from hospital and other microbiology laboratories and collated by the Public Health Laboratory Service (Fig. 2.10).

Registers

There are many registers of individual diseases affecting children including cancer, physical disability, hearing, speech and visual impairments. Because inclusion on all these registers is voluntary they are often incomplete.

INFORMATION: LITERATURE REVIEWS

Systematic vs. non-systematic reviews

Until comparatively recently the typical process for writing a review article or an editorial for a medical journal ran as described below.

An acknowledged expert in the field of interest would be invited to write an article; since there would be little dedicated time available for drafting, and since the writer would already be familiar with the subject, the writer would start with a clear idea of the article's conclusions, and then work backwards to support them with appropriate references. The non-systematic approach might come up with the right conclusions, but formal comparisons against the conclusions reached by systematic approaches showed that this was often not the case.

A systematic review starts by identifying a clearly focused question, then it makes strenuous efforts to identify all relevant studies, and finally it reviews the results of all relevant studies to see what conclusions can be drawn. Provided the studies were addressing similar questions in similar ways, their results can be combined to produce a quantitative summary of the original studies; this is called a *meta-analysis*.

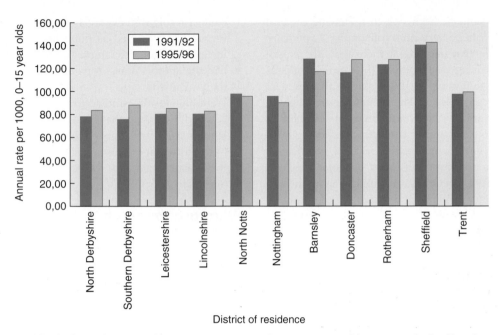

Fig. 2.9 Total finished consultant episodes (FCEs) per 1000 residents, 0–15-year-old age group by health authority: 1991–92 and 1995–96. From Patient Information System

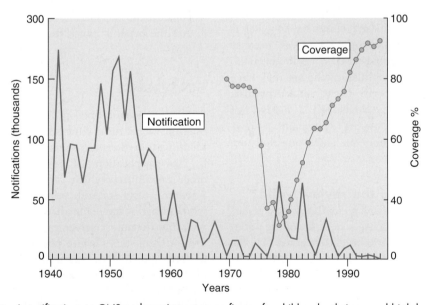

Fig. 2.10 Pertussis notifications to ONS and vaccine coverage figures for children by their second birthday: 1940–95, England and Wales. Reproduced with permission from Salisbury D, Begg N 1996 Immunisation against infectious disease. HMSO, London

This systematic approach to reviewing medical literature can be very time consuming. Experience has shown that even researchers who are experienced in using computerised literature databases are likely to find only half the studies that are relevant to a given issue. The remainder are likely to be found only by meticulous manual searching of relevant journals and by contacting research groups known to have an interest in that field. Fortunately the number of properly funded systematic reviews is increasing, and they are appearing more and more frequently in medical journals. The Internet is a very useful means of accessing good reviews. Two very useful websites are:

- The York Centre for Reviews and Dissemination at http://www.york.ac.uk/inst/crd/srinfo.htm
- The Cochrane library at http://www.cochrane.de/cc/cochrane/whatcdsr.htm

Critical appraisal of reviews

A well-conducted systematic review is an enormous asset; it vastly reduces the amount of time clinicians need to spend reading original studies, and produces an unbiased summary of what is known on a particular topic. However, because reviews can be influential articles, it is important to have a checklist for appraising whether they have been conducted properly. The Critical Appraisal Skills Programme has developed a helpful set of questions for appraising systematic reviews (adapted from Oxman 1994). These questions are detailed below.

Are the results of the review valid?

1. Did the review address a clearly focused issue? (An issue can be 'focused' in terms of the populations studied, the intervention given and the outcomes considered.)
2. Did the authors select the right sort of studies for the review? (The right sort of studies would both address the review's question and have an adequate study design.)
3. Were all the important, relevant studies included? (Did the authors use appropriate bibliographic databases; check reference lists;

contact recognised experts in the field; search for unpublished as well as published studies; and include non-English language studies?)
4. Did the authors assess the quality of the studies they included?
5. Were the results similar from study to study. (Consider whether the results of all the included studies are clearly displayed; whether the results of the different studies are similar; and whether the reasons that any variations in results are discussed.)

What are the results?

1. What is the overall result of the review? (Is there a clear 'bottom line' result expressed in appropriate units?)
2. How precise are the results? (Have confidence limits for the results been given?)

Can the results be used locally?

1. Can the results be applied to the local population? (Are the patients covered by the review sufficiently similar to those in the local population?)
2. Were all clinically important outcomes considered?
3. Are the benefits worth the potential harms and costs?

SCREENING

'Screening' was defined in 1951 by the US Commission on Chronic Illness as, 'The presumptive identification of unrecognised disease or defect by the application of tests, examinations or other procedures which can be applied rapidly. Screening tests sort out apparently well persons who probably have the disease from those who probably do not. A screening test is not intended to be diagnostic.' Once a person has been found to have positive or suspicious findings further tests are necessary in order to make the definitive diagnosis.

Screening is just one component of preventative child health care and is a form of *secondary prevention* of disease. This is the prevention of an impairment from progressing or its complete removal (or cure). The recognition of a raised thyroid-stimulating hormone (TSH) in the neonatal period following the heel-prick screening test enables definitive investigation and diagnosis of congenital hypothyroidism and subsequent thyroid hormone replacement therapy to be administered. *Primary prevention* occurs when the impairment is completely prevented from affecting the person, for example immunisation to prevent infectious diseases or traffic calming schemes to prevent road traffic accidents. *Tertiary prevention* is the minimising of handicap, once an impairment is well established and cannot be reversed or cured.

Screening is often confused with surveillance. Surveillance is the *ongoing* scrutiny of disease; in epidemiological terms, its main purpose is to detect changes in trend or distribution in order to initiate investigative or control methods. Child health surveillance is thus a combination of activities not just the application of specific screening tests.

Sensitivity and specificity

'Sensitivity' is the ability of the test to identify correctly those who have the disease. 'Specificity' is the ability of a test to identify correctly those who do not have the disease.

An ideal test would reach 100% sensitivity and 100% specificity. In practice, this combination is vir-

tually unobtainable. An improvement in one criterion is often associated with a deterioration of the other. Sensitivity and specificity vary according to the level which is chosen to separate normal from abnormal results. This is shown in Fig. 2.11, which plots the frequency distribution of the variable being measured and the results obtained when the cut-off point between 'normal and abnormal' is changed. Sensitivity and specificity are not of equal value (Fig. 2.12). A test which is 40% sensitive and 90% specific could not be compared with a test which is 90% sensitive and 40% specific. In the first case, 60% of those with the disease would not be detected. In the second case 10% of the diseased group would be missed, but 60% false positives would be generated. Specificity is made with the reference to the non-diseased group only, sensitivity with reference to the diseased group only.

In screening and diagnostic tests, the probability that a person with a positive test is a true positive (the person does have the disease) is referred to as the 'predictive value of a positive test' or 'positive predictive value'. The 'predictive value of a negative test' or 'negative predictive value' is the probability that a person with a negative test does not have the disease. Obviously, high predictive values are desirable. The value of the positive predictive value of a test is a/a+b and the value of a

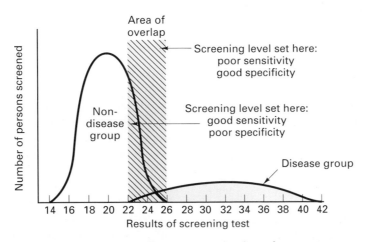

Fig. 2.11 Level set for the screening procedure will affect its sensitivity and specificity

SENSITIVITY = (a/a+c) The ability of the test to give a positive result in those individuals who have the disease

SPECIFICITY = (d/b+d) The ability of the test to give a negative result in those individuals who do not have the disease

PREDICTIVE VALUE This is a measure of the degree to which a positive test result predicts the presence of disease (may be positive or negative)

REFERENCE STANDARD

	True positives **a**	False positives **b**
TEST	False negatives **c**	True negatives **d**

Fig. 2.12 Calculating sensitivity and specificity

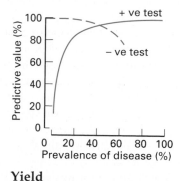

Fig. 2.13 Predictive value

negative test is d/c + d. The diagram shows the relationship between predictive value and prevalence when the test used has a high sensitivity (95%) and a high specificity (95%). Even with a screening test that has a high sensitivity and specificity, the predictive value will be low if the condition is rare (Fig. 2.13).

Yield

The yield of a screening test is the number of cases accurately identified by the test as a proportion of the total number of tests performed (= a/a + b + c + d).

The yield of a test can be improved by:

• Improving the test characteristics, i.e. increasing the sensitivity, e.g. by intensive staff training.

• Screening at the optimum time — this requires a knowledge of the natural history of the disease. For example, screening for 'glue ear' at school entry as opposed to the final year of primary school gives a higher yield of cases because of the tendency for this condition to spontaneously resolve with increasing age.

• Selection of high-risk groups or individuals — the prevalence of disease is higher in these categories so that hearing screening of very low birthweight babies using oto-acoustic emissions will yield a group of 6% of all babies born which will contain 60% of all sensorineural hearing losses. Similarly selective screening of disadvantaged children for language problems will yield much higher numbers than in the general population of children as a whole.

Other issues

Screening for disease within a community has its *costs*, not only in financial terms but also in emotional ones too. For example, if a test has a sensitivity of 90% (high by most standards) and a specificity of 98% and the true prevalence of the condition is 10% of the population ($n = 1000$), then at best the screen will pick up 90 patients. However, for every five 'true' patients identified there is one who will have a false-positive result and will be referred on for further investigation. This will mean not only additional costs of definitive tests, transport to the clinic, loss of employment but also more worryingly the additional concern and anxiety

Box 2.3
Criteria for appraising the viability, effectiveness and appropriateness of a screening programme (National Screening Committee 1998)

The condition:
- The condition should be an important health problem
- The epidemiology and natural history of the condition, including development from latent to declared disease, should be adequately understood and there should be a detectable risk factor, disease marker, latent period or early symptomatic stage

The test:
- There should be a simple, safe, precise and validated screening test
- The distribution of test values in the target population should be known and a suitable cut-off level defined and agreed
- The test should be acceptable to the population
- There should be an agreed policy on the further diagnostic investigation of individuals with a positive test result and on the choices available to those individuals

The treatment:
- There should be an effective treatment or intervention for patients identified through early detection, with evidence of early treatment leading to better outcomes than late treatment
- There should be agreed evidence-based policies covering which individuals should be offered treatment and the appropriate treatment to be offered
- Clinical management of the condition and patient outcomes should be optimised by all healthcare providers prior to participation in a screening programme

The screening programme:
- There should be evidence from high-quality randomised controlled trials that the screening programme is effective in reducing mortality or morbidity
- There should be evidence that the complete screening programme (test, diagnostic procedures, treatment/intervention) is clinically, socially and ethically acceptable to health professionals and the public
- The benefit from the screening programme should outweigh the physical and psychological harm (caused by the test, diagnostic procedures and treatment)
- The opportunity cost of the screening programme (including testing, diagnosis and treatment) should be economically balanced in relation to expenditure on medical care as a whole
- There should be a plan for managing and monitoring the screening programme and an agreed set of quality assurance standards
- Adequate staffing and facilities for testing, diagnosis, treatment and programme management should be available prior to the commencement of the screening programme
- All other options for managing the condition should have been considered (e.g. improving treatment, providing other services)

produced in a family because of the possibility of the patient having the disease itself. Similarly, if a person has the disease and the test is negative for that disease (10 of the total 100 patients will have such a result in the example given), then the costs of not obtaining early treatment may be very great, for example a false-negative phenylketonuria (PKU) or hypothyroidism test could have serious consequences in terms of late replacement therapy.

Any screening programme is only as good as the people who participate in it. One of the main issues around the *adequacy of cover* of many programmes is that the very people at highest risk are the ones who are not coming up to be screened. The prevalence of language and other developmental disorders is higher in the more deprived sections of our society and yet the services are not reaching them. There may be many reasons for this, including transport difficulties, financial restraints, organisational (the isolated single mother having to cope with four children under 5 years of age), and the value placed on the programme by the community. There is a significant advantage in being able to identify screening defaulters so that alternative approaches can be used, for example language stimulation programmes in day nurseries or 'captive' testing, i.e. the sweep hearing test or dental screening carried out for all school children soon after entry within the school itself (as opposed to a special clinic setting).

A distinction has to be made between screening tests and *case finding*. In the former, the screening test, if positive for a specific condition, is followed by more definitive tests. A McCormick toy discrimination test may be followed by free field audiometry in a controlled soundproofed room within an audiology clinic, or a positive Guthrie test will be followed by a full blood amino acid electrophoretic laboratory analysis. In the case of detecting testicular maldescent, the test used, careful physical examination of the groin, is diagnostic in itself and need not be followed by any other definitive tests in order to make a decision for the surgeon to treat.

Who is responsible for carrying out the procedure on any individual? Neglect of this essential aspect may cause a child not to be seen at all or result in chaotic overlap and waste of effort between groups such as health visitors, school nurses, community paediatricians and family practitioners. Confusion can result from different decisions on future management. A combination of better communication between practitioners and the application of routine clinical audit to this aspect of programme management should reduce the uncertainties in this area.

Criteria for appraising screening programmes (Box 2.3)

Since 1997 UK policy on screening programmes has been advised by a National Screening Committee, which has a child subgroup to consider screening issues specific to this age group. This Committee has published a checklist of criteria for appraising screening programmes that reflects current views regarding the range of issues that need to be considered (National Screening Committee 1988).

REFERENCES

Acheson D 1988 Public health in England. HMSO, London
Acheson D 1998 Independent inquiry into inequalities in health. The Stationery Office, London
Barker D J P 1994 Mothers, babies and disease in later life. BMJ Publishing Group, London
Butler N R, Golding J 1986 From birth to five — a study of the health and behaviour of Britain's five year olds. Pergamon Press, Oxford
Davey Smith G, Hart C, Blane D, Hole D 1998 Adverse socioeconomic conditions in childhood and cause-specific adult mortality: prospective observational study. British Medical Journal 316:1631–1635
Department of Social Security 1998 Households below average income 1979–1996/97. Corporate Document Services, Leeds
Doll R, Peto R, Wheatley K, Gray R, Sutherland I 1994 Mortality in relation to smoking: 40 years' observation on male British doctors. British Medical Journal 309:901–911
Hall S M, Plaster P A, Glasgow J F T, Hancock P 1988 Pre-admission antipyretics in Reye's syndrome. Archives of Disease in Childhood 63:857–866
Joint Health Survey's Unit. The Health of Young People '95–97. Summary of Key Findings. HMSO.
National Screening Committee 1998 First Report of the National Screening Committee. Health Departments of the UK, London
Office for National Statistics 1999 Social Trends 29. The Stationery Office, London
Oxman A D 1994 Users' guides to the medical literature

VI: how to use an overview. Journal of the American Medical Association 272:1367–1371

Salisbury D, Begg N (eds) 1996 Immunisation against infectious. HMSO, London

Schweinhart L, Weikart D 1993 A summary of significant benefits: the Highscope Perry pre-school study through age 27. High Scope Press, Ypsilanti

Stewart-Brown S 1998 Public health implications of childhood behaviour problems and parenting programmes. In: Buchanan A (ed) Parenting, schools and children's behaviour. Ashgate Publishing, Aldershot

Whitehead M, Dahlgren G 1991 What can be done about inequalities in health? Lancet 338: 1059–1063

Woodroffe C et al 1993 Children, teenagers and health: the key data. Open University Press, Buckingham

World Bank 1993 World development report: investing in health. Oxford University Press, Oxford

3 | Psychological needs of the community paediatrician

The work of the community paediatrician is inevitably stressful and at times unpredictable, but it is uncommon for the emotional effects of work to be discussed either amongst professionals or in research literature. It is equally uncommon to hear or see any discussion about ways in which a community paediatrician might look after his or her own emotional health. Indeed, recent evidence suggests doctors generally are not good at looking after their own physical or psychological health (McKevitt et al 1996), and neither are many of the professionals allied to medicine who all have in common the health care of other people.

Instead, it is common for those healthcare professionals to recommend to others ways of living more healthy lives whilst at the same time working within stressful environments themselves without making any plans or taking any action for looking after their own health. Often work stresses are played down or even ignored resulting in a professional and personal denial of one's own emotional needs. Whilst it is, of course, essential to identify the positive and rewarding aspects of a community paediatrician's job, it is as important to recognise and prepare for the inevitable work stresses and emotional difficulties associated with such work, and plan and implement functional ways of coping. Thus, in this chapter a review of work-setting pressures will be made, followed by an outline of common responses made by health professionals to such pressures. Finally, suggestions will be made about ways of looking after one's own emotional health.

WORK-SETTING PRESSURES

Expectations of others

Medical practitioners are still seen to be among the most trusted and reliable professionals and people are much more likely to disclose details of their personal lives to a doctor than to any other professional. Whilst this is undoubtedly a reflection of the respect afforded to the medical profession, it can result in patients and families expecting simple and swift answers to their problems. This is a particularly unrealistic expectation in much of the community paediatrician's workload, where the origins of child and family difficulties can result from a complicated mixture of medical, social and psychological issues. In many of these situations there is no simple solution, and families can present many times with chronic difficulties. The unrealistic expectations of others can, therefore, be a particular work pressure if they are internalised and become one's own unrealistic expectations.

Organisational stressors

In a recent study of the work stresses of hospital consultants three major sources were identified:

- The volume of work.
- The pressure from other peoples' expectations of them and demands made on them.
- The impact of work on personal lives (McKevitt et al 1996).

Psychological needs of the community paediatrician

An additional stressor was identified by junior hospital doctors which centred around decision-making and risk-taking associated with the job. This was obviously a function of inexperience and lack of confidence, but may also have been affected by the position of influence in which junior members of staff find themselves; they may have to meet both the patients' needs and senior colleagues and managers' requirements (Stoter 1997). Community paediatricians may find themselves in this intermediate position, in that there are often multiple competing demands from various sources (e.g. parents, child or teenager, school, social services, other health professionals).

Excessive workload and related time and organisational issues are the most commonly cited stressors by a range of health professionals. General practitioners, for example, list organisational unpredictability, time difficulties, interruptions and administration overload as their most stressful influences (Hambly & Muir 1997). Furthermore, significantly high levels of stress were identified in 50% of junior doctors where an excessive workload was combined with high levels of personal responsibility (Firth-Cozens 1987). Similarly, work overload was the major source of stress and tiredness for nurses at work (Dewe 1989), and a heavy workload was linked to high levels of anxiety, depression and psychosomatic disorders in a group of senior nurses (Baglioni et al 1990).

A list of common organisational pressures experienced by health professionals is shown in Box 3.1. These relate mainly to external influences connected with the work situation.

Psychological pressures

In addition to the organisational work pressures listed above, it is important to recognise the psychological pressures that are inevitably experienced by working with needy families. Many community paediatricians and other health professionals working with families are regularly exposed to emotionally draining situations in which they are attempting to help families who are in various forms of crisis or who are particularly demanding of the professional's resources. These families have

---

Box 3.1
Organisational pressures common to health professionals

Staff shortages and covering for colleagues

Professional isolation at work

Difficult team relationships

Lack of consultation and poor communication with colleagues

Lack of supervision, support and ongoing training

Unrealistic expectations by others

Feeling overwhelmed by volume of work and lack of time

Lack of preparation for the job

Frequent organisational changes

---

been labelled 'heartsink' patients (O'Dowd 1988) because of the emotional response that is evoked prior to seeing them. The important issue here is the psychologically stressful effect that constant contact with very needy families can have on the professional's emotional resources. Some of these particularly emotionally demanding family situations are shown in Box 3.2.

It is important to recognise that some families and young people evoke a more powerful emotional response in us than others. This is important for two reasons. Firstly, because we can only monitor our own emotional responses and needs if we are aware of how these emotionally demanding situations affect us. And secondly, because we need to be aware of how we respond to families who are in greatest emotional need so that we can remain professional. Stockwell's (1984) research with nurses is relevant here. She identified a relationship between the 'unpopular patient' who nurses labelled unhappy, more demanding, requiring regular attention and whom the nurses did not feel needed to be in hospital, and negative attitudes towards the patient and reduced levels of care.

Another feature of working with children and families in crisis is the extreme level and type of

---

Box 3.2
Emotionally demanding family situations

Dependent families requiring you to do something now

Families in crisis who are feeling out of control

Families where poverty and poor social conditions are the primary need

Families who are suspicious of help and/or vulnerable to feeling blamed

Parents who blame the child and label him 'evil, bad'

Children and teenagers who are anxious and/or suspicious of adults

Children and teenagers who are overly dependent on adults

---

emotions that can be presented within a consultation. Sometimes this can be emotionally overwhelming to the professionals concerned, who can respond either by experiencing many of the extreme emotions themselves, or by distancing themselves from the emotions. Some of these extreme emotions can include:

- grief and loss,
- sadness,
- anger and aggression,
- fear and anxiety,
- depression and hopelessness, and
- trauma.

In each case, hearing the family histories and seeing the exposed emotions in the family can be extremely sad and sometimes traumatising to the listener. The possible effects of this are summarised by Nichols (1994, p 174):

Emotional care . . . involves exposure to the emotions and distress of others . . . exposure to the emotions of others is, in itself, nothing more than normal life. Repeated exposure to particular types of intense emotion, perhaps several times a day on a daily basis, is a different issue.

COMMON RESPONSES FROM HEALTH PROFESSIONALS

Whilst research indicates that most health professionals report feeling that much of their working life is stressful, and that they feel under significant pressure for much of their time at work (McKevitt et al 1996, Nichols 1993), there appears to be significantly less awareness of how we respond emotionally to such pressures (Stoter 1997). Instead, many professionals tend to minimise their own needs and attempt to cope without reflecting on the effect of working under these conditions. This is not to say, of course, that work is not likely to be stressful. Rather, it is important to promote a self-acceptance that stressors will be present and suggests that self-knowledge of how we individually respond under such circumstances is an essential first step in developing an emotionally functional way of coping. In the remainder of this section there follows a discussion of a range of common responses to work pressures.

Lack of control

Feeling de-skilled and helpless is a particularly common response, especially for less experienced professionals who are seeing complex social problems and who feel under pressure to find swift solutions. These feelings of a lack of control over one's own working life and over the lives of patients are to be expected, but require some self-reflection about what is changeable and what is not.

Psychological stress

A helpful definition of the negative impact of stress is where the relationship between an individual and his environment is judged as exceeding his resources and causing difficulties for his emotional well being (Lazarus & Folkman 1984). This involves, therefore, an interaction between the individual's perception of the work situation and his perception of his own ability to cope. Whilst there is no doubt that some form of manageable pressure can be creative and produce adaptive responses, such as creativity, purpose and incentive

Psychological needs of the community paediatrician

Box 3.3
Psychological changes resulting from stress

Emotional: tense, irritable, agitated, unsettled, tearful, resentful of demands, emotionally fragile, increased anxiety, anger outbursts.

Physical: headaches, back and/or neck pain, excessive tiredness, increase in minor illnesses, skin problems

Behavioural: rushing, self-neglect, sleep problems, inefficiency, over/under-eating, difficulty starting new activities, changing appearance, reduced effectiveness

Cognitive: poor concentration, forgetfulness, distractible, thoughts of injustice, reduced motivation, thoughts of changing job

Relationships: difficulty coping with other people's needs, avoiding company, needing extra support, overcontrolling of others

---

to act (Health at Work in the NHS 1995), when this becomes out of balance then we can experience negative psychological symptoms. A range of these symptoms are shown in Box 3.3

Each person is likely to have a set of his own characteristic stress signs, which represent a change in usual functioning. There is also a set of possible longer term effects of ongoing stress which are sometimes described as signs of 'burnout'. These include: unresolved anger and resentment with the job; lack of interest in external activities; not being able to relax outside work; changes in relationships outside work; changes in weight; and longer-term illnesses. One possible effect of these longer-term stress responses on patient care has been described as four stages of disillusionment. These involve:

1. Over-identification with patients.
2. Stagnation where one merely conducts the work.
3. Frustration with the work.
4. Apathy used as a defence against frustration (Edelwich & Brodsky 1980).

(For more detailed discussions of the effects of stress on healthcare professionals see Chapter 12 in Rungapadiachy 1999.)

Physical ill-health

A recent study of hospital consultants identified a significant problem in the management of their own health (McKevitt et al 1996). In particular, in comparison to non-medical personnel the doctors were reluctant to take appropriate levels of short-term sick leave (i.e. 1–3 days), but had higher levels of longer-term sick leave (i.e. 7 or more days). Furthermore, they were less likely to consult a general practitioner when necessary in comparison to non-medical colleagues. In a further comparative study of sickness rates, a significantly reduced number of doctors in comparison to nurses reported taking time off work when ill (12% vs. 61%) (Glass et al 1993). This suggests that medical practitioners may not find it very easy to take a patient role and monitor their own health needs.

Behavioural responses

There are also a number of common actions taken by health professionals when under pressure which may offer some short-term relief but actually usually contribute to higher levels of stress. These include:

- Working longer, harder and faster in an attempt to keep on top of work levels.
- Overactivity, involving keeping busy with other activities as a way of avoiding the stressful activities.
- Addiction behaviours such as alcohol and drugs.
- Escapism, involving frequent changes in jobs and relationships, for example, and thus avoiding dealing with the difficulties.
- Taking out all frustrations on external sources by, for example, blaming others and/or expressing unresolved anger at others (Hambly & Muir 1997).

Emotional experiences

One aspect of the clinical work of the community paediatrician which is rarely discussed is the emotional impact of working with families and children. There are undoubtedly many positive features of this kind of work including feeling helpful to families and developing genuinely caring relationships

> **Box 3.4**
> **Common defence mechanisms used by health professionals**
>
> *Transference and counter-transference.* Transference involves the process of casting a current relationship in terms of past formative relationships due to some often superficial similarities between the two situations. For example, a doctor may be seen as similar to an influential and yet frightening, powerful figure of the past; this will affect the current ability to trust the doctor. Counter-transference is the unwitting reaction taken on by the doctor in response to this role, and can mean in this instance that the professional responds in an authoritative manner.
>
> *Projective identification.* Projective identification occurs when one transfers the emotions associated with a particular person or situation onto an alternative person. For example, a mother sees the violent father in her 8-year-old son and treats him accordingly. This defence mechanism can also be unwittingly applied by the health professional onto certain families who express superficially similar patterns.
>
> *Denial.* Denial occurs when one avoids or escapes unpleasant realities by believing or behaving as if they have not occurred. It can be an appropriate psychological protection to extreme events (e.g. trauma), but it can also be used as a way of avoiding painful emotional transactions between the health professional and the patient (e.g. denial by the doctor in discussing an emotionally charged diagnosis). During times of extreme stress and distress, some professionals can develop a form of professional detachment on a more widespread level by not engaging at an emotional level with families.

with them. We can also assume that it is periodically rewarding for most paediatric professionals to work with children and young people and see them develop appropriately. However, the other side of this kind of work is the painful, difficult feelings that professionals experience. Examples of these feelings include anxiety about childrens' and families' situations and anger at the injustices experienced by children (Stoter 1997). There is further evidence that professionals working with children experience particularly high levels of sadness when working with children who have experienced loss and bereavement (Scullion 1994, Downey et al 1995). Indeed, community paediatricians have a specific responsibility for assessing children where there have been allegations of abuse, and this must at times be traumatising for the professionals concerned.

Psychological defence mechanisms

A group of psychological processes, which are often unconsciously processed, can affect our understanding and attitude to families and their care. These may be acted out in front of us by families or taken on by ourselves as professionals. These individual defences usually protect us from becoming overwhelmed by anxiety, but can have a direct impact on our forms of care and on our own psychological health (Smith & Norton 1999). Some examples of the most common defence mechanisms used by health professionals are shown in Box 3.4.

Collective defences and prejudices

There are a series of global judgements that we can make when we are feeling under pressure which help us cope but do not accurately reflect the experiences of families. Collective defences can develop as teams or large organisations protect themselves against anxieties which are shared and where an organisation possesses unquestioned attitudes (Smith & Norton 1999). For example, some organisations have developed an ethos of refusing families the choice of professionals or the right to have a second opinion. Prejudices can occur where there is a risk of stereotyping families by utilising generalisations of psychological characteristics to large groups (Rungapadiachy 1999). For example, professionals may assume that all single parents are irresponsible. A final global judgement involves applying the fundamental attribution error in which we tend to see individuals in isolation and concentrate on what it is about the person that is causing the difficulty rather than looking at situational factors (Niven 2000). It is easy to slip into a tendency to blame parents when we are stressed or where families cannot act upon our advice, and this can lead to a depersonalised and detached view of families.

STRATEGIES FOR LOOKING AFTER OURSELVES

It is essential, then, that we take our own emotional health needs seriously, so that we are able to look after ourselves properly and act as professionally as possible. In order to do this, it is necessary to develop some self-awareness of how we function. This is about: 'recognising, acknowledging, accepting or challenging who we are, what we feel and what we can or cannot do' (Rungapadiachy 1999 p 18). It requires us to look at our own prejudices and defences, and recognise our strengths and question our weaknesses. Whilst it is often necessary to make organisational changes within the work environment to enable us to function more effectively, it is also essential to look after ourselves emotionally. This involves both identifying what we can do for ourselves at an emotional level, and seeking out how others can help us emotionally. Health professionals are good at giving support but are not always good at receiving support. Seeking support is still not seen as a strength, and we often fail to value disclosing our own feelings to others.

The following section discusses a range of organisational and personal coping strategies which can be individually adapted to each professional's needs.

Practical work-setting changes

There are a number of practical strategies which can be applied to the work setting to change personal expectations and alter working practices. One of these is to *set realistic targets* and to recognise that we cannot help everyone. It is sometimes the case that less experienced professionals can set unrealistic goals for themselves, although all staff can fall into this trap when under pressure (Niven 2000). It is often better to set oneself *short-term limited goals* and revisit them often. On occasions, some form of *limit setting* may be required in which an agreement of treatment length and type can be agreed with

families, although Smith & Norton (1999) suggest that specific treatment contracts can have complicated effects on the doctor–patient relationship. A further strategy involves an evaluation of the *capacity of the family to change*, bearing in mind the physical and emotional resources of the family involved. This is relevant because we can sometimes underestimate both the time required for change to take place, and the resources required for a family to adopt such changes.

Other changes to practical working strategies include *balancing workload over the day*, *taking short breaks* where possible, *working realistic hours* especially when there is a tendency to work longer when under pressure, and building in *regular holidays* and *short breaks* from work. Another useful strategy which is not often used by doctors is *rescheduling of work* when under pressure. Recent research evidence suggests that this is done significantly less often by doctors than nurses, resulting in lower feelings of control and higher levels of emotional exhaustion (Glass et al 1993). Finally, there is evidence that preparation for some of the frustrations and stressors of a job prior to starting can reduce staff turnover and increase work satisfaction. Thus, staff who were presented with a booklet containing the potential difficulties of the job in addition to benefits coped much better than staff who were shown a booklet which only showed the benefits (Weitz 1956 cited in Niven 2000).

Staff development, training and communication

Another area of practical support which has been shown to help with a professional's capacity to function effectively at work is the availability of appropriate staff development, training and communication (Niven 2000). Some of the particular themes that have been identified by health professionals as important include:

- Career planning and being able to identify future career requirements.
- Having time to develop ideas and projects of one's own.
- Having time to reflect on personal and professional issues.

There is also now an emphasis being placed within the NHS on the importance of ongoing professional development, and the need for planned training and education (e.g. Rughani 2000). This in part, reflects a recognition that professionals need to be able to identify their own training needs and have some say in how they are met. A further area which health professionals have identified as essential to their emotional health at work is the presence of good lines of communication. Research suggests that feeling consulted and listened to, receiving feedback from management and being involved in effective team working were all predictors of a rewarding working environment (McNeely 1995).

> **Box 3.5**
> ## Functions of self-expression and sharing
>
> Self-monitoring of feelings and stress signs
>
> Re-appraisal of one's way of coping
>
> Sharing of common problems
>
> Sharing of normal reactions to problems
>
> Opportunity to receive positive feedback
>
> Re-direction away from self-blame
>
> Opportunity to share positive ways of coping

Balance of personal and professional

There is clear evidence that being able to empathise with families is important in developing trusting relationships and bringing about change (Frankel 1995). However, it is also evident that we can become too enmeshed with the emotions of our patients, and begin to take these feelings home with us. While this form of emotional encroachment is inevitable at times, it is a sign of extreme stress if these feelings are following us home on a regular basis and we cannot switch them off. It is essential to have ways of switching off when away from work and it is helpful to have outside interests which are relaxing. However, this strategy of distancing oneself from work stressors is only palliative in the sense that it does nothing to deal with the stressors themselves. These active coping strategies are discussed in the next sections.

Social support

The function of social support is to utilise colleagues or other professionals in a supportive network to create a safe environment to explore one's feelings. It is distinctive from supervision in that its purpose is not fundamentally clinical but rather emotional and personal. Even though most people in caring roles have regular contact of some sort with colleagues, this may not be emotionally supportive contact. Thus, proper social support reduces emotional isolation, and is not used solely as a response to crises. Although crisis support certainly has its role, preventative support is ongoing and long term. The purpose of routine sessions enables some of the following themes to be discussed: how am I feeling, what has happened since we last met, how has this affected me and do I need to attend to any of these emotional issues? The potential benefits of this process of self-expression and sharing are shown in Box 3.5.

Social support can take a variety of forms. It can involve one to one reciprocal peer support, either in formal or informal settings. Sometimes the emotional benefits of this process are simply to be listened to. There is evidence, for example, from health professionals from the Kings Cross fire that colleagues who allowed them to talk and just listened were seen as the most emotionally supportive (Rosser et al 1991). Group support is another common form of social support, in which groups of work colleagues or professional groups meet in a supportive environment. Some of the types of group support are shown in Box 3.6.

An example of the effectiveness of group support was shown in a study by Maslach & Jackson (1982) in which doctors and nurses who were actively involved in peer support groups scored lower on measures of emotional exhaustion and depersonalisation. This group of professionals were also more likely actively to seek advice from other staff and were more likely to view situations from the patients' point of view.

Psychological needs of the community paediatrician

Box 3.6
Types of group support

A *small peer group* consisting of work colleagues

A *facilitator-led group* involving outside help

A *therapist-led group* concentrating on psychological issues

A *group providing forms of relaxation*, etc.

Box 3.7
Five step plan of emotional self-care

1. List work stressors and learn to identify and monitor your personal stress signs.

2. Identify unhelpful and helpful responses to stress.

3. Make an assessment of the context of work pressures and your ability to change them. Work pressures can be identified in three different ways:
   intrapersonal arising from within the individual
   interpersonal occurring between individuals
   extrapersonal exerted from outside the individual.
   Which stressors can be eliminated, which can be limited or reduced, which have to be accepted but need built-in support mechanisms?

4. Develop an intervention plan:
   take responsibility for self-monitoring and intervening to look after your own emotional state
   identify support facilities that are suitable for you and take it on as an individual responsibility to use them
   the plan needs to be preventative support, not crisis-driven support.

5. Evaluation:
   ongoing monitoring needs to be planned into your work schedule
   regular review of effectiveness of strategies.

Box 3.8
Five-step plan of emotional health care

1. Work stressors

2. Unhelpful and helpful responses

3. Assessment of context and ability to change

4. Intervention plan

5. Evaluation and effectiveness

skill rather than a weakness. Furthermore, participants need to feel a sense of safety and trust in their colleagues and therefore group support will not work if members are feeling under scrutiny or judged. Therefore a group's success is dependent on how it is set up and on the relationship between its members. (For further information on support groups see Owen 1990, Stoter 1997).

PUTTING SELF-CARE INTO PRACTICE

We need to be active in putting emotional self-care into practice and take responsibility for looking after our own emotional health. In fact Nichols (1993) believes that it is both unprofessional and a form of self-neglect to ignore our own emotional self-care. He stresses that it is not a sign of weakness to look after our emotional health within working hours, but rather a sign of strength and responsibility.

Box 3.7 shows a five step plan of emotional self-care which can be used as a guide to developing an awareness of one's own emotional needs and how to meet them. This can be put into practice using the form shown in Box 3.8.

REFERENCES

Baglioni L, Cooper C, Hingley P 1990 Job stress, mental health and job satisfaction among UK senior nurses. Stress Medicine 6:9–20

Dahlgren G, Whitehead M. 1991 Policies and strategies to promote social equity in health. Institute for Future Studies, Stockholm

Dewe P 1989 Stressor frequency, tension, tiredness and coping. Journal of Advanced Nursing 14:308–320

For social support to work, we have to be able to receive the time and attention of others. Thus, using social support needs to be seen as a strength and

Downey V, Benqiamin M, Heuer L, Juhl N 1995 Dying babies and associated stress in NICU Nurses Neonatal Network 14(1) 41–46

Edelwich J, Brodsky A 1980 Burnout: stages of disillusionment in the helping professions. Human Sciences Press, New York

Firth-Cozens J 1987 Emotional distress in junior house officers. British Medical Journal 295:533–536

Frankel R 1995 Emotion and the physician–patient relationship. Motivation and Emotion 19(3):163–173

Glass D, McKnight J, Valdimarsdottir H 1993 Depression, burnout, perceptions of control in hospital nurses. Journal of Consulting and Clinical Psychology 61:147–155

Hambly K, Muir A 1997 Stress management in primary care. Butterworth Heinemann, Oxford

Health at Work in the NHS 1995 Organisational stress in the NHS. OPUS Report. Health Education Authority, London

Lazarus R, Folkman S 1984 Stress, appraisal and coping. Springer, New York

Maslach C, Jackson S 1982 Burnout in health professional: a psychological analysis. In: Saunders S, Suis J (eds) The Social Psychology of Health and Illness. L Erlbaum Associates, Hillsdale NJ

McKevitt C, Morgan M, Simpson J, Holland W 1996 Doctor's health and needs for services. Nuffield Provincial Hospitals Trust

McNeely S 1995 Communication: another source of stress among nurses. The Occupational Psychologist 25:5–7

Nichols K 1993 Psychological care in physical illness. Chapman and Hall, London

Niven N 2000 Health psychology for health care professionals. Churchill Livingstone, Edinburgh

O'Dowd T 1988 Five years of heartsink patients in general practice. British Medical Journal 287:528–530

Owen G 1990 Support networks in the NHS. NASS. Occasional Papers No 1. National Association for Staff Support, Woking

Rosser R, Dewar S, Thompson J 1991 Psychological aftermath of Kings Cross Fire. Journal of Royal Society of Medicine 84:4–8

Rughani A 2000 The GP's guide to personal development plans. Radcliffe Medical Press, Oxford

Rungapadiachy D 1999 Interpersonal communication and psychology for health care professionals. Butterworth Heinemann, Oxford

Scullion R 1994 An identification of stress associated with accident and emergency departments, comparison of stress levels. Accident & Emergency Nursing (2) 79–86

Smith S, Norton K 1999 Counselling skills for doctors. Open University Press, Milton Keynes

Stockwell F 1984 The unpopular patient. RCN, London

Stoter D 1997 Staff support in health care. Blackwell Science, Oxford

Weitz J 1956 Job expectancy and survival. Journal of Applied Psychology 40:245–247

4 | Social science

WHAT IS SOCIOLOGY?

Sociology is the study of human social life, groups and societies. It is a dazzling and compelling enterprise, having as its subject matter our own behaviour as social beings. The scope of sociological study is extremely wide, ranging from the analysis of passing encounters between individuals in the street to the investigation of global social processes.

(Giddens 1997b p 2)

Sociology is a discipline in which we set aside our personal view of the world to look more carefully at the influences that shape our lives and others.

(Giddens 1997b p 14)

Sociology . . . is first and foremost a way of thinking about the human world; in principle one can think about the same world in different ways.

(Bauman 1997 p 12)

The raw material of social science is the interaction of people in their everyday lives and the social worlds within which these interactions occur. As Giddens points out, its scope is broad. Sociology embraces the contexts in which everyday encounters take place — the family, the school, the workplace. It also includes broader influences or structures which shape and pattern life in our society — 'class', 'gender', 'race', 'capitalism', 'democratic government'. It looks at a world with a history; a world that is constantly changing. This is reflected in the changing issues that concern social scientists.

As people go about their everyday business, they may be conscious of making choices about how they act that have impact on their own lives and the lives of others. At other times, they may act 'without thinking', in ways that have become routine or habitual, not of their conscious choosing. In some situations, they may be aware that their actions are constrained, they have little or no choice about what they say or do. In the course of a day people move between spheres with different 'rules' about what is or isn't appropriate behaviour as they deal with people at work, engage in family life or meet friends for a drink in the evening. Sometimes they may glide between these different roles, hardly noticing, involving themselves in patterns of behaviour they have observed or learned over many years. At other times they may feel uncertain about how to act or in conflict with what is expected of them. The ways people act are, thus, a product of the world they live in. Social behaviour follows patterns and is structured by constraints, learned behaviour and expectations — by the law, by custom, by the norms of different groups and so on. The actions of individuals combine to reproduce familiar routines, patterns and structures that recur and are recognised as a family, a school, a hospital, 'market economies', 'democratic government'. So, people live in a world which is 'structured', which has recognisable patterns of behaviour and recognisable institutions and structures within which these take place. At the same time, they have 'agency'. Within constraints, they make choices that conform to or challenge the social worlds which they inhabit. 'We create society at the same time as we are created by it.' (Giddens 1997a p 8).

This introduction has touched on a number of themes than run through writing in social science:

- There are many 'levels' of social life that the social scientist might be concerned with. For example, the level of individual actions and understandings; family life; the level of social institutions such as schools, hospitals; broader patterns of social life structured by class, race, gender.

- There is a tension between social 'structures' that pre-exist and constrain individual lives and 'agency' or individual choice or actions.
- Individual actions reproduce social institutions and social structures. They also have the potential to modify or change them.
- The social worlds and social structures within which people live may be seen as matters of consensus, reflecting shared values and interests. They may also be seen reflecting the interests and values of dominant groups, generating inequality and conflict.

Social science explanations aim to be different from commonsense understandings in a number of ways (Bauman 1997). Social scientists try to look beyond their own experience, to base their understandings on a wider view and to recognise that it is possible to question the 'obvious' and to see the familiar in very different ways. Social scientists are expected to support what they say with evidence and to be critical of the limitations of their evidence. As they reflect on and analyse the world they observe, social scientists arrive at competing explanations of what they see.

This chapter goes on to look at some questions social science engages with that might be relevant to people working in community paediatrics. It invites the reader to keep these questions in mind as they read this book and reflect on their work and experience.

MAKING SENSE OF SOCIAL LIFE: THE CONSTRUCTION OF MEANING

As social actors, people are constantly reflecting on and making sense of the world they inhabit. As the quote from Bauman at the start of this chapter points out, however, there are different ways of looking at the social world. 'Common sense' and experience may provide useful working knowledge for negotiating everyday life. Literature and poetry offer different kinds of accounts and insights. History offers competing explanations of how things have come to be as they are.

Social science offers yet another approach. It asks one to step back from the things that are taken for granted, to adopt the attitude of the 'sceptical stranger' (Clarke & Cochrane 1998) or to 'defamiliarize' the familiar (Bauman 1997). This involves looking more closely at 'commonsense' thinking, asking questions about the influences and interests that shape taken-for-granted ideas. It requires us to think more carefully about how the way things are labelled carries expectations which affect how people behave towards them (Clarke & Cochrane 1998). The label 'lone parent', for example, has come to carry powerful images and expectations. These expectations affect how lone parents are treated. They connect with the kinds of provisions seen as necessary to support lone parents, to encourage them to become independent and so on. The 'lone parent' is, in turn, aware of the ways in which lone parents are portrayed in our society, how others view them and the range of reactions this provokes. This has consequences for how they make sense of their own experience and how they see themselves (their 'subjectivity'). So, such labels carry complex associations, meanings and expectations. However, these meanings can change. 'Lone parent' in the 1990s links with a range of meanings and possibilities that are in some ways similar and in some ways different from the 'unmarried mother' of the 1950s. To be a 'lone parent' is more readily recognised as an option in Britain in the 1990s than in the 1950s. However, there are significant variations in how this possibility is viewed, both between groups within our society and between societies.

There has been a growing awareness of the power of language, the meanings and expectations that are attached to it and of how some labels and the identities they offer 'stigmatise'. For example, the diagnosis or label of 'mental handicap' carried a likelihood of being seen as 'different', facing rejection, marginalisation and exclusion in ways that have profound implications for individual identities and potential. This has led to attempts to apply a new label, 'learning difficulties', with changed meanings and implications.

Social science is interested in questions of how such ideas are produced and communicated, which groups in society have the ability to shape and influence how others think about particular issues and how dominant ideas come to be contested and challenged. Official surveys and statistics categorise people in ways that may not reflect the diversity of social life, for example, concealing same-sex relationships and households (Graham 1995). Professionals, those with 'expert knowledge', the media, those with political power are clearly groups with some power to influence how others see things. Social movements, such as the disability movement, feminism or the gay and lesbian movement, offer important examples of how 'dominant' ideas and 'commonsense' can come to be challenged and criticised.

'Discourse analysis' has become important in social science, involving the close analysis of how people talk or write about particular clusters of ideas. This raises awareness of different meanings that are in use. It focuses attention on where these appear and questions of what is implied or achieved by particular ways of talking or writing about something. '(Discourse includes) all forms of spoken interaction, formal and informal, and written texts of all kinds.' (Potter & Wetherell 1987 p 6)

Community is an example of a 'discourse' which has been widely used in social welfare and in everyday life. It is seen in phrases such as 'care in the community', community workers, community liaison, community development. There has been nostalgia about the decline of 'working class communities'. These suggest geographically bounded locations within which people know one another, share a culture, a sense of attachment and belonging, have 'roots' and offer mutual support in the face of poverty and disadvantage. However, commentators have highlighted the complexity masked by ideas of 'community'. In contrast to the rosy picture of 'belonging' and 'supporting', they may be marked by division and conflict, by hostility to outsiders and those who don't 'fit in'. They can be oppressive and restrictive as well as supportive and enabling (Hughes & Mooney 1998, Robb with Davies 1998). Modern life is mobile, fracturing family and community ties. People may pass through many places in their lifetime with some sense of their personal 'history', but shaped by diverse experiences that mean they don't quite 'belong' anywhere. 'Community' is a discourse which holds out possibilities of inclusion and belonging that fit uneasily with mobility and change.

Writers have identified 'communities of interest' in contrast to these 'communities of place'. Such communities need not be geographically bounded. They may be temporary, rather than having the longstanding 'roots' of the traditional community. For example, they may form as pressure groups to confront a threat such as the building of a road or the closure of a school. They may include self-help groups or support groups for people with conditions such as cancer, asthma or heart disease. There are even looser groupings such as 'the deaf community', 'the black community' or 'the gay community'. Communities of interest are thus more diverse. One person may belong to several such communities. They may be of temporary or lasting significance in a person's life. They vary in intensity of personal involvent and commitment. A person may choose to belong to some of these groups, others carry imposed identities. They may have little to do with geographical location, being evident in networks, newsletters or computer conferences. Thus, community may be a more complex and contested concept than might first appear. Recognising this complexity raises important questions for policy and practice that is 'community based'.

Similarly, Young (1999) raises important questions about the discourse of 'parenthood'. She suggests that this obscures awareness of the diversity of ideas and experiences of parenting in our society. Parenthood is often linked with assumptions of 'natural' behaviour and inclinations. However, within our society, people operate with very different notions of what 'being a parent' involves. At an individual level, parents work to reconcile conflicting ideas of children's needs for autonomy and supervision, for dependence and independence. They balance various pressures and viewpoints from peers, family, religion, cultural practice, professional and expert guidance as they 'construct' (and change) their understanding of what it means to be a 'parent'. Also, parenthood connects with and is reinforced by other powerful discourses of 'family', 'motherhood', 'childhood', 'learning and development', 'parental responsibility' and so on.

Such ideas, or 'discourses', carry judgements of what is 'normal' or 'acceptable' and implications for what should happen if these boundaries are crossed. However, this raises questions of who has the power to shape such judgements and whose ideas and experiences are excluded.

Patterns of family life in Britain today are diverse, yet an 'ideal' of 'normal' family life remains strong. This 'traditional family' coexists with a rise in divorce rates, 'serial monogamy', lone-parents, step-parents, same-sex parents and so on (Lentell 1998). Young (1999) argues that ideals of 'parenting', especially 'mothering' fail to recognise that these responsibilities are often shared amongst relatives, siblings, friends, paid carers and so on. This suggests a much wider range of 'informal' or 'unofficial' parents who fall outside the scope of many initiatives targeted at parents. Far from being 'natural', the 'family' and 'parenthood' are socially constructed. Ideals and patterns of 'family life' and 'parenting' are, in reality, variable and changing. With increasing diversity of family forms, cultural variations, changing patterns of employment and geographical mobility 'parenting' also has to adjust and change.

These examples suggest the importance of looking carefully at how such discourses are used in written materials, such as pamphlets and policy statements, in meetings where decisions are made, in professional practice and in everyday talk.

COMPETING EXPLANATIONS OF SOCIAL EVENTS AND ACTIONS

A problem with commonsense thinking is that often people work with contradictory ideas and draw on conflicting explanations of social problems without recognising or reconciling the discrepancies this generates. Social science helps clarify different ways of looking at and explaining social issues.

The disability movement has highlighted the significance of competing explanations for policy and practice by contrasting 'medical' and 'social' models of disability (Hughes 1998). In the medical model, to say someone is 'disabled' puts the focus on their individual limitations or impairment. Doctors, educationalists, psychologists, social workers and other professionals are involved in the assessment of the extent or nature of a person's impairment and in defining the kind of treatment, specialist help or rehabilitation that would be most beneficial. In this model, the disabled person is compared with a 'norm' of 'able-bodiedness' or 'health'. In the process, disability has been linked with varying degrees of dependence. Intervention, support and treatment has been aimed towards 'normalisation' (e.g. at one time, deaf people were encouraged to speak and lip-read rather than sign), segregation in institutions or provision for 'special needs'. The 'problem' and its solution, is focused at the level of the individual, their impairment and whether they can be helped to adapt to life in a 'normal' society.

The 'social model' challenges this by locating the problem of disability in the way society excludes and 'disables' certain people by making aspects of social life inaccessible to them. This model might point to public transport or buildings that are inaccessible to wheelchair users; television programmes without subtitles that deaf viewers have difficulty following; the 'invisibility' of disabled people and their experiences in the media; the exclusion of disabled people from decisions on policy and practice that affect them. This model challenges professional expertise by emphasising that disabled people themselves are a vital source of expert knowledge about living as a disabled person. It challenges the power of those making decisions that affect the lives of disabled people, calling on them to involve disabled people in decision-making, to recognise their viewpoint and their rights to self-determination. The association of 'dependence' and 'special needs' with disability are questioned. Most people are dependent on others who grow their food, deliver their post, clean their houses or drive trains they travel in. Everyone has needs for housing, transport, communication, education and employment which are met in many different ways. From this perspective, there is nothing 'special' about the needs of disabled people, they are 'normal' needs. Like everyone else, they have rights to housing, education and transport.

These contrasting models show that the way we explain the nature of disability leads to very different emphases in social policy and social intervention. These different models, or perspectives, have very different implications for where the 'problem' is located. This, in turn, has implications for how disabled people see themselves and how they are seen by others, for their identity as a group and as individuals. It also raises significant questions about the role of 'experts' and professionals in making decisions that affect the lives of disabled people. Such models are useful in thinking about and analysing particular practices and policies, and disabled people's reactions to them. However, it would be dangerous to assume that any one model captures the particular experiences and viewpoints of all disabled people (Hughes 1998).

COMPETING EXPLANATIONS, ALTERNATIVE POLICIES AND PRACTICE?

The two 'models' of disability outlined in the previous section show that different ways of explaining and looking at an issue can carry very different implications for policy and practice. This section looks more closely at how competing explanations of health inequalities are reflected in policy and practice.

Post-war Britain saw the introduction of the welfare state, intended to challenge the five great evils of want, ignorance, idleness, squalor and disease. This was to be achieved by welfare provisions such as public housing, the National Health Service (NHS), education and family allowances. National insurance and social security systems held out hopes of eradicating poverty, by the provision of minimum levels of income. However, it is clear that despite the provisions of the welfare state, children in Britain today grow up with very different standards of living and life chances. The risk of poverty is uneven, it is linked to social class, gender and ethnic origin. Unemployment, low pay, old age, disability, lone-parenting and family breakdown are also linked with poverty (Millar 1994, Oppenheim 1994). 'Poverty' is not easy to determine and can be defined in different ways. 'Absolute' poverty defines poverty as falling below a minimum income sufficient to secure basic necessities. Where this 'poverty line' should be drawn is debatable. In practice, it usually linked to the point at which people become eligible for state benefits

such as Income Support. 'Relative' poverty argues that poverty should be judged relative to the standards of a particular society. Thus, the threshold of poverty changes as average incomes and living standards rise. Relative poverty takes account of the changing income and resources necessary to participate in life in a particular society. This, therefore, tends to set the poverty threshold somewhat higher than measures of absolute poverty.

Not surprisingly, health and access to health care are also unequally distributed in society. (see Chapter 23). Class, in terms of occupational grouping, has been identified as a major factor structuring these patterns of inequality. Class affects the chances of being born of low birth weight, of growing up overweight, or being classified as having emotional or behavioral difficulties (Department of Health 1999). In later life, it connects with the likelihood of developing occupationally related illnesses, lung cancer or coronary heart disease or of dying early. The Black Report (Townsend & Davidson 1982) highlighted the impact of class and gender on health out-comes. It also pointed to differences between classes as 'consumers' of health services. Middle class patients have longer consultations, make greater use of preventative services and are more likely to seek medical attention for their children. During their consultations they were able to ask more questions and were given more information. Areas with the greatest health problems tend to have general practitioners with the longest lists and hospitals with less staff and equipment and less adequate buildings. These contribute to what Tudor Hart (1971) termed the 'inverse care law': the availability of good medical care tends to vary inversely with the need of the population served.

One of the Black Report's recommendations for tackling health inequalities was an increase in benefits to improve the material conditions of poorer social groups. However, there is little evidence of reductions in inequalities of income or health since the Black Report. The 1980s and early 1990s saw rising average incomes, yet at the same time a widening gap between the incomes of the richest and the poorest in this country (Hills 1996). The Acheson Report (Acheson 1998) reiterated the connection between health and class or income. The 'Health of Young People 95–97' (Department of

Health 1999a) highlighted class differences in health, diet and lifestyle amongst young people. Working class children were shown to be more likely to suffer from respiratory disease and to grow up to be smokers; they were likely to eat less fresh fruit and vegetables (Department of Health 1999a).

The factors producing these patterns are undoubtedly many and complex. Policy and practice aiming to tackle the problems of groups disadvantaged in terms of health draws on several levels of explanation. On the one hand, health inequalities are often presented as the outcome of particular lifestyles and patterns of behaviour which are, in turn, seen as matters within individual choice and control. This argues for programmes of health education which teach people about nutrition, the links between health and lifestyle, how to manage their budgets, their children, their time, their stress and so on. On the other hand, health inequalities are also explained in terms of material deprivation and inequality. Looking back to the nineteenth century, it has been argued that improvements in housing, living standards and sanitation were more important in explaining declining death rates from infectious diseases than medical advances in vaccination and drugs. However, the need for employment, higher incomes, better housing and better working conditions for the most disadvantaged in society have been less readily recognised as the bases for policies to deal with present-day health problems. 'The Health of the Nation' (Department of Health 1992) set targets for reducing death and ill health from common causes such as heart attacks and strokes, accidents, mental health and cancer. However, its emphasis was on achieving this through changes in lifestyle and individual responsibility, rather than by addressing the link between poverty and health.

Does this matter? Mears (1993) suggests that individualistic explanations have appeal at the political and policy-making levels. They shift attention away from dealing with more intransigent underlying structural issues of how certain groups come to be placed in situations of disadvantage because of their class, gender or ethnicity, for example. The focus on individual choices and lifestyles thus leads to 'blaming the victim'. Writers who focus on the importance of sociostructural forces argue that

health inequalities would be more effectively addressed by social reforms that improve the living standards of the poorest in our society. This approach would require policies to deal with underlying issues such as poverty and low incomes, housing, working conditions and other measures with direct effects on the conditions under which people live and work. For example, this might involve re-routing of traffic, provision of good food and milk in schools; legislation to tackle industrial accidents and disease; policies to increase stability of income and employment; improvements in housing and heating.

More recently, the Labour government has pledged its commitment to improving the health of the whole population and reducing health inequalities in its public health white paper, 'Saving Lives: Our Healthier Nation' (Department of Health 1999b). Again, different theories or explanations of health inequalities run through its proposals. It calls for partnership between people, communities and government to improve health. At an individual level, there is a strong emphasis on individual decisions people can make about their own and their families' health. These are supported by 'Healthy Citizens' programmes which include the much publicised telephone helpline service 'NHS Direct', and 'Expert Patients' programmes to help people manage their own illness. However, the White paper also emphasises the link between social, economic and environmental factors and ill health. It points to other government policies and initiatives in education, welfare-to-work, housing, neighbourhoods, transport and the environment as measures to deal with inequality. Thus, there is a recognition that the goal of reducing inequalities in health goes beyond the scope of the health service and health professionals.

However, in the short term, health professionals are given a major role in tackling health inequalities at an individual level, by changing the behaviour and lifestyles of people with limited resources and choice. This leaves those working in this field to reach their own understanding of how individual and structural factors combine to produce the health problems of the clients they meet and the implications of this for their own practice.

Edwards & Popay (1993) report a study that looks

at how community health and social workers view their role as service providers working with families with young children seen as 'in need'. The interviews conducted during this study revealed that these workers clearly saw poverty as the major negative influence on the welfare of young children. Most workers saw the income levels of those dependent on benefit as inadequate. Several commented that they themselves would be unable to manage on such a low income. However, at the same time, Edwards & Popay report how these workers also make observations about how individuals cope differently in similar situations. Thus, they see poverty not only as a matter of income level, but also in terms of ability to manage money, children and so on. They found that workers commented on their clients' low incomes, but at the same time on how they 'wasted money' on cigarettes, 'junk food', alcohol, taxis and so on. Similarly, on the one hand, they would point out the lack of safe play areas for children; on the other hand, they would also talk of some parents' reluctance to play with their children, or their lack of knowledge of how to. Edwards & Popay go on to look at how these workers use these different levels of explanation in ways that help them make sense of their own role, its boundaries and limitations.

The SPIDA project (Strategies for Practice in Disadvantaged Areas) set out to address the link between poverty and practice more directly. Its aim was to test a model of team learning about poverty in a GP practice in inner city Nottingham and to look at its impact on practice (Bond 1999). Team members gathered and shared information on poverty and found this changed their attitudes to clients. For example, they became less likely to see them as 'scrounging'. It also made them aware of their need for more information on issues such as housing. This, in turn, led to improved links with other agencies and awareness of the importance of enabling families to obtain their welfare entitlements.

These reports suggest that health professionals' personal understandings and explanations of the effects of poverty on individuals' lives can influence how they view and relate to their clients. They also show how these understandings can work to reinforce or challenge existing practice.

POWER

Running through the themes explored in this chapter are issues of power and influence. The chapter began by considering issues of personal choice or agency. It has touched on professionals' power to 'label' people in ways which have profound implications for how they see themselves or are seen by others and to determine what is in their 'best interests'. It has raised questions of how political and professional power can shape social policy and the scope for professional groups to influence how policy is interpreted or implemented in practice.

Some forms of power are more obvious than others. Lukes (1994) identifies different 'dimensions' of power. For example, the capacity to influence decision-making and to do things that affect change or affect other people are clearly aspects of power. However, interest groups and social movements, such as the disability movement or feminism, show that it is possible for collective action to increase the influence of groups that may have been excluded from decision-making processes that affect their lives.

Lukes then takes a step back to show that the ability to shape the decision-making agenda and the terms on which an issue is considered is an important dimension of power. His third dimension of power goes beyond issues of influence and agenda-setting, where conflict and grievance may be evident, to acknowledge the importance of 'the bias of the system ... the socially structured and culturally patterned behaviour of groups, and practices of institutions, which may indeed be manifested by individuals' inaction'. These 'biases' and structured patterns of behaviour operate to 'set the agenda' and terms of debate. The composition of decision-making bodies and their agendas mean that certain voices and viewpoints are silenced or are forever going against the bias of assumptions of how things operate and the terms on which they are debated.

The work of Michel Foucault has been influential in drawing attention to subtle and diffuse forms of power which work sometimes with, sometimes against, the dominant interests and influences in society. Power is not simply something 'held' by dominant actors or agents, or located in positions of influence and control. For Foucault, power is much more generally dispersed throughout social networks and relationships. For example, often power is not exercised directly, but through the everyday activities and behaviours of peripheral actors, who may perform their tasks in ways that support or resist the frameworks within which they are expected to work. For example, it is illegal to practise euthanasia. However, media reports have highlighted doctors who question this and who admit to having helped people to die. In turn, this raises complex questions about the boundaries between 'routine' decisions to withhold treatment and euthanasia.

An important concern in Foucault's work has been the power of knowledge and shifts in the kinds of knowledge viewed as credible or worthy of serious consideration. In matters of health, professional voices are amongst those recognised as 'intelligible', 'authoritative', as 'serious' contributors to debates. However, before this century, much knowledge of childbirth was the province of women and lay practitioners, which was based on practical experience, accumulated wisdom and folklore. This was challenged by medical knowledge and expertise, which transformed the process of birth. This is not to say that professional knowledge and expertise is uncontested. For example, the natural childbirth movement presented an alternative view of childbirth to the orthodoxy of the time which has had significant influence on how birth is organised in the NHS. This raises important questions about power in professional relationships and the many ways in which it is challenged. Patients increasingly take steps to increase their own knowledge (e.g. through self-help groups), and expect to be actively involved in decisions about their treatment. Some people choose to avoid consulting doctors or refuse treatment. Older relatives may sometimes have more influence than health visitors in matters of child care. Patients may adapt how they take a course of drug treatment. Gillespie (1995) looks at how inequalities of power and knowledge can shape the encounter between doctor and patient and at how doctors might deal with this differently. 'Doctor-centred' consultations are built around doctor's knowledge and expertise. The emphasis is on gathering information, probing and analysing to facilitate the doctor's diagnosis. 'Patient-centred' styles, on the other hand, aim to use the patient's knowledge and experience. The doctor makes greater use of silence, listening and reflecting to clarify and interpret the patient's account of their condition.

Beck (1992) takes a broader look at professional power. He looks at how professionalisation generates conditions under which knowledge can be produced without public consideration of its wider social implications. In the search for 'medical progress', techniques such as genetic engineering or in vitro fertilisation are developed. However, the moral and social consequences of such technological advances, the issues which tend to fuel debate in the public sphere, are 'talking about *unreal things, about what cannot yet be seen*'. Thus, much of the time, these developments proceed within environments which are professionally controlled and regulated.

Individual doctors are cut off from the socially transforming scope of their interventions. The latter do not even fall within their horizon of reference; they are shifted off in any case into the side effects of medical practice. What is of primary and central importance for physicians is 'medical progress', as internally defined and controlled within the profession . . . a relatively small group of researchers and practitioners of human genetics are promoting an upheaval in social circumstances, unconsciously and unplanned, in the apparent normalcy of their professional practice as employees.

(Beck 1992 p 212)

Beck presents 'professionalisation' as an aspect of risk in modern societies. It creates spaces within which professionals are entrusted to regulate and control research. In pursuit of medical progress and professional recognition, research with potentially enormous social implications may proceed, with limited external attention or control.

SOCIAL SCIENCE AND EVERYDAY LIFE

Social science may, at times, appear a somewhat detached, intellectual activity, more concerned with explaining and understanding the social world than with practical issues of social action and social change. However, as people make sense of the world they live in and explain it to themselves, they are engaged in constructing understandings, making sense of their society and their place in it. This, in turn, will have implications for how they act and how they interpret the actions of others.

This chapter is here in the belief that social science can connect with everyday lives, professional practice and social policy (Giddens 1997b) by:

- Increasing awareness of difference, seeing the world from other perspectives. 'Practical policies that are not based on an informed awareness of the ways of life of people they affect have little chance of success.' (Giddens 1997 p 13)
- Assessing the effects of policies and their failure to achieve their intended outcomes. Alerting practitioners and policy-makers to the unintended consequences of their actions. Helping them understand the limitations of particular interventions and what they are likely to achieve.
- Increasing awareness and self-enlightenment, encouraging critical reflection on everyday life and professional practice.
- Posing questions of whether actions contribute to reproducing social patterns and inequalities or to reform, social change and social justice.

REFERENCES

Acheson Sir Donald, (chairman) 1998 Independent inquiry into inequalities in health: report. The Stationery Office, London

Bauman Z 1997 Thinking sociologically. In: Giddens A (ed) Sociology. Introductory readings. Polity Press in association with Blackwell Publishers, Cambridge

Beck U 1992 Risk society. Towards a new modernity. Sage, London

Bond M 1999 Placing poverty on the agenda of a primary health care team: an evaluation of an action research project. Health and Social Care 7:9–16

Clarke J, Cochrane A 1998 The social construction of social problems. p.3–42. In: Saraga E (ed) Embodying the social: constructions of difference. Routledge in association with The Open University, London

Department of Health 1992 The health of the nation. The Stationery Office, London

Department of Health 1999a Health survey for England. The health of young people 95–97. The Stationery Office, London

Department of Health 1999b Saving lives: our healthier nation. The Stationery Office, London

Edwards J, Popay J 1993 Contradictions of support and self-help. Health and Social Care 2:31–40

Giddens A (ed) 1997a Sociology, introductory readings. Polity Press in association with Blackwell Publishers, Cambridge

Giddens A 1997b Sociology, 3rd edn. Polity Press in association with Blackwell Publishers, Oxford

Gillespie R 1995 The lay-professional encounter. In: Society and health. An introduction to social science for health professionals. Routledge, London, ch 7

Graham H 1995 Diversity, inequality and official data. Health and Social Care in the Community 3:9–18

Hills J (ed) 1996 New inequalities: the changing distribution of income and wealth in the United Kingdom. Cambridge University Press, Cambridge

Hughes G 1998 A suitable case for treatment? Constructions of disability. In: Saraga E (ed) Embodying the social: constructions of difference. London, Routledge in association with The Open University, London, ch 2, p 43

Hughes G, Mooney G 1998 Community. In: Hughes G (ed) Imagining welfare futures. London, Routledge in association with The Open University, London, ch 2, p 55

Lentell H 1998 Families of meaning: contemporary discourses of the family. In: Lewis G (ed) Forming nation, framing welfare. Routledge in association with The Open University, London, ch 6, p 227

Lukes S 1994 Power: a radical view. In: Anderson J, Ricci M (eds) Society and social science: a reader, 2nd edn. The Open University, Milton Keynes, ch 12, p 131

Mears R 1993 Debates about health inequalities. In: O'Donnell M (ed) New introductory reader in sociology, 3rd edn. Thomas Nelson, Walton-on-Thames, Reading, p 62

Millar J 1994 Lone mothers and poverty. In: Cochrane A, Clarke J (eds), Social problems and social welfare, block 4 readings, part II. The Open University, Milton Keynes, Reading 6, p 62

Oppenheim C 1994 The causes of poverty. In: Cochrane A, Clarke J (eds) Social problems and social welfare, block 4 readings, part II. The Open University, Milton Keynes, Reading 2, p 5

Potter J, Wetherell M 1987 Discursive psychology: beyond attitudes and behaviour. Sage, London

Robb M with Davies C 1998 Caring communities: fact or fiction? In: Understanding health and social care. The Open University, Milton Keynes

Townsend P, Davidson N (eds) 1982 The Black Report. In: Inequalities in health. Harmondsworth, Penguin

Tudor Hart J 1971 The inverse care law. Lancet i:405–412

Young V M 1999 Revealing parenthoods; some observations on theoretical, lay and professional experiences of parenting in contemporary society. Critical Public Health, 9:53–68

5 | Development

This section is concerned with milestones as they are currently used in child health practice with respect to gross motor and fine motor skills, cognitive and social development. Development of speech, vision and hearing are described in the appropriate chapters. The ability to assess the development of a child cannot be obtained from written accounts alone and indeed a written account is only a very minor part of such training. Although charts, such as the Denver Developmental Screening Chart, acknowledge the enormous range of normal that exists, it is impossible within a single scale to record all the individual variations in the quality of response obtained. Obtaining rapport with the child and recognising for example the shy, nervous or withdrawn child who is not performing to his real level of ability, are important skills which only come with practice and experience. In a way, what is needed is observation of the subtleties and fine detail of behaviour rather than testing for the crude gross milestones of development which are used in screening. If we are particularly concerned about a child, more detailed and graphic descriptions are certainly required in order to highlight areas of difficulty where particular help may be provided. Those using the standardised tests of developmental progress such as the Stanford Binet Intelligence Scale, the Wechsler Intelligence Scale for children, the Bailey scales of infant development and the Griffiths scales must ask themselves the reason for doing so. Is it to provide a clinical description of the child, his abilities and his difficulties which would aid diagnosis and management, or is it to provide a comparison of an individual child with his peer group?

Assessment of development depends upon accurate observation and interpretation of those observations in the light of our knowledge about 'normal' development. It must not be forgotten that parents are the ultimate authority on the development of their own child, supplemented in the school age child by teachers' observations. Formal developmental screening is no longer part of our child health surveillance programme, with the realisation that parental observation and anxiety will lead to earlier diagnoses than screening tests.

Descriptions of normal development, linked to a child's ability to perform particular tasks at a particular age, relate only to the performance of the 'average' child. For all milestones there is a very wide range of normal (Fig. 5.1). The developmental charts illustrated in this chapter show both the average and the range and are used to record a description of a child's progress, but should not be used as a pass/fail test. Allowance must also be made for prematurity in interpretation of developmental information. The initial age is the age at which the first few most advanced children display the skill; the median age is the age at which 50% of children display the skill; the limit age is the age at which nearly all children have acquired the skill. Failure to acquire a range of skills by the limit age signals the need for more detailed assessment. The development of individual children does not occur at a constant rate so that single observations of development, particularly in very young children, have little predictive value. Serial observations are much more valuable and will highlight children who 'fade' in their developmental progress compared to their peers and those who shine brighter and brighter with time.

Speech and language development are covered in Chapter 35.

Development

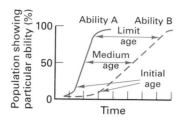

Fig. 5.1 Age range of ability

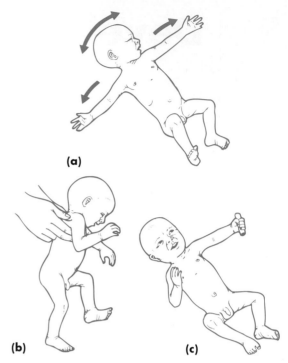

(a)

(b)   **(c)**

Fig. 5.2 (a) Moro reflex. (b) Stepping reflex. (c) Grasp reflex

ASSESSMENT OF REFLEXES

Reflexes in the newborn are a useful way of studying motor development. Exaggeration of reflexes, diminished reflexes, asymmetry of reflexes, persistence of primitive reflexes or delay in the acquisition of secondary reflexes form a useful body of knowledge in the study of developmental progress.

Moro reflex (Fig. 5.2a)

This is elicited in the supine position, with the head supported by one hand a little off the table. The head is then suddenly released, causing first abduction and extension of the arms with opening of the hands, followed by adduction of the arms and crying. This reflex is present very consistently at birth and disappears around 5 months. Persistence after 6 months of age must be considered abnormal. Because this reflex can be elicited so easily in its classic form, any variation from this should be considered with suspicion. An asymmetrical Moro reflex may be due to a fractured limb as well as to neurological causes.

Galant's reflex

With the baby held in ventral suspension, sharp stimulation with the fingernails of the skin down each side of the back results in flexion of the spine to the stimulated side. The Galant's response is present in very preterm babies and its persistent absence in the newborn may well indicate a poor prognosis. Asymmetry is also important, as in the Moro reflex.

The stepping reflex (Fig. 5.2b)

With the baby held vertically, contact of the soles of the feet on to a table causes reflex stepping movements of the legs. Persistence of the stepping reflex beyond the age of 6 months may indicate cerebral palsy.

The palmar grasp reflex (Fig. 5.2c)

Insertion of an object or the examiner's finger into the palm of the hand or on to the sole of the foot, produces reflex flexion of the fingers or toes. This produces a strong grasp with the palm and secondary contraction of the arm muscles sufficient to raise the baby from the supine position when traction is exerted by the examiner's finger. This reflex needs to be lost before voluntary grasping can occur. Abnormal persistence may indicate cerebral damage as may absence or asymmetry in the newborn period.

The asymmetrical tonic neck reflex (ATNR)

Turning of the head to one side leads to extension of the arm and leg on that side and flexion on the opposite side. This has been likened in boys to the position required to use a bow and arrow or in girls

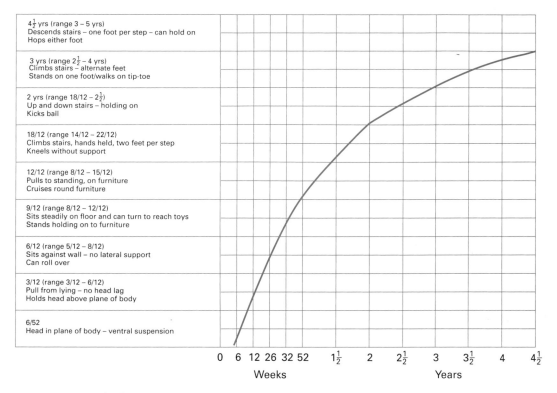

Fig. 5.3 Gross motor development

to the posture required to brush the hair holding a mirror in one hand and a brush in the other. In early life it may be useful in directing the hand towards objects in the visual field. However, it may prevent rolling over or the hands being brought to the face. Abnormal persistence of the ATNR, particularly in an exaggerated form, is very frequently found in infants with cerebral palsy.

Balance reactions

These are necessary in order for the child to develop ability in the sitting position. The response consists of extension of the arm to prevent falling when the child's body is displaced to either side in the sitting position. Similar saving reactions occur in the standing position.

The parachute reaction

The child is held in a ventral position and is rapidly lowered head first towards the table. The arms extend in order to 'save' the child. Failure to appear is frequently seen in children with neurological abnormalities.

POSTURE AND GROSS MOTOR
(Fig. 5.3)

The rate of development within an individual child varies depending upon his state of health, the degree of stimulation that he receives and such events as the arrival of a new baby, admission to hospital or a change of house. Allowance also needs to be made for prematurity. For this reason data related to a child's development cannot be taken in isolation from the environment in which he is living. Furthermore, the child's personality and temperament may distort his response to the test procedure.

Children follow different patterns of events leading to walking, including crawling, creeping and bottom-shuffling. Those who bottom-shuffle are usually late to walk because it is more difficult to get to the upright posture from the sitting position than from the crawling position. When assessing children who are slow to stand and walk it is obviously important to enquire about other methods of locomotion. Children who bottom-shuffle tend to dislike lying in the prone position and thus do not develop crawling. Some children go straight from sitting to walking without an intervening stage. Negro babies are generally more advanced in early motor development than other babies.

Six weeks

At the age of 6 weeks when lying prone, the baby is just able to raise his chin momentarily. When he is pulled to sit from the supine position the child still shows head lag but is able to show some ability to raise his head, particularly in the halfway position of this manoeuvre. When lying in the supine position the baby still adopts a pattern of flexion at the elbows, knees and hips. A pattern of extension at this age may be an indication of spasticity. Held in ventral suspension he can hold his head in line with the rest of the body. A large discrepancy in the performance of the baby in the prone and supine position with superior performance when prone may indicate a developmental abnormality such as cerebral palsy. However, some babies such as those who are bottom-shufflers, greatly prefer one posture to another. Others are not given the opportunity to develop their motor skills in a wide variety of postures.

Three months

By the age of 3 months there are some most impressive changes in the child's motor abilities. In the prone position, the child is able to lift the head and upper chest clear and is able to sustain this posture supported by the forearms. When pulled to sitting there is only minimal head lag. In ventral suspension the head is now above the level of the body. When held sitting, the back is straight and the head only occasionally drops forward. When held standing the child sags at the knees.

Six months

At 6 months of age, in the prone position, the baby can lift his head and chest clear, supporting his weight on extended arms, and can roll over. Rolling is a very complex motor activity involving coordination of right and left sides, arms, legs, head and trunk. If the child is able to execute such a complicated manoeuvre it is most unlikely that any motor deficit exists. In the supine position he is able to lift his head from the pillow and in this posture grasp his foot. When pulled to sit the head is erect and the back is straight. He is able to sit against a wall requiring no lateral support. When held standing the baby is able to bear weight on his feet.

Nine months

By the age of 9 months most children will be able to sit unsupported for 10–15 minutes. This posture will be stable and the baby is able to maintain balance as he reaches out to grasp nearby objects. By this age the child can also stand holding on and may attempt to take steps if supported. In the prone position some may be crawling and most should be making some attempt at this manoeuvre.

One year

At the age of 1 year the child can sit well and for an indefinite period of time. He can rise independently from the lying position to the sitting position and from the sitting position is able to crawl effectively on all fours. Some children get along by either hauling using the arms alone, or creeping on the hands and feet, or by bottom-shuffling: some miss out these stages altogether. The child is now able to get up and down from the standing position and is able to walk around the furniture, a manoeuvre known as 'cruising'. He may be able to stand alone for a few seconds.

Fifteen months

At 15 months the child can get to the standing position without the aid of nearby objects. He is able to walk unsteadily on a wide base but frequently falls due to minor obstructions. Additional hazards to safety occur as the child learns to crawl upstairs but is unable to get down. He is also able to kneel with or without support.

Eighteen months

By 18 months of age walking skills are well developed and falls are seldom though there is obviously wide individual variation. The child is now sufficiently stable to stoop and pick up an object from the floor without overbalancing. He can run for short distances and can push or pull toys around the floor. Carrying a large object does not result in falling over. He is able to sit down without help in a small chair. Getting upstairs can now be accomplished in an upright posture with the hand held and downward progression may occur by creeping backwards or by proceeding downwards step by step on the buttocks.

Two years

By 2 years of age the child can go up and down stairs holding on in the upright position. This is done step by step and does not follow the adult pattern of alternating feet on each step. Running is now more skilled and the child is able to change course to avoid obstacles. He may play in a squatting position from which he can easily rise to his feet. Climbing on and off furniture is performed with ease but often not with the approval of his parents. He is beginning to be able to both throw and kick balls without falling over in the attempt.

By the age of 2 the child can walk upstairs without holding on but cannot yet do this downstairs. He has now developed the ability to jump with both feet together and to stand on tiptoe following a demonstration of this.

Three years

At the age of 3 the child can walk upstairs with alternating feet but still has to use two feet on each step for descending. He can walk as well as stand on tiptoe and can also stand momentarily on one foot, a skill which many adults cannot demonstrate. The child can now pedal a tricycle as opposed to the previous manoeuvre of pushing it along with

his feet on the ground. Increasing agility enables the child to climb nursery apparatus and to jump down one step. Others may attempt more than this but are not likely to succeed.

Four years

By the age of 4 years the child can walk both up and down stairs using alternating feet. He can stand on one foot for 3–5 seconds and can also hop on one foot, though there is wide variation depending upon the opportunities and encouragement to develop these skills.

Five years

By the age of 5 years the child is able to skip on alternate feet and to run lightly on his toes. His wide repertoire of motor skills will be illustrated by climbing, sliding, swinging, etc. There is increased skill in kicking, throwing and catching balls. He is able in 90% of cases to walk heel to toe. By the age of 5 the child has developed a basic repertoire of gross motor skills. Following this there are improvements related to greater strength, greater precision, greater speed and length of performance.

FINE MOTOR SKILLS (Figs 5.4, 5.5)

The development of fine motor skills depends on normal vision and appropriate opportunities for learning. Deprivation of either will result in the delay of acquisition of such skills.

FOUR YEARS

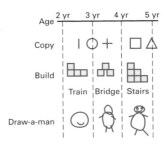

Fig. 5.4 Development of fine motor skills

Development

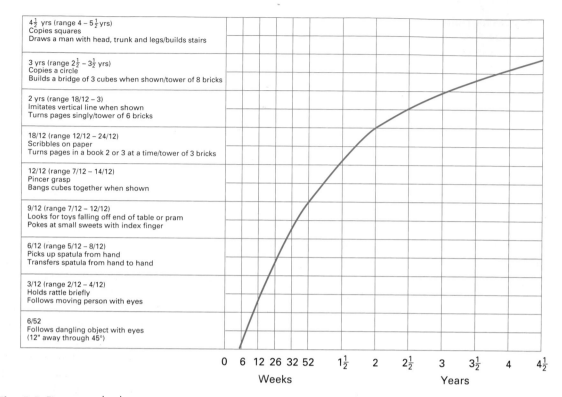

Fig. 5.5 Fine motor development

Six weeks

At 6 weeks the palmar grasp reflex operates but there are no voluntary fine motor movements.

Three months

At 3 months of age there is intense hand regard, in which the child stares continually at his own hand. This intense observation leads in the next few months to the development of voluntary use of the hand which is visually directed. At 3 months the child may reach out and hit objects such as pram beads.

Six months

By 6 months of age the child is able to pick up voluntarily any object such as a cube using a palmar grasp. Both the cube and his hand need to be within the same field of vision. At first this is only done with the greatest of difficulty and the cube is soon dropped. Lacking memory, the child does not look for the dropped object but seems to carry on unperturbed. Although voluntary grasp is established at this age, voluntary release is not seen for several months. At 6 months the child also begins to be able to transfer objects from one hand to another. However the child is not yet able to use this as part of a problem-solving exercise. So, if the child is offered a second cube, he is likely either to ignore this cube or to drop the first one and use the same hand to retrieve the second object. Once the child has learned the ability to grasp objects he soon learns to be able to bring them to his mouth, and to add these sensations to his other means of exploring and understanding objects.

Nine months

At 9 months of age the child has developed a mature grip between thumb and index finger and can also use his index finger to approach and poke at small objects. Toys that are dropped are now sought for. The child has a wide range of manipulative skills, objects can be shaken, bashed, pulled, pushed or held.

One year

By 1 year of age the practice of fine motor skills has enabled the child to pick up small objects such as crumbs. The child is able to use his fine motor skills to feed himself with a biscuit or hold his own bottle. He has developed the phenomenon of casting, in which toys are deliberately dropped and watched as they fall to the ground. Given two objects he may bring them together in the midline and match them or imitate a simple action such as banging two bricks together. If offered a third object, most children seem unable to transfer in order to grasp the third object but may become quite upset by this apparent dilemma and drop both of the original objects.

Fifteen months

At 15 months of age the index finger has developed as an organ for pointing to objects that he wants. Children are reported to be able to build a tower of two cubes though there is a wide variation between these abilities from various reports. This may well be highly dependent on the child's previous experience of bricks and his opportunity to practise. It cannot be assumed, as perhaps some developmental tests do, that most children grow up surrounded by one-inch cubes.

Eighteen months

By 18 months of age the average tower builder has progressed to a somewhat precarious edifice of three bricks. If given a crayon this will be used for spontaneous scribble usually in a preferred hand. The index finger may be used to point at objects in the book and the child can usually turn the pages two or three at a time, inflicting a variable degree of damage.

Two years

At 2 years of age the average tower builder is up to a tower of six cubes, again bearing in mind the wide variation in accomplishment in this task. Although performance with crayon and paper is still largely scribble, this may begin to assume a circular form and the child might also be able to draw dots and imitate a vertical line. Page turning one at a time is now achieved though it must be remembered that many children do not have books and cannot therefore develop the skill. Between 18 months and 2 years most children are able to complete simple jigsaws involving fitting a circle, square and triangle — initially by trial and error and only later by matching. Gains of skills and their level of development depend upon the availability of such toys as posting boxes, etc. Children may more readily demonstrate their fine motor skills in terms of manipulation of toys from activity centres up to small miniature toys, peg boards, jigsaws, dressing dolls, etc. than in more standardised tasks which do not hold the same degree of interest.

At 2½ years of age the child is able to build a seven-block tower. He is also able to construct a 'train' from three blocks placed horizontally in a row and one block placed on top for a chimney. With a pencil he is able to imitate a circle and a horizontal line if this is demonstrated. Only at the next stage are they able to copy the completed symbol without a previous demonstration.

Three years

By 3 years of age the child's tower has grown to nine bricks and using three bricks the child can copy a bridge design. He can draw a circle from a copy and can now draw a cross if this is first demonstrated. The child is, at this stage, beginning to produce recognisable pictures and will produce the first crude picture of a person plus a variety of assorted parts. The Goodenough draw a man test is a useful and reliable way of assessing development of children between ages 3 and 10. The child is asked to draw a man. He is left undisturbed and given as much time as he wants. The final drawing is scored using 51 criteria which record the degree of complexity and the anatomical details shown. The child is given a basal age of 3 years and is accorded an extra 3 months for each of the features recorded in his picture.

Four years

By the age of 4 years we have now reached the limits of tower building, bearing in mind the number of one-inch cubes the paediatrician can carry in his bag at any one time. The tower is now 10 or more cubes high. From about 4 the child is able to construct stairs with the one-inch cubes after an initial demonstration. He can now copy a cross without a previous demonstration and can also draw a square if the technique is shown first. The drawing of a man will now have a head and legs and the picture may or may not have a separate trunk. Most children will also be able to draw a very simple representation of a house. The child of 4 should be able to name the four primary colours in the one-inch bricks and is certainly able to match them. Some children may have been able to do this since the age of 3. A 4 year old can generally do buttons up, a useful practical skill which enables him to dress himself. However, absence of the skill probably indicates that the mother dresses the child because it is quicker.

Five years

The 5 year old can draw a square and a triangle from a copy. (He will need to be 7 to be able to copy a diamond and 9 to be able to copy a parallelogram.) He can also draw a house with door, windows, a roof and a chimney. Using one-inch cubes he can copy the step design without demonstration and also construct a 'gate'. Ideas of shape and copying ability have improved to the extent that the child can now learn to recognise and copy letters from the alphabet.

SOCIAL DEVELOPMENT AND PLAY (Fig. 5.6)

Although appropriate toys for each age group are inserted into the text, it must be recognised that to a large extent, the toys without the parent are useless. Also the importance of play such as peep-bo, round and round the garden, and nursery rhymes which do not require any toys are a very important aspect of stimulation.

Six weeks

At 6 weeks of age the child smiles in response to a friendly human face. The child is visually very alert and will fixate and stare at the mother's face for long periods. As well as crying he develops a whole range of sounds, coos, glugs, grunts and laughter, which indicate mood. An awake baby in a carrycot only receives the stimulation that is brought to him. This may be obtained from mobiles suspended above the cot, by carrying him around or by the use of a bouncing cradle in which the baby reclines.

Three months

At 3 months of age the child begins to react with excitement to familiar and pleasant situations such as feeding and bathing. Similar responses occur when he is played with. From 3 months the child may attempt to hit toys suspended on a string across the pram. Although the child can do very little with toys, things to listen to, such as a musical box, and things to look at, such as mobiles, are very useful.

Six months

At 6 months of age the child can successfully grasp suitable toys and transfer them to the mouth. He is capable of grasping a rattle and shaking it and may apply this strategy to many other objects. He is also able to play with his feet and take these to the mouth too. The child is now able to play with a wider range of toys of many different shapes and colours; they appear to enjoy those they can grasp or which make a noise like rattles and bells.

Nine months

At the age of 9 months the development of memory means that the child becomes much more wary of strangers and sensitive to separation from his

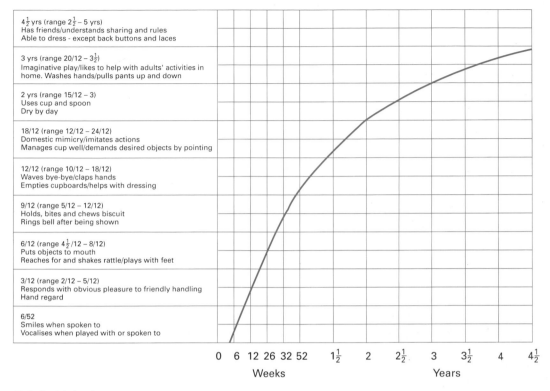

4½ yrs (range 2½ – 5 yrs)
Has friends/understands sharing and rules
Able to dress - except back buttons and laces

3 yrs (range 20/12 – 3½)
Imaginative play/likes to help with adults' activities in home. Washes hands/pulls pants up and down

2 yrs (range 15/12 – 3)
Uses cup and spoon
Dry by day

18/12 (range 12/12 – 24/12)
Domestic mimicry/imitates actions
Manages cup well/demands desired objects by pointing

12/12 (range 10/12 – 18/12)
Waves bye-bye/claps hands
Empties cupboards/helps with dressing

9/12 (range 5/12 – 12/12)
Holds, bites and chews biscuit
Rings bell after being shown

6/12 (range 4½/12 – 8/12)
Puts objects to mouth
Reaches for and shakes rattle/plays with feet

3/12 (range 2/12 – 5/12)
Responds with obvious pleasure to friendly handling
Hand regard

6/52
Smiles when spoken to
Vocalises when played with or spoken to

0 6 12 26 32 52   1½   2   2½   3   3½   4   4½

Weeks   Years

Fig. 5.6 Social development

mother. It also means that lost toys are looked for and he can play games such as peep-bo. He can feed himself with a biscuit, and attempts to hold his own cup or bottle. He may also try to grab the spoon. He can now handle toys which require a wider range of manipulative skills to make them work.

One year

At 1 year of age children who have been given the opportunity are able to drink from a cup. However, many parents feed their children as this is tidier, so that they do not develop the skill until somewhat later. The same applies to spoon feeding which children can manage with help at this age but not all get the opportunity. At 12 months children understand how to cooperate in dressing, recognising that shoes go on feet and arms go in the sleeves. However, although many children do

begin to cooperate with dressing at this stage, others who seem to dislike being dressed, develop the ability of doing the reverse of what is being required. The same can apply to nappy changing which can be a nightmare with a mobile unco-operative child. The child is now able to imitate gestures such as clapping hands and waving bye-bye. Some are able to produce this spontaneously in appropriate situations and others on demand. The child is also able to grasp quickly and imitate other actions such as ringing a bell or banging two bricks together. In play the child will often concentrate for long periods of time, putting objects in and out of boxes or quietly emptying mother's cupboards. Simple cooperative play is developing and the child will give a toy to the parent on request. Toys such as stacking beakers and pop-up men can be useful, though the child's skills are more directed towards taking apart rather than putting together. Rag books are also useful.

Fifteen months

At 15 months the curiosity and exploratory behaviour becomes more intense aided by the improved mobility and manipulative skills developed over this time. The child grasps anything within reach and cannot distinguish safe from dangerous objects. He will begin to be frequently told 'no' and reacts adversely if removed from unsuitable situations.

Eighteen months

The child of 18 months should be able to manage a cup without too much spillage and to be pretty adept at using a spoon independently. He may be able to take off shoes and socks, often in inappropriate circumstances. Negativism and the need for constant supervision are usually more marked than at 15 months. Domestic mimicry is seen in terms of the child copying mother sweeping. The beginnings of symbolic play are also seen, for example putting dolly to sleep or giving mother 'a cup of tea' in a toy cup. The child has progressed from toys that one pushes to trucks or cars, or fitting pieces into other types of shape fitting toys. Sand and water are most appreciated and the child will begin to be able to use drawing and painting materials in a chaotic uncoordinated and sometimes undesirable manner.

Two years

The 2 year old may be slightly less of a danger to himself than the child of 18 months. Greater awareness and knowledge and improved motor abilities may reduce some hazards but increase others. Negativism continues to be prominent and temper tantrums a common feature. The 2 year old should be pretty competent in eating and drinking. The 2 year old is also ready though frequently not willing to be toilet trained, however with greater or lesser difficulty, most children will become dry during the day around this age. The child's play shows further development in domestic mimicry. He begins to want to join in and 'help' with adult activities. Simple make-believe play is also developing. Children of 2 years are unable to share their belongings

and play alongside one another rather than with one another. Useful toys are replicas of adult materials such as tools, cups and saucers, toy cars, simple wooden trains and, of course, picture books and being told stories.

The 2 year old is usually pretty reliable with using the toilet during the day. However many need help in that they are unable to pull down their pants or replace them. Make-believe play is becoming increasingly elaborate with the child frequently talking to himself in play. Tray jigsaws may be very popular. Stories and picture books remain very popular. Scribbling with crayons and painting may just be beginning to emerge with some recognised form or pattern.

Three years

The 3 year old should at last be fairly independent with toileting and accomplish all the subsidiary functions such as pulling pants up and down and washing hands. He is also able to play together with other children and understands concepts such as sharing or taking turns. Many 3 year olds, and quite a number of younger children too, are confident enough to separate from their parents at nursery school or playgroup. Recognisable drawings of a human body or a house begin to be made. The 3 year old can begin to make real constructions out of bricks or construction toys of various types and can make sensible layouts using things like miniature animals, people, etc. The 3 year old is able to remember nursery rhymes and also stories. He is constantly asking questions about things that he sees.

Four years

The 4 year old continues to ask questions though they are now of the 'why' or 'how' variety rather than the 'what' or 'who'. He can dress and undress except for difficult buttons and laces, though the result may often be back to front or inside out. Imagination is shown strongly in play with such items as dressing up. He needs other children to play with and the idea of 'friends' becomes a well-established need.

Five years

The 5 year old is able to play games with increasingly complicated sets of rules. A wider time perspective occurs in play. Particular themes either in play or within school can be carried on over a prolonged period in time. A 5 year old can, but not always, be protective and responsible towards his younger brothers and sisters. The 5 year old can play and build constructively and copy or produce increasingly complicated designs. He has the ability to tell the time, recognise letters and numbers, beginning the process of learning to read.

EMOTIONAL DEVELOPMENT

There are many profiles of childhood describing behaviour at different ages. Theories based on these observations give us a means of understanding the process of learning, the development of reasoning and of emotional responses. Such theories have contributed towards educational progress and in our understanding abnormal or difficult behaviour. They provide a view of the child's world as the child perceives it, as opposed to our description of what the child does. The theories are not only clinically useful but also provide a fascinating insight into the world of a developing child. They are not mutually exclusive for each examines different aspects of child development and each makes its separate contribution towards our understanding.

GESELL

Arnold Gesell at Yale University first made detailed observations of normal child development which he classified into gross and fine motor, adaptive, language and personal/social.

On the basis of these observations, he drew three conclusions:

- That there is a defined sequence of development.
- That development proceeds in a cephalo-caudal progression.
- That development proceeds from gross undifferentiated skills to precise and refined ones.

The important implication of these findings for management in cases of developmental delay is that the child should be helped to acquire skills according to the sequence. Thus, it is inappropriate to teach a child to walk when he is yet unable to sit. Gesell thought that development reflected maturation of the central nervous system, rather than the results of learning. This theory was supported by observations that motor skills developed in a normal way in infants who were swaddled; however the quality of their performance was not studied.

Gesell also observed that it was not possible to induce the earlier development of particular skills by specific training and practice. He concluded from this again that central nervous system maturation was the dominant factor rather than training. It would be wrong to draw the conclusion from these relatively limited observations that nothing need be done or can be done for the young handicapped child on the argument that progress awaits brain maturation. This approach is too simplistic and although it must be accepted that damaged or delayed maturation will cause delay in development, it cannot be accepted that appropriate therapy and stimulation are not required. Some aspects of development are certainly dependent upon external stimulation; thus, the development of visual function depends on appropriate stimulation of the retina. Deprivation of this stimulation by opacities or gross uncorrected refractive errors results in the failure of development of visual function if these ophthalmic problems are corrected late. Similarly, cutting off the whiskers of mice results in defective development of the parts of the brain which control these sensitive organs. Others have developed the idea of critical periods for the acquisition of particular skills, which suggests that optimum learning occurs only if the required stimulation is obtained at a particular time in development.

In spite of these criticisms, Gesell has contributed an enormous amount towards our understanding of normal development, particularly motor development, and its clinical application to developmental diagnosis.

LEARNING THEORY

Learning theory and behaviour modification practice have wide application in many areas including

Development

the management of children with developmental delay. Learning theory is based upon the assumption that, with the exception of reflex responses, all behaviour is learned. It therefore stresses the role of experience in the environment rather than that of cerebral maturation. Certain responses are learned following specific stimuli and appropriate responses are reinforced. This has led to the therapeutic tool of behaviour modification whereby new responses may be learned and reinforcement withdrawn from inappropriate responses.

The theory on which behaviourism is based rests largely on animal experiments starting with Pavlov's classic experiments conditioning dogs to salivate when a bell was rung, through to the later experiments of Skinner and of Watson. The extreme point of view that all behaviour results from external learning cannot be accepted, but taken in conjunction with the other theories explaining child development, behaviour theory has an important application to our understanding of certain aspects of normal development and certain abnormalities in behaviour. For example, children probably acquire their gender identification by means of the type of stimulation they receive. Thus boys are encouraged to model themselves on their father's behaviour and are given trains and guns to play with whilst little girls are encouraged to model themselves on maternal behaviour and are given dolls and pushchairs to play with.

Animal experiments have shown that there are critical times for acquiring certain types of behaviour, for instance monkeys reared entirely away from their own mothers do not exhibit normal maternal behaviour and are aggressive and not protective towards their offspring. This animal model parallels that of early childhood deprivation and the failure of those individuals to bond or take care of their children.

Behaviour theory has been very useful in that it has identified how certain types of normal social behaviour are developed. Some understanding of the genesis of disturbed behaviour is gained and why within some families they recur. However, all external influences act upon some substrate. It is clear that babies have particular personalities right from birth, and that these personalities are to some extent independent of external factors.

ERIKSON

Eric Erikson's psychoanalytical theory covers the whole of human life from birth to old age. He describes each stage in terms of conflicts between two opposing forces. These conflicts arouse anxiety. Failure to resolve the particular conflicts of each stage in development results in maladaptive behaviours which continue into adult life.

Phase I: Infancy (the first year of life)

- acquiring a sense of basic trust
- whilst overcoming a sense of basic mistrust
- realisation of hope

In this phase, the child is entirely dependent. His satisfactions are in being fed and in the process of bonding to his parents. Absence of these results in anxiety. It is easy to see how important it is for the child to acquire, early on, a sense of confidence in the world around him. If he fails to do this and the world is seen as a hostile, unpredictable place, then he is likely to be a 'difficult baby' and to have feeding and sleeping problems. As adults, those severely deprived in this early stage are likely to be emotionally detached and aggressive, being unable to form deep and lasting relationships with others.

Phase II: Early childhood (1–3 years)

- acquiring a sense of autonomy (own will)
- whilst combating a sense of doubt and shame
- a realisation of will

In this stage the child acquires confidence in his own ability as opposed to self-doubt. He realises his own will and has the ability for independent action. He is, however, required to conform to certain behaviours and may feel guilty if he does not. Children of this age develop negativism, temper tantrums and toilet-training difficulties. He needs to learn to balance his own wishes against those of others. On the one hand, if he is unable to realise the strength of his will then as an adult he may be lacking in confidence and initiative. On the other hand, if he does not develop any form of censorship mechanism then he might have difficulty accepting the demands made by society.

Phase III: Nursery school age (3–5 years)

- acquiring a sense of initiation
- overcoming a sense of guilt
- realisation of purpose

From the self-confidence acquired in Phase II, a child goes on to initiate social behaviour which goes beyond himself into group situations. He must learn to share attention, affection and materials. In this phase conscience formation occurs and the child internalises previously external standards of behaviour. He may feel anxious that his separate autonomous behaviour is not always in accord with that of the group and guilt may result from this or from the fear of being found out.

With the greater sense of initiative the child begins to assume responsibility for himself as well. The child obtains his primary identification as male or female. Sexual curiosity and erotic feelings may arise and the Oedipus complex of attachment to the parent of the opposite sex is often seen. The child develops ideas of the future and can postpone satisfactions or pleasures till a later time.

Success in overcoming the conflicts of this stage results in a confident, outgoing person who is able to generalise his confidence into the group situation. Failure to do so at this stage may result in nightmares, fears of the dark, animals or physical injury.

Phase IV: Primary school age (latency) (5–11 years)

- acquiring a sense of industry
- whilst fending off a sense of inferiority
- realisation of competence

In this age group children acquire the drive to achieve whilst attempting to overcome a feeling of failure. This drive and competitive spirit applies in intellectual activities, physical activities and in social relationships. Success at these results in increasing self-esteem (and esteem from others), whereas failure or a sense of failure can result in difficulties in learning and impaired relationships. Those involved with school health will be very familiar with the child who finds himself isolated outside the competitive and energetic world of this age group.

Phase V: Adolescence

- acquiring a sense of identity
- whilst overcoming a sense of identity diffusion
- a realisation of fidelity

This description is perhaps best illustrated by Gauguin's picture *Ou venons nous ou sommes nous ou allons nous* — translated as 'where have we come from, where are we, where are we going to?' The child needs to acquire a firm sense of who he is, what he wants from life and where he is going. Failure to do this is described by Erickson as role diffusion.

In this stage the child acquires a time perspective and is able to work towards distant goals such as examinations. There is anticipation of particular achievements in the future. The role of leadership is further developed in this age group and for the first time ideological identification is seen in terms of political attitudes. Sexual identity develops further.

At this age the child should have acquired sufficient self-certainty in preparation for an independent life and decision-making. The drive towards decision-making is combated by a sense of doubt and uncertainty. Role experimentation in terms of jobs, ideology and allegiances may cause added conflicts with parents as the adolescent seeks to acquire his own individual identity. Understanding adolescent problems is understanding the balance between acquiring the self-certainty and anxiety about the ability to do so.

Phase VI

- acquiring a sense of intimacy
- avoiding a sense of isolation
- a realisation of love

This is the phase of courtship and marriage.

Phase VII

- acquiring a sense of generativity
- avoiding a sense of self absorption
- a realisation of care

This is Erickson's description of parenthood and the ability of parents to put the demands of their own child beyond that of their own.

Phase VIII

- acquiring a sense of integrity
- avoiding a sense of despair
- a realisation of wisdom

This is maturity!

PIAGET

Jean Piaget, a Swiss Zoologist, based his explanations of child development upon precise observations, particularly of his own children. His observations on cognitive development have been widely incorporated into teaching schemes in primary education.

The sensorimotor stage: 0–2 years

In this stage the child acquires a permanent image of himself and of the practical world about him. He learns to understand his separateness (dualism) from his mother.

1. Reflex action: 0–1 month

At this time Piaget describes all reactions as being simply reflex. For example, the child sucks in response to any object put into his mouth and he cannot distinguish between his own finger and the nipple.

2. Primary circular reactions: 1–4 months

By this time the child has formed motor habits which Piaget calls schema. Having developed these motor habits they can be wilfully repeated for their own sake, for example wilfully sucking the thumb.

3. Secondary circular reactions: 4–9 months

Now actions are produced not for the pleasure of their doing, but for the results they produce in the external world. Intentional acts are carried out. The child tries out all his various schemata on a new object until he finds one which produces the most satisfying results. Coordination of vision and movement develop, although the child only grasps an object if the hand and the object are seen simultaneously.

4. Coordination of schemata: 9–11 months

In this stage the child pursues a particular end rather than trying out all his various motor habits to look for a satisfying result. Therefore if the result is obtaining a particular object that he desires he might use his previous experience, such as tugging at the blanket on which the object is placed, to bring the object sufficiently near for it to be grasped.

Piaget describes memory developing at this time — the child realises that objects that have disappeared have not gone and that he should look to see where they have dropped or where they might reappear. A child will discover a block which has been hidden under a cup. He is able to imitate gesture and understand situational clues, for example preparations for a meal. With memory comes distress at separation from the parents. The child becomes much more discriminating in terms of adults and will not go willingly to a stranger. Children remember the child health clinic and immunising injections. Anticipatory crying occurs in the expectation of receiving a further injection.

5. Tertiary circular reactions: 11–18 months

At this age, the infant seeks new results by active experimentation. Thus if he is dropping objects from a pram he may vary the position of dropping the objects to observe the variation in effect that can be obtained.

6. Invention of new means through mental combinations: 18–24 months

In this stage, the child may be seen to solve problems not by physical experimentation but through mentally working out the solution and then applying this knowledge. Thus if a chain is in a small box, which does not admit the child's fingers, his first action may be to invert the box so that the chain is expelled rather than make unfruitful attempts to get his fingers into it to grasp it. These observations of Piaget can be readily repeated. They are a most worthwhile and rewarding part of a developmental assessment.

Infantile realism: 3–7 years

By 3 years of age, the child sees himself as the centre of the universe. He cannot conceive that others can have a different viewpoint (egocentrism). Animism describes the child's belief that everything is alive and has thoughts, feelings and wishes, just as he does. Dreams exist and thoughts and wishes are just as powerful as real events. In his pre-causal logic, nothing happens by chance. There is always a cause and causes are motivational. For example, balloons go up into the air because they want to. The child's beliefs are based not on what he perceives but on an internal model of the world which may bear little relationship to what his senses tell him. For instance the child is insensible to the contradiction that babies come from a baby shop even though he has never seen one. In the authoritarian morality of this age, the child believes that the punishment arises out of the crime. Bad events are explained as a punishment for something that he has done. It is easy for the child to feel responsible for events that have taken place, particularly in view of his egocentric stand-point.

It is during this period of infantile realism that the child may suffer excessive anxiety if he feels that his bad thoughts and wishes may actually have come true or that having such thoughts may result in some punishment following automatically. The pre-causal child will see teaching about heaven or hell or stories of Father Christmas coming down the chimney as very concrete and real. Rules are rigid and unalterable. Thus the child in the back seat is happy to point out the red light the parents have just crossed or the double yellow line at the kerbside!

Although there is a rapid expansion of language ability, Piaget observed that children mainly talk to themselves and that their 'conversations' are really a collective monologue.

Concrete operations: 8–11 years

At the time of his move to junior school the child acquires the ability to think logically. He realises that words, thoughts and rules are separate from concrete objects and activities. He is able to learn to compare and to contrast, and to understand the relationship of parts to the whole, to be able to group objects in time and space, and to understand the principles of conservation of mass, weight and volume.

Formal operation: from age 12 years

From 12 years of age the child acquires the ability for abstract thinking. This involves a systematic approach to problems and the ability to under-stand hypotheses. There is a progressive ability to acquire an understanding of concepts of space, time, causation, number, definition, order, shape, size, motion, speed, force and energy. It is only within the secondary school that such concepts can be properly understood and taught within the syllabus.

DEVELOPMENTAL ASSESSMENT

Developmental assessment is an important part of any paediatric evaluation. In most cases a brief question to the parents enquiring as to whether they have any concerns about the child's developmental progress, together with informal observation of the child's activities during the appointment, will be sufficient.

In other circumstances, a more detailed assessment will be necessary. This may be because there is already concern about a developmental problem, or because the child is felt to be at increased risk of there being developmental delay, for example in follow-up of high-risk infants, assessment of children with other disabilities (physical or sensory impairment) or in socially deprived children. Sometimes it will be necessary as part of an assessment of special educational need, or as part of an evaluation of the needs of children in the care of social services.

The developmental assessment is just part of the whole evaluation which should also include a developmental history, an account from the parents of the child's current functioning and a medical examination. It may also include reports of the child's functioning in other environments, for example family centre, nursery or school. It may be helpful to directly observe the child, not just in the clinic, but also in one of these settings, and/or in the home.

Development

METHODS OF DEVELOPMENTAL ASSESSMENT USED BY PAEDIATRICIANS

Informal

In many cases, it is sufficient for the paediatrician to carry out an informal assessment in the clinic. An experienced paediatrician will be able to use a range of toys, books and simple tests (e.g. drawing shapes and building with bricks) that they are familiar with to build up a picture of the child's developmental level. With experience, they will have become familiar with the range of responses to a particular task at any given age, and can therefore compare the child being assessed with this. It is useful to consider a few skills in each area of development, for example gross motor, fine motor, social development and play, and communication. The paediatrician can then give an approximate developmental age at which the child is functioning for each parameter. When expressed in this way it is easily understandable to parents, who will be able to discuss their own view of the child's development and whether the paediatrician has got what they consider to be an accurate picture. In other cases it may serve to illustrate to parents the degree of difficulty the child has in a specific area or alternatively may reassure them about their child's progress.

Formal

Sometimes it is necessary to use a more formal, standardised assessment. This will give a quantitative assessment, resulting in a test score. Providing it is carried out with appropriate skill, the results should be reproducible. Such tests are used to compare the performance of groups of children, as may be necessary in research. For clinical purposes, they can be useful to get a deeper insight into an individual child's pattern of strengths and weaknesses, helping with diagnosis, planning interventions and monitoring progress over time.

There are many different tests available; some used for screening and others for detailed assessment. Most require specific training and a set of equipment. The use of some tests is restricted to particular professional groups, usually psycholo-

gists. The tests described here are those commonly used by paediatricians in the UK.

Denver II (Frankenberg et al 1992)

Age range 0–6

Previously known as the Denver Developmental Screening Test, this is widely used in clinical practice. In some areas, it has been introduced as a universal screening tool used by health visitors. The assessor completes a form, which represents graphically the developmental profile with boxes showing the 25th, 50th, 75th and 90th centile for children attaining each ability.

This test is best used as a screening test. It can be performed quickly, in 10–20 minutes in a clinic. Its use is not restricted to any professional group and no specific training is required.

Schedule of growing skills
(Bellman et al 1996)

Age 0–5 years

This test is also primarily designed as a screening test, but is more detailed and can therefore be used as a more in-depth assessment. A record form is completed, looking at nine skill areas — passive postural, active postural, locomotor, manipulative, visual, hearing and language, speech and language, interactive social and self-care social. A skills score is calculated for each area, which is then converted to a developmental age. An additional cognitive skills score is derived from selected items in the other nine areas.

The schedule takes about 20 minutes to complete. No specific training is required, and its use is not restricted.

Griffiths Scales of Mental Development (Griffiths 1970, 1976)

0–8 years

This is a British test, widely used by UK paediatricians. Its use is restricted to those who have been on an accredited training course. The scales are divided into six areas — A, locomotor; B, personal social; C, hearing and speech; D, eye and hand coordination; E, performance; F, practical reasoning (for those over 2 years). Results are scored as a mental age in months for each area which is divide by chronological age to give a developmental quotient (DQ). General quotient (GQ) can also be obtained by the average of the subquotients, but the meaning of this is limited, the real value of the test being not just levels attained, but the profile of the child's skills across the six areas. The Griffiths scales take about an hour to complete.

Other tests to consider

The paediatrician should also be aware of some of the many other tests that may be appropriate in particular circumstances, or to look at specific areas of development. Details of these are beyond the scope of this text but are discussed in detail elsewhere (Pollak 1993)

Examples of other tests include Reynell–Zinkin scales (Reynell & Zinkin 1979), for assessment of children with visual impairment, and the Leiter International Performance Scale Battery, which assesses non-verbal ability, and can be useful for those with no language, including deaf and autistic children. There are many specific language assessments, for example Reynell Developmental Language Scale (Reynell 1969) and developmental coordination problems can be usefully assessed using the Movement Assessment Battery for Children (Movement ABC)(Henderson & Sugden 1992).

The Wechsler Intelligence Scale for Children (WISC) and the Wechsler Preschool and Primary Scale of Development (WPPSI) (Wechsler 1974) are primarily used by psychologists. They cover the ranges 4–17, and have separate verbal and non-verbal sections. They are likely to be used for educational purposes in older children, where assessment is beyond the skills or the remit of most paediatricians.

REFERENCES AND FURTHER READING

Bayley N 1965 Comparisons of mental and motor test scores for ages 1–15 months by sex, birth, order and race, geographical location and education of parents. Child Development 36:379
Bellman M, Lingam S, Aukett A 1996 Schedule of growing skills. NFER–Nelson Publishing Company, Windsor
Bryant G M, Davies K J, Newcombe R G 1974 The Denver developmental screening test: achievement of test items in the first year of life by Denver and Cardiff infants. Developmental Medicine and Child Neurology 16:475–484
Buckler J M H 1979 A reference manual of growth and development. Blackwell Scientific, Oxford
Egan D, Illingworth R S, McKeith R 1971 Developmental screening 0–5. Clinics in Developmental Medicine No 30. Spastics International Medical Publications and Heinemann, London
Erikson E H 1967 Childhood and society. Penguin Books, Harmondsworth
Frankenberg W K, Dodds J, Archer P, Shapiro H, Bresnick B 1992 The Denver II: a major revision and restandardisation of the Denver Developmental Screening Test. Pediatrics 90:477–479
Gessell A 1948 Studies in child development. Harper and Row, London
Gessell A 1966 The first five years of life. Metheun, London
Griffiths R 1970 The abilities of young children. Association for Research in Infant and Child Development, Amersham, Bucks
Griffiths R 1976 The abilities of babies. Association for Research in Infant and Child Development, Amersham, Bucks
Henderson S, Sugden D A 1992 Movement assessment battery for children. The Psychological Corporation, Harcourt Brace, London.
Holt K S 1991 Child developments, diagnosis and assessment. Butterworth Heinemann, London
Illingworth R S 1979 The normal child, 10th edn. Churchill Livingstone, Edinburgh
Maier H L 1969 Three theories of child development. Harper and Row, London
Piaget J 1929 The child's conception of the world. Routledge and Kegan Paul, London
Piaget J, Inhelder D 1969 The psychology of the child. Routledge and Kegan Paul, London
Pollak M 1993 Textbook of developmental paediatrics. Churchill Livingstone, Edinburgh.
Reynell J 1969 Reynell Developmental Language Scales. NFER–Nelson Publishing Company, Windsor
Reynell J, Zinkin P 1979 Manual for Reynell–Zinkin Developmental Scales for young visually handicapped children. NFER–Nelson Publishing Company, Windsor.
Robson P 1970 Shuffling, scooting and sliding; some observations on 30 otherwise normal children. Developmental Medicine and Child Neurology 12:608–617
Sheridan M 1973 Children's developmental progress. National Foundation for Educational Research, Windsor
Terman L M, Merril M A 1961 Stanford Binet Intelligence Scale. LM Harrap, London
Wechsler D 1974 Manual for the Wechsler intelligence scale for children. Psychological Corporation, New York

6 | Clinical genetics and genetic services: principles and practice

INTRODUCTION

The specialty of clinical genetics represents an interface between advanced technology and the family. Community paediatricians will often encounter genetic disease and will work with clinical geneticists as part of the essential multidisciplinary approach to complex paediatric problems. Genetics — beyond modified tomatoes and cloned sheep — is beyond the realm of experience of most people; the issues raised within a family by the discovery of genetic disease are wide-ranging and therefore demand an experienced and sensitive approach.

The aim of this chapter is to give a brief overview of current clinical paediatric genetic practice. No discussion about clinical genetics can take place without a reference to basic science. There are already many excellent texts dealing with the fundamentals of DNA structure and function. The first part of the chapter, therefore, deals with contemporary *principles* of paediatric genetic disease. The second part deals with the *practice* of clinical paediatric genetics in the service setting, with reference to community practice where possible, and with careful consideration to ethical issues. Clearly, in such a rapidly evolving speciality, published reference material is rapidly outdated; regularly updated electronic media is referred to as often as possible. For example, Online Mendelian Inheritance in Man (OMIM) is an up-to-date catalogue of genetic disorders and is available at no cost at http://www.ncbi.nlm.nih.gov/omim/. The disease reference numbers used throughout this chapter come from OMIM. A glossary of genetic terms is offered at the end of the chapter.

PRINCIPLES

A note on genetic nomenclature

A series of nomenclatures have been devised to standardise the notation of chromosome abnormalities, genes and proteins. The aim is not to confuse, but to simplify!

Size

The smallest DNA subunit is the *base* (Guanine, Cytosine, Thymine or Adenine). The size of a DNA segment is commonly expressed in *kilobases* (kb; =1000 bases) or *megabases* (Mb; =1 000 000 bases).

Chromosomes

Chromosomal regions are labelled according to the standard International System for Human Cytogenetic Nomenclature defined in Paris in 1971. Each chromosome has a short arm ('p': *'petit'*), a centromere (cen) and a long arm ('q': *'queue'*). The ends of the arms are refered to as 'telomeres' ('pter' and 'qter'). In cytogenetic terms, 'proximal' means towards the centromere (also refered to as 'centromeric') and 'distal' means towards the telomere (i.e. 'telomeric'). Chromosome bands are labelled numerically from the centromere towards the telomere. For example, the first band on the short arm of chromosome 1 is labeled 1p1. This is subdivided into three subregions labelled, from centromere to telomere, 1p11, 1p12 and 1p13. In turn, band 1p13 is further subdivided into 1p13.1, 1p13.2 and 1p13.3. This increasing resolution enables precise localisation of genes and accurate description of cytogenetic abnormalities.

A further standard nomenclature is used to described abnormal chromosomes. The *karyotype* is a short-hand description of the chromosome constitution of an individual or cell. It contains the number of chromosomes, followed by a description of the sex chromosomes and then a description of any abnormalities. Normal male and female karyotypes are written as 46, XY and 46, XX respectively. *Numerical* abnormalities are known as *aneuploidy*: 47, XX +21 describes a female with trisomy 21; 47, XXY describes an individual with a sex chromosome aneuploidy known as Klinefelter's syndrome; 45,X describes an individual with monosomy X (Turner's syndrome). Cytogenetic terminology can be very complex. Terms used to describe common *structural* abnormalities are:

- 't' (reciprocal translocation), e.g. 46, XX, t(2;3)(p16;q27) — this describes a female with a reciprocal exchange between chromosomes 2 and 3, with breakpoints in bands 2p16 and 3q27.
- 'del' (deletion), e.g. 46, XY, del(22)(q11.2) — this describes a male with a deletion of band q11.2 of chromosome 22.
- 'dup' (duplication), e.g. 46, XY, dup(15)(q12q14) — this describes an individual in which a region of chromosome 15 between bands q12 and q14 is duplicated.
- 'inv' (inversion), e.g. 46, XX, inv(12)(q21.2q24.1) — this describes a female in which a region of chromosome 12 between bands q21.2 and q24.1 has become inverted.
- 'mar' (marker), e.g. 47, XX, +mar — this describes a female in whom there is an extra, unidentified chromosome fragment known as a marker.
- 'r' (ring), e.g. 46, X, r(X)(p22.3q28) — this describes a female in whom the terminal bands of each arm of one X chromosome have been lost, resulting in the formation of a ring-shaped structure.

Genes and proteins

Genes are allocated a symbol of up to six characters by the Genome Database Nomenclature Committee (see http://www.gene.ucl.ac.uk/nomenclature/). Gene symbols are written in upper case and italics. The protein product of the gene is written in normal, lower case script. For example, the *FBN1* gene on chromosome 15 encodes a protein known as fibrillin (mutations in *FBN1* cause Marfan's syndrome) and the *TCOF1* gene on chromosome 5 encodes a protein known as treacle (mutations in *TCOF1* cause Treacher–Collins syndrome, a form of mandibulofacial dysostosis). Many genes have previously been identified in other species such as the fruit fly *Drosophila melanogaster*, and may also have rather unusual names. *SHH* on chromosome 7, for example, encodes a protein known as sonic hedgehog; mutations in *SHH* cause holoprosencephaly in humans.

The nomenclature used to describe variations in DNA sequence within or around a gene — whether a disease-causing mutation or a polymorphism — is very complex and interested readers should refer to Strachan & Read (1999) for detail. For example, the common cystic fibrosis gene mutation in Caucasians is written as ΔF508: this means that mutation results in the deletion (Δ) of the 508th amino acid (F = phenylalanine) from the mature cystic fibrosis transmembrane conductance regulator protein. Another example is the 35delG mutation in *GJB2*, a common cause of autosomal recessive non-syndromal hearing loss, which describes the deletion (del) of the 35th base (G: guanine) from the start of the gene.

The spectrum of genetic pathology

How common is genetic disease? It has been estimated that at least 50% of all conceptions are lost in the first trimester as the result of a genetic or cytogenetic fault. Of those who survive to term, 2% will manifest a chromosome or single gene disorder as a neonate; by the age of 25, at least 5% of the population will be living with a disease in which genetics plays a significant role (Baird et al 1988). After the age of 25, around 1.6% of the population will develop a late-onset single gene disorder, 0.2% will learn that they have a chromosome abnormality (e.g. presenting as recurrent miscarriage or infertility), 60% will develop a common 'multifactorial' disorder with a genetic component and 25% will develop a somatic cell genetic disorder such as cancer (data from Rimoin et al 1997). This, together with the fact that all of us are thought to carry at least two (different) recessive genes, means that 'genetics' impacts on *all* of us and may have implications for our healthcare system from the moment we are conceived to the moment we die. Much of this burden impacts directly on community practice. It is also clear that the community paediatrician will see many children manifesting genetic disease and many thousands more who appear phenotypically normal but who are genetically 'programmed' to develop disease in adult life.

Strictly, the word 'gene' is a general term that should perhaps only be used in the context of what is considered to represent a normal (*consensus*) DNA sequence. Differences in the sequence may either be disease-causing *mutations* or may simply represent normal variation in the population (*polymorphism*). Each of the two copies of the DNA sequence is known as an *allele*. Thus, when we refer to the parents of a child with cystic fibrosis (CF) as carriers of a cystic fibrosis 'gene', what we really mean is that they are heterozygous for a disease-causing allele of the *CFTR* gene which when present in the homozygous state causes CF.

A seemingly bewildering number of genetic mechanisms can cause genetic disease or predispose to common disease. Essentially, however, all of these affect a single molecule, DNA, and can be placed on a *spectrum* ranging from point mutations to chromosome rearrangements and aneuploidy. It is useful to retain this concept in relation to genetic tests. The reader is referred elsewhere for a more detailed discussion of human DNA structure and function (Strachan & Read 1999) and of some of the concepts within this section (Mueller & Young 1998).

A single gene can be mutated in a number of ways (Fig. 6.1). *Point mutations* in the coding sequence, for example, are well-known causes of disease. They may be inherited or may arisen de novo. Point mutations in the *FBN-1* gene, for example, cause Marfan's syndrome and approximately 25% of cases have no antecedent family history. *Deletion* of DNA sequence within a gene ('intragenic' deletion) is also a well-recognised mutational mechanism and is seen particularly in many cases of Duchenne and Becker muscular dystrophies, as the result of intragenic deletion within the *DMD* gene. In recent years, two novel causes of human genetic disease have been characterised: *triplet repeat expansion* and *genomic imprinting*. These mechanisms serve to reinforce both the dynamic nature of the genome and the role of sex specificity in non X-linked genetic disease.

Duplication of single genes is an unusual mechanism, which is responsible for a common form of

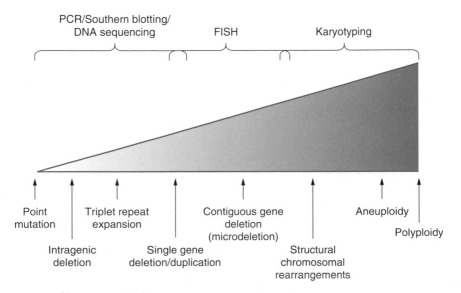

Fig. 6.1 The spectrum of human genetic disease.

hereditary motor and sensory neuropathy. *Deletion* of a single gene is rarely encountered, but deletion of a number of adjacent genes has become a well-recognised phenomenon giving rise to a '*contiguous gene*', or '*microdeletion*', syndrome. The exact phenotype of a child with a microdeletion syndrome largely depends partly on the genes lost in the microdeletion.

Deletion or duplication of large chromosome segments — much larger than is seen in a microdeletion syndrome — are a significant cause of recurrent miscarriage and multiple congenital abnormality/mental retardation (MCA/MR) syndromes. Although a number of rearrangements are associated with clearly recognisable phenotypes — deletion of the short arm of chromosomes 4 in Wolf–Hirshhorn syndrome and 5 in cri-du-chat syndrome for example (Jones 1997) — many have unique or very rare phenotypes. A full search of the literature and cytogenetic databases may be necessary to find previously documented cases. The commonest of these chromosomal rearrangements encountered in clinical practice is the *translocation*, which can either be balanced (when no chromosome material is deleted or duplicated) or unbalanced. The largest scale genetic imbalance is *aneuploidy*. Down's syndrome is a familiar example of aneuploidy in which there are three copies of chromosome 21 in each cell; monosomy implies the loss of a chromosome, as illustrated by classical Turner's syndrome (45, X). Most autosomal aneuploidies (i.e. involving non-sex chromosomes) are incompatible with extrauterine life and are commonly seen in spontaneous miscarriage material. Trisomies, for example, account for about 60% of chromosomally abnormal abortuses (Gardner & Sutherland 1996). Trisomy 21 also accounts for many spontaneous pregnancy losses but in addition is compatible with survival into adulthood, whereas long-term survival in liveborn infants with trisomies 18 and 13 (Edwards' syndrome and Patau syndrome) is exceptional. Aneuploidy of sex chromosomes is, however, commonly associated with survival into adulthood with the notable exception of monosomy X, a frequent cytogenetic abnormality in early miscarriage material. Sex chromosome aneuploidy may cause so few problems that it is only detected when, for example, an individual presents to an infertility clinic. This is often the case with Klinefelter's syndrome (47, XXY).

Autosomal dominant disease

Key features of autosomal dominant inheritance
- Disease features manifest in heterozygotes (i.e. only one allele is mutant).
- The recurrence risk for an affected individual is 50%.
- New mutations give rise to apparently sporadic autosomal dominant disease with no antecedent family history.
- Some heterozygotes may have very mild disease features ('*reduced penetrance*') or none at all ('*non-penetrance*').
- The same mutant allele can cause different disease features in different individuals ('*variable expressivity*').
- A single mutation may give rise to several apparently unrelated disease features in the same individual ('*pleiotropy*').

Marfan's syndrome (OMIM 154700)
Marfan's syndrome is an autosomal dominant multisystem connective tissue disorder affecting mainly the skeleton, the cardiovascular system and the eye. Most cases are caused by mutations in the *FBN-1* gene on chromosome 15q21.1, which encodes a structural protein known as fibrillin. Fibrillin deficiency results in weakness and possible mechanical failure of connective tissue. Twenty-five per cent of cases represent a new mutation arising from either a spontaneous mutational event in a parental gamete or as a consequence of parental *gonadal mosaicism*. This term refers to a clone of cells within a parent's gonad (usually the father) which harbours a disease-causing mutation and produces mutant gametes.

Making a confident diagnosis of Marfan's syndrome in children can be very difficult, since the phenotype can take many years to develop (Lipscomb et al 1997) and tends to vary considerably both within the family and between different families. Diagnosis of possible new mutations is especially difficult, since a positive family history is a diagnostic criterion (de Paepe et al 1996). In addition, tall, slim build and high-arched palate are both common traits in the general population and are difficult to interpret in the absence of other signs of connective tissue disease. Marfan's syndrome therefore creates practical clinical problems relating to *pleiotropy, variable penetrance, variable expression* and the overlap with normal population traits. DNA testing for Marfan's syndrome is not yet available within the service setting, and the diagnosis is still made on clinical grounds over one hundred years after its initial description.

All children with a suspected diagnosis undergo an initial multidisciplinary diagnostic work-up including skeletal, cardiac and ophthalmological assessment. Regular surveillance of *clearly affected* children should continue well into adulthood, with particular attention during puberty, during which time a number of disease features may accelerate (scoliosis, pectus deformity, aortic root dilatation). Adolescents are particularly vulnerable to psychosocial problems relating to the diagnosis of Marfan's syndrome (Van Tongerloo & De Paepe 1998) and supportive counselling can be provided by the genetic counselling team if necessary. It is also important to reassess those children with *suspected* Marfan's syndrome periodically, aiming to avoid over-medicalisation and undue anxiety. The introduction of consensus multidisciplinary guidelines will set the minimum standards for the management of individuals with confirmed or suspected Marfan's syndrome and will encourage equitable service provision. Although no such guidelines have yet been ratified on a national (UK) level, this is an area of intense activity which has already produced some early encouraging results in Scotland (see 'Tuberous sclerosis' below).

Tuberous sclerosis (OMIM 191100 and 191092)

Tuberous sclerosis (TS) is an autosomal dominant condition affecting at least 1 in 10 000 live births. It is characterised by the age-dependent development of hamartomas in a number of tissues, for example the skin and central nervous system, and is often associated with epilepsy and learning disability. A good clinical review is presented by Huson & Rosser (1997). Unlike Marfan's syndrome, most

cases of TS are sporadic (between 60% and 70%), with no phenotypic manifestations in either parent; some of these cases represent new dominant mutations in a TS gene, although parental gonadal mosaicism certainly accounts for sibling recurrences in apparently sporadic cases (Rose et al 1999). Most TS is caused by mutation in one of two genes: *TS1* on chromosome 9q34, whose gene product is known as hamartin, and *TS2* on chromosome 16p13.3, whose gene product is known as tuberin (a simple example of *genetic heterogeneity*). It is currently thought that the hamartin and tuberin proteins interact as tumour suppressors. *TS1* mutations appear to account for around one in six cases, the remainder being *TS2* (Jones et al 1999). This genetic heterogeneity is reflected in the clinical difference between the two subtypes of TS. Broadly, children with TS2 tend to have more aggressive disease, and are more likely to have significant learning disability. They may also have severe renal cystic disease in addition to the characteristic — and common — renal angiomyolipomatosis, since the gene responsible for autosomal dominant polycystic kidney disease is adjacent to *TS2* and both genes can be deleted or disrupted as part of a contiguous gene syndrome. Genetic testing in TS is now possible, although because no clinically useful genotype–phenotype correlation has emerged to date prognostic predictions are very limited. Testing may however be warranted if it enables parents to opt for prenatal diagnosis in subsequent pregnancies. The Scottish Clinical Genetics Guidelines Working Group has recently reported its evidence-based care pathway for tuberous sclerosis (Bradshaw et al 1998), which permits coordinated assessment and care of affected individuals and enables the patient or parent to feel more involved in the care process.

Autosomal recessive disease

Key features of autosomal recessive inheritance

- Disease features manifest in homozygotes (i.e. both alleles have the same mutation).
- Disease features may also manifest in compound heterozygotes (i.e. both alleles are mutant, but the mutations are different).

- Heterozygotes are disease free and are referred to as 'carriers'.
- A male and female carrier have a 25% chance of having an affected child, a 50% chance of having a child who is also a carrier and a 25% chance of having a child who has two normal alleles.

Cystic fibrosis (OMIM 219700)

Cystic fibrosis (CF) is the commonest autosomal recessive genetic disorder affecting caucasians. Around 1 in 22 caucasians carry a single mutant allele of the *CFTR* gene (Cystic Fibrosis Transmembrane Regulator) in addition to a normal ('wild-type') allele. The 'carrier frequency' is different in other racial groups and this should always be remembered when calculating genetic risks in such individuals. At the time of writing, nearly 900 *CFTR* mutations and 120 or so polymorphisms have been documented (Cystic Fibrosis Mutation Database 2000). This is termed *allelic heterogeneity*. In practice each racial group has a number of common mutations: the ΔF508 (deletion of phenylalanine from amino acid position 508) mutation, for example, accounts for 75–88% of *CFTR* mutations in Northern Europeans, whereas the G542X nonsense mutation is more typical in Africans.

Individuals with CF are either *homozygotes* for a single CFTR mutation or are *compound heterozygotes* for two different mutations. The relationship between an affected individual's genotype and phenotype is complex and difficult to predict (Cutting 1997). Some features are clearly related to the genotype. Homozygosity for the 'severe' allele ΔF508 present with classical CF characterised by pancreatic insufficiency, increased sweat chloride excretion and chronic lung disease. 'Atypical' forms of CF are associated with 'milder' CF alleles. For example, compound heterozygosity for ΔF508 and R117H (a 'mild' allele) causes pancreatic sufficient CF. The phenotype can also be modified by different factors. The 'mild' R117H allele, for example, may be converted into a 'severe' allele capable of causing pancreatic insufficient CF by a well-characterised polymorphism on the *same CFTR* allele. Polymorphisms in the *mannose-binding lectin* gene increase the severity of CF lung disease by impairing the immune response to *Staphylococcus*

aureus and *Pseudomonas aeruginosa* (Gabolde et al 1999). A further modifier on chromosome 19 also appears to increase the risk of meconium ileus (Zielenski et al 1999) but at the time of writing the gene has not been characterised. The concept of CF as a simple autosomal recessive disease is therefore being challenged; in the future genotype–phenotype correlations will become accurate as the role of modifiers is better understood. Similar advances in pharmacogenetics may have a profound effect on the management of this disease.

Hyperphenylalaninaemia (OMIM 261600)

Hyperphenylalaninaemia is an autosomal recessive aminoacidopathy resulting from mutations in the *PAH* gene encoding phenylalanine hydroxylase (see http://www.mcgill.ca/pahdb/). A severe form, associated with greatly reduced enzyme function, manifests as phenylketonuria (PKU), while a milder form is associated with relatively preserved enzyme levels and is known as non-PKU hyperphenylalaninaemia. Genotype–phenotype data has been presented by Tyfield (1997). Some *PAH* alleles are 'severe', with low residual enzyme activity, and individuals who have two severe *PAH* alleles are likely to have PKU. Conversely, milder *PAH* alleles are associated with higher residual enzyme activities and individuals with two mild alleles are likely to have non-PKU hyperphenylalaninaemia. Phenotype prediction in compound heterozygotes is more difficult. The precise phenotype does not appear to be a function simply of genotype, however, and other factors have been proposed (Tyfield et al 1995). Although routine genotyping is not common practice at present, recent data has suggested that genotype data may influence decision-making with regard to dietary control (Greeves et al 2000); further work is clearly needed in this area.

X-linked recessive disease

Key features of X-linked recessive inheritance

- Disease features manifest in males.
- Milder disease features may also occasionally manifest in females ('*manifesting carriers*') as the result of *skewed X inactivation*.

- 'Full-blown' disease features may manifest in homozygous females.
- Male-to-male transmission does not occur (males only pass on their Y chromosome to their sons).
- Each son of a carrier female has a 50% chance of being affected.
- Each daughter of a carrier female has a 50% chance of also being a carrier.

Fragile X syndrome (OMIM 309550)

Fragile X syndrome is the commonest cause of inherited learning disability. The clinical features are well summarised by de Vries et al (1998). A cytogenetically detectable fragile site at Xq27 is seen in a proportion of X chromosomes in affected males when their lymphocytes are grown in folic acid-deficient medium (Lubs 1969, Sutherland 1977). This forms the basis of a insensitive diagnostic test which is no longer generally used. Fragile X syndrome was the first 'triplet repeat expansion' disorder to be reported (Oberlé et al 1991, Verkerk et al 1991) and is caused by an expansion of a CGG trinucleotide repeat at one end of the *FMR-1* gene (*Fragile X Mental Retardation-1*). The modern diagnostic test looks specifically at CGG repeat expansion in the *FMR-1* gene (Fig. 6.2).

The following scenarios are commonly encountered in clinical genetic practice:

1. A male or female *premutation* carrier — may have mild learning disability which is currently thought to represent background population risk and is not believed to be attributable to *FMR-1* mutation.
2. A male premutation carrier transmitting to his daughter — expansion into the full mutation range does not usually occur and the daughter therefore carries the premutation.
3. A female premutation carrier transmitting to her children — expansion usually occurs, although contraction has also been reported. The risk of expansion to a full mutation increases with the size of the premutation (Fisch et al 1995).
4. A male with a full mutation — has fragile X syndrome. Up to 20% of affected males are mosaic for cells with the premutation and cells with the full mutation, giving rise to phenotypic variation in males.
5. A female with a full mutation — the phenotype depends on X chromosome inactivation patterns within the brain; if X inactivation is adversely 'skewed' (see adrenoleukodystrophy), the likelihood of learning disability is increased but is impossible to quantify.

Triplet repeat expansion disorders (Table 6.1)

A number of genes contain triplet repeats — a sequence of three bases repeated over and over, written as $(CTG)_n$ for example. These may be either in the coding sequence, usually encoding *polyglutamine tracts* (e.g. Huntington's disease) or in the non-transcribed part of the gene (e.g. myotonic dystrophy). Several human diseases are caused when the triplet repeat length increases ('expands'), disrupting gene structure or function in some way. These diseases are generally autosomal dominant neurodegenerative disorders, but the important exceptions in paediatric practice are fragile X syndrome (X-linked) and Friedreich's ataxia (autosomal recessive).

Many of these diseases display *anticipation* — the disease increases in severity and/or symptoms start earlier with each successive generation due to increases in the size of the triplet repeat. Some diseases also have a 'premutation' stage whereby the 'carrier' is not affected but may have a child who is; the best example is fragile X syndrome.

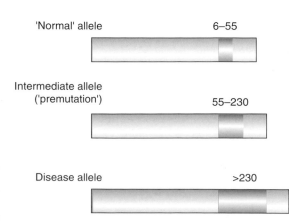

Fig. 6.2 Triplet repeat expansion in the *FMR-1* gene causes fragile X syndrome

Clinical genetics and genetic services: principles and practice

Table 6.1
Childhood triplet repeat expansion disorders

Disease	Repeat	Site
Fragile X syndrome	$(CGG)_n$	5'UTR of FMR-1
Friedreich's ataxia	$(GAA)_n$	intron 1 of FRDA
Myotonic dytrophy	$(CTG)_n$	3'UTR of DMK
Juvenile myoclonus epilepsy	$(CCCCGCCCCGCG)_n$	promoter of JME gene

UTR = untranslated region (a controlling region either at the beginning (5') or end (3') of the gene)

Myotonic dystrophy (OMIM 160900)

Myotonic dystrophy is a classical autosomal dominant triplet repeat expansion disorder principally causing progressive myotonia and weakness. It results from expansion in a CTG repeat situated in an untranslated region at the end of the DMK gene on chromosome 19, encoding the myotonin protein kinase. Normal alleles have 5–35 CTG repeats, whereas disease alleles have from 36 up to 4000.

Myotonic dystrophy displays anticipation perhaps more clearly than any other genetic disease. Individuals with small expansions may only develop premature cataracts or frontal baldness; as the expansion increases in size with each generation, the age of onset of muscle symptoms and signs decreases. Marked expansion is likely to occur if an affected *female* passes on her disease allele: this induces prenatal onset muscle weakness, leading to fetal akinesia, polyhydramnios and congenital myotonic dystrophy with respiratory insufficiency.

Friedreich's ataxia (OMIM 229300)

Friedreich's ataxia is the commonest inherited childhood ataxia syndrome. It usually presents with gait ataxia between the ages of 8 and 15 and rapidly progresses to areflexia, pyramidal leg weakness, loss of distal joint position and vibration sense and dysarthria in most patients (Harding 1997). Some patients develop optic atrophy, cardiomyopathy, diabetes mellitus, deafness or scoliosis. It is an autosomal recessive disease: most affected individuals are homozygous for an expanded GAA triplet repeat in the first intron of the FRDA gene on chromosome 9 (encoding frataxin). Point mutations in FRDA have also been described. Disease alleles contain between 200 and 900 repeats, compared to 7–20 in normal individuals.

Chromosomal microdeletions and microduplications

CATCH phenotype (OMIM 188400)

Submicroscopic deletion of band q11 of chromosome 22 results in a number of related phenotypes known collectively by the acronym 'CATCH' (Cardiac anomalies, Abnormal facies. Thymic hypoplasia, Cleft palate and Hypocalcaemia; Ryan et al 1997) (Table 6.2). Many genes lie within the deleted region but their contribution to the CATCH phenotype is poorly understood. The phenotype is caused, at least in part, by impaired neural crest cell migration into the developing pharyngeal pouches and cardiac outflow tract during embryogenesis. At the 'syndromic' end of the phenotypic spectrum lie Di George syndrome (DGS), velocardiofacial syndrome (VCFS) and conotruncal anomaly–face syndrome (CTAFS); at the other end, 22q11 microdeletion may cause isolated cleft palate, hypernasal speech, isolated or familial non-syndromic heart defects, psychiatric disorders or may indeed have no apparent phenotypic associations at all.

22q11 microdeletions usually arise de novo. Many families have been reported, however, in which a 22q11 microdeletion is inherited as a

Table 6.2
Clinical features associated with 22q11 microdeletion

Clinical feature	Frequency (%)
Congenital heart malformation[a]	
Total	75
Otolaryngeal abnormalities:	
Total	50
Velopharyngeal insufficiency	30
Cleft palate	15
Other	5
Neonatal hypocalcaemia	
Total	60
Thymic aplasia	
Total	b
Significant immune defect	~1
Urogenital anomalies	
Total	36
Renal aplasia, dysplasia, cysts	17
Obstructive uropathy	10
Vesicoureteric refux	4.5
Other renal anomalies	4.5
Undescended testes	8
Development	
Short stature: <3rd centile	30
Moderate–severe learning problems	18
Adult psychiatric illness	~3

Source: Ryan et al 1997; Vantrappen et al 1999
[a] See Table 6.7
[b] Data on the frequency of thymic aplasia is difficult to ascertain; although a feature of Di George syndrome it is not seen in other patients with 22q11 microdeletions

Table 6.3
Clinical features of Williams syndrome.

Clinical features	Approximate frequency (%)
Dysmorphic facies	100
Characteristic personality ('cocktail party manner')	100
Learning difficulties (moderate–severe)	Most
Growth retardation (<10th centile)	80
Infantile hypercalcaemia	45
Cardiovascular anomalies	
SVAS	45–75
PPAS	20–35
Other[a]	unknown
Hyperacusis	>90%
Gastrointestinal	
Hernias	40
Constipation	25
Rectal prolapse	10
Renal anomalies	18
Skeletal abnormalities	45

For definition of abbreviations see Table 6.7
[a] Includes peripheral arterial stenoses, e.g. coronary, renal and cerebral
Source: Metcalfe 1999

dominant Mendelian trait, often with marked intrafamilial variability. Molecular diagnosis relies on FISH studies.

Williams syndrome (OMIM 194050)

Williams syndrome is caused by microdeletion of a 2-Mb region of chromosome 7q11.23. As with 22q11 microdeletion, 7q11.23 microdeletions also usually arise de novo, although a few families with dominant inheritance have been described. Within the deleted region lie a number of contiguous genes; one such gene is *ELN*, encoding elastin: deletion or mutation of one *ELN* allele is known to cause familial supravalvar aortic stenosis and peripheral pulmonary stenosis, malformations which are a common feature of Williams syndrome (Table 6.3). Laboratory confirmation of this diagnosis is with FISH analysis.

Smith–Magenis syndrome (OMIM 182290)

Microdeletion of chromosome 17p11.2 results in a childhood syndrome with a characteristic *behavioural* phenotype (Winter & Baraitser 1998). Dysmorphic features are reminiscent of Prader–Willi syndrome; deafness, scoliosis, cardiac, brain and renal anomalies and immune impairment may also be found. Children with Smith–Magenis syndrome often have grossly disturbed sleep patterns and display self-destructive behaviour.

Hereditary motor and sensory neuropathy (OMIM 118220)

The term 'hereditary motor and sensory neuropathy' (HMSN) refers to a group of inherited peripheral neuropathies also known by the eponym 'Charcot–Marie–Tooth disease'. The commonest form of HMSN — type 1 — is characterised by low nerve conduction velocities caused by peripheral nerve demyelination. The major subgroup, HMSN1A, accounts for 75–80% of HMSN1 and is caused by a duplication of a 1.5-Mb segment of chromosome 17 containing the peripheral myelin protein 22 (*PMP22*) gene (the same region that is deleted in Smith–Magenis syndrome). A small number of HMSN1A families have a point mutation in *PMP22*. HMSN1B is caused by point mutations in the P_0 gene which encodes a major component of the myelin sheath; a further variant is caused by mutations in the *early growth response 2* (*EGR2*) gene (Warner et al 1999), and mutations in the X-linked *GJB1* gene (OMIM 302800) may mimic autosomal dominant HMSN since female carriers may manifest owing to skewed X inactivation.

Imprinting

Males and females differ in the way they inactivate certain chromosomal segments using DNA methylation. This complex process of *genomic imprinting* occurs in the gonad: in the testis, a male removes the 'female' imprint from chromosomes derived from his mother and applies a male imprinting pattern; the opposite occurs in the ovary. Some genes inherited from a male are silenced by imprinting and only the corresponding female-derived genes are 'switched on', and vice versa. Two diseases in particular illustrate the consequences of imprinting in a region of proximal chromosome 15q (15q11–q13).

Angelman's syndrome (Fig. 6.3)

Among the many genes in this region is *UBE3A* (ubiquitin-protein ligase E3A). Only the *maternally derived* copy of *UBE3A* is 'switched on'; loss of maternal *UBE3A* expression causes Angelman's syndrome, characterised by hypotonia, epilepsy, neurodevelopmental delay, absence of speech and a characteristic facial appearance (OMIM 105830).

Prader–Willi syndrome (Fig. 6.3)

This region also contains a cluster of genes, of which *SNRPN* (small nuclear ribonucleoprotein N) and *NDN* (necdin) are well characterised. Only *paternally derived* genes in the *SNRPN* cluster are 'switched on'. Loss of *paternal* expression of genes in the *SNRPN* cluster causes Prader–Willi syndrome (PWS), a childhood disorder characterised by neonatal hypotonia, neurodevelopmental delay, hypogonadism and hyperphagia (Nicholls 1999; OMIM 176270).

Genetic heterogeneity

Hearing impairment

Over 1 in 1000 children are affected by severe or profound congenital deafness. At least 50% of cases have a genetic cause; environmental factors contribute to a proportion of the remainder, and in some the cause remains unknown. Approximately a third of sensorineural deafness is seen as part of a chromosomal, single gene or idiopathic childhood syndrome, of which there are over 300 (Winter & Baraitser 1998) (Table 6.4).

More commonly, however, sensorineural deafness is an isolated trait ('non-syndromic hearing loss': NSHL) and is largely considered to be genetic, especially if congenital and bilateral. Around 85% of prelingual NSHL is autosomal recessive, 15% is autosomal dominant, 1–3% is X-linked and mitochondrial inheritance is rare. By contrast, postlingual (late onset) deafness is usually autosomal dominant or mitochondrial (Kalatzis & Petit 1998). At the time of writing nearly 70 loci associated with NSHL are known with gene identification for 17 of these (Table 6.5); this undoubtedly represents a fraction of all single gene causes of NSHL. Some gene mutations known to cause *syndromic* hearing loss can also cause NSHL in some individuals:

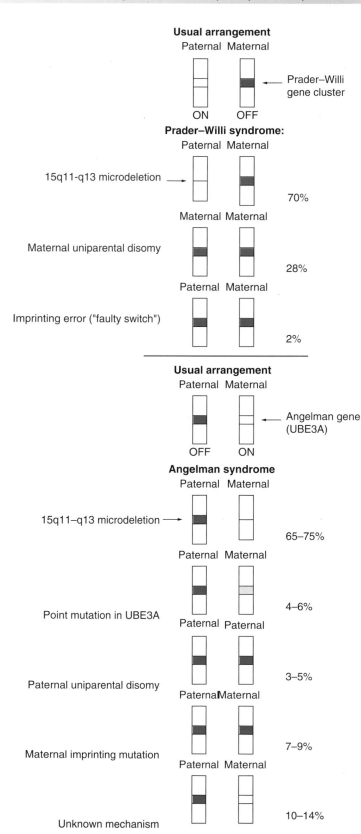

Fig. 6.3 Molecular mechanisms underlying Prader–Willi and Angelman's syndromes (percentages refer to the approximate proportion of cases accounted for by each mechanism)

Table 6.4
Associations of sensorineural deafness: Mendelian syndromes

Syndrome	Gene(s)	MIM number
Alport's syndrome	COL4A5 COL4A3 & 4	104200
Branchio-oto-renal syndrome	EYA1	113650
Pendred's syndrome	PDS	274600
Stickler's syndrome	COL2A1 COL11A1 & 2	108300
Treacher–Collins syndrome	TCOF1	154500
Usher's syndrome[a] Type 1B Type 2A	MYO7A USH2A	276903 276901
Waardenburg's syndrome type I type II type III type IV	PAX3 MITF PAX3 EDNRB EDN3 SOX10	193500 193510 148820 277850

[a] There are three types of Usher's syndrome: type 1 (at least six subtypes, in only one of which the gene is known), type 2 (at least three subtypes, one gene known) and type 3 (only one form known, gene unknown)
From Van Camp & Smith (1999)

Table 6.5
Single gene basis of non-syndromal sensorineural hearing loss

	Loci (no.)	Genes cloned (no.)
Autosomal recessive	29	7
Autosomal dominant	35	11
X-linked	7	1
Mitochondrial	–	2

From Van Camp & Smith (2000)

instances), looking for syndromic associations and evidence of subclinical hearing impairment. If autosomal recessive inheritance is suspected, GJB2 testing may be offered. Given an apparently sporadic case of unexplained NSHL an empirical recurrence risk may be offered to the parents. A figure of 10% is considered appropriate in this context (Parker et al 1999). Further advances in genetic technology will permit detailed genotyping and accurate genetic counselling.

Visual impairment: retinitis pigmentosa

Inherited retinal diseases are a common cause of visual impairment in childhood, often leading to severe visual loss in later life. The most frequent form of inherited/genetic retinopathy is retinitis pigmentosa (RP), which affects around 1 in 3500 individuals worldwide. RP is characterised by progressive degeneration of the mid-peripheral retina, causing night blindness, tunnel vision and ultimately leading to total visual loss. The hallmark physical finding is that of 'bone spicule' retinal pigment deposits and the 'gold standard' clinical test is the electroretinograph (ERG), which shows reduced or absent evoked potentials.

RP occurs as a feature of over 170 syndromes (Winter & Baraitser 1998). More commonly, however, RP is an isolated feature and in that context is considered to be genetic in origin, particularly if bilateral. Isolated RP is genetically heterogeneous,

mutations in MYO7A, for example, can cause Usher's syndrome type 1B and either autosomal recessive or autosomal dominant NSHL. Of particular relevance is the GJB2 gene, encoding the gap junction protein subunit connexin26. Mutations in GJB2 account for up to 50% of autosomal recessive NSHL in caucasians, with a single mutation (35delG) comprising a significant proportion of these cases.

Clinical genetic assessment of a child with hearing impairment begins, as always, with a detailed family history and clinical phenotyping of the child and his parents (including an audiogram in many

Table 6.6
Childhood syndromal associations of retinitis pigmentosa

Condition	Inheritance	MIM number
Adrenoleukodystrophy (neonatal)	AR	202370
Alström's syndrome	AR	203800
Angelman's syndrome	microdeletion	234400
Alagille's syndrome	AD	118450
Ceroid lipofuscinosis	AR	204200, 204500
Cockayne's syndrome	AR	216400
Cohen's syndrome	AR	216550
Cystinosis	AR	219800
Congenital infection (CMV, Rubella, HSV, VZV)	–	–
Hereditary spastic paraplegias	AR/AD	Numerous
Homocystinuria	AR	236200
Infantile Refsum's disease	AR	266510
Kearns–Sayre syndrome	mt	165100
Laurence–Moon–Bardet–Biedl syndrome	AR	245800, 209900
Leigh's disease	AR/XR/mt	256000
MCAD deficiency	AR	201450
Sjögren–Larsson syndrome	AR	270200
Usher's syndrome[a]	AR	276900
Zellweger's syndrome	AR	214100

AD = autosomal dominant; AR = autosomal recessive; XR = X-linked recessive; mt = mitochondrial; CMV = cytomegalovirus; HSV = herpes simplex virus; VZV = varicella zoster virus; MCAD = medium chain acyl-coA dehydrogenase
[a] See also Table 6.4

with autosomal dominant, recessive and X-linked recessive forms recognised (Table 6.6). Disease-causing mutations in several genes have been identified, but most of the genes have not been cloned and only their chromosomal location from linkage studies is known (see Retinal Information Network at http://www.sph.uth.tmc.edu/Retnet/).

If the pedigree shows clear Mendelian inheritance it is possible to provide meaningful risk counselling with the possibility of genetic linkage analysis (at the time of writing, mutation analysis is not commonly available). More commonly a child presents with RP and no family history of eye disease: this presents a difficult challenge. Non-genetic and syndromic causes should be excluded. If the proband is male, X-linked recessive inheritance is most likely and the parents, particularly the mother, should be offered carrier testing in the form of fundoscopy and ERG. Absence of features does not, however, completely exclude carrier status. Carriers for autosomal recessive RP do not generally show any abnormality even on ERG and it is therefore often impossible to distinguish an isolated recessive case from a new dominant mutation. In addition, non-penetrance is recognised in autosomal dominant RP, so that a parent may well 'carry' a dominant RP gene but have normal eye investigations. For these reasons, genetic counselling in isolated cases of RP is difficult and empirical recurrence risk figures are used in many cases (Harper 1998). Full genetic assessment is, however, strongly recommended in anticipation of future technological advance.

THE GENETICS OF COMMON CHILDHOOD DISEASE

Many common childhood diseases cluster within families but do not obey the rules of Mendelian inheritance. They are not caused by mutations in single genes but result from a complex and poorly understood interaction between a number of inherited 'susceptibility genes' and environmental factors. This is known as multifactorial inheritance. A single susceptibility gene — or *polygene* — does not cause disease on its own, but interacts with other susceptibility factors (genetic or environmental) to increase an individual's *liability* to disease. Such polygenes are distributed throughout the population and are present in all of us. An individual develops disease when his liability exceeds a particular *threshold*. This is known as the *liability threshold model*. Familial clustering of many common paediatric diseases is thought to reflect this model (e.g. congenital malformations, asthma, autism). The liability threshold model predicts a much lower recurrence risk for this group of diseases, usually around 2–5% (this corresponds to the

square root of the population incidence of a given polygenic disorder). However, Mendelian (i.e. single gene) forms of the condition should always be carefully excluded in a given family before 'polygenic' counselling is offered. This may involve detailed assessment of apparently phenotypically normal parents for subtle signs of disease.

Congenital heart malformation

Congenital heart malformations (CHMs) represent the commonest group of birth defects, comprising some 6–8 per 100 live births. The aetiology of CHMs is extremely heterogeneous, with a large number of syndromic and teratogenic/environmental associations (see Brennan & Young 2001 for a more detailed account) (Table 6.7). *Isolated* CHMs may be inherited as Mendelian traits (autosomal dominant supravalvar aortic and peripheral pulmonary stenoses, for example, caused by mutations in the *elastin* gene); this possibility must always be taken into account in the genetics clinic and a full cardiovascular assessment of the parents may be warranted to exclude forme frustes (e.g. left axis deviation in autosomal dominant atrioventricular septal defect). A multifactorial basis has been proposed for the majority of CHMs and this has been confirmed in large population studies which have confirmed that most isolated CHMs have a low recurrence risk (Ferencz et al 1997, Burn et al 1998). At the time of writing no 'polygenes' for isolated CHM have been identified, although at least one susceptibility locus has been identified on chromosome 1 for atrioventricular septal defect (Sheffield et al 1997).

Neural tube defects

The term 'neural tube defect' encompasses a spectrum of malformation ranging from anencephaly and myelomeningocoele to subtle lumbar spine malformations such as terminal lipomeningocoele and lumbosacral sinus. Early epidemiological studies found recurrence risk data compatible with a multifactorial model of inheritance (Bonaiti-Pellié & Smith 1974). As with other multifactorial disorders a number of syndromic and teratogenic associations exist which should always be excluded before coun-

Table 6.7
Common syndromic, teratogenic and environmental associations of congenital heart malformations

	Major heart defect	Genetic mechanism
Chromosome aneuploidy syndromes		
Turner	CoAo, AS, HLHS	Monosomy X
Down	VSD, AVSD, ASD	Trisomy 21
Cat-eye	TAPVR, ToF	Partial tetrasomy 22
Chromsome microdeletion syndromes		
Di George	CTD, IAA	22q microdeletion
Williams	SVAS, PPAS, SAS	7q microdeletion
Single-gene syndromes		
Noonan	PS	AD, chromosome 12
Alagille	PPAS	AD mutations in JAGGED
Holt–Oram	ASD	AD mutations in TBX5
Ellis–van Creveld	ASD, CA, AVSD	AR mutation in EVC
Teratogen exposure syndromes		
Fetal rubella	PDA	
Fetal alcohol	VSD, ASD, ToF	
Idiopathic syndromes		
Kabuki	CTD	Unknown
Rubinstein–Taybi	Wide variety	Unknown
3C	AVSD, CTD	Unknown

3C = craniocerebellocardiac syndrome; AD = autosomal dominant; AR = autosomal recessive; TAPVR = total anomalous pulmonary venous return; CA = common atrium; ASD = secundum atrial septal defect; AVSD = atrioventricular septal defect; VSD = ventricular septal defect; CTD = conotruncal defects; ToF = tetralogy of Fallot; AS = aortic valvular stenosis; SVAS = supravalvar aortic stenosis; CoAo = coarctation of the aorta; IAA = interruption of aortic arch; HLHS = hypoplastic left heart syndrome; PDA = patent ductus arteriosus; PS = pulmonary valvular stenosis; PPAS = peripheral pulmonary artery stenosis; SAS = systemic arterial stenosis

selling (Table 6.8). X-linked inheritance of isolated neural tube defects (NTDs) has also been reported (OMIM 301410). A well-recognised *environmental* susceptibility factor is maternal folic acid intake. Periconceptual folic acid supplementation has been shown to reduce both the occurrence and recurrence of NTDs (MRC Vitamin Study Research Group 1991, Czeizel & Dudas 1992). The first *genetic* susceptibility factor to be described is a defect in homocysteine metabolism: a common polymorphism in the *MTHFR* gene (5,10-α-methylenetetrahydrofolate reductase: OMIM 236250.0003) reduces enzyme activity and impairs homocysteine metabolism. Homozygosity for this polymorphism increases plasma homocysteine levels; both have been shown to be more common in children with NTDs and their mothers than in controls, as has low maternal red blood cell folate (Christensen et al 1999). Folic acid

Clinical genetics and genetic services: principles and practice

Table 6.8
Syndromic and teratogenic associations of neural tube defects

Condition	Inheritance	MIM number
Meckel–Gruber syndrome	AR	249000
Waardenburg's syndrome type III	AD	193500
X-linked laterality sequence	XR	304750
Maternal diabetes	–	–
Embryonic exposure to Cocaine Sodium valproate Vitamin A/retinoids Thalidomide	–	–

Box 6.1
Syndromic causes of autism

Fragile X syndrome
Tuberous sclerosis
Angelman's syndrome
Mat dup 15 q[a]
Untreated phenylketonuria
Rett's syndrome
Sanfilippo's syndrome (MPS III)
Adenylosuccinate lyase deficiency

[a] Maternally-derived duplication of proximal chromosome 15q

appears to interact with the mutant enzyme and greatly reduces the risk of NTD, although the mechanism for this is not clear. Mutations or polymorphisms in genes encoding other enzymes involved in homcysteine metabolism may also function as susceptibility factors for NTDs.

Autism

A specific cause can only be found in a minority (<20%) of autistic children. A significant genetic cause for the remaining children is supported by twin studies, which show an increased concordance in monozygotic twins compared to dizygotic twins, and family studies, which demonstrate a sibling recurrence risk 50–100 times greater than the general population. A liability threshold model has been proposed, and genome-wide searches for susceptibility genes have been undertaken in large numbers of families (International Molecular Genetic Study of Autism Consortium 1998, Barrett et al 1999). Such studies have suggested a large number of race-specific susceptibility genes but further work is needed to refine the data. At the time of writing, no susceptibility genes have been identified from this work. In the genetics clinic, therefore, empirical counselling statistics are currently used once a syndromic cause has been carefully excluded (Box 6.1).

LABORATORY TESTS: HOW THEY ARE DONE

The spectrum of DNA pathology demands a set of laboratory tools able to operate with different degrees of resolution. The following sections give an overview; more detailed accounts are reported in Mueller & Young (1998) or Strachan & Read (1999).

Cytogenetic analysis

Chromosomes range between 2 and 10 μm in size at metaphase (the stage at which they are typically examined in the laboratory). Numerical chromosome abnormalities are therefore easily detectable by examining a *metaphase spread* (the chromosomes from individual cell nuclei, fixed and spread onto a microscope slide) using light microscopy. Chromosomes are identified by the specific banding pattern generated by the combination of denaturation and staining with a DNA-specific dye (e.g. Giemsa, resulting in a G-banded karyotype). Structural changes below several Mb in size are often not possible to resolve with 'routine' karyotyping; a technique known as *FISH* (Fluorescence In Situ Hybridisation) is employed for this (Fig. 6.4). FISH is mainly used to detect microdeletions but can also be used to characterise chromosome

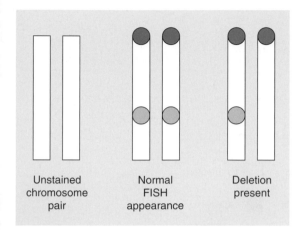

Unstained chromosome pair

Normal FISH appearance

Deletion present

Fig. 6.4 Fluorescent in situ hybridisation (FISH) is a powerful technique mainly used in clinical laboratory practice to detect microdeletions. Two fluorescent DNA probes are used; each one fluoresces a different colour under ultraviolet light. One probe corresponds to DNA sequence from within the microdeletion interval (shown as green) and the other is a marker probe (shown as red). The probes are allowed to hybridise with chromosomes fixed to a microscope slide. If the chromosome is intact, both probes will hybridise; if a microdeletion is present, only the marker probe will hybridise. The fluorescent signals are easily visualised using microscopy

rearrangements such as reciprocal translocations or the complex rearrangements found in tumour cells.

Molecular DNA analysis

FISH techniques overlap a little with molecular DNA techniques in terms of resolution. However, resolution down to a single base requires extraction and purification of DNA. DNA is not visible by light microscopy so a variety of indirect techniques have been developed.

Often, the clinician is interested in identifying a specific gene mutation, either one which has already been identified in the family, a common mutation (e.g. the G380R mutation in the fibroblast growth factor receptor 3 [FGFR3] gene known to cause most cases of achondroplasia) or as part of a 'mutation screen' (e.g. cystic fibrosis). A technique known as the *polymerase chain reaction* (PCR) is usually employed to amplify the genomic segment containing the putative mutation, giving sufficient material for further analysis. Each individual has

two copies (*alleles*) of the genomic segment under investigation; if one allele contains a mutation, its mass and/or charge will change. Electrophoresis of the PCR reaction products can then be used to differentiate between the normal allele and the disease-causing allele on the basis of size/charge. More complex PCR-based techniques have been developed to allow simultaneous screening for multiple mutations, as in cystic fibrosis.

A variety of other techniques, including automated DNA sequencing, are increasingly employed to look for gene mutations in situations where no common mutation exists. At the time of writing, however, these techniques remain time consuming, expensive and of limited availability in the service setting.

If mutation testing is not possible, it may still be possible to offer DNA diagnostic testing if there is a suitable family history and structure. This employs a gene tracking technique known as *linkage*, or *segregation*, *analysis*. The principle involves generating a 'fingerprint' — or *haplotype* — of both alleles of interest using a series of polymorphic DNA markers spaced within or around the disease gene. The 'high-risk' haplotype can be determined in affected family members and this can be tracked through the family, allowing genetic testing in other family members.

PRACTICE

This section concerns issues of contemporary clinical genetic practice. Particular attention is paid to the use and interpretation of genetic tests, as this area has seen major advances since the last edition of this book.

Recording a family tree

An accurately drawn pedigree forms the initial component of most clinical genetic assessments. It helps the clinician establish the mode of inheritance, reach a diagnosis and calculate the risk to other family members. It also records many other aspects of family structure such as adoption, marriage histories and reproductive histories (Fig. 6.5).

A useful practical guide to recording family histories is given by Rose (1999). A standard

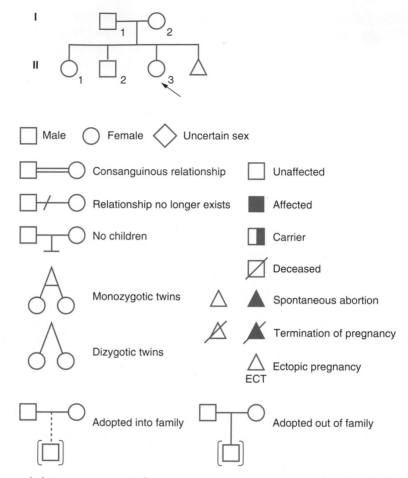

Fig. 6.5 Pedigree symbols in common use. Each generation is given a roman numeral, and each individual in a generation is given an arabic numeral, so that all family members have a 'coordinate' (e.g. II:2). The proband is marked with a small arrow below and to the right.

nomenclature has been developed for pedigree drawing (Bennett et al 1995). In practice it is rarely possible to draw a neat, accurate pedigree at the first attempt, and it is advisable to use a 'working draft' while you collect detailed family data. A number of potentially sensitive pieces of information should be sought if possible (it is not always appropriate to address these issues in one sitting):

- Do the siblings of a given individual share the same biological parents?
- Consanguinity: this is not always predictable from the family's cultural background. If present,

what is the degree of relationship (e.g. first cousins, uncle–niece)?

- Assisted conception: this is particularly relevant if donated gametes have been used.
- Adoption.
- Miscarriages, stillbirths, terminations of pregnancy or ongoing pregnancies.
- If a relative has died, what was the cause of death and age at death? This is especially important in adult practice when considering a family history of cancer.
- If an affected family member has received treatment in hospital, it is often useful in the assessment of a pedigree to record the full name, date of

birth and hospital of that individual. Consent may then be obtained if necessary to access medical records in order to confirm or refute diagnoses.

Clinical genetic assessment of the dysmorphic child

A dysmorphic child presents a unique diagnostic challenge. Reaching a syndromic diagnosis is important not just for the child, but for the wider family. There is no magic to diagnostic genetic assessment; the same techniques are used as elsewhere, but attention is paid to every tiny detail.

History

Assessment always begins with a detailed history and a pedigree. The mother's past obstetric history may detail miscarriage or stillbirth, and these may also be present elsewhere in the family, suggesting a recurrent cause such as an inherited chromosome rearrangement. The pregnancy history relating to the child being assessed may reveal fetal exposure to maternal disease — such as diabetes mellitus — or teratogenic agents, including drugs and alcohol. Fetal ultrasound findings will be located in the mother's maternity records and may be of use. All other sources of documentation relating to the child should be examined: surprisingly often, a vital clue is a yellowed laboratory report tucked away in a dark recess of the child's hospital record!

Examination

Examination of the child should be as thorough as circumstances allow. A key part of the diagnostic process is to simply *look* and to recognise when a feature is abnormal. It should be possible to record any dysmorphic features (Aase (1990) has written an excellent handbook defining dysmorphic features). It is often helpful to adopt an hypothetico-deductive approach by initially examining anatomical regions such as the face or hands, and to extend to other organ systems if abnormalities are found. For example, the finding of low-set ears and down-slanting palpebral fissure may lead directly to cardiac auscultation (a possible diagnosis being Noonan's syndrome), or the discovery of conical teeth may prompt examination of other ectodermal appendages such as hair and nails (a

possible diagnosis being ectodermal dysplasia). Some 'soft' signs such as fifth finger clinodactyly and Brushfield spots may contribute little to the diagnostic debate (2% of normal children have Brushfield spots). It is also helpful to examine the parents as well since they may be manifesting subtle dysmorphic signs themselves. In addition, many seemingly unusual features may simply be a separate family trait: pre-auricular pits are a good example.

Much useful information can also be gained from *measuring* anatomical features. While the height, weight and occipitofrontal circumference are useful, a clinical geneticist is often more interested in relative proportions. For example, the ratio of upper segment to lower segment length is essential to characterise short stature, or in the assessment of a child thought to have Marfan's syndrome. Furthermore, detailed measurements around the eyes will distinguish between *hypo*telorism, *hyper*telorism and telecanthus. Standard tables and graphs of normal measurements are widely available for comparison (Hall et al 1989).

Investigation

A diagnosis may be reached simply on the basis of a recognisable 'gestalt'. Often, however, further work will be required. Chromosome analysis may be warranted (consider this in all dysmorphic children). Sometimes DNA testing is required if the phenotype suggests a single gene disorder. A host of other blood or urine tests may be ordered, depending on the phenotype. Radiological investigations may be requested to characterise suspected skeletal dysplasia or assess skeletal maturity. Colleagues in other paediatric subspecialities may provide futher diagnostic information (paediatric ophthalmology, for example).

A further diagnostic tool is the genetic database, many of which are listed at the end of this chapter. Targeted interrogation of electronic databases may yield rare syndromic diagnoses, or may certainly prompt further investigation of the child in order to obtain futher phenotypic information. A wider search of the medical literature may be required to locate similar case reports of rare conditions.

A final diagnostic technique used not infrequently in dysmorphology is to 'wait and see'.

Many dysmorphic syndromes evolve with time, and as the phenotype changes it may be possible to make a diagnosis.

Ethical framework: genetic testing in children

While an individual's genetic information is unique to that individual, it also reflects a common heredity that extends out into the wider family. Clinical genetics services therefore operate both at the level of the individual and of the entire family. Furthermore, a single individual may be encountered at any point from conception to death. This wide and complex remit demands a clear ethical framework. Many of the ethical issues involved will be familiar to a community paediatrician, but genetic testing in children deserves particular attention.

The Clinical Genetics Society, a professional body of clinical geneticists in the UK, has produced a document detailing the recommendations for genetic testing in children (Clarke 1994a; see also http://www.bshg.org.uk/testchil.htm). An independent view has also been expressed by the Genetic Interest Group (GIG), a national alliance of charities, voluntary organisations and support groups whose aim is to support families affected by genetic disease (Dalby 1995). The central themes emerging from these two documents and from the debate which ensued following their publication form 'ethical guidelines' for genetic testing in childhood:

1. Genetic testing in childhood is appropriate in a *diagnostic* context.
2. *Predictive* genetic testing in childhood may be appropriate if the disease onset is during childhood or if there are useful medical interventions such as dietary modification, medication or clinical surveillance for complications.
3. *Predictive* testing for *adult-onset* disorders is often not appropriate if the child is well and there are no useful medical interventions. Such testing is felt to challenge the child's autonomy and right to confidentiality, and is generally felt to be better undertaken when the child is mature enough to consider the full implications of testing for himself. However, predictive testing

of this nature may at times be requested on non-clinical grounds such as to alleviate anxiety — as a test result may well be negative — and to facilitate the establishment of the best psychosocial environment for the child and his family. In situations such as this, professionals should remember that '. . . parents are responsible for the welfare of their children, and at the end of the day most of them are better equipped to decide what is in the best interest of a particular child, and the family as a whole than are outsiders. Denying them the right to cope in a way they see as best may have the opposite effect to that intended.' (Dalby 1995).

It is also worth remembering that presymptomatic testing is also possible in some instances *without* DNA analysis: for example, a child at risk from retinitis pigmentosa or familial adenomatous polyposis coli may have retinal changes detectable with fundoscopy long before the symptomatic phase.

4. Testing for *carrier status* (for a recessive or X-linked condition, or a balanced chromosome rearrangment, for example) during childhood is conceptually similar to presymptomatic testing. Knowledge of carrier status is of *reproductive* significance and is rarely associated with ill-health, however. Accordingly, most carrier testing is deferred until puberty or until the child becomes sexually active, but it may be appropriate to test earlier for similar non-clinical reasons to those outlined above. Carriers are sometimes identified by prenatal testing. Although the arguments are similar to carrier testing in childhood, a fetus has no legal rights at the time of the test. Careful discussion with the parents is therefore required *before* the test is performed to determine whether or not this information should be disclosed, since a prenatal test is usually performed to specifically detect an affected fetus, allowing the parents to opt for termination of pregnancy if they wish.

Essentially, therefore, each request for genetic testing in childhood should take account of the context in which the request is made. There are few cases in which testing is absolutely contraindicated; careful dialogue between parents and professionals will determine the correct way to proceed. The issues surrounding consent for genetic testing are the same as in any other branch of paediatrics; 'Gillick competent' children should be given the opportunity to give their own informed consent. It is also worth reinforcing the notion that parents *and* professionals have an ongoing committment to both the tested and untested child; both should be given access to genetic counselling in their own right when 'mature enough'. In the case of a tested child, updated testing may be available.

A final point relates to healthy but genetically 'at-risk' children being considered for adoption placement. The same arguments for and against testing apply to this group, with an additional consideration being the impact of inherited disease on the placement. Each case must be carefully considered, balancing the child's autonomy with the prospective adoptive parents' wishes and with appropriate consultation between the medical advisor to the adoption agency and clinical genetics services. The same 'rules' apply to children in foster care or residential care, in which case the social services department may assume parental responsibility.

Interpretation of laboratory tests

Cytogenetic tests

The main practical problems posed by cytogenetic testing are *limited resolution, mosaicism* and *polymorphism*. The resolution of cytogenetic analysis by light microscopy is limited. Small, subtle chromosome rearrangements (known as '*cryptic*' rearrangements) may escape detection. For example, a child with 'idiopathic' dysmorphism and neurodevelopmental delay may have an unbalanced cryptic reciprocal translocation resulting from malsegregation of a balanced translocation carried by one of the parents. Failure to identify such a karyotypic abnormality may result in incorrect counselling with respect to prognosis and recurrence risks. Recently it has been reported that cryptic microdeletions in the subtelomeric regions of some chromosomes (i.e. just proximal to the end of a chromosome arm) account for unexplained neurodevelopmental delay in some children (Knight et al 1999). At the moment FISH remains the only means of detecting truly cryptic rearrangements and subtelomeric micro-

deletions. Its widespread use as a diagnostic 'screening' tool in children with unexplained, non-specific neurodevelopmental delay with or without dysmorphic features remains a subject of debate.

Demonstration of a mosaic karyotype in a child often poses considerable interpretive difficulties. In this situation, more than one cell line is found in the same individual. This is usually demonstrated either antenatally in cultured amniocytes or post-natally in peripheral blood lymphocytes. The proportions of each cell line in these tissues give no clue to the distribution in other tissues and it is not usually possible to accurately predict the phenotypic effects of such mosaic findings, particularly with respect to neurodevelopmental delay in an apparently structurally normal fetus/child. A common example in paediatric practice is Turner mosaicism: approximately 10% of girls with a Turner phenotype are mosaic, with one monosomy X cell line and at least one other, usually 46,XX. Other more unusual karyotypes are also seen, such as 45,X/46,XX/47,XXX. The phenotype in such individuals can vary from normality to short stature, infertility and pubertal delay. This poses a prognostic dilemma, particularly in the prenatal context.

Human genetic variation may manifest as differences in chromosome structure that have no phenotypic consequences and simply represent chromosome polymorphism. Accurate assessment of variant chromosomes by an experienced cytogeneticist is vital, since most karyotypes are requested on the basis of abnormal phenotype. Many structural variants are recognised, the commonest of which is variation in the appearance of pericentromeric heterochromatin on chromosome 9 (Gardner & Sutherland 1996). They are rarely reported by cytogenetic laboratories unless there are difficulties in interpretation.

DNA tests

Molecular DNA tests are usually more focused than most cytogenetic tests — after all, a karyotype examines the entire genome — and the main practical problems encountered are somewhat different: *residual risk* and *interpretation* with respect to *penetrance* and *expressivity*.

Residual risk is a concept that refers to the inability of a test to *exclude* a disease or carrier status in certain clinical contexts and is perhaps best illustrated by *CFTR* mutation testing. A standard genetic *carrier* test for cystic fibrosis looks for 12 different known disease alleles which together account for approximately 90% of disease alleles in a typical UK population. A *negative* carrier test *does not exclude* carrier status, but leaves a small residual risk. Equally, further testing in a neonate who is identified through screening as a carrier of the common delta F508 allele may not identify a second allele but that will not remove the chance of cystic fibrosis entirely. In such cases, a careful analysis of other evidence is warranted (immunoreactive trypsinogen measurement in a dried blood spot, sweat testing and stool pancreatic enzymes) and more detailed molecular analysis may be undertaken (Box 6.2).

DNA test results sometimes pose considerable interpretive difficulties. The main challenge is to predict the likely phenotype from a given genotype. This is rarely possible with any degree of confidence since most genetic diseases exhibit intrafamilial variability in terms of *penetrance* and/or *expressivity* (see Marfan's syndrome above for a practical illustration). At the time of writing such difficulties are mainly encountered in adult practice where *presymptomatic* testing for delayed-onset autosomal dominant neurodegenerative disorders like Huntington's disease is common. In paediatric genetic practice, presymptomatic testing of this nature is largely restricted to hereditary tumour predisposition syndromes where the gene test result may either exclude the diagnosis or clarify ongoing management issues such as clinical screening (examples include familial adenomatous polyposis coli (FAPC), Von Hippel–Lindau syndrome and type 2 neurofibromatosis). In no case is it possible to accurately predict the phenotype. Presymptomatic genetic testing is certainly possible for other disorders (e.g. autosomal dominant spinocerebellar ataxia (SCA)) that may impact on aspects of early adult life, not just in terms of health but also lifestyle and career planning. Such testing should, however, occur within the correct ethical framework. In all cases, interpretation remains problematical.

In most instances, genetic testing is undertaken for diagnostic or prognostic reasons in a child with a phenotypic abnormality. Again, interpretive difficulties may arise when there is no clear genotype–phenotype correlation. For example, although cystic fibrosis gene mutations may be broadly classified as 'severe' or 'mild', it is not currently possible to predict the likely disease course in a neonate or child who is a compound heterozygote for a severe allele and a mild allele. In addition, genetic testing for Marfan's syndrome is likely to be available within the next 5–10 years in children presenting with a 'Marfanoid habitus'. Identification of a fibrillin-1 mutation in such children will have limited use as a predictor of disease course and the absence of a mutation will not necessarily exclude the diagnosis. This situation is likely to improve with the identification of other causative genes and genetic modifiers that may also act to influence the phenotype, but service application of this knowledge is many years away.

Box 6.2
Risk calculation using Bayes' theorem

A caucasian individual has a negative genetic carrier test for cystic fibrosis that detects 90% of disease alleles. He/she has a prior risk of being a carrier of 1/22 (the carrier frequency in a UK caucasian population), and a 21/22 chance of *not* being a carrier. A negative test result leaves a *residual risk* of being a carrier of 10%, since only 90% of alleles are examined. The chance of being a non-carrier is thus 9/10. These risks are multiplied down the columns to give joint risks, and the ratio of these risks gives the posterior risk of being a carrier. This test has reduced the individual's risk of being a CF carrier from population risk to 1/190. See Young (1999) for further detail.

	carrier	non-carrier
prior risk	1/22	21/22
conditional risk (negative test)	1/10	9/10
joint risk	1/220	189/220
posterior risk	1/190	

Genetic counselling

The aim of genetic counselling is to enable individuals with genetic disease to live normal lives and to enable informed decision-making around issues such as reproductive choice. A useful overview is presented by Clarke (1994b). Genetic counselling requires at least two major components: *information giving* and *support*. Some individuals are 'information seekers' and have many questions, others are more specific, and others may not have any particular questions. Some patients and families will accept devastating information with surprising ease and may need little in the way of support; others may benefit from the sort of supportive counselling that can be provided by a skilled genetic nurse specialist or genetic associate. More advanced counselling techniques may be offered to the few patients who struggle to come to terms with genetic disease.

A useful way to start a genetic consultation is therefore to set the scene by asking what information the consultand is expecting ('agenda setting'). In some centres, the consultation will be preceded by a home visit, during which the genetic nurse specialist or genetic associate will place the referral in a psychosocial context and will already have told the family what to expect. Information about genetic disease is often extremely complex — how would you describe a chromosome to someone with no previous exposure to genetics? — and should be delivered clearly, non-directively and at a level appropriate to the family. Genetic risk, for example, can be communicated in different ways and is certainly perceived in different ways: a risk of disease of 1 in 9 is the same as 11% or odds of 8:1 against; or you could say that the chance of health is 8/9, 88% or odds of 8:1 in favour. There are no rights and wrongs here: different ways of expressing the same idea may be required. It might be advisable in some situations to cover the material over more than one session, and in the case of children it is sensible to repeat the process when the child has reached adulthood to enable discussion about reproductive choice. Throughout this process it is important to offer support and a clear line of communication with the clinical genetics service.

Careful, sensitive consideration should also be given to minority groups. The religious beliefs of an individual will dictate the type of information offered (a discussion about prenatal diagnosis and termination of pregnancy, for example, may be inappropriate and even offensive). It should also be remembered that disability is usually defined by able-bodied individuals, and that some groups of people may not perceive any particular disability in themselves. Work with some people — those with hearing impairment or skeletal dysplasias such as achondroplasia, for example — should therefore take account of these sensitivities.

Clinical genetics services in the UK

The central clinical responsibilities of specialist genetics services in the UK are to provide accurate genetic diagnoses, genetic counselling to affected individuals and their families and expert advice to other healthcare professionals. Clinical genetics services are therefore delivered in a truly multidisciplinary context, interfacing with most other medical specialities. Additional activities include teaching at undergraduate and postgraduate levels, training, research and development and close liaison with laboratory genetic services. Raeburn et al (1997) have reviewed the development and structure of genetic services in the UK.

Although the local organisation of clinical genetics services differs from region to region, they have generally adopted a 'hub and spoke' structure with one central centre providing both outpatient clinics and laboratory services with 'satellite' clinics in district general hospitals providing equitable service delivery across the population. This system has been in place for many years and appears to work well, although future developments may involve an increase in locally based services while central clinics focus particularly on specialist and joint clinics (Harper et al 1996). Genetics directorates are often incorporated into larger directorates such as family care (including paediatrics and obstetrics) or laboratory diagnostics.

Clinical genetics services are provided by a team of professionals with different training backgrounds and therefore different, but complementary, skills. Clinical geneticists undertake postgraduate training in clinical genetics and often hold higher degrees in genetics; they work closely with nurses who have undertaken further postgraduate training in medical genetics and/or genetic counselling, genetic associates (in some centres) who hold basic degrees in science and have completed further training in genetic counselling, and (in some centres) counsellors who have trained in social sciences or psychology before specialising in genetic counselling.

The commissioning of clinical genetics services has proved difficult for a number of reasons including the complexity of the services provided and the relative lack of public health medicine consultants with specific experience of genetics services who can advise regional commissioning groups (Davies et al 1998). In addition, measures of quality and outcome are difficult to define in such a speciality (Fryer et al 1998), although considerable progress has been made in parallel with more widespread changes within the National Health Service.

RESOURCES

Web resources
British Society for Human Genetics.
http://www.bshg.org.uk
Contact a Family on-line. http://www.cafamily.org.uk
Jablonski's Online Multiple Congenital Anomaly/Mental Retardation (MCA/MR) Syndromes.
http://www.nlm.nih.gov/mesh/jablonski/syndrome_title.html
On-line Mendelian Inheritance in Man (OMIM).
http://www.ncbi.nlm.nih.gov/omim

CD ROM clinical databases
Bankier A 2000 Pictures Of Standard Syndromes and Undiagnosed Malformations (POSSUM). The Murdoch Institute for Research into Birth Defects, Melbourne
Winter R, Baraitser M 1999 London Dysmorphology Database (LDDB). Oxford University Press, Oxford
Winter R, Baraitser M 1999 London Neurogenetics Database (LNDB). Oxford University Press, Oxford

General texts
Harper P S 1998 Practical genetic counselling, 5th edn. Butterworth-Heinemann, Oxford
Jones K L 1997 Smith's recognizable patterns of human malformation, 5th edn. WB Saunders, Philadelphia

Mueller R F, Young I D 1998 Emery's elements of medical genetics, 10th edn. Churchill-Livingstone, Edinburgh
Rimoin D L, Connor J M, Pyeritz R E (eds) 1997 Emery and Rimoin's principles and practice of medical genetics, 3rd edn. Churchill Livingstone, Edinburgh
Rose P W, Lucassen A 1999 Practical genetics for primary care. Oxford University Press, Oxford
Strachan T, Reid A P 1999 Human molecular genetics, 2nd edn. Bios Scientific, Oxford
Young I D 1999 Introduction to risk calculation in genetic counselling, 2nd edn. Oxford University Press, Oxford

GLOSSARY

The following is an abbreviated glossary of terms commonly used in clinical genetic practice. The National Human Genome Research Institute at the National Institutes of Health in the US has a very useful online glossary at http://www.nhgri.nih.gov/DIR/VIP/Glossary/pub_glossary.cgi.

allele: the DNA sequence on one chromosome corresponding to a single gene.
aneuploidy: deviation from the normal diploid human chromosome number (46).
anticipation: a phenomenon observed in some autosomal dominant diseases whereby the disease worsens with each successive generation.
autosome: chromosomes 1–22, the non-sex chromosomes.
Bayes' theorem: a risk calculation which combines the prior and conditional probabilities of an event to allow derivation of the posterior probability.
centromere: the junction between a chromosome's p and q arms, and the point to which the spindle attaches during cell division.
chromosome: a complex of supercoiled DNA packaged with proteins and located in the cell nucleus.
disomy: the presence of a pair of chromosomes, one maternally derived and the other paternally derived.
DNA: deoxyribonucleic acid, the nucleic acid in which genetic information is encoded.
exon: a segment of DNA within a gene whose code is translated into an amino acid sequence.

expressivity: the severity of a phenotypic feature in an affected individual.

gamete: a reproductive cell (ovum or spermatozoon).

genotype: an individual's genetic constitution.

haploid: the chromosome number in a normal gamete (i.e. 23).

haplotype: term used to describe the variation in DNA sequence within or around a given gene — a type of DNA fingerprint.

heterozygous: different alleles at the same locus on a pair of homologous chromosomes.

homologous chromosomes: chromosomes containing the same loci.

homozygous: identical alleles at the same locus on a pair of homologous chromosomes.

intron: a segment of DNA within a gene which is removed during RNA processing and is not translated into amino acid sequence.

locus: the position of a gene on a chromosome.

Mendelian inheritance: single gene inheritance which obeys the laws of segregation and independent assortment described by Gregor Mendel.

microdeletion: the submicroscopic deletion of a series of contiguous genes from a chromosome segment.

mitochondrial inheritance: disease caused by mutation in mitochondrial DNA and exclusively inherited through the female line.

mosaicism: the existence of more than one cell line within an individual, each with a different genotype.

mutation: an alteration in an individual's genetic code.

obligate carrier: an individual who must be a carrier on pedigree grounds.

penetrance: the proportion of individuals with a given disease genotype who develop disease features, however mild.

phenotype: the features in an individual arising from an interaction between genotype and phenotype.

pleiotropy: disease manifestations at a number of different sites arising from a single mutant gene.

polymorphism: non-pathogenic variation in DNA sequence within a population.

reciprocal translocation: a chromosome rearrangement in which material is exchanged between two non-homologous chromosomes.

Robertsonian translocation: a chromosome rearrangement in which two acrocentric chromosomes become fused at their centromeres, with loss of the satellited 'p' arms (the acrocentric chromosomes are numbers 13, 14, 15, 21 and 22).

telomere: the highly specialised sequences at each end of a chromosome.

zygote: the fertilised ovum.

REFERENCES

Aase J M 1990 Diagnostic dysmorphology. Plenum Medical, New York
Baird P A, Anderson T W, Newcombe H B, Lowry R B 1988 Genetic disorders in children and adults: a population study. American Journal of Human Genetics 42:677–693
Barrett S, Beck J C, Bernier R et al 1999 An autosomal genomic screen for autism. Collaborative linkage study of autism. American Journal of Medical Genetics 88:609–615
Bennett R L, Steinhaus K A, Uhrich S B et al 1995 Recommendations for standardized human pedigree nomenclature. American Journal of Human Genetics 56:745–752
Bonaiti-Pellié C, Smith C 1974 Risk tables for genetic counselling in some common congenital malformations. Journal of Medical Genetics 11:374–377
Bradshaw N, Brewer C, FitzPatrick D 1998 Guidelines and care pathways for genetic diseases: the Scottish collaborative project on tuberous sclerosis. European Journal of Human Genetics 6:445–458
Brennan P, Young I D 2001 Congenital heart malformations: aetiology and associations. Seminars in Neonatology (in press)
Burn J, Brennan P, Little J et al 1998 Recurrence risk in offspring of adults with major heart defects: results from first cohort of British collaborative study. Lancet 351:311–316
Christensen B, Arbour L, Tran P et al 1999 Genetic polymorphisms in methylenetetrahydrofolate reductase and methionine synthase, folate levels in red blood cells, and risk of neural tube defects. American Journal of Medical Genetics 84:151–157
Clarke A 1994a The genetic testing of children. Report of a working party of the Clinical Genetics Society (UK). Journal of Medical Genetics 31:785–797
Clarke A (ed) 1994b Genetic counselling. Practice and principles. Routledge, London
Cutting G R 1997 Cystic fibrosis. In: Rimoin D L, Connor J M, Pyeritz R E (eds) Emery and Rimoin's principles and practice of medical genetics, 3rd edn. Edinburgh: Churchill Livingstone, Edinburgh
Cystic Fibrosis Mutation Database June 2000

http://www.genet.sickkids.on.ca/cftr/Cystic Fibrosis Resource Centre

http://www.cysticfibrosis.co.uk/cystic.htm

Cziezel A, Dudas I 1992 Prevention of the first occurrence of neural tube defects by periconceptual vitamin supplementation. New England Journal of Medicine 327:1832–1835

Dalby S 1995 GIG response to the UK Clinical Genetics Society report 'The genetic testing of children'. Journal of Medical Genetics 32:490–491

Davies S J, Farndon P, Harper P S 1998 Commissioning clinical genetic services. A report from the clinical genetics committee of the Royal College of Physicians of London. Royal College of Physicians, London

de Paepe A, Devereaux R B, Dietz H et al 1996 Revised diagnostic criteria for the Marfan syndrome. American Journal of Medical Genetics 62:417–426

de Vries B B A, Halley DJ , Oostra B A et al 1998 The fragile X syndrome. Journal of Medical Genetics 35:579–589

Ferencz C, Loffredo C A, Correa-Villasnor A C et al (eds) 1997 Genetic and environmental risk factors for major cardiovascular malformations: the Baltimore–Washington infant study: 1981–1989. In: Perspectives in cardiology, vol 5. Futura Publishing, New York

Fisch G S, Snow K, Thibodeau S N et al 1995 The fragile X premutation in carriers and its effect on mutation size in offspring. American Journal of Human Genetics 56:1147–1155

Fryer A E, Lister Cheese I A F 1998 Clinical genetic services. Activity, outcome, effectiveness and quality. A report from the clinical genetics committee of the Royal College of Physicians of London. Royal College of Physicians, London

Gabolde M, Guilloud-Bataille M, Feingold J, Besmond C 1999 Association of variant alleles of mannose binding lectin with severity of pulmonary disease in cystic fibrosis: cohort study. British Medical Journal 319:1166–1167

Gardner R J M, Sutherland G R 1996 Chromosome abnormalities and genetic counselling. Oxford University Press, Oxford

Greeves L G, Patterson C C, Carson D J et al 2000 Effect of genotype on changes in intelligence quotient after dietary relaxation in phenylketonuria and hyperphenylalaninaemia. Archives of Disease in Childhood 82:216–221

Hall J G, Froster-Iskenius U G, Allanson J E 1989 Handbook of normal physical measurements. Oxford Medical Publications, Oxford

Harding A 1997 Hereditary ataxias and paraplegias. In: Rimoin D L, Connor J M, Pyeritz R E (eds) Emery and Rimoin's principles and practice of medical genetics, 3rd edn. (pp2225–2234) Churchill Livingstone, Edinburgh

Harper P S 1998 Practical genetic counselling. Butterworth-Heinemann, Oxford

Harper P S, Hughes H, Raeburn J A 1996 Clinical genetics services into the 21st century. A report from the clinical genetics committee of the Royal College of Physicians. Royal College of Physicians, London

Huson S M, Rosser E M 1997 The phakomatoses. In: Rimoin D L, Connor J M, Pyeritz R E (eds) Emery and Rimoin's principles and practice of medical genetics, 3rd edition. (p.2269–2292) Churchill Livingstone, Edinburgh

International Molecular Genetic Study of Autism Consortium 1998 A full genome screen for autism with evidence for linkage to a region on chromosome 7q. Human Molecular Genetics 7:571–578

Jones A C, Shyamsundar M M, Thomas M W et al 1999 Comprehensive mutation analysis of TSC1 and TSC2 — and phenotypic correlations in 150 families with tuberous sclerosis. American Journal of Human Genetics 64:1305–1315

Jones K L 1997 Smith's recognizable patterns of human malformation, 5th edn. WB Saunders, Philadelphia

Kalatzis V, Petit C 1998 The fundamental and medical impacts of recent progress in research on hereditary hearing loss. Human Molecular Genetics 7:1589–1597

Knight S J, Regan R, Nicod A et al 1999 Subtle chromosomal rearrangements in children with unexplained mental retardation. Lancet 354:1676–1681

Lipscomb K J, Clayton Smith J, Harris R 1997 Evolving phenotype of Marfan's syndrome. Archives of Disease in Childhood 76:411–416

Lubs H A 1969 A marker X chromosome. American Journal of Human Genetics 21:231–261

Metcalfe K 1999 Williams syndrome: an update on clinical and molecular aspects. Archives of Disease in Childhood 81:198–200

MRC Vitamin Study Research Group 1991 Prevention of neural tube defects: results of Medical Research Council Vitamin Study. Lancet 338:131–137

Mueller R F, Young I D 1998 Emery's elements of medical genetics, 10th edition. Churchill Livingstone, Edinburgh

Nicholls R D 1999 Incriminating gene suspects, Prader–Willi style. Nature Genetics 23:132–134

Oberlé I, Rousseau F, Heitz D et al 1991 Instability of a 550 base-pair segment and abnormal methylation in fragile X syndrome. Science 252:1097–1102

Parker M, Fortnum H, Young I D, Davis A C 1999 Variations in genetic assessment and recurrence risks quoted for childhood deafness: a survey of clinical geneticists. Journal of Medical Genetics 36:125–130

Raeburn S, Kent A, Gillot J 1997 Genetic services in the United Kingdom. European Journal of Human Genetics 5 (suppl 2):188–195

Rimoin D, Connor J M, Pyeritz R E 1997 Emery and Rimoin's principles and practice of medical genetics, 3rd edn. Churchill Livingstone, New York

Rose P 1999 Taking a family history. In: Rose P, Lucassen A (eds) Practical genetics for primary care. Oxford general practice series. Oxford University Press, Oxford

Rose V M, Au K S, Pollom G et al 1999 Germ-line mosaicism in tuberous sclerosis: how common? American Journal of Human Genetics 64:986–992

Ryan A K, Goodship J A, Wilson D I et al 1997 Spectrum of clinical features associated with interstitial chromosome 21q11 deletions: a European collaborative study. Journal of Medical Genetics 34:798–804

Sheffield V C, Pierpont M E, Nishimura D et al 1997 Identification of a complex congenital heart defect susceptibility locus by using DNA pooling and shared segment analysis. Human Molecular Genetics 6:117–121

Strachan T, Read A P 1999 Human molecular genetics, 2nd edn. Bios Scientific, Oxford

Sutherland G R 1977 Fragile sites on human chromosomes: demonstration of their dependence on the type of tissue culture medium. Science 197:265–266

Tyfield L A 1997 Phenylketonuria in Britain: genetic analysis gives a historical perspective of the disorder but will it predict the future for affected individuals? Molecular Pathology 50:169–167

Tyfield L A, Zschocke J, Stephenson A et al 1995 Discordant phenylketonuria phenotypes in one family: the relationship between genotype and outcome is a function of multiple effects. Journal of Medical Genetics 32:867–870

Van Camp G, Smith R J H. Online. Hereditary Hearing Loss Homepage. World Wide Web URL: http://dnalab-www.uia.ac.be/dnalab/hhh/June 2000

Van Tongerloo A, De Paepe 1998 Psychosocial adaptation in adolescents and young adults with Marfan syndrome: an exploratory study. Journal of Medical Genetics 35:405–409

Van trappen G, Devriend K, Swillen A et al 1999. Presenting symptoms and clinical features in 130 patients with the vell-cardio-facial syndrome, the Leuven experience. Genetic Counselling 10:3–9

Verkerk A J, Pieretti M, Sutcliffe J S et al 1991 Identification of a gene (FMR-1) containing a CGG repeat coincident with a breakpoint cluster region exhibiting length variation in fragile X syndrome. Cell 65:905–914

Warner L E, Mancias P, Butler I J et al 1999 Mutations in the early growth response 2 (EGR2) gene are associated with hereditary myelinopathies. Nature Genetics 18:382–384

Winter R M, Baraitser M 1998 Oxford medical databases: London dysmorphology database (CD ROM). Oxford University Press, Oxford

Young I D 1999 Introduction to risk calculation. Oxford University Press, Oxford

Zielenski J, Corey M, Rozmahel R 1999 Detection of a cystic fibrosis modifier locus for meconium ileus on human chromosome 19q13 [letter]. Nature Genetics 22:128–129

7 | Nutrition

Good nutrition is essential for all but it is difficult to overemphasise the importance of early nutrition particularly in newborn infants who do little more than feed, sleep and grow. Parents recognise that an increase in weight indicates that their child is thriving, whereas doctors know that loss of weight is often the first sign of underlying illness. Good growth in the early months of life not only promotes early success, but may also have a major impact on adult size, well being and longevity. In Western countries where food is plentiful and the food industry is able to prepare and present foods in many forms and to add whatever 'extras' might be thought to be beneficial, the question on what to feed infants and children becomes more challenging.

NATIONAL ADVICE

It is, and has been, the advice of all authorities, national and international, that breast feeding is the best way to feed healthy infants, but that is not to say that infants cannot be reared successfully without breast milk. Weaning is not recommended before 4 months of age, but healthy infants do not appear to come to any harm if they are given weaning foods earlier. Young children should be given an interesting and varied diet, but some appear to thrive on 'junk foods' hurriedly swallowed. Clearly if we are to give advice it has to be based on sound nutritional knowledge and to be realistic within the lifestyle and culture of the child and his family. In the UK, we are fortunate in having regular national surveys and reports. Those relating to this chapter are given in Box 7.1.

Government reports do not make easy reading but offer advice based on the best available information. Not infrequently there is insufficient data on which to make specific recommendations. It is important that health professionals do not give contradictory advice. However, we may have no option but to express an opinion based on the information that is available.

DIETARY REFERENCE VALUES (DRVS) (Box 7.2)

In 1987 an expert panel was set up to review the original recommended daily amounts (RDAs) of food, energy and nutrients for groups of people in the UK. The most obvious change was the increase in nutrients covered, from 10 to around 40, and the change in nomenclature. The term recommended daily allowance suggests the minimum required for good health. In reality, for the vast majority of people the RDA was substantially more than individual needs. It was set as a population figure where if the average was near the RDA, deficiency was very unlikely. The panel decided to set a range of figures based on the distribution of requirements for each nutrient. These figures have been published as dietary reference values (Department of Health 1991). They have been set for most nutrients assuming a normal distribution of intake, where a notional mean has been called the estimated average requirement (EAR). The reference nutrient intake (RNI) has been set at a notional 2SDs above the mean and the lower reference nutrient intake (LRNI) at a notional 2SDs below the mean (Fig. 7.1).

For many nutrients it was not possible to establish DRVs with any confidence so a safe intake was set. For fats, carbohydrates and fibre recommendations were set within healthy eating guidelines. All

> ### Box 7.1
> #### National surveys and reports
>
> DH 1991 Dietary reference values
>
> Mills A, Tyler H 1992 Food and nutrient intakes of British infants aged 6–12 months
>
> DH 1994 Weaning and the weaning diet
>
> DH 1994 Nutrition aspects of cardiovascular disease
>
> Gregory J R et al 1995 National diet and nutrition survey: children aged 1½–4½ years
>
> Foster K, Lader D, Cheesbrough S 1997 Infant feeding 1995
>
> Thomas M, Avery V 1997 Infant feeding in Asian families
>
> Gregory J, Lowe S 2000 National diet and nutrition survey: young people aged 4–18 years

> ### Box 7.2
> #### Definitions of dietary reference values (DRVs): the term used to cover LRNI, EAR, RNI and safe intake
>
> EAR — estimated average requirement of a group of people for energy[a] or protein or a vitamin or mineral. About half will usually need more than the EAR, and half less
>
> LRNI — lower reference nutrient intake for protein or a vitamin or mineral. An amount of the nutrient that is enough for only the few people in a group who have low needs
>
> RNI — reference nutrient intake for protein or a vitamin or mineral. An amount of the nutrient that is enough, or more than enough, for virtually all people in a group. If the average intake of the group is at the RNI, then the risk of deficiency is very small
>
> Safe intake — a term used to indicate intake or range of intakes of a nutrient for which there is not enough information to estimate RNI, EAR or LRNI. It is an amount that is enough for almost everyone but not so large as to cause undesirable effects
>
> [a] As excess energy leads to obesity only an EAR has been set.

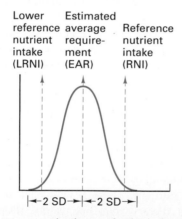

Fig. 7.1 Frequency distribution of individual requirements

DRVs should be applied with an understanding of their background and not applied indiscriminately to individual children, particularly sick children. There is wide variation in need between children of similar age, weight, activity and feeding patterns due to differences in food absorption, utilisation and metabolic efficiency. For some nutrients, an intake below the LRNI may not lead to a deficiency state, and for others an intake above the RNI may

cause no harm. It is helpful to read the evidence on which the values are based (Department of Health 1991).

MILK FOR THE NEWBORN

Breast feeding

All experts are agreed that breast feeding is the correct way to nourish an infant over the first months of life. There are very few absolute contraindications, for example galactosaemia and alactasia which are both extremely rare. There are situations when it is not ideal to breast feed where breast milk contains traces of maternal drugs — see list of those to avoid (BNF 2001, Appendix 5) or where there is a risk of transmitting HIV. Many books have been written on the benefits of breast feeding to the mother and the infant. The advantages and disadvantages can relate to both the

Table 7.1 **Composition of mature human milk**	
Mean values for pooled samples of expressed milk per 100 ml	
Energy (kcal)	70
Protein (g)	1.3
Lactose (g)	7
Fat (g)	4.2
Sodium (mg)	15
Potassium (mg)	60
Calcium (mg)	35
Phosphorus (mg)	15
Iron (µg)	76
Source: Department of Health and Social Security (1977)	

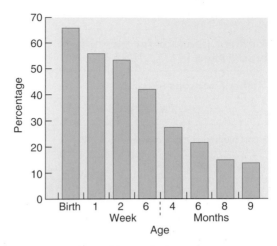

Fig. 7.2 Prevalence of breast feeding at ages up to 9 months in UK (1995). (Reproduced with permission from Foster et al (1997))

mother and infant physically, emotionally and socially, though they will not be discussed here.

Breast milk contains a range of nutrients which meet all the requirements of the great majority of infants (Table 7.1). The sugar is lactose, which is bound to protein, and the protein is 60% whey and 40% casein. The whey protein is an interesting mixture of many different proteins including IgA, which is probably not digested, lactoferrin and lysozyme, which probably protect against infection, and lactalbumin. It also contains traces of the protein from the mother's own diet, so hypersensitivity can develop to protein the mother has digested. The fats more directly reflect what the mother has eaten.

The debate becomes a little fraught when we consider the vitamins A and D and iron. Breast milk contains little vitamin D, and vitamin A levels depend on maternal stores and diet during lactation. At present in the UK it is recommended that breast-fed infants are not given supplements of vitamins A and D until 6 months, unless there is any concern that the maternal supply is inadequate when they should be given from 1 month. Routine iron supplementation is not recommended as the low levels in breast milk are compensated for by better absorption (Department of Health 1994a).

Human milk has the advantage that it is ready to feed, sterile, at the correct temperature, has varying constituents and is convenient for the mother. But this last point, in a two-income family, or a single working mother is its disadvantage, for it needs the mother to be in attendance. It is a target for the World Health Organization (WHO) and for many countries including the UK that a larger percentage of infants should be breast fed. The number of mothers starting to breast feed has not really increased in the last 15 years despite a National Breast Feeding Initiative started in 1993 and an annual National Breast Feeding Awareness Week each year since (Fig. 7.2). The UK Baby Friendly initiative is part of the UNICEF initiative which aims to promote infant and child health through protecting and supporting breast feeding. Though the incidence in the UK as a whole was 66% in 1995 (compared with 62% in 1990) this may be attributed to the sample surveyed, which was characterised by a greater proportion of older, well-educated mothers of higher socioeconomic group, all positive indicators for breast feeding. The reasons why mothers choose to breast feed or not are instructive and particularly relevant if we wish to promote breast feeding (Table 7.2). The 5-yearly national surveys provide invaluable information.

Nutrition

Table 7.2 **Mothers' reasons for planning to breast feed in UK, 1995**	
Mothers' reasons	**%[a]**
Breast feeding is best for the baby	83
Breast feeding is more convenient	37
Breast feeding is cheaper	21
Closer bond between mother and baby	20
Mother's own experience	17
Breast feeding is natural	12
Breast feeding is good for mother	12
Influenced by medical personnel	3
Influenced by friends or relatives	2
Other reasons	2

[a] Percentages do not add up to 100 as some mothers gave more than one reason
After Foster et al (1997)

Box 7.3
Successful breast feeding is facilitated by

- Putting the baby to the mother's breast very soon after birth
- Correct positioning at the breast
- Feeding on demand rather than at set times
- Not giving complementary feeds
- A positive and relaxed atmosphere
- Supportive and consistent advice

Samples of infant formula should not be given to mothers nor advertised to them

The reasons why mothers give up breast feeding are many and complex (Table 7.3). Support of breast-feeding mothers from experienced health professionals is essential if the large drop-out rate is to be reduced. Demand feeding should be encouraged with realistic expectations of feed duration and frequencies. Newborn infants do not generally 'sleep through the night' and may be expected to feed 8–12 times in 24 hours and are unlikely to fall into a regular feeding pattern for the first few weeks. This should not be seen as the mother failing to satisfy, but the natural process of establishing feeding. The bouts of erratic and frequent feeding seen in the previously settled infant should be explained as the natural process of 'supply and demand' as the infant sucks more to ensure more milk is produced. It is not quite so easy as 'making up another ounce', but is completely normal. The Royal College of Midwives has produced an excellent book on 'Successful Breast Feeding' which gives practical advice and is essen-

tial reading for those involved (Royal College of Midwives 1988) (Box 7.3).

Formula feeding

Whilst we may wish, where possible, for an infant to be breast fed, we must also accept that every mother has a right to choose what she feels is best for her and her baby and support her in this decision (Table 7.4). In this country bottle feeding is a safe and satisfactory alternative providing there is adequate parentcraft teaching.

The first decision facing a mother will be which milk to choose from the 12 normal infant formulas currently available in the UK. They must all meet the national guidelines which implement an EC Directive in order to be marketed as infant formulas. They are all prepared from cows' milk with modifications to mimic human milk as closely as possible and, as technology has improved, so has the profile of these formulas (Table 7.5).

The first category historically are those known as the 'modified' or 'casein-dominant' formulas, which are essentially cows' milk diluted to reduce the excess protein, with added fat, sugar, vitamins and minerals to levels slightly higher than found in human milk to compensate for poorer absorption. The second group are the 'highly modified' or 'whey-dominant' formulas which are further modified to alter the ratio of whey:casein to appro-

Table 7.3
Reasons given by mothers for stopping breast feeding at different ages in UK, 1995

Reasons for stopping	% Stopping breast feeding[a]		
	< 1 week	6–12 weeks	> 8 months
Insufficient milk/baby seemed hungry	32	59	13
Baby would not suck/rejected breast	29	10	22
Painful breasts or nipples	28	8	3
Breast feeding took too long/tiring	11	18	12
Mother was ill	11	8	3
Did not like breast feeding	10	3	2
Baby was ill	7	5	–
Domestic reasons	6	6	2
Difficult to judge how much baby had drunk	4	2	–
Baby could not be fed by others	3	4	6
Mother had inverted nipples	2	0	–
Embarrassment	1	3	1
Returning to work	1	19	18
Had breast fed as long as intended	1	2	28
Not convenient[b]	–	6	5
Baby was teething/biting[b]	–	–	28
Other reasons	10	5	11

[a] Percentages do not add up to 100 as some mothers gave more than one reason
[b] Code only introduced at later waves of study
From Foster et al (1997)

ximate that found in human milk (60:40), giving an easily digested protein with a more similar balance of amino acids. The formulas also have reduced electrolytes making hypernatraemia less likely. The 'whey-dominant' formulas are recommended as an alternative to breast feeding from birth.

All infant formulas are available as sterile powders which require only addition of water, the standard for all being to add 1 level scoop of powder to 1 fluid ounce (30 ml) of cooled boiled water. Some companies now market ready measured sachets which only need addition to a predetermined volume of cooled boiled water. Good hygiene is essential and all equipment used for feeding must be sterilised. All new parents must be taught the correct practice if the increased incidence

Nutrition

Table 7.4
Mother's reasons for planning to bottle feed in UK, 1995

Mother's reason	%[a]
Other people can feed baby with bottle	36
Mother's own previous experience	30
Did not like the idea of breast feeding	27
Would be embarrassed to breast feed	7
Can see how much the baby has	6
Expecting to return to work soon	6
Bottle feeding is less tiring	4
Medical reasons for not breast feeding	4
Persuaded by other people	3
No particular reasons	1
Other reasons	6

[a] Percentages do not add up to 100 as some mothers gave more than one reason
After Foster et al (1997)

Table 7.5
Normal infant formulas marketed in the UK

Brand	Whey dominant	Casein dominant
SMA Nutrition	SMA Gold	SMA White
Cow & Gate	Premium	Plus
Farleys	First Milk	Second Milk
Milupa	Aptamil First	Aptamil Extra Milumil
Boots	Formula 1	Formula 2
Hipp Organic	Infant Milk	–

of gastroenteritis in bottle-fed infants is to be reduced.

Once a formula is chosen and correctly made then the question arises as to how much is required. Bottle-fed infants should be demand fed in much the same way as breast-fed infants, enabling them to regulate their own intake. An average guide of 150–200 ml/kg/day of correctly made infant formula will meet the nutritional needs of most infants but should not be used prescriptively. In theory the total volume can be divided out over 6–8 feeds a day. The number will depend on the individual but will tend to decrease with age as the stomach capacity increases, allowing larger volumes to be taken at a time. A guide is given to show average volumes which might be taken at different ages (Table 7.6).

There are currently six companies marketing infant formulas in the UK and there is little to

choose between the different brands. How the industry markets breast milk substitutes is subject to an international code. These are particularly relevant to the developing countries, but apply to all. In the UK the promotion is primarily directed at health visitors as the advertising of formulas to parents is a breach of the code aimed at promoting breast feeding. Each product vies at being most like human milk. As we know this to be a variable feast, this argument presents difficulties of interpretation. When it was discovered that taurine and carnitine were abundant in human milk but not found in cows' milk, they were added and used as a promotion feature. Current 'interest' is in the addition of nucleotides for immunological benefits, long chain polyunsaturated fatty acids (LCPs) for brain and retinal development, and to manufacture human whey proteins like lactoferrin to add to infant formula. They may also be added under the general requirement that infant formula should be as like human milk as possible. The authorities will have to reassure themselves that they are safe.

A new 'normal' infant formula has been designed 'for the 56% of babies who present every month with minor feeding problems'. Omneo Comfort 1 (Cow & Gate) features partially digested whey protein for 'easy digestion', reduced lactose and added starch to thicken for 'comfortable digestion', prebiotics for 'healthy gut flora and softer stools', a unique fat blend 'which is closer to breast milk' for

Table 7.6 Feed volume and number by age[a]		
Age	**Volume**	**No.**
1–2 wk	50–70	7–8
2–6 wk	75–110	6–7
2 mth	110–180	5–6
3 mth	170–220	5
6 mth	220–240	4

[a] These figures are a guide only; the needs vary from day to day and feed to feed

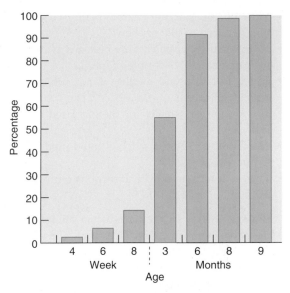

Fig. 7.3 Age at introduction of solid foods in UK (1995). (Reproduced with permission from Foster et al (1997))

'improved calcium and fat absorption and softer stools' and claims to be the 'all-round milk for digestive comfort and overall well being for use from birth onwards'. It even has a follow-on milk — Omneo Comfort 2 — for use from 6 months. Mothers reading this will surely wonder how any other formula should be considered?

Whilst health professionals will be concerned about the content, mothers are also influenced by the physical presentation (packet or tin, powder or granules) and the convenience and cost. A recently introduced 'organic' formula (Hipp Organic Infant Milk) may be preferred by some mothers.

Ready to feed liquid formulas are now available which would alleviate the common problem of overconcentration of feeds found in a number of clinical trials and shown to result in excessive weight gain (Lucas et al 1992). However the increased cost would make them unacceptable to most.

One factor commonly affecting the mother's choice of milk is her perception of whether it will satisfy. Studies have shown 'switching' rates, i.e. the number of mothers wishing to change their infant from one milk to another, of 25% in infants up to 6 weeks of age. In the UK the main reason given is 'a hungry baby'. The fact that the casein-dominant formulas are marketed as being more satisfying, 'for the hungrier bottle-fed baby', leads to the natural progression from whey- to casein-dominant

formulas, despite the fact that there is no evidence to support these claims. On the contrary, there is evidence to show there is no difference (Taitz & Scholey 1989). However, it is likely that this misconception leads to a delay in the early weaning that might result if the placebo effect of this change was disputed!

FOOD FOR THE WEANLING

Weaning

Weaning is the transition from an all-milk liquid diet to a varied diet using solid foods. The term means 'to accustom to' and this suggests a slow process of adaptation and not milk today and solids tomorrow.

Weaning does not need to start at the same age or weight in all infants. 'The majority of infants should not be given solid foods before the age of 4 months, and a mixed diet should be offered by the age of 6 months' (Department of Health 1994a). Nevertheless, the 1995 national survey showed that 91% of infants had solid food before the minimum recommended age (Foster at al 1997) (Fig. 7.3). The early introduction of solids is undesirable for a number of reasons:

Nutrition

- Most infants lack the neuromuscular coordination required to bite or chew.
- Nutritional requirements are best met by breast milk or a suitably adadpted formula.
- Gut maturation and motility is not sufficiently developed.
- The kidney isn't ready for the increased solute load.
- The use of energy-dense foods could predispose to obesity.
- There is interference with absorption of minerals from milk.

However, delay in the introduction of solids is undesirable because infants may not achieve an adequate nutritional intake on milk alone after 6 months of age. The infant by this age has developed a biting/chewing action, which should be encouraged. It is also at about this age that the store of iron laid down in fetal life diminishes.

In 1995 7% of infants were being given solids by the age of 6 weeks. Although this is a drop from previous years (9% in 1990, 11% in 1985), this is still a concern. Of these infants only 5% had been offered home-made food, suggesting that the easily available commercial products have a role to play in this very early weaning.

Commercial babyfoods are used for the majority of infants at 4–5 months, with only 41% using any home-made food at all. This may be because of lack of knowledge as to what foods can be given, or the feeling that the manufacturer knows best, and possibly because of advertising statements such as 'F— — — — is the natural transition from milk to real food', suggesting that use of 'real' food is not acceptable!

Weaning is the process of changing from breast or bottle to spoon, liquid to solid, smooth to texture, warm to a variety of temperatures and milk to a variety of tastes. In other words a process of adopting a new way of eating which should be carried out in a slow, gradual manner. The following guidelines are useful:

- The spoon can be offered first, smooth and plastic, with a small amount of milk.
- Never add solids to the bottle.
- Offer 1–2 teaspoons of pureed fruit or vegetables, or gluten-free cereal mixed with milk.

- Do not add sugar, other than to sour fruits.
- Do not add salt or use salty convenience foods intended for adults.
- Offer one new food at a time, enabling any dislikes or intolerance to be seen.

The amount given should be very small starting at one feed and slowly building up. These initial stages should take a few weeks to introduce new tastes, textures and temperature and then the quantities offered slowly increased. The baby will start to cut down on milk as the amount of solid food increases. At this stage, small quantities of protein foods, for example meat or fish, should be included to replace that lost from the decreasing milk. Using commercial babyfoods as a convenience is sensible, but the use of suitable family food is important so that the taste and texture of home-made food is introduced to the infant early on, reducing the chance of problems when trying to change from one texture to the range found in family food.

The question of what is 'suitable family food' is very difficult to answer. The family living on ready-prepared convenience foods would be well advised to use the convenience foods designed specifically for infants, due to the large quantities of salt added to many ready-made meals. The ability of the kidney to concentrate urine and therefore handle a higher solute load increases with age, but other than the RNI there are no concrete recommendations on what is a dangerous level of salt at any given age. However, advice on not adding salt when preparing foods for infants is also good advice for the future as a means of preventing hypertension in later life by not getting accustomed to salty foods.

'Mashed potatoes and gravy' is a very commonly described meal in early weaning as it is already a suitable texture. However, it is unlikely to be a home-made boiled potato mashed with gravy made from meat or vegetable juices! It is much more likely to be a reconstituted dried mash product with reconstituted dried gravy with a sodium level many times higher! Soup is another commonly used food, which is easily eaten by infants. Again it is much more likely to be a dried or tinned variety with a salt level considerably higher than its home-made equivalent.

After Milk

what's next?

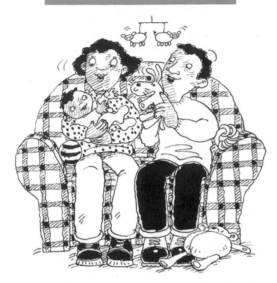

Fig. 7.4 Leaflet on weaning. (Cover reproduced with permission from British Dietetic Association)

Table 7.7			
Composition of cows' milks per 100 ml.			
Component	**W**	**S-S**	**S**
Energy (kcal)	66	46	33
Protein (g)	3.2	3.3	3.3
Carbohydrate (g)	4.8	5.0	5.0
Fat (g)	3.9	1.6	0.1
Vitamin A (µg)	52	21	1.0
Riboflavin (mg)	0.17	0.18	0.18
Vitamin D (µg)	0.03	0.01	tr
Calcium (mg)	115	120	120
Iron (µg)	50	50	50

W = whole; S-S = semi-skimmed; S = skimmed
From Holland et al (1989)

Finger foods should be introduced from 6 to 9 months providing the infant can sit well. Drinks should be offered from a cup from 6 months. The aim of weaning is to have the child eating normal chopped family food by 9–12 months. These stages are given in more detail in the British Dietetic Association leaflet 'After milk — what's next?' (British Dietetic Association 1999) (Fig. 7.4).

Milks

The onset of weaning does not mean that breast milk or formula should stop. An extended period of mixed feeding is to be encouraged. There are advantages in continuing breast milk or infant formula throughout the first year (Department of Health 1994a).

Doorstep cows' milk should not be the main milk drink until after the age of 1 year due to its low level of iron and vitamin D. However, it can be used from 6 months of age when it is more convenient to make sauces, desserts, etc. for the whole family. When used it should be full cream (Table 7.7).

Follow-on milks have been designed to replace cows' milk from the age of 6 months, for example Step Up (Cow & Gate), Forward (Milupa). They are lower in protein and higher in iron and vitamin D and have been shown to decrease iron deficiency in this vulnerable group. Whether there is any advantage in changing from a normal formula is not known, but they offer an option which is seen by many mothers as 'the next step' and are used by about 25% of infants at 8–9 months. They are not available on milk tokens. Cow & Gate now market a milk for use after follow-on milk, known as Next Steps.

Goats' or sheep's milk are unsuitable for infant feeding as they are low in iron, vitamin D and folic acid. Goats' milk is also low in vitamin A. If used after the first year they must be pasteurised or boiled before consumption. Infant formula based on modified goats' milk is available in the UK, but use is minimal.

Soya formulas were initially made available for use by the medical profession in the treatment of proven cows' milk intolerance, for example Wysoy (SMA Nutrition), Infasoy (Cow & Gate). They are now generally available and so can be used by anyone without medical advice. They have no obvious advantage over normal formulas. There has been concern over high aluminum levels and more recently phyto-oestrogens, so their use is not advocated by the Department of Health except in the treatment of cows' milk intolerance under medical supervision. A hydrolysed protein formula, for example Nutramigen, is increasingly preferred. Soya formulas have been modified to provide full nutrition and the soya milks found in supermarkets are not suitable for infants and young children.

Preterm formulas are intended for use with low birthweight (LBW) infants in hospital. However, they are sometimes continued after discharge in infants who are well enough to be at home but have a lot of catch-up growth to make. They are higher in most nutrients, particularly protein, energy and sodium. Recently follow-on formulas have been introduced for LBW infants at discharge, Nutriprem 2 (Cow & Gate) and Premcare (Farleys). Their use is currently small due to their high cost, but they will soon be prescribable.

Infant drinks

A wide range of infant drinks, fruit and herbal varieties, are available for infants. Most breast- and bottle-fed infants in this country do not need extra fluid until solids are used and milk intake drops, nevertheless they are popular. Concern over the effect of sugar on teeth has resulted in a range of drinks being marketed as 'no added sugar'. Some have no sugar at all. Others have as much as 10% which though not 'added' is naturally present from the concentrated fruit juice used and are still very sweet. Some may have the pH increased by the addition of buffers. If used, they are best given in small quantities as a flavouring for water along with meals, when the sugar and acid will be buffered by other foods. Water or milk only should be given outside of mealtimes.

Water

In normal circumstances there is no advantage in using bottled water in preference to boiled tap water taken from the first tap on the mains supply (usually the cold tap in the kitchen). Bottled waters, other than those labelled 'natural mineral water', are expected to conform to essentially the same standards as the public water supply and they are therefore suitable for giving to infants or

for preparing feeds. As with tap water, bottled water should be boiled and cooled before use. 'Natural mineral water' is covered by less comprehensive regulations and must not be used as it may contain high levels of substances such as nitrates as well as sodium. Water that has been artificially softened should not be used for infants because of high sodium levels. Effervescent waters are not suitable for infants (Department of Health 1994a).

Vitamins

Clinical manifestation of vitamin deficiency is extremely rare in Europe. Many of the foods marketed for infants contain added vitamins and conventional household diets properly prepared also contain a variety of vitamins, apart from vitamin D. The main source of this vitamin is from the effect of sunlight on the skin.

Poor intake of vitamins may occur in children who have delayed weaning, bizarre eating patterns, food aversion and improperly treated food intolerance. Vitamin D can be deficient in Asian children because of their dark skin and prolonged bottle feeding with early use of unmodified cows' milk. Currently the Department of Health recommendation acts as a safety net by recommending the use of supplementary vitamins, 5 drops daily to breast-fed infants from 6 months, or from 1 month if the mother's vitamin status is suspect, and for bottle-fed infants once the intake of formula drops below 500 ml. They should be continued until 5 years unless adequate vitamin status can be assured. Appropriate vitamin supplements are made available at low cost to all (Table 7.8).

Fluoride

When fluoride is added to water at levels of 1 ppm there is a decrease in the incidence of dental caries by 50–60%. Despite the evidence, some areas do not have a fluoridation programme. However there is considerable debate as to whether systemic fluoride should be recommended where water is not fluoridated, due to the risk of excess causing enamel opacities. Local policies exist and parents are advised to discuss it with their dentist.

FEEDING PROBLEMS IN INFANTS

Most of the following problems relate to feeding. Parents may often blame the feed and be tempted to try an alternative. It is highly unlikely that such a change would lead to improvement in any of these problems, so the practice of switching formulas should not be advocated by health professionals.

Wind

Wind is air that has been swallowed and causes more problems in some babies than others. Some air is swallowed with feeding and infants swallow a lot of air when crying. Feeding too quickly or too slowly may be the cause of excessive wind, as may vigorously shaking the bottle just before feeding. It is not a serious problem but is distressing for mother and infant. Advice should be offered on an appropriate sized hole in the teat to ensure feeding isn't too fast or slow. The infant should be positioned so that the teat is always full of milk and feeding should be interrupted occasionally to allow winding. With the breast-fed infant, check that a good seal is made while sucking.

Possetting

Regurgitation of small quantities of feed soon after feeding is quite common in infants. It is not usually a serious problem, however it is messy and families vary in how much they can tolerate. The problem may be due to overfeeding or incompetence of the sphincter at the end of the oesophagus. Reflux usually only occurs when the stomach is full so oesophagitis is uncommon. It usually resolves with age as the diet becomes more solid, the sphincter becomes stronger and the child more upright. Feed thickeners may be required with more serious reflux and a wide range are now available for addition to feeds, from those based on alginic acid (for example Gaviscon Infant (Reckitt and Colman)) or carob bean gels (for example Instant Carobel (Nutricia)) which are not absorbed, to starch-based thickeners (for example Vitaquick (Vitaflo Ltd)) which contribute to the total energy intake and should not be used unless this is required (Table 7.9).

Table 7.8 **Department of health vitamin drops**	
	5 drops daily provide
Vitamin A	200 µg
Vitamin C	20 mg
Vitamin D	7 µg

Table 7.9 **Feed thickeners**		
Product	**Quantity**	**Comments**
Gaviscon Infant	1 dose to 4 fl oz (120 ml)	Alginic acid acts as thickening agent and is not absorbed. High in sodium
Instant Carobel Nestargel	0.5–1% (1–2 scoops to 2 fl oz (60 ml) 0.5–1%	Gel from carob bean which is not absorbed As for Carobel but requires heating to thicken before mixing
Nutilis, Thick n Easy, Thixo D, Vitaquick	Approx. 3%	Thicken instantly. Are absorbed so give 4 kcal/g = 12 kcal/100 ml @3% May be beneficial in failure to thrive
Enfamil AR	1 scoop + 1 oz (30 ml) water	A thickened infant formula
Omneo Comfort 1	1 Scoop + 1 oz (30 ml) water	A thickened infant formula

There is a thickened formula on the market, Enfamil AR (Mead Johnson), which offers an easy solution. It thickens at low pH in the stomach as does Gaviscon Infant (Reckitt and Colman), unlike the others which thicken in the bottle, making it easier for the infant to take and less likely to block the teat. The main drawback is that mothers may try to adjust the degree of thickness, which will alter the nutritional composition. Omneo Comfort 1 (Cow & Gate) works in a similar way.

Colic

Three-month or evening colic is the common term used to describe the harmless but distressing condition when infants, usually in the evening, cry for long periods of time, drawing up their legs as if in pain. The cause is unknown but various feeding practices have been incriminated. It is obviously uncomfortable for the baby and causes considerable parental anxiety. The use of a non-alcoholic gripe water is sometimes beneficial as are some of the herbal infant drinks (e.g. fennel) which are said to be soothing. Remedies such as Infacol (Pharmax) are said to disperse wind and may help. Many remedies have been tried but health professionals have little to offer other than reassurance that the infant is not seriously ill and that it will eventually resolve.

Constipation

The passage of hard stools causes straining and discomfort and needs correcting. The passage of a normal soft motion once a week is not uncommon and does not require intervention. Constipation is more common in formula-fed than breast-fed infants. Increasing the volume of fluid by offering cooled boiled water is often sufficient. If not, diluted fresh fruit juice or even prune juice may help (1 : 10–1 : 5 dilution). Once the infant is taking solids use of fruit and vegetable usually helps. If stool softeners such as lactulose are used, they are more likely to help if given in small divided doses rather than one daily dose.

Gastroenteritis

This is a fairly common problem in infancy, more so in bottle-fed infants. It is characterised by the frequent passage of watery stools with or without vomiting. It is usually of short duration, but can be critical due to fluid and electrolyte losses particularly in young infants who have higher fluid requirements and less mature renal compensation. It should always be treated with oral rehydration solutions (ORS) to replace fluid and electrolyte losses with resumption of normal nutritional intake as soon as possible.

Breast-fed infants should continue to breast feed with ORS supplements by bottle. Infants who are bottle feeding should have ORS solution only for 24 hours and then resumption of full-strength formula, with solids if appropriate when formula is tolerated. ORS solutions can be continued along with milk feeds if necessary. Occasionally there is a transient lactose intolerance which will require a short-term avoidance of lactose, necessitating the use of a low lactose formula, for example Galactomin 17 (Cow and Gate) or SMA LF (Wyeth Nutrition), and lactose free solids. This is uncommon and should always follow a number of failed regradings and stool chromatography for confirmation.

There is a formula marketed for infants with diarrhoea (HN 25, Milupa), which is low in lactose and has added cereals and is said to allow more rapid return to feeding with a shorter duration of loose stools and less hunger and weight loss. This is generally an unnecessary product. It was developed for use when regrading with 1/4, 1/2 and 3/4 strength feeds was recommended after 24 hours on ORS only. This is no longer the case.

DIETARY HABITS OF THE PRESCHOOL CHILD

The pre-school years represent a transition from total dependence and an all-milk diet to some independence and a diet based on family foods. An increasing number of children will also receive meals as part of another family, be that a childminder or nursery. Emphasis has been placed on finding out more about the eating habits of this age group in the last few years. Until publication of the National Diet and Nutrition Survey (Gregory et al 1995) there had been nothing since the survey of 1967–68. From these and a number of smaller studies we now have an insight into the way this age group eat which can be used in conjunction with the DRVs to make recommendations for future health.

Energy

There has been a reduction in overall energy intake of children in the UK presumably because of a more sedentary lifestyle and heated homes. For each age group the mean energy intakes were below the EARs. This was not thought to be due to inadequate intakes as children in this survey were on average significantly taller than in 1967–68, but more likely that the reference value is too high.

At all ages cereal and cereal products made the largest contribution to energy intake (average 30%, varying from 27% in the youngest to 32% in the oldest). This was closely followed by milk and milk products (average 20%, varying from 26% in the youngest to 16% in the oldest) as might be expected. It is interesting to note that on average children were obtaining one-fifth of their energy away from home, making the need for good nutrition in nurseries and other childcare facilities a priority for local authorities.

Fat

The diet in early infancy provides about 50% of dietary energy from fat, allowing children to meet their high energy requirements from manageable volumes of milk. The proportion of energy from fat decreases with age as milk is replaced with other foods containing less fat.

There has also been a downward trend in the total fat intake and proportion of energy derived from fat, in the UK, USA and other countries. Where there has not been an equivalent drop in total energy, the fat has been replaced by an increase in carbohydrates and refined sugars and is probably one of the causes of childhood obesity.

On average the proportion of energy from fat has dropped to about 36% between the ages of 1 and 4 years in the recent survey, a drop of 3–4% on 25 years ago. This is close to the recommendations on fat for the adult population as a whole of 35% of dietary energy from fat (Department of Health

1994b). This may be seen as healthy, but was compensated for by an increase in non-milk extrinsic sugars.

Fat is a major source of energy and in the toddler years where energy requirements are approximately three times higher than adults on a weight basis, it plays an important role in meeting these requirements.

Carbohydrate

Total carbohydrate intakes in the survey increased with age but there was no significant difference in the proportion of energy derived from carbohydrate, which was about 51% for all ages. However there was large individual variation. The major source was cereals (39%) as would be expected, although 14% was obtained from drinks which would obviously be sugar.

Non-milk extrinsic sugars is the term used to describe the sugars not found within the cell structure, excluding milk sugars. These are the most likely to cause dental caries (e.g. honey, sucrose, fruit juices), and because of this the national recommendation is that no more than 10% of dietary energy should come from these foods (Department of Health 1991). This includes young children, although the survey showed that less than a tenth of children in all age groups were achieving this and on average they were obtaining 19% of their energy intake from these sugars.

The dental survey carried out concomitantly (Hinds & Gregory 1995) showed the strong link between consumption of these sugars and dental caries. For example, 40% of 3–4 year olds who had sugar confectionery most days or more often had caries, compared with 22% of those who consumed it less frequently. The consumption of drinks in bed every night was seen in nearly a third of all children. Of these, caries was seen in 29% who had drinks containing non-milk extrinsic sugars as opposed to 11% of those who drank milk.

Fibre

High fibre foods are more bulky and have a lower nutrient and energy density and it has therefore

Nutrition

been suggested that children on high fibre intakes may not be able to consume adequate nutrition. High fibre foods may also contain phytates which decrease mineral absorption. What exactly constitutes an appropriate fibre intake in children is not known, as there are no data on the physiological effects in children. The panel on DRVs, who more correctly define fibre as *non-starch polysaccharides* (NSP), suggest that children need proportionally less NSP in relation to their size, and children under 2 years should not take NSP-rich foods at the expense of more energy-dense foods required for growth.

The national survey showed an average intake of 6.1 g daily which increased with age, but with considerable variation. When considered in relation to number of bowel movements there was a positive correlation. This survey provides some of the first data on both fibre intake and bowel habit in this age group. Although there is no specific DRV for fibre in children in the UK, the recommendation in the USA is that 'American children over 2 years of age should consume a minimum amount of dietary fibre equivalent to age (in g) plus 5 g daily'. Therefore a 4 year old should consume a minimum of 9 g fibre daily, which is considerably more than the average intake seen in the UK survey. A maximum safe limit was set at 'age (in g) plus 10 g daily' (Williams et al 1995).

WHAT SHOULD THE PRE-SCHOOL CHILD EAT?

Individuals vary a great deal in their nutrient intake and requirements, so in the non-obese child, appetite is a good indicator of when the child has had enough. There is no one food that must be eaten or must be avoided from a healthy diet, but a good mixed diet should be based on milk, lean meat, poultry, fish, eggs, cheese, fruit, vegetables, bread and cereals (preferably whole grain). These foods have a good nutrient density and will provide the necessary energy, protein, vitamins, minerals and fibre.

Sugary foods and drinks should be restricted as they play a major role in dental caries and provide only energy. Fried foods and high fat foods such as chips, pastry, fatty meat products and crisps should be limited. It would be unrealistic to expect children to totally avoid these foods. There should

be a gradual transition over to lower fat and sugar containing foods from the age of 2 years. See the section on 'Eating for the future' (Fig. 7.5).

Milk is an important source of calcium, riboflavin and protein and children should normally be having the equivalent of one pint of full cream milk daily. Children who dislike milk as a drink can have it in puddings or sauces or as equivalents where one-third of a pint (200 ml) milk is equivalent to a carton of yoghurt or 1 ounce (30 g) of cheese. The Department of Health recommend full cream milk up to the age of 5 years, but accepts that semi-skimmed milk may be appropriate in children over 2 years who are growing well, where the rest of the family are using it. Fully skimmed milk is not recommended before 5 years due to its low energy density (Table 7.7):

Department of Health vitamin supplements should be continued until 5 years as a 'safety net' unless there is no doubt about the adequacy of the child's diet.

This age group is renowned for food fads and refusals. These should be seen as a natural part of child development and parents advised to ignore them. They should never 'give in' and replace a refused meal with a packet of crisps or equivalent. This purely reinforces the wrong behaviour. The child will eventually get hungry and eat if replacements are withheld.

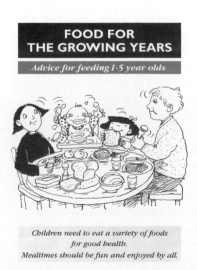

Fig. 7.5 Leaflet providing advice on feeding 1–5 year old. (Cover reproduced with permission from British Dietetic Association)

COMMON PROBLEMS IN THE PRE-SCHOOL CHILD

Toddler diarrhoea

A small number of children pass frequent loose stools containing particles of undigested food three or more times each day. Whilst the diarrhoea may be profuse and unpleasant, the child continues to grow and gain weight adequately. The problem usually presents during the second half of the first year until early childhood.

Two dietary adjustments may help. If the child is on a low fat intake, which often occurs if milk has been reduced after weaning or if full cream milk has been replaced by skimmed milk, adding fat to the diet may increase the bowel transit time. Secondly, a decrease in fruit and vegetables may help, particularly if taken in excess. Parents should be reassured that the problem is self-limiting and that the child is not ill. Toilet training, though difficult, may help.

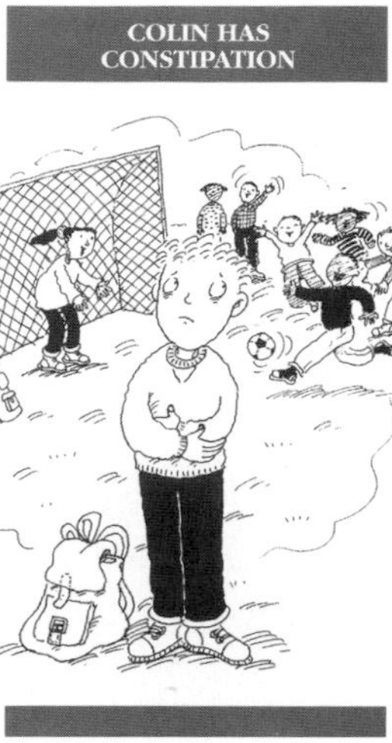

Fig. 7.6 Leaflet providing advice on management of constipation. (Cover reproduced with permission from British Dietetic Association)

Constipation

This is a common problem and may be treated simply with sound dietary advice to increase foods high in cereal fibre, fruit and vegetables and not forgetting to increase fluid intake. In some children an increased fluid intake alone may be sufficient, but there is no point increasing fibre without fluid, as there will be inadequate fluid for the fibre to absorb.

More severe constipation however, will probably need dietary advice and a prescribed stool softener along with advice on increased exercise and regular 'toiletting', particularly after meals when increased gut motility will help. Stool softeners should hopefully only be necessary in the short term to help establish proper eating and bowel habit. Improvement is more likely if the whole family takes on the new healthier way of eating rather than singling out one child.

Poor dietary habits

Failure to thrive is considered in more detail in other chapters. Here it is considered in relation to the child who is not obtaining sufficient nutrition to grow. Poor dietary habits are likely to be the main problem.

Some infants fail to transfer from bottle to mixed feeding and continue to consume large quantities of milk which often fails to meet energy and nutrient requirements. If the milk used is not an infant formula or follow-on milk they are also likely to become anaemic. This is more common in some Asian families (Thomas & Avery 1997).

The solution is simple in theory, but in practice difficult to carry out. Reducing milk intake to an acceptable level and not giving in to demands is not easy for either parent or infant, especially in the short term. The child will demand what he has been used to receiving, leading to distressing days and disturbed nights. However, this is short lived and usually results in a more appropriate diet for age. Parents will need support from health professionals and other members of the family if this is to be successful. Reassurance that the child will eat when hungry and not starve or dehydrate is essential.

Excessive use of drinks other than milk can also be a big problem in this age group. There has been

Nutrition

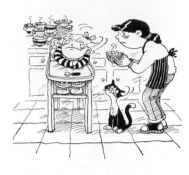

HELP
MY CHILD WON'T EAT!

A GUIDE FOR FAMILIES

Fig. 7.7 Leaflet providing guidance on children who are poor eaters. (Cover reproduced with permission from British Dietetic Association)

a seven-fold increase in fruit juice consumption in the last 20 years probably because of the increased availability and choice, but also the 'healthy' image they assume. The concerns are many, including links with dental health because of the high natural sugar and acidity, non-specific diarrhoea because of the malabsorption of large amounts of fructose, and failure to thrive due to a decreased appetite for other more nutrient dense foods. Conversely obesity, along with short stature is also more common in children with high fruit juice intakes of greater than 12 fluid ounces (360 ml) daily (Dennison et al 1997).

Establishment of good eating habits is important and parents should be given guidance before problems 'set-in' (Fig. 7.7).

- Offer a variety of foods of different taste, colour and texture.
- Give food at regular and frequent mealtimes, e.g. 4-hourly meals and 2-hourly snacks.
- Offer drinks only with meals and snacks to limit fluid intake.
- Present small amounts in an appealing way, allowing for second helpings.
- Try to eat as a family using the same foods.
- Allow plenty of time and do not have distractions from the meal such as television.

- Don't insist on a clean plate every time.
- Keep desserts out of sight and don't use as a reward.

Anaemia

Iron deficiency anaemia is the most commonly reported nutritional disorder in the UK. The Diet and Nutrition Survey reported an incidence of 12% in children aged 1–2 years reducing slightly with age. Little data is available for children under this age other than for at-risk groups where incidence is as high as 30%. As well as causing anaemia, iron deficiency may also lead to tiredness, apathy, lack of capacity for exercise, increased risk of infection, impaired development in infancy, adverse effects on IQ in pre-school children and poor educational achievement in school children.

From the age of 6 months when in utero iron stores are depleted, a dietary source of iron is essential. This is potentially a period of great risk for iron deficiency because of high requirements and a small capacity for food. Continued breast feeding, infant formula or follow-on milk throughout the first year will help and many commercial weaning foods are supplemented with iron.

Red meat, offal and products made from them are the richest sources of the most easily absorbed form of iron in the diet, *haem iron*, although these foods provided only about 14% of the total iron intake in the national survey of 1–2 year olds. Cereals and cereal products provide almost half (48%) of their dietary iron intake from fortified breakfast cereals and fortified white bread. However, iron from cereals, pulses, eggs and green vegetables is in the form of *non-haem iron* which is not so well absorbed (Box 7.4).

Certain factors will influence the absorption of non-haem iron from foods and knowledge of these can make a big difference to whether a diet provides sufficient iron. For example orange juice, because of the high vitamin C content, can double the absorption of non-haem iron, whereas tea, because of the tannins, can reduce it by 75% (British Nutrition Foundation 1995). So the British practice of giving tea to infants and young children should be actively discouraged!

> ## Box 7.4
> ### Dietary sources of iron
>
> - Haem — red meats, offal, burgers, sausages, pork, turkey, chicken
> - Non-haem — egg yolks, wholemeal bread and cereals, fortified breakfast cereals, pulses, dark green vegetables, dried fruits
>
> Factors which increase absorption of non-haem iron include foods containing haem iron and vitamin C. Those which inhibit its absorption include tannins, phytates and vegetable fibre

Excessive weight gain

Obesity is an easier problem to prevent than treat. It is relatively uncommon in young children and does not necessarily persist into adulthood. Where it does, the parents are also likely to be obese. It is unusual for the obese child to come from a family with good eating habits and it is an essential part of treatment that the whole family's way of eating is changed.

General guidelines for the child would also apply to the rest of the family:

- Avoid foods high in fat, e.g. fried foods, crisps and similar snacks.
- Reduce the use of butter and margarine.
- Avoid foods high in sugar, e.g. confectionery, preserves and sweetened drinks.
- Eat only at mealtimes, which may include suggested snacks.
- Use low calorie drinks and low fat spreads, cheese, etc.
- Increase the intake of fruit and vegetables.
- Use skimmed or semi-skimmed milk in place of full cream milk. Limit to 300–500 ml daily.
- Remove fat from meats and use more lower fat meats, poultry and fish.
- Avoid severe calorie restriction and rapid weight loss.

In general children should aim to control their rate of weight gain by 'growing into their height'. However, in order to motivate the child it is often beneficial to allow some loss, in which case a slow gradual loss is desirable. This should be done in conjunction with an exercise programme with a sensible increase in activity for the whole family. The aim should be for a sustained change in family lifestyle rather than a short sharp improvement with resumption of previous habits.

Food intolerance

This is a fashionable diagnosis ranging from intolerance to one food, for example strawberries, through to multiple intolerance of many nutritionally important foods. There is usually no way of making a diagnosis other than withholding the suspected food, leading to relief from symptoms, followed by re-introduction of the food and the return of symptoms.

Dietary exclusion should never be attempted without referral to a suitably experienced paediatric dietitian, unless the culprit is obvious and nutritionally unimportant, for example prawns. The dietitian will advise exclusion of the likely foods and design an appropriate nutritionally adequate diet around what is left. This may necessitate the use of prescribed supplements to ensure an adequate intake. It is not uncommon for the diet to be more of a problem that the initial symptoms. Treatment must include a suitable challenge as most children grow out of their intolerance.

Peanut allergy

Peanut allergy is particularly in vogue at the moment and symptoms include vomiting, diarrhoea, urticaria, angiodema, acute abdominal pain, exacerbation of atopic eczema, asthma and anaphylactic shock. The prevalence is unknown but there has been an increase in reported cases. It is a true food allergy which is thought to be a lifelong condition. The pattern of previous reactions in an individual does not always predict the severity of a future attack. Treatment includes being prepared for the next attack as total avoidance of peanuts is very difficult, so accidental exposure is always a concern. Treatment may include rapidly acting oral antihistamines for mild reactions, inhaled adrenaline (epinephrine) or for those with potential anaphylaxis, intramuscular or subcutaneous adrenaline (epinephrine).

Nutrition

Avoidance of peanuts from food is very difficult. Foods most likely to contain peanuts include: cakes, biscuits, pastries, ice cream, desserts, toppings for desserts, cereal bars, peanut butter, nut spreads, satay sauce, ground nuts, mixed nuts, confectionery, vegetarian products, curries, salad dressings, breakfast cereals, Chinese, Thai or Indonesian dishes.

Goods sold loose or unwrapped are generally unlabelled and best avoided.

For manufactured foods with labels, check the ingredient list for:

- ground nuts, earth nuts, monkey nuts, mixed nuts and peanut butter.

Avoidance of *refined* vegetable oils, which could be peanut is probably not necessary in most peanut-sensitive individuals, as any residual peanut protein is undetectable. However, there is still conflicting opinion, so if refined oils are being avoided, check also for:

- Peanut, arachis, vegetable or ground nut oils, any of which could be derived from peanuts.
- Hydrolysed vegetable protein, food additives E471 and 472 (a–e) and lecithin.

New labelling will hopefully begin to include the statement 'contains unrefined peanut oil' on products where this may be the case.

Eating out is difficult and most severe reactions are caused by eating foods away from home.

Advice on prevention exists, but is under regular review as more information becomes available. At the present time the British Dietetic Association recommends the following (British Dietetic Association 1999):

- For infants from a non-atopic family, there is no need to specifically delay the introduction of peanuts, i.e. peanuts of a suitable texture can be introduced from 6 to 8 months of age.
- For infants and young children with atopy, e.g. eczema, hayfever, asthma, other proven food allergy, or from a family with a clear history of atopy, the introduction of peanuts is best delayed until at least 3 years of age (or until an age advised by their medical practitioner).

- For pregnant or breast-feeding women with atopy or from a family with a clear history of atopy, it seems prudent that they also avoid peanuts.

These recommendations are for peanuts only.

With the possible exception of vegans, avoiding peanuts is unlikely to nutritionally compromise most children.

Behaviour

Food intolerance and behaviour have been linked ever since the Feingold diet was introduced from the USA. This diet involves avoiding some artificial colourings and preservatives, which claims to improve the behaviour of overactive children. The validity of this has been questioned and trials do not support any link. Despite this the Hyperactive Children's Support Group (HACSG) has continued to recommend it. They have also linked it to other diets which may lead to nutrient deficiencies making referral to a dietitian essential.

Food additives can be avoided by:

- Eating more fresh, natural food.
- Looking at food labels.

To make labelling easier, additives used in the European Economic Community (EEC) have been given a number ('E' number).

OLDER CHILDREN AND ADOLESCENTS

Once the child starts school a number of changes take place which have an effect on diet. Most children will now eat one meal in a different environment either as a school meal or packed lunch away from home. Trends in the way we eat tend to be revealed in the older school child and adolescent, when peer pressure exerts a great effect. In general, eating has become less formal and eating out and take-aways have become more common.

Getting to school in the morning is often a rush and breakfast can be missed altogether or eaten on the move. Breakfast is an essential meal for all children because of their high nutritional requirements and should not be missed. Omission of breakfast following an overnight fast seems to affect performance in the classroom, particularly in tests requiring the use of memory (Pollitt 1995). It has also been shown that the contribution made by breakfast to overall nutrient intake is not made up elsewhere in the diet, where breakfast is missed (Ruxton & Kirk 1997) (Fig. 7.8).

Although children are taller and heavier than in the past, it does not follow that the diet is healthier. The survey of British schoolchildren in 1983 (Department of Health and Social Security 1989) showed a knowledge of healthy eating principles, which was not reflected in their diets. When looking at the proportion of energy derived from fat, three-quarters had intakes over the 35% maximum recommended (Department of Health 1994b) and nearly a third over 40%. Most children had adequate amounts of most nutrients but 1 in 3 girls had iron intakes and 1 in 4 had calcium intakes below the LRNI. They ate less fruit and vegetables and more chips than desirable. In summary their diets were too high in fat, particularly saturated fat, too high in sugar and too low in iron, calcium and fibre (Department of Health and Social Security 1989).

A more recent survey of the diets of 4–18 year olds in Britain published as part of the Food Standards Agency National Diet and Nutrition Survey programme, shows that some improvements have taken place, but that there is still a long way to go in achieving healthy eating targets with young people (Gregory & Lowe 2000). There was a decrease in mean energy intakes in all age groups, which were consistently below the EAR. As children were again found to be taller and heavier than previously, it suggests that recommendations are too high for the current activity levels, which were lower than HEA advice.

The total amount of fat consumed was on average less than in 1983, which is consistent with trends seen in the National Food Surveys for the population as a whole. This can partly be accounted for by the decrease in overall energy, but the remainder may well be replaced by an increase in non-milk extrinsic sugars, which contributed a mean of over 16% of energy, compared to the maximum 11% recommended. Some children are receiving a quarter of their energy from these sources, particularly carbonated drinks and chocolate confectionery.

Although intakes of most vitamins and minerals were adequate for most children, there were still deficiencies of vitamin A, iron and zinc in some groups. During the 7-day recording period over 70% of children had not eaten any citrus fruit and about 60% no leafy green vegetables.

At the launch of this report, the Minister for Public Health promised action to include these issues in the National Plan for the NHS and be a priority for the Department for Education and Employment.

School meals

School meals should be an ideal time to introduce or reinforce healthy eating to a captive population, particularly the younger school child. Sadly, this is not usually the case. Following the 1980 Education Act there was no requirement for local authorities to provide any meal at all. Some continued to do so, but with no nutritional standard to aim for. Prior to 1980 a meal conforming to prescribed nutritional standards was provided for all children who wanted it.

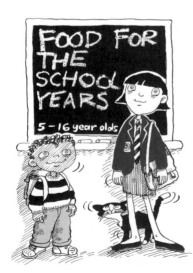

Fig. 7.8 Leaflet providing advice on food for school age children. (Cover reproduced with permission from British Dietetic Association 1999)

Following this change in policy the government agreed to review the diets of British school children (Department of Health and Social Security 1989) and, as already stated, found that although they usually met intakes for protein and energy, their diets were high in fat and sugar and as such unhealthy. This was particularly so in those children who skipped school lunch (over 10% of older children) and ate out in local cafes. Their overall diets were poor, as the deficiencies in the midday meal were not made up at other mealtimes.

Health promotion groups have been lobbying the Departments of Health and Education to re-introduce nutritional standards for school meals to meet recommended intakes within current healthy eating guidelines. In 1997 an assurance was given by the Secretary of State for Education that minimum nutritional standards would be intro-duced. In October 1998 'Ingredients for success', the consultation document on those standards, was published and a number of initiatives are underway to produce the most fundamental changes to school meals since de-regulation in 1980 (Department for Education and Employment 1998a). This followed another Department for Edu-cation and Employment (1998b) consultation docu-ment called 'Fair funding — improving delegation to schools', which recommended delegation of the responsibility for school meals to individual gov-erning bodies. However it was acknowledged that they would also be required to meet the forthcom-ing nutritional standards.

The implementation is likely to include a 'whole school, whole day' framework, linking food pro-vided with the taught curriculum. While laying down regulation, it will avoid banning popular foods, but will work towards educating children to make informed choices. Standards will be expressed in terms of foods rather than nutrients. They will be based on the concepts of balance and variety illustrated by the 'Balance of Good Health'. (See 'Eating for the future', below).

Vegetarianism

Adolescents often want to try out new ways of eating and it is not uncommon to see a phase of vegetarianism, particularly in girls. Vegetarian diets vary considerably as to the extent of avoidance of animal products. The greater the avoidance, the more likely the risk of nutritional deficiency. However, vegetarians as a group have been shown to have a lower incidence of certain chronic dis-eases, presumably due to the higher intake of un-saturated fats, fibre and antioxidants. It is essential that the likely nutritional deficiencies are known and avoided by inclusion of suitable alternatives. (Table 7.10).

Nutrients most likely to be lacking include:

- *Iron* — The absorption of iron will be increased to a limited extent when the dietary provision is low. Iron from non-haem sources is better absorbed when eaten together with a source of vitamin C.
- *Calcium* — This is likely to be deficient only where milk is avoided, in which case a nutri-tionally adequate substitute should be used.
- *Vitamin B$_{12}$* — This is only likely to be a problem in vegan diets where children should be re-ceiving sufficient from a suitable soya formula. Where this is not the case a supplement should be given.

A vegetarian diet is generally more bulky and less nutrient dense than a non-vegetarian diet which may cause problems during periods of rapid growth, such as weaning and adolescence. National vegetarian and vegan societies can offer good nutri-tional advice. Details and more information can be found elsewhere (Wardley et al, 1997) (Fig. 7.9).

Drinks

Milk and water are the drinks favoured by health professionals for children (Department of Health 1994b). However, there is a decline in milk drink-ing which is of great concern, particularly as it is being replaced by fruit juices and fizzy drinks. The consumption of milk in 11–16 year olds has decreased from 40% of drinks consumed in 1982 to 16% in 1993 (National Dairy Council 1996). Milk is

Table 7.10
Characteristics of vegetarian diets

Group	Foods excluded	Possible nutrient deficiencies	Suitable food substitutes
Partial vegetarian	Red meats: beef, pork, lamb, meat products, offal	Iron	Poultry, fish, eggs, milk, cheese, yoghurt, beans, lentils, nuts, seeds
Lacto-ovo vegetarian	Meat, fish, poultry	Iron, zinc, vitamin B_6	Eggs, milk, cheese, yoghurt, beans, lentils, nuts, seeds
Lacto vegetarian	Meat, fish, poultry, eggs	Iron, zinc, vitamins D, B_6	Milk, cheese, yoghurt, beans, lentils, nuts, seeds
Vegan	Meat, fish, poultry, eggs, milk, yoghurt, cheese	Protein, energy, iron, calcium, zinc, vitamins, D, B_6, B_{12}	Beans, lentils, nuts, seeds, soya milk,[a] rice milk[a]

[a] Fortified with calcium
Reproduced with permission from Oxford University Press

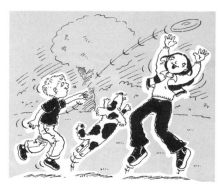

FOLLOWING A VEGETARIAN DIET

ADVICE FOR 5 TO 16 YEAR OLDS

A vegetarian diet is one which does not include any meat or fish

A vegetarian diet can be very healthy, but you need to find suitable alternatives to meat. It is important to choose the right variety of foods to provide all the essential nutrients to stay fit and healthy.

Fig. 7.9 Leaflet providing advice on vegetarian diets for children age 5–16 years. (Cover reproduced with permission from British Dietetic Association)

a major source of calcium which is particularly important in the growing child and for prevention of bone disease in later life.

The increased use of both fizzy drinks and fruit juices is of concern not only because of the corresponding drop in milk consumption but also because they are often high in sugar. Even if 'diet' versions are used, the acidity is very high and both sugar and acid are major factors in dental decay. Canned drinks are often drunk as a snack along with sweets and chocolate which only serves to increase the detrimental effect on teeth. The increase in these drinks of high energy, poor nutrient density has been highlighted as a cause of poor weight gain in young children due to suppression of appetite for proper meals (Hourihane & Rolles 1995).

EATING FOR THE FUTURE

In 1993 the UK government adopted a White paper entitled 'The health of the nation' (Department of Health 1992). As good nutrition was seen to be an important factor in many of the key objectives, a Nutrition Task Force was established in order to give guidance on nutritional issues. A number of initiatives have sprung from this including the publication of 'The eight guidelines for a healthy diet':

1. Enjoy your food.
2. Eat a variety of different foods.
3. Eat the right amount to be a healthy weight.
4. Eat plenty of foods rich in starch and fibre.
5. Don't eat too many foods that contain a lot of fat.
6. Don't eat sugary foods too often.
7. Look after the vitamins and minerals in your food.
8. If you drink alcohol, keep within sensible limits.

These guidelines have formed the basis for healthy eating messages for the whole population

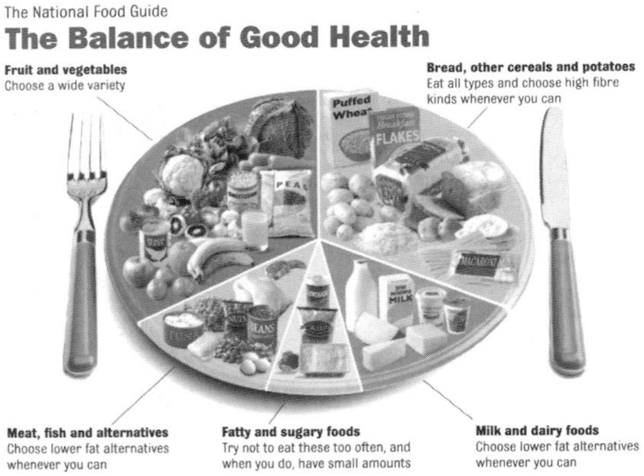

Nutrition

The National Food Guide
The Balance of Good Health

Fruit and vegetables
Choose a wide variety

Bread, other cereals and potatoes
Eat all types and choose high fibre kinds whenever you can

Meat, fish and alternatives
Choose lower fat alternatives whenever you can

Fatty and sugary foods
Try not to eat these too often, and when you do, have small amounts

Milk and dairy foods
Choose lower fat alternatives whenever you can

Fig. 7.10 Five commonly accepted food groups. (Reproduced with permission from the Health Education Authority 1994)

and, other than the advice on alcohol, can be used for children with certain provisos. To ensure a consistent method of teaching the task force developed a pictorial guide called 'The Balance of Good Health'. This is simply a version of the food groups which have been used in a variety of formats by nutritionists and dietitians for many years. As always, not all health professionals like the system chosen, some preferring the American Pyramid Model, or other systems which do not incorporate a plate. There has been criticism of the plate as it might suggest that all food groups must be present in the proportions the plate suggests at every meal.

The Balance of Good Health is based on the five commonly accepted food groups (Fig. 7.10). One of the most important messages given is that no one food is 'good' or provides all the nutrients we need and no one food is 'bad' so must be avoided. The concept of balance is essential, requiring a variety of foods from each food group over each meal, day or even longer. Emphasis needs to be placed on eating plenty from the bread and cereal, and fruit and vegetable groups, a moderate amount from dairy and meat groups and small amounts from the fat/ sugar group. The Balance of Good Health applies to most people; however when used for children the following information must be included:

- Use full fat milk and dairy products for children under 2 years, with a gradual transition over to lower fat products from 2 to 5 years

- Include one pint of milk, or equivalent, daily in growing children
- Gradually introduce wholegrain cereals and bread, but not if this results in refusal

The Health Education Authority (HEA) has used this plate model in a number of publications and is happy for it to be used by health professionals in producing literature for teaching.

When dealing with the general public one of the key issues has to be consistency of information, as nothing annoys the consumer more than conflicting messages. We live in an age where the media latch onto medical and nutritional research as soon as it is published and present it to the public without the background knowledge to be able to interpret it. Scares such as BSE (bovine spongiform encephalopalty) and the link with CJD (Creutzfeldt–Jakob disease), genetically modified produce and its safety, and topics such as lycopenes in tomatoes and the suggestion that tomato ketchup is therefore good for you, do nothing to support the idea that we know what we are doing. The links between diet and adult disease are very complex and cannot be summed up in simple messages such as 'butter is bad for you'.

However, the messages need to be clear and simple as well as consistent. Health professionals may know that there are different types of fat in the diet and that although we are looking for an overall reduction in total fat, we mainly want a reduction in saturated fats and more use of monounsaturated and polyunsaturated fats. This is meaningless to most people. Cholesterol and the difference between low density lipoprotein (LDL) and high-density lipoprotein (HDL) cholesterol means very little to the general public. In school, children are taught about the feeding habits of the honey bee or how to bake scones, but do they get taught how to eat healthily and why? The school curriculum is beginning to include healthy eating under health education, but there is still a long way to go. It is also essential that the food industry takes on board these messages, so that in these days of ready prepared and convenience meals, the food we buy contains the appropriate types of fat.

It is not known when changes in diet begin to affect the development of adult disease but Professor Barker and colleagues in Southampton suggest that nutritional factors which affect the fetus and young infant may have long-lasting effects and are important indicators for adult disease such as coronary heart disease and cardiovascular disease (Barker 1997).

Links between diet and adult disease are very complex and there are many different views which have led to conflicting messages to the public. There is little doubt that certain aspects of diet are linked to adult disease, for example high fat intakes and heart disease, low fibre intakes and bowel cancer. However, there are other risk factors which may be more relevant for example smoking and heart disease or lung cancer.

Diet is only one of the risk factors in coronary heart disease, but an important one as its consequences are potentially preventable (Box 7.5). When considering preventive strategies for children, direct extrapolation of results from intervention studies in adults is not appropriate as most children are at low risk of cardiovascular events and the

potential risks may outweigh the long-term health benefits (Gaziano 1998). In the light of this and the work of Professor Barker suggesting that poor growth both pre and post birth predisposes us to adult disease, there has been a strong held, though not unanimous belief that the most important issue in infants and young children is ensuring optimum growth through adequate nutrition and not reduction of fat and increase in fibre as for the rest of the population.

DIET IN DISEASE

Modifying the diet may be central to the treatment of some diseases and relevant to the management of many. It is important that all who have care of the child or advise the family understand the principles involved. Diets are prescribed treatments and should not be altered without discussion with the prescriber and dietitian. Here is a brief summary of some of the diets used by families for the benefit of their children. For detailed information on the dietary treatment of clinical conditions see Shaw & Lawson (2001).

Diabetes mellitus

Diabetes in children is invariably of the insulin dependent type and treatment involves insulin injections and control of diet with the aim of normalising blood glucose. Dietary treatment aims to provide a balanced diet, incorporating healthy eating principles, which gives optimal growth and weight gain. Current healthy eating principles of reduced fat and sugar with higher fibre apply very well to the diabetic diet so there is no reason why the child with diabetes should eat any differently to the rest of the family, providing the family diet is healthy. Carbohydrate intake is not so much restricted as tailored to requirements and the insulin adjusted to control blood glucose levels.

The child needs normal amounts of carbohydrate but in an unrefined form, so an accurate diet history is taken from each child and/or parents and used as a baseline for dietary advice. The current aim is to provide 50% of energy as carbohydrate, but in practice this is rarely possible in children without resorting to refined carbohydrates.

Box 7.5
Diet and cardiovascular disease

For adults, the report on diet and cardiovascular disease (Department of Health 1994b) made the following recommendations:

- Population average intake of protein should remain at 15% food energy

- Population average intake of carbohydrate should increase to 50% food energy

- Population average intake of fat should decrease to = 35% food energy
  = 11% of food energy from saturated fatty acids
  7–10% of food energy from polyunsaturated fatty acids
  13% of food energy from fat as monounsaturated fatty acids

- An increase in average consumption of fibre-rich foods to give about 18 g non-starch poly saccharides daily

- Population average intake of salt should be 6 g daily

These % refer to food energy excluding alcohol

Nutrition

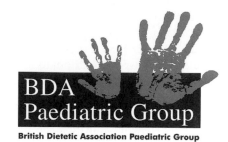

Fig. 7.11 Specialised formula leaflet. (Cover reproduced with permission from British Dietetic Association)

The British Diabetic Association exists to offer advice and support and children are strongly recommended to join. Diabetic camps are organised to take children out of the home situation for a holiday with other diabetics of similar age, with support from doctors, dietitians, nurses and other interested volunteers.

Cows' milk protein intolerance

There are few symptoms that haven't been attributed to cows' milk intolerance and estimates of incidence vary considerably. True protein intolerance is not common. The promotion of soya formulas for the prevention of cows' milk intolerance and their easy availability are why some mothers make their own diagnosis and begin treatment before they seek advice.

When cows' milk intolerance is diagnosed a totally cows' milk free diet is required. If the baby is breast feeding this should continue, otherwise a nutritionally complete milk substitute is necessary. Two groups of products are available — soya formulas or hydrolysed protein formulas (see Fig. 7.11).

Soya formulas which have been adapted for infant feeding are available on prescription for proven milk intolerance, for example Soya formula (Farleys), Infasoy (Cow & Gate). There are other soya 'milks' available in liquid or powder form which purely consist of diluted soya beans and

are not suitable for infant feeding, for example Plamil (Granose). As already stated a hydrolysed protein formula such as Nutramigen is usually recommended in preference to the soya formulas due to the high levels of phyte-oestrogens in soya products.

The remainder of the diet must also exclude cows' milk, so the advice of a dietitian should always be sought, as milk is widespread amongst manufactured foods, including the commercially prepared baby foods. Parents should be given advice on how to safely exclude milk from the diet and how to identify the milk-containing items to avoid, by checking ingredient labels, for example hydrolysed whey, lactose, casein, etc.

Children tend to become more tolerant of cows' milk protein as they grow older. The time to introduce a 'challenge' will vary from child to child. Often it happens in error when a child gets hold of chocolate or a drink that contains milk. The introduction should be slow over a period of about a week. Some specialists advise hospital admission for the initial challenge in case there is anaphylaxis, which though rare is very dangerous.

Children who do not take a nutritionally adequate milk substitute in amounts of approximately 500 ml daily will require calcium supplementation until the diet reverts to normal.

Nutritional support

Many medical conditions in children disturb the normal homeostasis resulting in disturbances of eating and reduced appetite. If prolonged, this is obviously going to affect growth, the younger the child the more dramatic will be the result. Involvement of a paediatric dietitian is essential if nutritional intake is to be optimised in order to maintain a normal growth rate, or in some cases catch-up growth.

Nutritional support may be required in a wide variety of children including those born prematurely or growth retarded, those with physical inability to feed (e.g. cerebral palsy), those with increased requirements and poor appetite (e.g. bronchopulmonary dysplasia), increased requirements and malabsorption (e.g. cystic fibrosis), those with poor appetite due to nausea (e.g. children with cancer) and a huge range of others (e.g. renal disease, gastrointestinal and liver disease and HIV infection.).

Table 7.11
Religion and diet

Religion	Pork	Beef	Other meat	Non-scaly fish	Eggs	Milk	Canned foods
Buddhist	No	No	No	No	No	?	
Hare Krishna	No	No	No	No	No		No
Hindu[a]	No	No			?		
Jain	No	No	No		No		
Jewish[a]	No			No			
Muslim[a]	No						
Rastafarian	No	No	No	No	No	?	No
Seventh Day Adventist	No	No	No	No			
Sikh[a]		No					
Zen (Macrobiotic)	No	No	No	No	No	No	No

[a] Dietary restrictions may be greater if foods are not prepared in acceptable way

Dietary advice on including foods of high nutrient and energy density is essential and the expertise of the dietitian in helping to incorporate any other dietary prescription is essential, for example restricted protein, phosphate and potassium in a renal child with no appetite. There is also a large range of manufactured products designed specifically to meet the dietary needs of different medical conditions. Many are designed mainly for adults and require modification by a dietitian to make them suitable for use with infants and children.

However, the manufacturers are beginning to listen to the pleas from paediatric dietitians for products designed specifically to meet the nutritional requirements of infants and young children. A recent development has been to market a feed suitable for use with infants who have increased requirements. This may be due to poor intake, as in congenital heart disease, or need for catch-up growth as in growth restricted infants. Previously their increased needs have been met by the addition of energy supplements, which may lead to weight gain, but due to an inadequate protein intake will not give good growth. The new ready-to-feed products, Infatrini (Cow & Gate) and SMA High Energy (SMA Nutrition), provide the appropriate nutritional requirements without any adaptation. They are ideal for use in tube-feeding infants where previous practice was to use infant formulas with an increased risk of contamination, particularly with overnight feeding. They are available on prescription for certain clinical conditions but there is potential for abuse if not used appropriately. They should be used in conjunction with a dietitian and not just prescribed by doctors when other dietary intervention may be more appropriate.

Products suitable for children who are tube feeding are also available in cans or bottles of sterile ready to use feeds, Nutrini and Nutrini Extra (Cow & Gate), Paediasure (Abbott) and Frebini (Fresenius). These have different nutritional profiles and should only be used under dietetic supervision.

Much more is expected of parents of children with medical problems these days. Infants and children are discharged with nasogastric tubes,

Nutrition

gastrostomy buttons and even intravenous feeding. Although, the health professional needs to ensure the family is able to cope, in reality they do much better in many ways. Infection rates at home are lower for gastrostomy buttons and intravenous lines, and the child is usually much happier and less like a 'sick child' when at home. However, we must not forget the extra pressure being placed upon the whole family and appropriate community liaison and respite care is essential. It is essential that the growth and changing nutritional requirements are not forgotten because the child is out of sight, so regular dietetic input is required.

The Advisory Committee on Borderline Substances (ACBS)

Many childhood conditions require the use of special dietary products in order for the diet to be nutritionally adequate and acceptable to the child and family. These products are often very expensive, but in some cases the diet would be impossible to follow without them, for example phenylalanine free amino acid mixtures in the treatment of phenylketonuria (PKU), lactose-free infant formulas in the treatment of alactasia, gluten-free pasta in the treatment of coeliac disease.

The Committee meets regularly to decide which food items are necessary to the dietary treatment of a particular condition. A full list of those accepted for use in prescribed diets can be found in the British National Formulary, Appendix 7 (BNF 2001). The Committee recommends products on the basis that they may be regarded as drugs for the management of specified conditions. Prescriptions issued in accordance with the Committee's advice and endorsed ACBS will normally not be investigated. However, if a prescription does not meet the criteria of the ACBS, the prescriber may be charged for the items prescribed. At about £300 a month for amino acids alone, the GP with a child with PKU on his list is usually very careful!

REFERENCES AND FURTHER READING

Barker D J P 1997 Fetal nutrition and cardiovascular disease in later life. British Medical Bulletin 53:96–108

British Dietetic Association 1999 Peanut allergy — information for dietitians. BDA, Birmingham

BNF 2001 British National Formulary 41. British Medical Association and Royal Pharmaceutical Society, London

British Nutrition Foundation 1995 Iron: nutrition and physiological significance. British Nutrition Foundation, London

Dennison B A, Rockwell H L and Baker S L 1997 Excess fruit juice consumption by pre-school children is associated with short stature and obesity. Pediatrics 99:15–22

Department for Education and Employment 1998a Ingredients for success. A consultation paper on nutritional standards for school lunches. DfEE, Sudbury

Department for Education and Employment 1998b Fair funding. A consultation paper on improving delegation to schools. DfEE, Sudbury

Department of Health and Social Security 1977 The composition of mature human milk. Report on health and social subjects no 12. HMSO, London

Department of Health and Social Security 1989 The diets of British school children. HMSO, London

Department of Health 1991 Dietary reference values for food energy and nutrients for the United Kingdom. HMSO, London

Department of Health 1992 The health of the nation. Strategy for health in England. HMSO, London

Department of Health 1994a Weaning and the weaning diet. Report on health and social subjects no 45. HMSO, London

Department of Health 1994b Nutrition aspects of cardiovascular disease. Report on health and social subjects no 46 HMSO, London

Foster K, Lader D, Cheesbrough S 1997 Infant feeding 1995. Office for National Statistics, London

Gaziano J M 1998 When should heart disease prevention begin? New England Journal of Medicine 338:1690–1692

Gregory J, Lowe S 2000 National diet and nutrition survey: young people aged 4 to 18 years. Vol 1: Report of the diet and nutrition survey. TSO, London

Gregory J R, Collins D L, Davies P S W, Hughes J M, Clarke P C 1995 National diet and nutrition survey of children aged 1–4 years. Vol 1: Report of the diet and nutrition survey. HMSO, London

Hinds K, Gregory J R 1995 National diet and nutrition survey of children aged 1–4 years. Vol 2: Report of the dental survey. HMSO, London

Holland B, Unwin I D, Buss D H 1989 Milk products and eggs. Royal Society of Chemistry, Cambridge

Hourihane J O'B, Rolles C J 1995 Morbidity from excessive intake of high energy fluids: the 'squash drinking syndrome'. Archives of Disease in Childhood 72:141–143

Lucas A, Lockton S, Davies P S W 1992 Randomised trial of a ready to feed compared with a powdered formula. Archives of Disease in Childhood 67:935–939

Mills A, Tyler H 1992 Food and nutrient intakes of British infants aged 6–12 months. HMSO, London

National Dairy Council 1996 Milk and children. NDC, London

Pollitt E 1995 Does breakfast make a difference in school? Journal of the American Dietetic Association 95:1134–1139

Royal College of Midwives 1988 Successful breast feeding. RCM, London

Ruxton C H S, Kirk T R 1997 Breakfast: a review of associations with measures of dietary intake, physiology and biochemistry. British Journal of Nutrition 78:199–213

Shaw V, Lawson M 2001 Clinical paediatric dietetics. Blackwell, Oxford

Taitz L S, Scholey E 1989 Are babies more satisfied on casein based formulas? Archives of Disease in Childhood 64:619–621

Thomas M, Avery V 1997 Infant feeding in Asian families. HMSO, London

Thompson J M 1998 Nutritional requirements of infants and young children. Blackwell, Oxford

Wardley B L, Puntis J W L, Taitz L S 1997 Handbook of child nutrition, 2nd edn. Oxford University Press, Oxford

Williams C L, Bollella M, Wynder E L 1995 A new recommendation for dietary fiber in childhood. Pediatrics 96:985–988

Useful literature for families and professionals

After milk, what's next 1999. Leaflet on weaning

Food for the growing years 1999. Advice leaflet for feeding 1–5 year olds

Food for the school years 1993. Healthy eating for schoolchildren

Following a vegetarian diet 1999. Advice for 5–16 year olds

HELP my child won't eat! Advice leaflet for food refusal in young children

All the above are produced by the Paediatric Group of the British Dietetic Association and can be purchased from:

BDA Paediatric Group
Unit 21, Goldthorpe Industrial Estate
Goldthorpe
Rotherham
S63 9BL

The Balance of Good Health. A pictorial guide to healthy eating using food groups

Feeding your Child from 1–3
Weaning your baby

All of the above are produced by the Health Education Authority and are available free of charge in limited quantities from local health promotion units or from:

HEA Customer Services
Marston Book Services
PO Box 269
Abingdon
Oxon OX14 4YN

Colin has constipation. An educational story for children

Available free of charge from:
Solvay Healthcare Ltd
Gaters Hill
West End
Southampton
SO18 3JD

Specialised Formulas Leaflet. A summary of the composition of specialised formulas designed for use in infants with cows' milk intolerance or malabsorption. Updated annually.

Available free of charge from:
Cow & Gate Nutricia Ltd
Whitehorse Business Park
Trowbridge
Wiltshire
BA14 0XQ

8 | Health promotion

Health promotion is an important component of community paediatrics. To some degree it is included in every chapter of this book, but it is particularly highlighted in Chapters 7, 20, 22, 25 and 36. Every consultation provides opportunities for health promotion and every programme for health care should have health promotion as one of its components. This chapter sets out to define health promotion, track important landmarks in its development, explore two main approaches to practice and activity in one key setting: the school. Finally, comments about the evidence base and data available will be made before moving on to look at some examples of evidence-based practice.

DEFINITIONS AND HISTORICAL PERSPECTIVE

The concept of health promotion is now an integral part of strategic planning for health. In the context of this book, it is clear that the promotion of a baby's and child's positive health is dependent on, and inseparable from, that of the mother, the family and the community in which he is conceived, nurtured and develops through childhood and adolescence to adulthood. Concepts of health promotion crystallised during the 1970s, although some of the elements of what we now term 'health promotion' were in place long before, for example, health education with which most community paediatricians will be familiar (Ewles & Simnett 1992) (Fig. 8.1).

Concepts were built around 'health' being seen as a positive attribute, involving social and personal resources, as well as physical capacities. The World Health Organization (WHO) in its Constitution (WHO 1946) stated that health is 'a state of complete physical, mental and social well-being (Ewles & Simnett 1992), and not merely the absence of disease or infirmity'. This definition has been criticised as over-idealistic and failing to include emotional, spiritual and societal well being, but it is still the most frequently used definition. Such thinking emerged over much the same time as the realisation that existing public health measures and health education were inadequate to protect people from preventable ill health and premature death: people simply do not do what they are told is in their best interests.

THE WORLD HEALTH ORGANIZATION

In 1977 WHO overtly adopted a perspective on health promotion, as published in the Alma Ata Declaration (http://www.who.int/hpr/docs/almaata.html). In 1981 the influential WHO's 'Health For All by the Year 2000' initiative was launched (WHO 1981) and by 1984, WHO had established its European Office's health promotion programme. At that time it produced its widely adopted definition of health promotion as a realm of health-enhancing activities creating a 'process of enabling people to increase control over and improve their health' (WHO 1984). Successfully established WHO programmes, such as 'Healthy Cities' and 'Health Promoting Schools', based on various conceptual models of influences on positive health, (Downie et al 1990, Kemm & Close 1995), underline the global acceptance that childhood conditions have an impact in later life, and that ill health is, at least in part, the result of non-medical factors, such as access to care, personal behaviour, the prevailing culture and environmental conditions. Complementary activities at structural and organisational levels, internationally, nationally, community wide and individually, are needed to prompt change if health outcomes are to improve. The main determinants of health and inequalities in health are illustrated in Fig. 8.2 (Chief Medical Officer's Health of the Nation Working Group 1996).

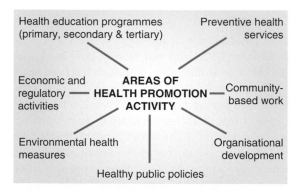

Fig. 8.1 A framework for health promotion activities. From Ewles & Simnett (1992)

While our understanding of the complexity of conditions conducive to child and family health has evolved, there are prerequisites before health promotion activities can flourish: freedom from the fear of war, equal opportunities for all, the treating of basic physical and psychological needs and political will supported by the public (WHO 1979). It is not difficult to see that the notion of promoting health is still subsumed by meeting much more basic survival needs among many millions of children, for example in war-torn and developing countries. However, it would be wrong to be overpessimistic. The successes of preventive programmes, such as the smallpox eradication programme, polio protection, clean water initiatives, together with simple and practical rehydration education, should be acknowledged. In less troubled parts of the world, widening gaps in inequalities in health, family break-up and relative poverty, increasing levels of smoking and alcohol consumption among school-age pupils, illegal drug use and the failure to prevent the spread of AIDS will continue to result in unnecessary death and

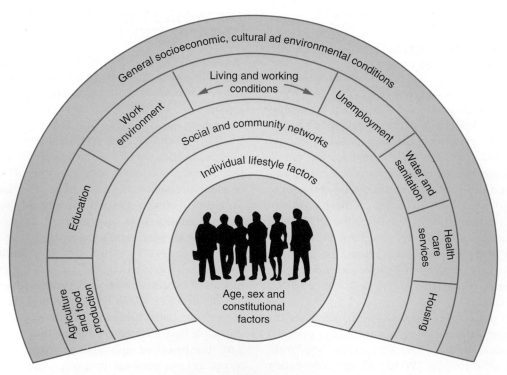

Fig. 8.2 The main determinants of health. (Dahlgren and Whitehead 1991).

suffering for many children. Yet here too there is cause for optimism, at least in the UK, based on three factors: recent Government policies, the adoption of theory-driven practice and a growing evidence base.

RECENT UK GOVERNMENT POLICIES

Policies of successive UK Governments have moved health promotion from a marginal to a central health strategy with, in the late 1990s, the appointment of the first Minister for Public Health. Policy shifts have put less stress on biomedical models of health and much more on those derived from socio-economic evidence of inequalities in health (Acheson 1998). Health-related policies for a wide range of ages have been rapidly introduced by a number of government departments, for example: 'Making a Difference', strengthening midwifery and health visiting; 'School Travel', promoting safe, healthy and sustainable travel to school; 'Me, Survive, Out There?' for children living in care.

Even more recently 'Saving Lives' (Secretary of State for Health 1999), a follow-up to the 'Health of the Nation' initiative, takes a radically different approach to its predecessor. It urges far-reaching changes, based on 'joined up thinking', to be achieved though interagency partnership and collaboration between health services and other providers. These policies will have a profound influence on the status of health promotion, and practice. High priority has been given to policies designed to improve health among women of childbearing age, expectant mothers and young children, including: reducing poverty, improving nutrition, increasing the prevalence of breast feeding, reducing smoking prevalence during pregnancy and increasing social and emotional support, improving the availability of social housing, traffic controls, high-quality pre-school education and increasing the network of health promoting schools. The Government has set 'tougher but attainable long-term targets in priority areas': cancer, coronary heart disease and stroke, accidents and serious injury, and mental illness. Progress will be assessed through interim milestones in the four priority areas by 2005, the setting of local targets for improving health, performance management and an assessment framework. At a local level, proactive community paediatricians will have the opportunity to be part of the process whereby local targets are set. Full details of policies cited above may be found on the Department of Health website: http://*www.official-documents.co.uk/cgi-bin/empower*

THEORY-DRIVEN PRACTICE

The second cause for optimism is that, as the specialisation of health promotion has developed, so underpinning theories of practice have evolved, informed by psychosocial theories of health-related behaviour change and thinking around community participation linked to community development.

Models of behaviour change

Theoretical models have become particularly influential in health promotion practice (Perkins et al 1999). Early ideas tended to emphasise psychologically orientated models that focus on the individual (Becker 1974). More recently, models have introduced socio-psychological elements that allow for the individual's social context (Ajzen & Fishbein 1980, Tones et al 1989). Others have emphasised the need to enhance the individual's self-efficacy, viewed as the major determinant of behaviour change in social and cognitive learning theory (Bandura 1986). It has also been argued that changes in social structures and cultural processes that prompt intentional or unintentional change have been neglected by those who also suggest that health promotion practitioners need to develop strategies, closely allied to research, that recognise the cultural context and use people's own beliefs and practices to inform and implement projects (Bunton & Macdonald 1992). The model shown in Fig. 8.3 summarises key stages in a more recent theory of change, linked to change processes.

Existing conceptual theories do not wholly explain or predict actual behaviour change, reflecting the difficulties of testing such theories. Put simply, in practice, how do you examine children's psychological processes and obtain data over time

Health promotion

	Stages of change				
	Pre-contemplation	Contemplation	Preparation	Action	Maintenance
Processes	Consciousness raising Dramatic relief Environmental re-evaluation Self-re-evaluation		Self-liberation	Contingency management Helping relationship Counter-conditioning Stimulus control	

Fig. 8.3 Stages of change in which change processes are most emphasised. From Systems of psychotherapy: a transtheoretical analysis, by JO Prochaska & JC Norcross. Copyright © 1994, 1984, 1979 Brooks/Cole Publishing Company, Pacific Grove, CA 93950, a division of International Thompson Publishing Inc.

from families and in school or social settings where relationships are dynamic and children are inevitably exposed to uncontrolled factors present in the real world?

Principles locked into theories of behaviour change are complex (Tones et al 1989), but generally suggest that persuasive information is the prime method of changing attitudes. In turn, attitudes determine behaviour. The presentation of the message and the characteristics of the audience determine the appropriateness of the information for prompting change. In particular, existing knowledge and social values influence the acceptability of information to the individual. Most theories integrate 'cues', or stimuli, that disrupt or challenge the existing belief system (Mullen et al 1987). Change may or may not take place as a result of any one particular 'cue' when, for example, emotional issues block action or fear is aroused. Sometimes the individual will not have the financial resources or skills to implement change, for example, to the family's diet. However, the more the exposure to acceptable cues, the more likely change is to take place (Tones et al 1989). Community paediatricians can consider capitalising on pre-existing cues, and introducing their own opportunistically and systematically in their practice. They may also consider how naturally forming social networks and other institutions, such as nurseries, can be harnessed to provide cues. They are of the following types.

Internal cues

Internal cues, such as illness, can occur when carers respond to what the child is experiencing by seeking your advice. For example, a parent with a child with diabetes will want to understand the nature of the condition, the management techniques and to develop new skills. Sustained support will be needed in such a case to ensure that changes are adopted as routine practice: 'one-off' changes are more easily prompted, for example, a mother upset by seeing another child with whooping cough may have her own child immunised.

External but personalised cues

An example of these cues is, verbal information from health professionals. Evidence suggests that doctors are seen as reliable sources of information (Worsley 1989). However patients are — understandably — often anxious in consultations, and may forget 50% of what they are told. Parents and children start with very different levels of knowledge of general English and medical terms. Parents and children often take on the 'sick role' and are not able to be assertive in a medical consultation. Many will leave with an incomplete understanding of what has been said, rather than ask further questions or admit to their failure to understand the 'explanations' given. It is good practice to develop the habit of defining terms and checking that the information we have given has been understood by obtaining feedback from the patient, and to repeat information in a different way if necessary. Writing down important points legibly, possibly in a formal record kept by the parent, and reading them back is also constructive. Information needs to be discussed openly and translated into small practical steps which can be measured and supported. For example, advice such as 'take more exercise' or 'you must lose weight' could be modified as 'try walking to school rather than take the bus' or 'see if you can stick to one sweet a day'. These behaviours can be recorded by the child and the children seen, supported and possibly rewarded over a period of time. In these processes listening is as important as talking. Face to face work with groups with similar needs is not only an efficient use of resources, but also provides much needed peer group support.

When a carer or child's lack of skill in speaking English inhibits communication, you will need to use a skilled translator. A video recording of one of our own consultations can be an educational and sometimes a disturbing experience!

External and impersonalised cues

Example of these cues are leaflets, posters and the media.

Leaflets and posters

While the written word can be very useful in supplementing the information given in a consultation, a well-stocked wall of pamphlets should complement, not substitute for, face to face discussion: leaflets and other impersonal media have been shown to be relatively ineffective in themselves (Whitehead 1989). However, leaflets and posters may be used effectively to set the health agenda, and to reinforce messages from other sources. They should give consistent messages over time, for example over smoking in pregnancy or breast feeding being one element within a planned, professionally directed programme. You therefore need to find the time to read them, and agree with what they say, before allowing them to be used. A cynical observer might feel that posters form part of the permanent interior decoration, to cover the cracks in the walls, or may look to see how many leaflets are used as entertainment for young children.

Readability is an important consideration. Although they often have the intellectual capacity to do so, an estimated 10–15% of adults and teenagers are not skilled readers and have difficulty with texts above the level of a tabloid newspaper (around the level of an average 11–12 year old). Materials demanding advanced reading skills will therefore be of very limited benefit, but there are standarised ways, such as the Flesch and Smong indices, by which you can check how easy or difficult a text is to read (Flesch 1951, Nicoll 1985). There may also be a need for literature in minority languages. Before developing your own, ask colleagues practising in other areas where those languages may be more common if they can help. You will need to check that the recipient can read in their mother tongue.

The mass media

Most teenagers and parents obtain health-related information from mass media outlets, including printed materials, radio and television (Nicoll 1985). There is no doubt that soap operas that deal with, for example, teenage emotions and behaviour, are widely watched by youngsters. Messages may be mixed. Newspapers and magazines have an unprecedented interest in reporting and advising, ranging from the highly personalised, sensationalist and irresponsible to balanced and informed discussion. Adults may not approve of their approach, but the teenage magazine market, particularly among girls, is 'street-wise' about style, language and presentation, which health education materials sometimes try to emulate — and are very lucrative. A quick look at any magazine stand will show that the commercial market capitalises on the selling-power of articles and stories about sex, although many young people still come to clinics not knowing basic facts about their bodies, how contraception works or the possible results of risk-related behaviour.

Significant others

Significant others include family members or peer groups where information, cultural norms and strong role models are all influential (Marcoux et al 1990, Michell & West 1996). For example, the behaviour of men and women when they become fathers and mothers is known to be influenced by the parenting they themselves experienced as children,

Health promotion

and have observed within their families. Perhaps the most extreme, and disturbing, example of this is the pattern of generational child abuse, whether sexual, psychological or physical. Another example may be seen in the new mother, who may be given a great deal of support from her own mother, some of it unhelpful, for example, out of date information, passing on habits such as not putting babies on their backs to sleep, weaning too early or bottle feeding. Resisting this advice in favour of that given by health professionals may be difficult! Risk-related behaviour such as smoking, poor diet and lack of exercise are known to be related to family patterns, while peer influence is associated with decisions about risk-taking behaviour, such as smoking and illegal drug taking as children move into adolescence. Altering risk-related behaviour inculcated from birth or learned within the prevailing culture is exceptionally difficult: working with families is often not only intensive but also long term, yet working with individuals in isolation will not necessarily uncover or address directly some of the important contextual influences.

Barriers to effectiveness

In general, it seems that those most needing support to reduce health-related risks are least likely to act on the impersonal messages of mass media health education; for example, parents who go on smoking in the full knowledge of the harm it may do their children; those in the lower social classes and school pupils who are frequently absent (Charlton & Blair 1989). It also seems that children wanting advice have poor knowledge of where to obtain it, or are reluctant to do so by, for example, going to the family doctor for advice about contraception.

Community paediatricians may have to accept that in some 16% of cases change will never be adopted, whatever the incentive (Rogers & Shoemaker 1983). While it may be relatively easy to influence some people, there is a point when the same — or alternative — programmes are unlikely to produce the desired outcome in others. This may result in more realistic expectations of health promotion targeting of programmes.

COMMUNITY PARTICIPATION AND COMMUNITY DEVELOPMENT

The term 'community participation' has been used to describe many kinds of activities and processes (Kroutil & Eng 1989). It is beyond the scope of this chapter to examine in any detail the complexities and conflicting views that are associated with it. Briefly, it was originally applied only to the organisation and delivery of health care in the developing world, but it is now being used to describe community-based activities generally. WHO has embraced the concept of 'Community Action for Health' as part of the original 'Healthy Cities Initiative' (Fig. 8.4).

Community participation in health may be defined as a process by which various groups within the community engage in the provision and delivery of health care, both formally and informally and with varying degrees of power. Population groups, such as parents, and individuals within those groups, such as mothers with handicapped children, are enabled to some greater degree to understand, influence, share or control decisions effecting the provision and delivery of health care.

Here, the term 'community participation' encompasses notions of 'pure' community development: the latter term is sometimes used to mean only the former. In community participation activities that seek to 'develop the community', professionals are seen as having a supportive but non-directive role. They act as resources as the community itself identifies issues of concern, decides on actions to remedy problems and takes control of decision making and resources, developing its capacity to do so during the process.

There is now a growing conviction amongst some health workers in the UK that a 'quiet revolution' is taking place whereby participation by groups in disadvantaged communities can, and should, be stimulated for ethical reasons of equity (Watt & Rodmell 1988). This is a reversal of the traditional 'medical model' where community needs have been determined by professionals. However, it has been argued that the language of community participation has been adopted without health professionals taking on board the ultimate outcome

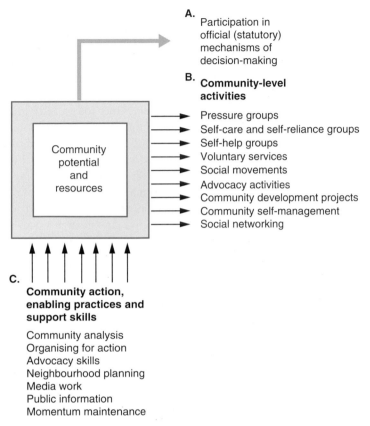

A. Participation in official (statutory) mechanisms of decision-making

B. Community-level activities

Pressure groups
Self-care and self-reliance groups
Self-help groups
Voluntary services
Social movements
Advocacy activities
Community development projects
Community self-management
Social networking

Community potential and resources

C. Community action, enabling practices and support skills

Community analysis
Organising for action
Advocacy skills
Neighbourhood planning
Media work
Public information
Momentum maintenance

Fig. 8.4 Community action for health at city level. From Tsouros (1987–90)

of the community controlling the definition of its own health needs, and their solutions (Farrant 1991).

Within communities there are groups that share a common bond by meeting needs, such as social, educational, economic or health needs. They focus on, but are not confined by, geographical boundaries. Social networks link groups and act as a structural basis for social support and information. For example, a mother may know local people because she was brought up locally, has been to school there, works in a local shop and belongs to a mother and toddler group. Such networks have the potential to be used to spread information, especially when local 'opinion leaders' are engaged in the process. The extent of these types of social networks is closely related to familial and community ties and their strength has a positive or negative impact on lifestyle, health practices and health. It is not diffi-

cult for community paediatricians to see the impact of weak ties among isolated single mothers or children frequently moved from school to school.

Models of community development use differing terminology but tend to explore notions of progression or intensity of participation, as shown in the early model of a 'Ladder of Citizen Participation' (Arnstein 1969) (Fig. 8.5).

Participation ranges from marginal to substantive, structural participation (Arnstein 1969, Broadly & Hedley 1989). Low participation — starting with non-involvement — progresses to high participation through the community: receiving information, being consulted, advising joint planning, obtaining delegated authority and having control over the setting and achievement of goals. Participation may develop spontaneously within a community, be induced — this is the most common type found in community-based work

8 Citizen control	Degrees of citizen power: negotiation, decision making and managerial power
7 Delegated power	
6 Partnership	
5 Placation	Degrees of tokenism: enable people to hear and be heard, but have no power to ensure views are acted upon
4 Consultation	
3 Informing	
2 Therapy	Non-participation: these levels enable power-holders to 'educate' or 'cure' participants
1 Manipulation	

Fig. 8.5 The ladder of citizen participation. From Arnstein (1969)

with families and is discussed below — and, finally, imposed or compulsory participation.

Induced participation

This has been described as 'facipulation': a mix of facilitation and manipulation which occurs when professionals have an existing or hidden agenda (Tones et al 1989). It may be seen in various activities such as professionally prompted and supported groups, sometimes associated with specific, immediate and shared problems, such as loneliness, handicapped children or carers of children with debilitating diseases or conditions (Orr 1987, Unell 1996). Induced participation may fluctuate between either very low or very high degrees of involvement and is usually at the point of delivery. For example, professionals have:

- Built on existing social structures, strengthening naturally occurring helping networks to increase social ties and mobilise support, for example, through summer school health initiatives.
- Worked with existing groups to enable the group to take some limited and specific control over some aspects of its health, for example in self-help groups.
- Set up new groups by drawing together those with similar needs, such as those for women with postnatal depression.

This is all a great deal more difficult in practice than it sounds on paper: the underlying assumption is that people within the community, including within schools, form homogeneous groups: the 'haves' and 'have nots' (Kroutil & Eng 1989). In reality groups within the community are fragmented and difficult to 'find'. Once found, individuals may be unwilling to co-operate. It is a very real problem for those wishing to work with 'hard to reach' groups. Those whose views are not overtly sought, those who do not respond to individual approaches or who are marginal to, or do not join, groups may be the people whose views and participation in programmes are most needed, for example, bullied children, school truants, drug takers and abusing parents.

Despite the difficulties, health workers have played a key role in participatory initiatives. Projects are usually small and fragile, being seen as experimental, usually underfunded and overambitious and marginal to core health activity (Farrant 1991). It has been argued that the health of women and children may best be promoted through co-operative ventures that unite and integrate the home, community agents and services, and the school (Schiller et al 1987, Allensworth & Wolford 1988). 'Facipulation' based on collaborative efforts by healthcare teams, including health visitors, community paediatricians, school nurses and local doctors with school staff, social services, other local authority departments, voluntary groups and so on will be required for this to be achieved.

Barriers to community participation

Some of these have been intimated above. In addition there is a tendency for people to be interested in health only when they — or someone close to them — is ill, and then only when they relate to specific problems. Many other concerns occupy parents, such as work and financial constraints. Secondly, it is recognised that inducing participation is slow, yet many community projects have short-term funding — pump-primed projects supposed to act as models of good practice, but in practice having little chance of doing so, come and go. Finally, participatory activities are fraught with opportunities for challenge and conflict as power is sought or devolved (Rodmell & Watt 1986). Overcoming these barriers demands sustained commitment, patience and resources from those who plan health strategies.

This chapter now moves on to consider a specific setting that provides opportunities for health promotion for young people.

SCHOOLS AND HEALTH PROMOTION

School health programmes have been transformed since the 1970s, despite being relatively poorly funded, not having high status within many schools and operating in the face of the other demands of the National Curriculum. Even so, they are in the front line in combating the complex influences on change, outlined above, and — not least — the powerful commercial interest in accessing the youth market and establishing brand loyalty. The rising levels of risk factors, such as smoking among teenage girls, underage intercourse and unwanted pregnancies, simplistically suggest that schools have simply got it all wrong. More plausible, and based on theories of behaviour change, is the argument that schools are just one agent for change in what needs to be a multifaceted and unified approach: they cannot be blamed for not solving all the problems single handed.

Health concerns such as smoking, HIV/AIDS and personal safety require individual attention, but none should be dealt with in isolation. Comprehensive programmes, employing the model of a spiral curriculum approach, explore health topics and themes as they are needed, then return to them and develop learning at different stages as the child grows and matures. Teaching and learning packs have been written for pupils in mainstream schools, but variations have also been developed for pupils with mild and moderate learning difficulties, together with support for teachers (Coombes & Craft 1989). Common to all schools is the health National Curriculum based on a comprehensive vision whereby the subject is a cross-curricular theme. Nine components form a framework: substance use and misuse; sex education; family life education; safety; health-related exercise; nutrition; personal hygiene; environmental aspects of health education; psychological aspects of health education.

The health education programme should not rest on information-giving alone. It is encouraging that staff use experiential learning, such as demonstrating restricted lung function in smokers, oral history from local people suffering from preventable illnesses, and develop skills in pupils to go alongside knowledge through, for example, role play enabling them to resist unwelcome influences.

Schools cannot support children who are not in school, and of concern to health promotion are school truants. Truancy is a high-risk occupation being associated with crime, sexual abuse, smoking, alcohol and illegal drug taking, demoralisation and pregnancy. The National Child Development Study found that 20% of children aged 16 were truants at some time and that, by the age of 23, had fewer qualifications, less stable careers and lower status occupations which have little future (Hibbert & Fogelman 1990). Some local authorities provide alternative centres for those who drop out of the school system in an attempt to reach them, such as the Nottingham Health Authority's 'Base 51' project.

The role of the school medical service

There are a number of ways in which members of the school medical service can make a contribution to school and individual health promotion.

Teacher support

Very few teachers get specific training in health education, although they may have had opportunities to attend in-service training events. Teachers may ask for advice about individual pupils and their families. They may also need to update and refresh their own knowledge about health topics. The school nurse or doctor, easily approachable on the teacher's territory of classroom or school, is

Health promotion

likely to be the first and most important point of contact. If necessary, links can be made between the teacher and other health professionals.

In the classroom

Many school nurses and doctors take an important part in classroom teaching, usually in tandem with the class teacher. Sometimes this is confined to specific topics in sex education, for example menstruation, contraception, sexually transmitted infections, HIV/AIDS. However some schools have felt that this 'medicalises' the topics concerned in an unhelpful way and have preferred either to use members of the school medical service as supporters and providers of information outside the classroom (see section above), or to co-teach the whole of the health or sex education programme with the school nurse. Much depends on personal preferences and the amount of time available for such a regular commitment.

Individual counselling

This is carried out either at a school medical, or as the need arises, the school nurse or doctor can play an important part in counselling on individual or family health-related problems. Often the school nurse will be well known and well trusted by the pupils. They may seek her advice on a whole range of topics, from the relatively trivial (although not to the pupil concerned) to the very serious, such as a disclosure of sexual abuse.

Links to the community

As staff of the health authority, members of the school medical service will have ready access to people and resources which may not be so easily available to the teacher. For instance, health authority colleagues will include staff in family planning clinics, the HIV/AIDS information officer and health promotion officers. The health promotion unit will have free posters and leaflets and a collection of teaching resources for loan to schools and school medical service staff. Outside speakers and resources can enliven the school health education programme and suggestions are likely to be welcomed. Training for school medical service staff on helping with health education programmes in schools may be available locally.

EVIDENCE-BASED PRACTICE

The debate about whether health promotion 'works' has been lively, with accusations of a failure to show impact one of the major criticisms of health promotion programmes. Views about how to generate evidence of effectiveness have polarised at one end around demand for rigorous techniques using, for example, classic case-control study designs and, at the other, around unsubstantiated rhetoric based on the claim that individuals and communities, unlike laboratory specimens, are open to influences from many uncontrollable sources. It may be that, generally, the measures that are taken are those that are relatively easy and acceptable, such as routine immunisation uptake rather than the factors that prevent carers from taking part in such proven programmes.

The adoption of social scientific research methods and the use of complementary quantitative and qualitative data has become increasingly accepted in health research, giving researchers a more varied choice of practical approaches (Pope & Mays 1995). Even so, it is clear that there is an on-going need for interdisciplinary cooperation both within medicine and between disciplines to enable practitioners and researchers to 'understand, learn to respect and work with each others' models' (Stacey 1988). The evaluation of community participation projects seems to have been particularly difficult: little is yet understood about its dynamics and impact. As in other fields, it is likely that little will reach the printed page about what does not work!

Data measuring the impact of methodologies used in community participation is scant (Schiller et al 1987). It may be that many community workers are more concerned with achieving success than measuring it (Tones et al 1989). Where evidence of success is available it tends to be descriptive, come only from those whom the scheme has continued to engage, and not those untouched — or indeed alienated — by initiatives. Evidence that participants are genuinely receiving a new, rather than alternative, service is also apparently unavailable, as is good research data about changes in self-esteem or behaviour using methods that do not introduce recall bias.

In terms of monitoring behaviour internationally,

the WHO publishes data by which to measure changes in basic health status, such as neonatal and infant morbidity and morality. The WHO's comprehensive website home page is: *http://www.who.int/home/info.html*. In the UK there are now comparative data available through Government-funded national school-based surveys (see the Department of Health website: *http://www.doh.gov.uk/stats/hypmain.htm*), while the Health Behaviour Survey run by the Exeter School Health project generates evidence on a rolling programme (see website: *http://omni.ac.uk/umls/detail/C0001578.html*). Both rely on the cooperation of children within the school setting, a practice that has been questioned for ethical reasons (Denscombe & Aubrook 1992). The Adolescent Health Trust produces annual data drawing together data from a wide range of sources (Coleman 1999). More locally, 'one-off' studies reflect local concerns and priorities. While these are not always published, they should be accessible, often through local health departments.

Again in the UK, the Health Education Authority is the central agency which is responsible for an overview of the nation's health education programmes and produces many of the materials that are used. It is a useful source of information about tested and current initiatives. An overview of its activities can be seen on its website: http://*www.hea.org.uk/index.html*. Other national voluntary organisations such as the Child Accident Prevention Trust (email: *safe@capt.demon.co.uk*.) have an important influence in their area of interest. In each health authority there will be a health promotion advisor linked to providing units able to advise on materials for schools, playgroups and other organisations. In addition, the local authority will provide services to support accident prevention, in particular road safety.

REFERENCES

Ajzen I, Fishbein M 1980 Understanding attitudes and predicting social behaviour. Prentice Hall, New Jersey
Allensworth DD, Wolford CA 1988 Schools as agents for achieving the 1990 health for all objectives for the nation. Health Education Quarterly 15:3–17
Arnstein SR 1969 A ladder of citizen participation. American Institute of Planners Journal July:216–224
Bandura A 1986 Social foundations of thought and action: a social cognitive theory. Prentice Hall, New Jersey
Becker MH 1974 The health belief model and personal health. Health Education Monograph 2:326–473
Broadly M, Hedley R 1989 Working partnerships: community development and local authorities. National Council for Voluntary Organisations, London
Bunton R, Macdonald G 1992 Health promotion: disciplines and diversity. Routledge, London
Charlton A, Blair V 1989 Absence from school related to children's and parental smoking. British Medical Journal 298:90–92
Chief Medical Officer's Health of the Nation Working Group 1996 Variations in health. What can the Department of Health do? Department of Health, London
Coleman J 1999 Key data on adolescence. Trust for the Study of Adolescence, Brighton
Coombes G, Craft A 1989 Special health: a professional development programme in health education for teachers and pupils with mild or moderate learning difficulties. Health Education Authority, London
Dahlgren G, Whitehead M. 1991 Policies and strategies to promote social equity in health. Institute for Future Studies, Stockholm
Denscombe M, Aubrook L 1992 'It's just another piece of schoolwork': the ethics of questionnaire research on pupils in schools. British Educational Research Journal 18:113–131
Downie RS, Fyfe C, Tannahill A 1990 Health promotion: models and values. Oxford Medical Publications, Oxford
Ewles L, Simnett I 1992 Promoting health: a practical guide to health education, Scutari Press, London
Farrant W 1991 Addressing the contradictions: health promotion and community health action in the United Kingdom. International Journal of Health Services 21:423–439
Flesch RF 1951 How to test readability. Harper & Bros, New York
Hibbert A, Fogelman K 1990 Future lives of truants, family formation and health-related behaviours. British Journal of Educational Psychology 60:171–179
Kemm J, Close A 1995 Health promotion: theory and practice. Macmillan Press, Basingstoke
Kroutil LA, Eng E 1989 Conceptualising and assessing potential for community participation: a planning method. Health Education Research 4:305–319
Marcoux BA, Trenkner LL, Rosenstack M 1990 Social networks and social support in weight loss. Pateint Education and Counselling 15:229–239
Michell L, West P 1996 Peer pressure to smoke: the meaning depends on the method. Health Education Research 11:39–49
Mullen PD, Hersey JC, Iverson DC 1987 Health behaviour models compared. Social Science and Medicine 24:973–981
Nicoll A 1985 Written material concerning health for parents and children. In: Macfarlane A (ed) Progress in child health. Livingston, London, pp 89–102
Orr J 1987 Women's health in the community. Wiley, Chichester

Health promotion

Perkins ER, Simnett I, Wright L 1999 Evidence-based health promotion. Wiley, Chichester

Pope C, Mays N 1995 Reaching the parts other methods cannot reach: an introduction to qualitative methods in health and health services research. British Medical Journal 311:42–45

Rodmell S, Watt A 1986 Conventional health education: problems and possibilities. In: Rodmell S, Watt A (eds) The politics of health education: raising the issues. Routledge and Keegan Paul, London, pp 1–16

Rogers EM, Shoemaker FF 1983 The diffusion of innovations. Free Press, New York

Schiller P, Steckler A, Patton F 1987 Participatory planning in community health education: a guide based on the McDowell County, West Virgina Experience. Third Party Publishing Company, Oakland

Secretary of State for Health 1999 Saving lives: our healthier nation. The Stationery Office, London

Stacey M 1988 Epilogue. Health behaviour and health promotion research. In: Anderson R, Davids JK, Kickbusch I, McQueen DV, Turner J (eds) Oxford University Press, Oxford, pp 271–279

Tones BK, Tilford S, Robinson YK 1989 Health education: effectiveness and efficiency. Chapman Hall, London

Tsouros AD 1987–90 WHO Healthy Cities Project: a project becomes a movement. Review of progress. SOGESS, Milan

Unell J 1996 Help for self help: a study of a local support service. National Council for Voluntary Organisations, London

Watt A, Rodmell S 1988 Community involvement in health promotion: progress or panacea? Health Promotion 2:359–368

Whitehead M 1989 Swimming upstream: trends and prospects for education for health, Kings Fund Institute Research, London, p 42

WHO 1946 Constitution of the World Health Organization. WHO, New York

WHO 1979 Formulating strategies for health for all by the year 2000. Health for all Series 2. Geneva, WHO

WHO 1981 Global strategy for health for all by the year 2000. Geneva, WHO

WHO 1984 Health promotion: a discussion document on the concept principles. Geneva, WHO Regional Office for Europe

Worsley A 1989 Perceived reliability for sources of health information. Health Education Research 4:367–376

9 | Growth

Growth represents the summation of all the processes that convert fetus through childhood to a sexually mature adult. The study of growth is therefore at the heart of paediatrics and serial measurement must be a priority in child health programmes. Primary care staff need instruction in careful measurement of the main growth parameters, length or height, weight and head circumference, and there should be procedures for checking reliability of measurements. An individual child's readings should be part of his health record, and need to be assessed in comparison with valid population standards so that significant variation from the normal range or deviation from acceptable growth rates may be recognised. Poor growth may be the first sign of an environmental or health restraint. Organic disorders of sufficient severity to alter growth are usually conspicuous, for example asthma or cardiac disease, but others such as autoimmune hypothyroidism, coeliac disease and chronic inflammatory bowel disease are sometimes more insidious. Serial growth review is also valuable for the recognition of growth hormone deficiency and Turner's syndrome. Growth measurement is an essential tool in monitoring the progress of children with already identified chronic disorders. At a population level, growth monitoring can be used as an index of the general health and nutrition of that population, and may be useful in comparing the impact of social and economic policies. Last but by no means least, parents are interested in how their children are growing.

NORMAL PATTERNS OF GROWTH

The height–growth curve can be broken down into three components — infancy, childhood and puberty — and this serves to highlight the main control of each phase. Infancy is a continuation of rapid fetal growth and is primarily dependent on nutrition, while childhood reflects the increasing contribution from growth hormone and other endocrine pathways. Puberty is a time of superimposed growth acceleration due to the combined effects of growth hormone and sex steroids; as a general rule the sex hormones modify the tempo of adolescent growth but have minor impact on final stature.

After birth, the rate of growth decelerates quickly and during the first 18 months many healthy babies change their centile position for both length and weight (see 'Influences on growth', 'Genetic' below). Through childhood the velocity of growth decelerates further before the onset of the adolescent growth spurt. As a rule pubertal acceleration is an early component of female puberty but is delayed until the second half of male puberty (testicular volume >8 ml).

Growth charts

The UK cross-sectional reference data charts (1996) provide contemporary standards by which to assess growth from 30 weeks' gestation to age 20 years. The data has been transformed to a nine-centile format to facilitate more discriminatory criteria for community use. The 0.4th centile is obviously more specific than the previous 3rd centile for the detection of disordered growth but the challenge of growth surveillance is to develop guidelines for the recognition of growth failure in children who still exceed the lower centile limits.

The distribution of height and weight centiles reminds us that, whereas height is normally dis-

Growth

tributed, weight in industrialised countries is biased towards obesity (Fig. 9.1). Each intercentile height band is equivalent to 0.67 SD so that the 2nd and 0.4th centiles match −2.0 and −2.67 SD respectively.

The current standards derived from cross-sectional data do not attempt to illustrate the considerable variation in peak height velocity during puberty. The criticism has been made that the charts are less useful in the management of individual children in late childhood (prepubertal deceleration) and adolescence (girls typically showing early pubertal acceleration and boys mid and late pubertal acceleration). Most growth specialists continue to use cross-sectional charts despite this problem; however charts incorporating longitudinal data and attempting to encompass peak growth rates are available.

INFLUENCES ON GROWTH
Genetic

Family information about stature, body weight and timing of puberty are all relevant to the assessment of a child's growth. In deriving mid-parental height attention should be paid to the possibility that a parent with exceptional short or tall stature may have an inherited disorder, for example skeletal dysplasia and Noonan's syndrome causing short stature, or Marfan's syndrome responsible for tall stature. It is also possible that both generations are victims of deprivation. The impact of maternal growth on the size and health profile of her offspring has been given renewed emphasis by epidemiological research highlighting the intergeneration effect of fetal programming.

The current growth standards take account of secular trend with the 50th centile having increased by 0.8–1.7 cm compared to the original Tanner charts. Northern European data suggest that the secular increase in height is reaching a plateau but unfortunately this is not true for weight gain. Children of Asian origin are showing a greater secular change, and this is one of the reasons why the standards currently exclude non-white populations. As a general rule, the shape of the height–growth curves is consistent between racial groups and the UK standards can be applied after taking account of parental heights.

Nutritional

The effects of malnutrition on growth are well known. 'Catch-up' growth is more likely to occur after acute starvation than after chronic malnutrition. A baby born with intrauterine growth retardation occurring in the later stages of pregnancy usually grows more rapidly than normal after birth and 'catches up' by the second year of life. However a baby who has suffered chronic malnutrition in utero (usually symmetrically small in weight, length and head circumference) tends to remain small. Small for gestational age (SGA) infants are a heterogeneous group but approximately 15% fail to show catch-up growth by 18 months and are destined to remain small. Intrauterine malnutrition also programmes endocrine pathways, notably insulin release and growth factor production, and this may explain the greater risk of type 2 diabetes and adverse lipid profiles in later life when dietary excess becomes a greater challenge.

For the clinic doctor it is useful to appreciate that the symmetrically small child is less likely to be amenable to nutritional correction than the child who has discrepant loss of weight alone. It is a striking feature of some SGA infants who go on to deviate further through infancy that they have very difficult feeding behaviour. Russell–Silver and Noonan's syndrome infants often fall into this category.

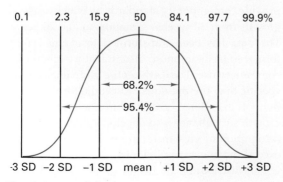

Fig. 9.1 Normal distribution

In industrialised societies over-nutrition is a considerable public health challenge. Standards are available for childhood Body Mass Index (BMI = weight (kg) (BMI = weight (kg)/height (m)^2) height (m)^2) with values over the 91st centile defined as overweight and over the 98th centile as obese. Children with a short or stocky build and well-developed musculature may have a misleadingly high BMI. The infancy component of the chart is not a predictor of future obesity, however early childhood increase in BMI is more suggestive. Relative over-nutrition promotes growth in stature and advance in skeletal maturation with earlier sexual maturation.

Emotional

Unhappy stressed children tend to grow less well. This may result from decreased appetite or disorganised meal patterns as well as from disordered neurohormonal control of growth. It is sometimes difficult to separate emotional factors from socio-economic ones, and there is often a relationship with nutritional and feeding difficulties. Removal from the stressful relationship or environment may have a dramatic beneficial effect on growth. In later childhood, disordered eating behaviour or exceptional commitment to physical exercise may result in delayed puberty and growth.

Endocrine

Growth is regulated by a complex interplay of endocrine pathways (Fig. 9.2). While we have a reasonable understanding of the classical hormonal pathways, we are only at the threshold of comprehending and investigating hormonal signalling at cellular levels.

Growth hormone

Growth hormone (GH) is secreted by the anterior pituitary gland, its release being mediated by the hypothalamus, which integrates release of growth hormone releasing hormone (GHRH) and inhibitory somatostatin. Normal GH release is pulsatile with the main peaks occurring 1–1.5 hours after the onset of sleep. An appropriately suppressed baseline component is also necessary for normal growth. Disordered growth may arise when the amplitude of pulses are reduced, or when the distinction between basal and pulse levels is lost. The usual investigative approach is to measure peak GH levels after a provocation test, for example intravenous glucagon or oral clonidine. Unfortunately provocation tests have high false positive rates, and this is especially true for tests conducted in late childhood or early puberty. An alternative approach is to measure growth factors that are

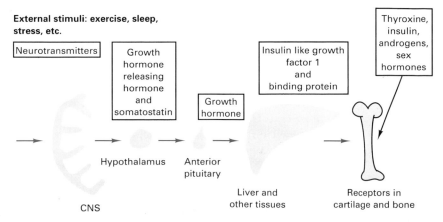

Fig. 9.2 Endocrine factors influencing growth

downstream of GH, insulin-like growth factor-1 (IGF-1) and IGF binding protein-3 (IGFBP-3). While potentially useful, there is also a substantial effect of nutritional status on IGF-1 and IGFBP-3.

It is relatively easy to recognise classical severe GH deficiency in children with early growth failure, immature facies, relative obesity and marked bone age delay. Investigation of the growth axis is unequivocally abnormal and there is a clear indication for GH therapy. However such children are relatively rare and are becoming more infrequent, possibly as a consequence of improved obstetric practice with less recourse to instrumental delivery. It is also relatively easy to justify GH investigation and treatment when there are recognised anatomical or physiological disorders of the hypothalamic–pituitary axis. Panhypopituitarism is almost universal after craniopharyngioma surgery, and there is a growing population at risk of GH insufficiency after cranial irradiation administered in the management of leukaemia and brain tumours. The challenge in contemporary practice is to determine what degree of partial GH deficiency in otherwise normal children merits intervention with GH therapy, and this opens up the debate as to whether society should detect and treat children who are healthy apart from having short stature.

Thyroid hormone (thyroxine)

This hormone acts synergistically with GH and has a critical role in brain development. Children with congenital hypothyroidism (incidence about 1 in 3000 births) are at risk of severe learning problems unless detected and treated promptly. Neonatal thyroid stimulating hormone (TSH) screening linked to a rapid confirmation and treatment process enables affected children to start thyroxine replacement by 14–21 days, and this has been successful in ensuring that the majority achieve normal or near normal developmental status. Infants with congenital hypothyroidism are typically post-mature with greater than average birthweights, but without replacement early infancy growth failure is conspicuous.

Acquired primary hypothyroidism is usually autoimmune, and needs consideration in children and adolescents with subnormal growth. A low thyroxine or free thyroxine, with an elevated TSH level, establishes the case for thyroxine replacement. Some laboratories abbreviate thyroid function tests to TSH measurement alone; this is sensitive for detecting primary hypothyroidism but may result in pituitary or hypothalamic hypothyroidism being overlooked.

Cortisol

Cortisol in therapeutic dosage is obviously growth suppressing, but steroid-induced growth failure is fortunately uncommon, or is anticipated as an inevitable penalty of essential treatment. High dosage inhaled and topical steroids may however be overlooked as causes of growth failure or impaired adrenal function, the latter manifesting as delayed recovery after coincidental illness or as fasting-induced hypoglycaemia. Adrenal insufficiency, Addison's disease, is a rare but not to be forgotten cause of weight loss, gastrointestinal symptoms and potential collapse. Endogenous cortisol excess, Cushing's syndrome, is even rarer in childhood despite the misconception that it may account for the all too common problem of late childhood obesity.

Androgens, produced primarily by the adrenal zona reticularis of the prepubertal child, appear to have a role in skeletal maturation and the modest growth acceleration seen normally between ages 6 and 8 years. Some children have a more conspicuous 'adrenarche' with a pronounced late childhood growth spurt and relatively early pubic hair growth (pubarche). This is usually an innocent event that does not lead to early true puberty (gonadarche). There is overlap between adrenal and ovarian androgen metabolism, and girls with androgen excess may be at higher risk of subsequent ovarian dysfunction and polycystic ovarian syndrome.

Testosterone

The Leydig cells of the testis secrete testosterone under the control of luteinising hormone (LH). In the male fetus, testosterone and its derivative dihydrotestosterone (DHT) are key factors in the differentiation of internal and external genitalia. Following delivery and during early infancy there are surges in testosterone release but the overall trend throughout childhood is for levels to be low or undetectable by usual assays. The pubertal increase follows the greater amplitude of LH pulses and increasing testicular volume, and stimulates the appearance of sexual characteristics and the peak height velocity, with the emphasis being on trunk growth.

Female sex steroids

At the onset of puberty a complex hypothalamic process determines the cyclical release of follicle-stimulating hormone (FSH) and LH that in turn regulate ovarian production of oestrogens, progestogens and androgens. The endocrine ovaries are inactive until age 6–8 years, after which ultrasound imaging shows increasing follicular development, followed by detectable increase in plasma oestradiol levels. In addition to causing maturation of the internal and external genitalia and other sexual changes, oestrogens have a substantial role in mineralisation and maturation of the skeleton.

MEASURING GROWTH

Height and supine length

The principle is to accurately measure the distance between flat surfaces applied to the top of the head and the soles of the feet.

Supine length is measured in children below age 2 years, and in older children who are unable to stand. Equipment is available for both infants (the neonatometer) and longer subjects based on a supine table with fixed headboard and a moving baseplate. Two staff are necessary, an assistant to hold the head in firm contact with the headplate, and the measurer to straigthen the legs and to manoeuvre one or both feet flat against the calibrated footplate.

Height is measured from the age of 2 years. The child must be barefoot and stand erect with heels, buttocks and shoulder blades against a firm vertical surface or backplate. There is a standard position for the head with the lower border of the orbit on the same horizontal plane as the external auditory meatus (Fig. 9.3). The measurer applies gentle upward pressure on the mastoid processes while ensuring that the heels remain on the baseplate. The calibrated headplate should ideally be weighted to make firm contact with the scalp. Stretching is ineffective in correcting for diurnal variation, up to 2 cm shortening in the day, and serial measurements should be made at around the same time.

The 'gold standard' for height measurement is provided by a stadiometer, regularly calibrated against a 1-metre standard rule, and operated by a trained individual. The less expensive magnimeter is a reliable alternative for static use. Minimetre (Castlemead) and Leicester Height Measure (Child Growth Foundation) are more suitable devices for portable application. In a specialist growth clinic, sitting height or crown–rump length are measured for comparison with total length as an index of body proportion.

Weight

Weight is the most frequently recorded measure of growth in the first months of life. It is easily

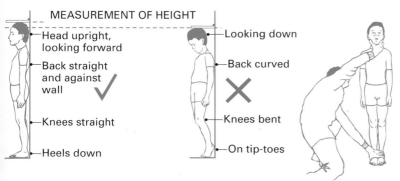

MEASUREMENT OF HEIGHT

Head upright, looking forward

Back straight and against wall

Knees straight

Heels down

✓

Looking down

Back curved

Knees bent

On tip-toes

✗

Five points of correct technique

1 Child's hands by sides

2 Child looking forward

3 Your hand under child's chin with fingers on mastoid processes, exert gentle upward pressure

4 Your other hand on child's feet to keep back straight and to prevent heels rising

5 Keep Microtoise against wall

Fig. 9.3 Measuring height

performed but potentially laden with errors. Accurate electronic scales provide reliable tools given co-operative subjects.

Body mass index (BMI) is defined above (p 137).

Skinfold measurements are seldom performed other than for specialist and research reasons.

Head circumference

Head circumference or occipito-frontal circumference (OFC) should be measured with a narrow tape placed in the horizontal plane encompassing the midpoint of the forehead, between eyebrows and hairline, and the occipital prominence.

Puberty

Puberty is recorded by the changes in pubic hair, external genitalia in boys, and breast development in girls using the five-stage scheme described by Tanner. The volume of the testes may be gauged against a calibrated orchidometer.

Measurement reliability

In any measurement accuracy is essential if the observations are to be of use, and this is especially true if serial measures are to provide the basis for deriving growth velocity. Instruments, observers and, least predictably, subjects introduce errors. Instruments need to be correctly installed and regularly calibrated. Observers should be trained and reassessed to determine their error of measurement, ideally no more than 2–3 mm for repeated height measures of an individual child. The greater challenge is to provide consistent reliability over time in an attempt to minimise errors that will otherwise deny useful interpretation of height velocity. The Wessex Growth Study has highlighted the problems facing community evaluation of growth rate; errors in two measurements over time are amplified by the calculation of height velocity, and it is the nature of normal growth for there to be phases of faster and slower growth.

Measurements are worthless unless recorded accurately, preferably both as dated text and on appropriate charts. Age calculation may be duo-decimal (e.g. 5 years 6 months) or decimal (e.g. 5.5 years). Prematurity, less than 36 weeks' gestation, requires correction on infancy growth charts and it may reduce confusion if dates are also included on the chart. Plots of discrete dots provide clearer growth lines than overlapping blobs and circles. It is seldom necessary to plot height velocity on dedicated height velocity charts; deviation across population centiles is a clear enough message.

When to measure?

The extent to which growth monitoring should be incorporated in child health surveillance has stirred considerable controversy. On the one hand serial measurements between birth and, at least, school entry are claimed to be potentially valuable for the detection of disorders that might otherwise be overlooked. On the other hand there is little supporting evidence for this proposition from actual community surveys that have encountered problems with both sensitivity and specificity using height velocity criteria.

Hall (2000) drawing on the 'Coventry Consensus' Meeting, 1998, has suggested the following:

1. Single height measurements with a cut-off at the 0.4th centile come closest to satisfying the criteria of screening.
2. School entry provides a reasonably effective and low-cost option for the application of universal growth screening. This requires reliable measurement and careful records.
3. Height measurement at other ages, using the 0.4th centile to trigger action, is good practice and should be undertaken when children present to health services. However on current evidence, and because there is no validated protocol for children under the 0.4th centile, this should not be part of total population screening.

EVALUATION OF SUSPECTED GROWTH FAILURE

Community and hospital based paediatric staff should agree local guidelines for assessment and investigation. Primary care and community teams can deal with the majority of otherwise healthy short children without recourse to laboratory investigations. A relatively straightforward agenda of tests will usually resolve uncertainty when underlying disease needs to be excluded. A minority will need specialist referral because of unexplained growth failure or because there may be a role for treatment intervention.

A comprehensive history and examination will identify the majority of health or environmental restraints sufficient to impair growth. Dysmorphic features may provide clues in SGA infants with persistent growth failure. Girls with Turner's syndrome may have escaped recognition despite attending ENT and eye clinics. Children with short stature due to a milder skeletal dysplasia, for example hypochondroplasia, may not have striking trunk limb disproportion; review of short parents may be more revealing. The examination should include examination of visual acuity, fields and fundoscopy. Optic chiasma and pituitary area tumours are rare but the penalty for overlooking them is severe.

Parental heights should be obtained, by direct measurement if possible, and plotted with the necessary adjustment on the child's chart, i.e. 12 cm is added to the mother's height for a boy, or subtracted from the father's height for a girl. The midparental centile ± 8 cm demonstrates the child's target height. A child whose height appears to be inappropriate for this target requires review; a common explanation for discrepancy, especially in late childhood or early adolescence, is constitutional delay of growth and puberty (CDGP). A family history of delayed puberty obviously helps to consolidate this explanation (Fig. 9.4).

Basic investigations

A left hand and wrist X-ray provides a standardised basis for assessing skeletal maturity or bone age, and this provides a guide as to future growth potential. Either the method of Greulich and Pyle or that of Tanner and Whitehouse may be used; both are based on X-rays of normally growing children, and there are reservations regarding application to disordered growth or abnormal skeletons.

Depending on the clinical findings, it may be justified to carry out basic blood tests, looking for evidence of chronic bowel disease (full blood count (FBC), C-reactive protein (CRP), antigliadin and endomysial antibodies), thyroid dysfunction (free thyroxine, TSH), renal disease (electrolytes, creatinine) and chromosomal abnormalities (e.g. Turner's syndrome).

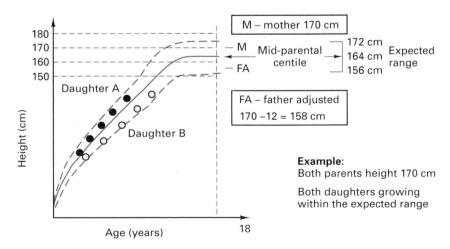

Fig. 9.4 Interpretation of measurements

Growth

SHORT STATURE (Table 9.1)

The majority of children with short stature and/or growth failure fall into one of the following categories.

Familial or constitutional short stature (Fig. 9.5)

A growth record confirming height increase parallel to normal centiles suggests that the child is achieving his growth potential. This is reinforced if he is healthy and the predicted growth pattern fits the target height. Difficulties arise when serial heights deviate across centile channels, and calculated height velocities are at or less than the 25th centile for age. Short children have low normal height velocities, and phases of subnormal growth reflecting relative GH insufficiency compared to normally growing children. These findings, together with parental ambition for improved stature, may necessitate referral to a specialist centre. The therapeutic reality is that GH has a limited role in such children, and available evidence suggests that they are no happier as the result of being given modestly improved height.

Constitutional delay in growth and puberty (Fig. 9.6)

This is a common cause of declining height velocity in late childhood, and is paralleled by delayed puberty and bone age delay of 18 months or more. A healthy child with a family history of CDGP does not require further investigation. Explanation and reassurance about an acceptable final height prediction satisfies most such youngsters. The combination of genetic short stature and CDGP does however present a greater challenge to diagnosis and counselling.

Some boys react adversely to their predicament with behavioural problems, and may warrant specialist supervision of short-term low-dosage androgen, oxandrolone or testosterone. Low-dosage androgens accelerate height, especially if the tests have reached 8 ml or more, but do not alter adult stature. There is clearly a large placebo effect with such intervention but the benefit has been confirmed by randomised control studies.

Intrauterine growth retardation

The heterogeneous aetiology of intrauterine growth retardation (IUGR) and persisting infancy growth failure has been discussed. In the absence of a recog-

Table 9.1 **Classification of short stature**	
Non GH deficient	**GH deficient**
• Idiopathic (short normal)	• Idiopathic

• Delay
• Intrauterine growth retardation
• Syndromes:
    chromosomal, e.g. Turner's, Down's
  other, e.g. Noonan's
• Diseases of other systems
    malabsorption
    renal, respiratory, cardiac
	• Organic, i.e. known cause
	  congenital, e.g. septo-optic dysplasia, pituitary stalk lesions
	  pituitary/hypothalamic tumours, e.g. craniopharyngioma
	  cranial irradiation
	  other acquired, e.g. trauma, CNS infection

• Skeletal dysplasias, e.g. hypochrondroplasia Other endocrine disorders	

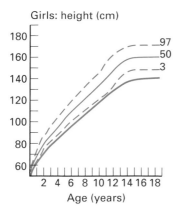

Fig. 9.5 Constitutionally short

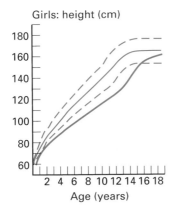

Fig. 9.6 Delayed maturity

growth and café au lait areas. The majority does not have a demonstrable genetic basis although some familial cases have been associated with maternal uniparental disomy of chromosome 7, an area linked to candidate growth factor genes. Affected infants have difficult feeding behaviour and may be susceptible to hypoglycaemia. Infants without syndromatic features may have identical growth patterns.

Nutritional management is the priority but there is current interest in the potential role of GH treatment to correct persistent infancy and early childhood growth failure. These children are not GH insufficient by conventional criteria but they appear to have relative GH resistance. Carefully conducted research suggests that short- to medium-term high-dosage GH can promote catch-up growth and restore normal growth trajectories. The long-term implications of such intervention have yet to be resolved.

Turner's syndrome

Turner's syndrome occurs in approximately 1 in 2500 live-born girls, about 60% having the karyotype 45,X and the remainder a spectrum of partial X chromosome deletions, ring forms and mosaics. Under 5% have mosaic karyotypes incorporating a portion of Y chromosome and are at risk of mixed gonadal dysgenesis with potential malignant transformation.

Girls may present at birth with low birthweight, dysmorphic features and coarctation of the aorta. In others, residual fetal lymphoedema results in characteristically puffy hands and feet. The classical features in childhood are short stature with a mean adult height of 143 cm (4 ft 8 in), absent or incomplete puberty, and a range of dysmorphic features including a wide neck, low hairline, broad chest, cubitus valgus and narrow nails. As in normal girls, height is influenced by parental stature and the 25% with taller parents have heights above the 2nd centile until late childhood. The dysmorphic features may be subtle and are often overlooked despite attendance at clinics because of recurrent otitis media, refractory errors and squints. A substantial minority of girls are diagnosed late as a result. General intelligence is usually intact but the

nised maternal cause, it is convenient to classify IUGR as syndromatic or non-syndromatic. Turner's syndrome is an obvious example of the former and readily confirmed by chromosomal analysis. Dysmorphology databases and genetic studies have generated an extensive differential diagnosis.

Russell–Silver syndrome

This syndrome refers to the combination of growth failure with relative preservation of the head circumference, triangular facies with micrognathia, clinodactyly and, in some, asymmetrical limb

Growth

girls have more difficulty with spatial and abstract areas. Some have impaired body language and social skills, and are susceptible to behavioural and emotional problems. Early recognition and proactive measures can minimise some of the potential school consequences.

Priorities in management include counselling and support, a realistic appraisal of future height, and a positive view regarding hormone replacement for puberty and adult life. For some girls and their families short stature is acceptable and intervention is inappropriate; in others height is a major issue and they may choose the option of long-term GH therapy. Turner girls are not GH deficient but they can achieve modest final height gain with sustained high-dosage GH. In UK studies the median gain is 5–8 cm with 30% reaching final height above 150 cm, compared to about 10% of untreated girls. Girls who start GH before mid-childhood gain more height but the responses are variable.

Approximately 20–30% of girls enter puberty spontaneously with breast changes but few sustain pubertal progress and reach menarche. The usual practice is to introduce an escalating programme of oestrogen replacement from age 12 to 14 years, the aims being to match normal sexual maturation and optimise skeletal mineral content. Turner girls are prone to obesity in adolescence; they are also at increased risk from autoimmune hypothyroidism and type 2 diabetes. The issue of infertility must be discussed but there is now the realistic option of ovum donation. These are some of the challenges facing adult Turner women and there is a place for regional clinics offering multidisciplinary support.

Noonan's syndrome

This syndrome, with an incidence of 1 in 1000 to 1250 live births of both sexes, is a relatively common cause of short stature. Diagnostic features include the facial appearance, chest deformities and congenital heart disease, especially pulmonary stenosis. Autosomal dominant inheritance with variable expression occurs but many cases are sporadic. Unfortunately there is no readily available genetic test. Recognised individuals gave a wide range of IQ and of verbal-performance discrepancy.

Skeletal dysplasia

Skeletal dysplasia definition and management is usually best served by a clinic offering the combined services of paediatrician, clinical geneticist and orthopaedic surgeon. Some of the milder forms, for example hypochondroplasia, may not show obvious body disproportion during childhood but present with growth failure in an otherwise healthy child. An affected parent will be relatively short with stocky limbs. It is a feature of hypochondroplasia and allied conditions that the pubertal growth phase is blunted. The evidence that GH treatment makes a worthwhile difference to final height remains unconvincing.

Other genetic causes of short stature

Growth failure may be a component of a wide spectrum of dysmorphic syndromes and it usually reflects programmed small stature or associated skeletal abnormality rather than endocrine insufficiency. Priorities are to define the disorder in liaison with a clinical geneticist, review disorder-related growth patterns in published studies, and check for reversible components, notably suboptimal nutrition.

Endocrine disorders

Hypothyroidism and GH deficiency are the two main endocrine causes of short stature.

Hypothyroidism in childhood is sometimes insidious in onset so that short stature with markedly delayed bone age may be the first recognised manifestation. Thyroid function tests comprising both free thyroxine and TSH will differentiate primary and secondary hypothyroidism, the latter usually being one component of hypopituitarism. Primary hypothyroidism arising in childhood is usually due to autoimmune thyroiditis, and once established it is likely that thyroxine replacement will be a lifelong requirement.

Growth hormone deficiency is not a distinct entity but refers to a spectrum of defects in the complex pathway linking brain centres to the GH receptors of the liver (Fig. 9.7). There is then a secondary axis comprising IGF-1 and other growth factors that act on growth plate chondrocytes.

Severe congenital GH deficiency is usually associated with high-resolution magnetic resonance imaging (MRI) evidence of partial or complete interruption of the pituitary stalk. It is uncertain whether the interrupted stalk represents developmental failure or acquired injury. These infants are more likely to have associated panhypopituitarism.

Septo-optic dysplasia comprises developmental failure of midline structures including septum pellucidum, optic chiasma and pituitary. The gene HESX-1 has been implicated. This disorder together with hypopituitarism must be considered in infants with visual impairment or nystagmus, hypoglycaemia, prolonged jaundice, electrolyte disturbance and growth failure.

Acquired causes of GH deficiency and panhypopituitarism include craniopharyngioma, hypothalamic and optic nerve glioma. Most children with craniopharyngioma come to medical attention because of deteriorating vision or headaches and raised intracranial pressure; it is only subsequently that pre-existent growth failure is recognised. It is mandatory to check visual acuity and fields as well as to perform fundoscopy in children with growth failure. Skin pigmentation or a positive family history may signal the likelihood of neuro-fibromatosis. Cranial irradiation as part of the management of leukaemia or brain tumours may result in partial GH deficiency; craniospinal irradiation adds a component of impaired trunk growth, and cytotoxic therapy may further depress tissue response to growth factors.

Children with severe GH deficiency or panhypopituitarism are relatively easily identified, and GH therapy is clearly justified. The greater and more common management challenge is to define those children with partial isolated GH deficiency (IGHD), especially those who are destined to have unacceptable final height that might be amenable to GH therapy. IGHD overlaps with so-called normal short stature, and it is a matter of debate whether health resources should be targeted at children who suffer more from society's attitude to height than they do from health risk. It is relevant that considerably more boys than girls are diagnosed as having IGHD.

The biochemical confirmation of GH deficiency is usually the final step after excluding other causes of growth failure. GH provocation tests such as glucagon or clonidine should be performed in experienced centres supported by laboratory services with validated GH assays.

In the UK licensed indications for synthetic human growth hormone (Somatropin) in childhood are insufficient secretion of GH, Turner's syndrome and chronic renal insufficiency. GH is administered as a daily subcutaneous injection and requires shared care guidelines, careful supervision recognising that poor compliance is an issue, and close monitoring of the growth response. The first year height response is compared to predicted targets; a good response with for example doubling of height velocity from below 4 cm per year up to 8 cm per year justifies continuation; a poor response requires reappraisal of the diagnosis, dosage regimen and compliance. GH treatment is usually continued until near final height or a height increment of less than 2 cm per year. Patients with severe GH deficiency may be candidates for adult replacement using a lower-dosage regimen.

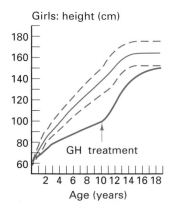

Fig. 9.7 Growth hormone deficiency

TALL STATURE (Table 9.2)

Parents and children who seek advice because of tall stature are far fewer than those who are concerned about being short. Being tall is seen as an advantage in our society. However excessive tallness can be as much of a handicap as being small. A 5 year old who is as tall as an average 8 year old is expected to behave as the older child, and may be labelled as clumsy or aggressive. In teenage years particularly, being very tall may cause problems with forming relationships and emotional difficulties are common.

Familial tall stature

Tall parents, especially those who found their own adolescence challenging, may seek advice about the future growth patterns of tall daughters. Final height is likely to be acceptable if puberty and menses occur relatively early, or childhood bone age advance supports a pattern of constitutional advance in growth and puberty. Of greater concern are slender, long-limbed girls with no bone age advance and a familial predisposition to late puberty and hence delayed epiphyseal fusion. Established methods of height prediction can be used to determine whether adult height is likely to exceed 180 cm (5 ft 11 in), but the error may be 4–5 cm, a figure that almost matches the reduction claimed for drug intervention. Treatment to reduce height gain needs to be introduced near the onset of puberty so that it subtracts from late childhood growth; the component linked to puberty is inevitable. Families need careful counselling with a realistic evaluation of the benefits and risks of moderate dosage oestrogen therapy given for 1–2 years.

Nutritional obesity and growth advance

A high-energy food intake in infancy and early childhood promotes modest growth acceleration and relatively early puberty. The combination of tall stature and obesity is only rarely linked to definable endocrine pathology, but a minority of obese adolescent girls develops hirsutism and menstrual problems as part of the spectrum of polycystic ovary syndrome. This complex entity is linked to obesity-driven hyperinsulinism and adrenal androgen excess. The long-term health implications become even more threatening if there is a familial predisposition to type 2 diabetes.

Pathological tall stature

Marfan's syndrome

This syndrome should be considered in tall thin children especially if accompanied by thoracic deformity and scoliosis. Supportive features of this autosomal dominant condition are a positive family history, joint laxity, eye problems and heart murmurs. Approximately 30% have echocardiographic evidence of aortic root enlargement or mitral valve prolapse. It is important not to apply the label too readily to children with long limbs and joint laxity without other supportive criteria.

Homocystinuria

Homocystinuria, due to deficiency of cystathionine synthetase, is an autosomal disorder that produces some of the physical features matching Marfan's

Table 9.2
Classification of tall stature

| Not dysmorphic | | Dysmorphic |
Normal velocity	Increased velocity	
• Familial	• Hypothalamic/pituitary disease	• Marfan's syndrome
• Obesity	• Hyperthyroidism ·	• Klinefelter's syndrome
• Growth advance	• Adrenal disease Gonadal disease	• Cerebral gigantism (Sotos' syndrome)

syndrome but with high myopia including a risk of lens dislocation, learning and behavioural problems, epilepsy and an increased risk of thromboembolic disease. Specialist laboratory advice is required for confirmation.

Chromosomal syndromes with tall stature

Klinefelter's syndrome (XXY)

This syndrome has an incidence of 1.3 per 1000 male births but only a minority is diagnosed in childhood. Boys may be diagnosed at amniocentesis, or present because of hypogonadism, developmental delay or gynaecomastia. Their relative tall stature due to disproportionate leg growth is seldom a presenting issue.

XYY

XYY occurs in 1 per 1000 male births and it is estimated that 85% remain unrecognised. Childhood growth is accelerated with an average final height of 188 cm. Temper tantrums, an increased antisocial score and other behaviour problems are reported in nearly 50% of XYY boys.

Other overgrowth syndromes

A recent review commented on nearly 300 conditions that incorporated macrocephaly, obesity, increased birthweight or excess stature. In addition as many as 50% of children with these features do not fit recognised diagnostic categories. Two of the most frequently diagnosed are Beckwith–Wiedemann and Sotos' syndromes.

Beckwith–Wiedemann syndrome (BWS) comprises exomphalos, macroglossia and growth acceleration during fetal life and infancy, and it appears to be linked to overexpression of the growth factor, IGF-II. A majority arise as sporadic mutations with 15% following autosomal dominant inheritance.

Sotos' syndrome, a mainly sporadic condition, has a phenotype of fetal and childhood overgrowth, advanced bone age, developmental delay, and a facial gestalt of dolichocephaly, tall bossed forehead and long jaw. Final height is usually at the 98th centile.

Endocrine disorders

Childhood tall stature may result from precocious puberty, or oversecretion of adrenal or thyroid glands. Pathological overproduction of growth hormone by a pituitary adenoma is exceptionally rare. Key factors in initial assessment are to review the growth record for evidence of growth acceleration, and to check for signs of early puberty or adrenal overactivity (obesity, hirsutism, acne and hypertension). Bone age advance beyond normal limits raises the probability of an endocrine disorder.

Precocious puberty (Table 9.3)

Unacceptable early puberty is difficult to define, as it depends as much on the attitude of child and family as it does on age. The usual lower age of puberty onset is 8 years in girls and 9 years in boys. As a general rule early puberty is commoner in girls and less likely to have a pathological basis. Early

Table 9.3 **Causes of early puberty**	
Physiological	**Pathological**
• Familial	• Intracranial tumours, e.g. of hypothalamus, pineal area
• Tall obese girls	• Extracranial tumours, e.g. of adrenal glands, gonads
• Isolated adrenarche Isolated thelarche	• Others such as hypothyroidism, mental retardation, cranial radiotherapy, drugs

female puberty that follows a normal sequence of events, growth acceleration matched by breast development and pubic hair growth, is likely to have a central origin based on early reactivation of the hypothalamic centres that control pulsatile secretion of gonadotrophins. In the majority of girls with borderline early puberty it is unnecessary to arrange cranial imaging unless there are other risk factors, for example recent onset headaches, visual signs or skin pigmentation suggestive of neurofibromatosis. By contrast, the less frequent, boys with early onset central puberty characterised by matching testicular and penile growth, always merit cranial imaging as they have a high likelihood of midline tumours such as germinoma.

Premature adrenarche

Children, girls more than boys, may present at age 6–8 years with pubic hair, skin changes linked to increased apocrine activity, and modest height acceleration. The usual explanation is enhanced but innocent maturation of the adrenal production of androgens, reflected by pubertal levels of plasma androstenedione or DHAS. The bone age is advanced by 1–2 years and remains in keeping with the height adjusted for parental range. Experienced clinicians seldom have difficulty in distinguishing early adrenarche from adrenal pathology such as late-onset congenital adrenal hyperplasia or adenoma/carcinoma. Boys with non-salt-losing congenital adrenal hyperplasia present with dramatic early childhood growth acceleration and bone age advance. Typically their penile enlargement and pubic hair contrasts with prepubertal sized testes.

Isolated premature breast development (thelarche)

This is relatively common, both in infancy and in mid-childhood. The fluctuating and usually modest breast growth typically resolves without other features of puberty such as growth acceleration. Isolated thelarche reflects transient pulsatile secretion of FSH and oestrogen. Total puberty usually occurs at an acceptable age, although a small minority of girls may have an interrupted slow progression to full early puberty.

FAILURE TO THRIVE

Children, particularly infants who gain weight slowly, are seen commonly in community paediatric clinics. The difficulty for the paediatrician and child health team is to decide which of these is growing normally, and which are failing to thrive. This is important because failure to thrive (FTT) is associated with long-term effects on development, growth and family relationships. FTT is also a condition of high prevalence, affecting approximately 5% of the under fives population, depending on definition.

Definitions

FTT is not a syndrome or disease, but is a description of a pattern of weight gain which is at one extreme of the normal range. Deciding where normality ends, particularly allowing for the phenomenon of regression to the mean, and abnormality (with need for action) begins, has been aired often in the literature over the last 10 years (Cole 1998b, Wright et al 1998a, Raynor & Rudolph 2000).

The value of any anthropometric index of FTT must lie in its usefulness in identifying the child at risk, and of predicting the severity of other developmental and nutritional problems also present. To date, no one method has proven better than another. What seems to be crucial is that the identification and early assessment of faltering weight gain in infancy includes a clinical team expert in reviewing growth over time, development, dietary and nutritional status, as well as psychosocial and family factors.

Does FTT matter?

FTT children as a group have cognitive abilities 1–1.5 SDs below population or control group means measured at the age of 20–22 months (Skuse et al 1994, Reif et al 1995, Wilensky et al 1996). They are shorter at long-term follow-up (Tse et al 1989, Reif et al 1995, Wilensky et al 1996), particularly when impaired growth occurs during the critical nutritionally dependant infantile phase of growth, in the early postnatal period.

Causal factors in FTT

Understanding of the many factors that can contribute to a child's FTT is crucial both in evaluating the benefits of different interventions, but also in planning preventative strategies. It is unhelpful to divide FTT into 'organic or non-organic'. The proportion of babies suffering from major organic conditions is very small (1–5%), and even when present, other non-organic factors may be operating. The routine use of blood investigation without pointers on history or examination is likely to yield positive results in under 1% of babies (Frank & Zeisel 1998).

FTT has a multifactorial aetiology with complex interactions between child, parent, family and environmental factors. It is beyond the scope of this book to consider them in detail, but the following should be considered in the assessment and interventions planned.

A. Child factors
- Small appetite, with reduced demands for feeds.
- Subtle oral–motor problems.
- Oral hypersensitivity.
- Level of responsiveness of the infant.
- Communication skills, both verbal and non-verbal, particularly at mealtimes.
- Developmental status.
- Illness.

There may be a history of feeding difficulties, sometimes in association with early vomiting.

B. Carer factors
- Parents ability to compensate for any difficulties a child has in feeding.
- Maternal IQ, with poorer interactions, less compensatory parenting.
- Eating attitudes.
- Eating habits.
- Eating disorders.
- Maternal history of abuse.

C. Parent–child interactions
- Disrupted parent/child relationships and stressful social environments are common in FTT. This interaction is complex, with the anxious attachments sometimes seen resulting from characteristics of both the child and parent, together with characteristics of the social environment.
- A very small subgroup of children failing to thrive do so as a result of abuse or neglect.

What interventions are effective in FTT?

As children with FTT are not a homogeneous group, assessment and intervention programmes must be flexible. The 'FTT team' involved must be multidisciplinary, and may include a paediatrician, a health visitor and a dietician, with access to psychological and social work expertise. It must allow the nutritional and psychosocial perspectives to be addressed.

Any approach must include an understanding of parental beliefs and attitudes to food, and to the child's FTT. Nutritional interventions must be more than simply the giving of nutritional advice. Feeding problems need to be identified on history, by observation at mealtimes (perhaps including video recordings) and should be home based. Completion of a 3- to 5-day food diary is also helpful. Behavioural approaches using ignoring and positive reinforcement of behaviour are also helpful, particularly when this is supported at home by a keyworker.

Management in hospital/clinic or at home?

There is increasing evidence that effective community-based management in FTT is cost effective. The relative efficiency of clinic-versus home-based work is the subject of a recent review (Wright et al 1998b). Both achieve beneficial effects on weight gain. Interventions that are home based, particularly in young infants, also have advantages for cognitive and language development. In addition, parents at home may be more receptive to the changes required to increase calorie intake if they feel they are involved collaboratively. A better understanding of parents' views is also more likely at home, with an active partnership reached when

Growth

agreeing what work needs to be undertaken. Hospitalisation should be reserved for babies whose weight is at a dangerously low level.

OBESITY IN CHILDREN

Paediatricians face problems of overweight in around one in four of their patients. Studies consistently report a high prevalence of obesity in children and adolescents and rates are on the increase (WHO 1998). National studies from 1972 to 1990 of health and growth in Scottish and English children showed a twofold increase in excessive weight for height in all age groups and both sexes (Chinn & Rona 1994).

Ethnic minority groups in Britain show different patterns of obesity, with Afro-Caribbean children maintaining their tall slim build, whilst other groups, such as Urdu-, Punjabi- or Gujarati-speaking Indians, showing a trend towards greater obesity (Chinn et al 1998).

Overweight children may be identified by routine school nurse's or health visitor's measurements, by parental or teacher concern or by the child himself. There may be difficulties with peer relationships, reluctance to take part in games and unhappiness related to bullying.

Definitions

Definitions of obesity are usually based on measurements such as skinfold thickness or body mass indices calculated from weight and height. None of these is entirely satisfactory. Skinfold thickness is measured using Holtain skinfold calipers in standard positions on the triceps and subscapular areas. These measurements are not easily reproducible.

Body mass indices are indirect measures of obesity (weight/height, weight/height^2 for age). There are times when body fatness does not change with age as height does and therefore the indices can be misleading. These indices should therefore be used with caution.

A recent international survey has attempted to develop an acceptable definition of childhood overweight and obesity, using body mass index (weight/height^2) and drawing centile curves to provide age- and sex-specific cut-off points for childhood obesity from 2 to 18 years (Figs 9.8, 9.9). These should help to provide internationally

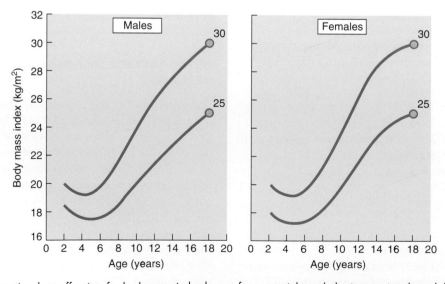

Fig. 9.8 International cut-off points for body mass index by sex for overweight and obesity, passing through body mass index 25 and 30 kg/m^2 at age 18 (data from Brazil, UK, Hong Kong, Netherlands, Singapore and USA). From Cole et al (2000)

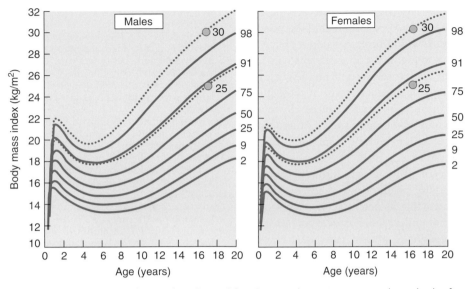

Fig. 9.9 Centiles for body mass index for British males and females. Centile curves are spaced two-thirds of z score apart. Also shown are body mass index values of 25 and 30 kg/m² at age 18, with extra centile curves drawn through them. From Cole et al (2000)

comparable prevalence rates of overweight and obesity in children (Cole et al 2000).

Aetiology

Uncommonly there is a pathological cause for obesity. Useful clues are associated short stature and/or mental retardation. However obesity is seldom the presenting feature of these disorders, for example dysmorphic syndromes such as Down's or Prader–Willi syndromes, endocrine disorders such as GH deficiency, hypothyroidism. In these disorders being overweight can be an additional handicap and part of the management should be weight reduction/control.

Other risk factors such as those for cardiovascular disease, cancer, diabetes, orthopaedic disorders and psychological problems should also be evaluated.

'Simple obesity' is the result of mismatch between calorie intake and energy expenditure. These children are tall for their age and for their parents. There are complex social and psychological factors involved. The rapid rise in childhood obesity has been mirrored by an explosion of sedentary leisure pursuits for children such as computers, video

games and television watching (Anderson et al 1998).

Interventions

The most successful weight reduction programmes are those that combine diet and exercise within a framework of behaviour modification. The child and family must be motivated to lose or control weight, otherwise treatment failure rates are high.

Treatment of obesity is most successful if realistic goals are set; a balanced diet is emphasised; a safe reduction in weight loss of about 0.5 kg a week is achieved through a moderate reduction in energy intake (about 20–25% decrease); increased physical activity is emphasised; parental support is strong and behaviour therapy is provided to help both child and parents achieve the diet, exercise and behaviour goals.

On an individual basis, support of the child from parents, teachers, school nurse and doctor, GP and dietician is essential. On a wider scale, education and national policies regrading nutrition and health have their part to play (Department of Health 1992).

Growth

Garrow (1991) has suggested that one of the strategies to reduce the proportion of obese people in the population would be to develop a policy in primary schools to identify school entrants who are above the 90th centile for weight for height and provide facilities for weight control in these children between the ages of 5 and 12 years. However, implementing and maintaining such a programme in the school curriculum in the long term may prove to be difficult.

The delivery of programmes through primary care or community paediatrics has received little formal assessment and its potential role seems to be undervalued and underused. Frequent contact with healthcare professionals from an early age has been identified as an important strategy for the effective management of obese children through the provision of advice, encouragement and support for adopting healthy household eating and exercise patterns at an early stage in life (Pronk & Boucher 1999).

REFERENCES AND FURTHER READING

Anderson R E, Crespo C J, Bartlett S J, Cheskin L J, Pratt M 1998 Relationship of physical activity and television watching with body weight and level of fatness among children. Results from the Third National Health and Nutrition Examination Survey. JAMA 279:938–942

Betts P R, Butler G E, Donaldson M D C et al 1999 A decade of growth hormone treatment in girls with Turner syndrome in the UK. Archives of Disease in Childhood 80:221–225

Chinn S, Rona R J 1994 Trends in weight-for-height and triceps skinfold thickness for English and Scottish children, 1972–1982 and 1982–1990. Paediatric and Perinatal Epidemiology 8:90–106

Chinn S, Hughes J M, Rona R J 1998 Trends in growth and obesity in ethnic groups in Britain. Archives of Disease in Childhood 78:513–517

Cole T J 1994 Do growth chart centiles need a facelift? British Medical Journal 308:641–642

Cole T J 1995 Conditional reference charts to assess weight gain in British infants. Archives of Disease in Childhood 73:8–16

Cole T 1998a Annotation: growing interest in overgrowth. Archives of Disease in Childhood 78:200–204

Cole T J 1998b Conditional reference charts to assess weight gain in British infants. Archives of Disease in Childhood 78:8–16

Cole T J, Freeman J V, Preece M A 1995 Body mass index

reference curves for the UK, 1990. Archives of Disease in Childhood 73:25–29

Cole T J, Bellizi M C, Flegal K M, Dietz W H 2000 Establishing a standard definition for child overweight and obesity worldwide: international survey. British Medical Journal 320:1240

Department of Health 1992 The Health of the Nation, a strategy for health in England. CM 1523. HMSO, London

Donaldson M D C 1997 Growth hormone therapy in Turner syndrome — current uncertainties and future strategies. Hormone Research 48:35–44

Downie A B, Mulligan J, Stratford R J, Betts P R, Voss L D 1997 Are short normal children at a disadvantage? The Wessex Growth Study. British Medical Journal 314:97–100

Frank D A, Zeisel S H 1988 Failure to thrive. Paediatric Clinics of North America 351:187–206

Freeman J V, Cole T J, Chinn S, Jones P R M, White E M, Preece M A 1995 Cross-sectional stature and weight reference curves for the UK, 1990. Archives of Disease in Childhood 73:17–24

Garner P, Panpanich R, Logan S 2000 Is routine growth monitoring effective? A systematic review of trials. Archives of Disease in Childhood 82:197–201

Garrow J 1991 Importance of obesity. British Medical Journal 3003:704–706

Hall D M B 1995 Growth monitoring in the next five years. Journal of Medical Screening 2:174–178

Hall D M B 2000 Growth monitoring. Archives of Disease in Childhood 82:10–14

Pronk N P, Boucher J 1999 Systems approach to childhood and adolescent obesity prevention and treatment in a managed care organisation. International Journal of Obesity 23(suppl 2):S28–S42

Raynor P, Rudolf M 2000 Anthropometric indices of failure to thrive. Archives of Disease in Childhood 82:364–365

Reif S, Beler B, Villa Y, Spirer Z 1995 Longterm follow up and outcome of infants with non organic failure to thrive. Israeli Journal of Medical Science 31:483–489

Skuse D, Pickles A, Wolke D, Reilly S 1994 Postnatal growth and development: evidence for a sensitive period. Journal of Child Psychology and Psychiatry 35:521–545

Skuse D, Albanese A, Stanhope R, Gilmour J, Voss L 1996 A new stress-related syndrome of growth failure and hyperphagia in children, associated with reversibility of growth hormone insufficiency. Lancet 348:353–358

Tse W Y, Hindmarsh P C, Brook C J 1989 The infancy–childhood pubertal model of growth: clinical aspects. Acta Paediatrica Scandinavia Supplement 356:38–45

Voss L 2000 Standardised technique for height measurement Archives of Disease in Childhood 82:14–15

Voss L D, Mulligan J, Betts P R, Wilkin T J 1992 Poor growth in school entrants as an index of organic disease: the Wessex growth study. British Medical Journal 305:1400–1402

WHO 1998 Consultation on obesity. Global prevalence and secular trends in obesity. In: World Health Organization (ed) Obesity preventing and managing the global epidemic. WHO, Geneva: pp 17–40

Wilensky D S, Ginsberg G, Altman M, Tulchinsky T, Yishay F B, Auerbach J 1996 A community based study of failure to thrive in Israel. Archives of Disease in Childhood 75:145–148

Wright C M, Avery A, Epstein M, Burks E, Croft D 1998a New charts to evaluate weight faltering. Archives of Disease in Childhood 78:40–43

Wright C M, Callum J, Birks E, Jarvis S 1998b Effect of community based management in failure to thrive: randomised controlled trial. British Medical Journal 317:571–574

10 | Health economics

The rapid growth in expenditure on health care is an international problem fuelled by demographic changes, technological advance and changing expectations. The UK currently invests around £50 billion a year in the National Health Service (NHS), which constitutes approximately 7% of the nation's wealth (Gross Domestic Product (GDP)). Interestingly this is comparatively low relative to most other Organization for Economic Cooperation and Development (OECD) nations and especially the USA, which invests twice this level at nearly 15% of GDP. In all developed countries, however, one thing is clear — the 'health economy' is very large and hugely important. Decision-makers in health care face a great deal of difficult choices, the subject of economics aims to help with some of these.

THE ECONOMICS PERSPECTIVE
What is economics?

"The study of how men and society end up choosing *to employ* scarce resources *that could have* alternative uses"

(Samuelson 1980)

Simply, economics is about allocating scarce resources. Any introductory economics textbook will have a quote similar to the one above, which contains three elements fundamental to understanding the economics perspective: choosing, scarce resources and alternative uses.

Firstly, 'choosing' or decision-making is what the discipline of economics strives to analyse and ultimately assist with. Indeed, economics has been labelled the 'science of choosing'. It aims to provide a framework of choice so that the full implications of all choices are clearly identified before they are made.

Secondly, scarcity is known as *the* economic problem. Scarcity exists since needs, wants, demands or desires will always be greater than resources available to meet them. This is a fundamental starting point for the economic perspective.

Thirdly, economists differ to, say, accountants in the way that they conceptualise cost. They think about the possible alternative use of any resources, the notion that economists call 'opportunity cost'. Opportunity cost is a key concept underpinning the economics perspective.

The real cost of doing one thing is not actually the pounds you spend but the opportunity of doing something else with this money. Yes, it is important to know the financial implications of a certain action you choose to do but it is the benefits that you could have derived from what you did not choose to do that is the real cost of this action. Now, choosing to use resources one way will always mean giving up the chance to use them in other desirable ways. So, the question that economists ask is: 'are the benefits from what is "chosen" greater than what is "forgone"?' Thus opportunity cost can be defined as the benefits given up in the best alternative use of the resources.

Economics of health

So why is this economics perspective useful in the context of health care? Health economics examines the problem of scarcity as it arises with respect to health and health care. It examines how we as individuals and societies confront the fact that while the resources available to us are limited, the alternative uses for these resources are unlimited. Thus health economists are interested in some very important questions. How is health produced? What role does health care play in its production? What is the value of health? How do we go about measuring health status? What influences demand for health and health care? What influences the supply of health care? How can equilibrium between demand and supply be achieved? The discipline of health economics is the study of these questions and the answers to them which individuals and societies have put forward.

Scarcity demands that choices must be made as to what health care should be provided, how it should be provided, in what quantities and how it might be distributed. Economic evaluation is the area of health economics used to help address these issues. It is also what occupies the bulk of many health economists' time.

ECONOMIC EVALUATION

So, economic evaluation of healthcare programmes aims to aid decision-makers with their difficult choices in allocating healthcare resources, setting priorities and moulding health policy. But it might be argued that this is only an intermediate objective. The real purpose of doing economic evaluation is to improve efficiency: the way inputs (money, labour, capital, etc.) can be converted into outputs (saving life, health gain, improving quality of life, etc.)

The choice of what health care to provide is about what economists call allocative efficiency. This means that we strive for the maximisation of benefits (however we decide to measure this) subject to given available resources. So, from a fixed resource we aim to get as much out of a range of healthcare programmes as possible. This will mean we will need to compare very different interventions, say surgery for tonsillectomy versus outpatient clinics for asthmatics. Thus allocative efficiency is about finding the optimal mix of services that deliver the maximum possible benefit in total. Resources will be directed to interventions that are relatively good (i.e. efficient) at converting inputs into health benefits and away from those that require larger input for relatively low health gain. This approach may

of course be constrained by certain equity consideration, to ensure that certain groups do receive health care.

The choice of how to provide health care is about what economists call technical efficiency. This means that we might strive for minimum input for a given output. For example, if we have decided that performing tonsillectomies on children is worthwhile, part of an allocatively efficient allocation of resources, then we may need to examine the efficiency of how we do this. So, if the output we wish to achieve is to successfully remove a child's tonsils then we might choose between, say, a day-case procedure or an inpatient stay. This is an issue of technical efficiency since the output or 'outcome' is fixed but the inputs will differ depending on which policy we adopt. The day-case approach may perhaps require more intensive staff input and more follow-up outpatient visits. If this were the case then inpatient tonsillectomy may be the more technically efficient strategy.

Thus with any given healthcare programme an economic evaluation is aiming to make explicit the total resources consumed specifically by that programme (i.e. attributable to it) and the total benefit generated specifically by that programme. Drummond et al (1997) defines economic evaluation as 'the comparative analysis of alternative courses of action in terms of both their costs and consequences'. It differs from other forms of analysis because it considers both costs and consequences and is comparative.

Evaluation needs to be comparative, as an intervention can only be labelled as good or bad relative to some benchmark or alternative even if this alternative is a 'do nothing' strategy. If an evaluation is not comparative and does not consider both costs and consequences, then it is only a partial evaluation. It is a description of either just the costs or just the benefits of one intervention in isolation. This is most uninformative since it is one-dimensional and without a context by which to judge relative performance (efficiency). If both costs and consequences are considered but no comparator is provided, then the study is again only a partial evaluation, described as a cost–outcome study. It lacks context and is of limited use. If alternatives are compared but only in terms of costs or benefits and not both, then again the study only provides a partial evaluation and can be labelled an effectiveness study or a cost analysis. It would be comparative but only across one dimension. Hence, an economic approach can be considered a full evaluation technique.

Costs and consequences

Costs can be defined in many ways but generally can be considered as direct, indirect and intangible. Direct costs are those immediately associated with an intervention such as staff time, consumables, etc. Indirect costs might include a patient's work loss due to treatment. Intangible costs may be things like pain, anxiety, quality, etc. All types of economic evaluation deal with costs in the same way or at least in the same units (i.e. monetary).

Benefits, however, can be analysed in three different ways reflecting the different types of economic analysis used in evaluation. Firstly, benefits can be examined in terms of the immediate (direct) effects on health, these are usually clinically defined units appropriate to the area of study, such as 'lives saved', 'reduction in tumour size', etc. Secondly, benefits from an intervention can be considered in more generic terms such as the impact on general well-being/happiness/satisfaction, these are more generally labelled as 'utilities'. The utility of an intervention to an individual is its benefit. Measures such as the quality adjusted life year (QALY) are used to quantify this. Thirdly, benefits might be considered in the same terms as costs, which means that benefits must be valued in monetary terms by some means.

Whatever the approach, the same three-stage process for the assessment of all costs and benefits can be applied. All relevant cost and benefit variables must be: (i) identified, (ii) quantified and (iii) valued.

There are several issues to consider in the assessment of costs and benefits. Externality costs and/or benefits may arise since interventions do not just affect the patient receiving care. For example, if I receive treatment for a contagious disease you will benefit as well as me, any evaluation needs to account for this.

The differential timing of costs and benefits must also be considered in an evaluation.

The effects of health treatments do not always occur at the same point in time. Costs may be incurred today but benefit may not arrive until next year (i.e. preventative treatments, health promotion), part of this future benefit might be that future costs will be avoided. £100 spent today may not have the same value as £100 spent next year because of inflation, interest on savings and not least a positive rate of time preference. People may just prefer to have £100 in their pocket today rather than £100 in a week or a month or a year, because it offers them more choices. This can be incorporated into economic evaluation by the notion of discounting future costs and benefits to their present-day value. A simple formula can be applied to do this for any chosen discount rate, normally within the range of 0–10%.

One further issue to consider in any evaluation is sensitivity analysis. Whilst all evaluations strive to be rigorous and systematic in their approach they will inevitably be subject to some uncertainty. The measurement of key cost and benefit variables is crucial to the result of an economic evaluation (i.e. this is the best use of resources). A change in the value of any of these variables might in fact reverse this result (i.e. one variable may be slightly lower than our observed measurement and in fact it is not the best use of resources, our result would be wrong). Results are sensitive to the deterministic variables in the analysis, the crucial issue is just how sensitive? To test the level of uncertainty of our measured variables' sensitivity analysis should be performed. For example, we might want to vary the amount of nurse time we have estimated for a certain procedure, say double it from 1 hour to 2 hours, what effect does this have on our result, if any? It is wise to vary the most important and most uncertain variables within a plausible and justifiable range in order to test the robustness of the evaluation carried out.

Types of economic evaluation

The different ways of looking at benefits combined with cost analysis represent the different techniques of economic evaluation: cost–effectiveness analysis (CEA), cost–utility (CUA) and cost–benefit analysis (CBA). When to use each of the above techniques will depend on the nature of the question to be addressed, which may be a choice between alternative clinical strategies for a condition; timing of an intervention; settings for care; types and skill-mix of personnel proving care; programmes for different conditions; scale or size of a programme; or other ways to improve health.

Cost–effectiveness analysis

Cost–effectiveness analysis (CEA) is concerned with technical efficiency issues, such as: what is the best way of achieving a given goal or what is the best way of spending a given budget? Comparisons can be made between different health programmes in terms of their cost–effectiveness ratios: cost per unit of effect. In a CEA, effects are measured in natural units. So, if the question to be addressed was: what is the best way of treating renal failure, then the most appropriate ratio with which to compare programmes might be 'cost per life saved'. Similarly, if we wanted to compare the cost-effectiveness of programmes of screening for Down's syndrome the most appropriate ratio might be 'cost per Down's syndrome fetus detected'. In deciding whether long-term care for the elderly should be provided in nursing homes or the community, the 'cost per disability day avoided' might be the most appropriate measure.

The advantage of the CEA approach is that it is relatively straight forward to carry out and is often sufficient for addressing many questions in health care. However, it is not comprehensive — the outcome is unidimensional under this analysis but often health programmes generate multiple outcomes. For example, in Down's syndrome screening, fetuses detected is one outcome, but miscarriages avoided might be another very relevant outcome measure, especially if, say, blood testing is being compared to amniocentesis. But this cannot be incorporated into this form of analysis. So CEA not only assumes that the outcome of the health programme is worthwhile per se but also that it is the most appropriate measure. A further problem with CEA is comparability between very different

health programmes. Cost per fetus detected may be a useful way to compare the efficiency of blood testing versus amniocentesis, but how would these be compared to drugs aimed at reducing cholesterol. Health programmes with different aims cannot be compared with one another using CEA: cost per unit reduction in cholesterol cannot meaningfully be compared with fetuses detected. Hence CEA is useful when comparing programmes within like areas, where common 'currencies' can be used.

Cost–utility analysis

Cost–utility analysis (CUA) is concerned with technical efficiency and allocative efficiency (within the healthcare sector). It can be thought of as a sophisticated form of CEA, since it also makes comparisons between health programmes in terms of cost–effect ratios. However, CUA differs in the way it considers effects, these are multidimensional under this form of analysis. CUA tends to be used when quality of life is an important factor involved in the health programmes being evaluated. This is because CUA combines life years (quantity of life) gained as a result of a health programme with some judgement on the quality of those life years. It is this judgement element that is labelled utility. Utility is simply a measure of preference, values can be assigned to different states of health (relevant to the programme) that represent individual preferences. This is normally done by assigning values between 1.0 and 0.0, where 1.0 is the best imaginable state of health (completely healthy) and 0.0 is the worst imaginable (perhaps death). States of health may be described using many different instruments (SF-36, Nottingham Health Profile, Sickness Impact Profile, EuroQol EQ-5D), these provide a profile of scores in different health domains. EuroQol EQ-5D, for example, simplifies health into just five domains: mobility, self-care, usual activities, pain/discomfort and anxiety/depression. Each domain is given a score from 1 to 3, so the health profile would read 11111 for the best scores in all domains and 33333 for the worst. EuroQol EQ-5D has 243 possible health profiles, all of which have been assigned a utility value by general population surveys.

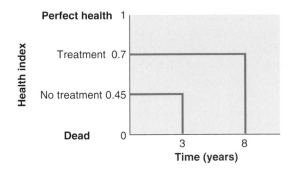

Fig. 10.1 Quality-adjusted life years

These utility values are then combined with survival data to derive quality adjusted life years (QALYs) for different health programmes. For example, assume that a patient who receives no treatment has a life expectancy of 3 years and their quality of life has a value 0.45. Now, if this patient receives a certain intervention then it is expected that life expectancy will be 8 years and the quality of those years will have a value of 0.70. The multi-dimensional gain from the intervention can then be summarised. With no treatment 1.35 QALYs (3 × 0.45) are produced, with treatment 5.60 QALYs (8 × 0.70) are produced, thus the gain is 4.25 QALYs. Figure 10.1 shows this graphically.

This approach of using utility is not restricted to similar clinical areas but can be used to compare very different health programmes in the same terms. As a result 'cost per QALY gained' league tables are often produced to compare the relative efficiency with which different interventions can turn resources invested into QALYs gained. Comparability then is the key advantage of this type of economic evaluation. For a decision-maker faced with allocating scare resources between competing claims, CUA can potentially be very informative. However, the key problem with CUA is the difficulty of deriving health benefits. Can a state of health in fact be collapsed into a single value? If it can then whose values should be considered in these analyses? For these reasons CUA remains a relatively underused form of economic evaluation.

Cost–benefit analysis

Cost–benefit analysis (CBA) is concerned with allocative efficiency. Under this form of economic evaluation, costs and benefits are measured in commensurate units (normally money). While the other forms of economic evaluation deal with relative efficiencies, CBA can be used to evaluate health programmes in a more absolute way. So we can ask is intervention X worthwhile per se? Are the benefits greater or less than the costs? CBA can reveal the net economic impact of an activity: gain or loss. Only activities that generate a net economic gain might then be considered further by comparing the magnitude of the gain under different activities.

CBA can be used to consider allocative efficiency in its widest sense because once benefits have been converted into monetary terms then the net economic impact of very different activities can be compared. The gain to society from, for example, building a new bridge might be compared with prescribing a new pharmaceutical. Resources might be reallocated based on the results of CBA until the point when any further reallocation of resources cannot make anyone better off without making at least someone else worse off. This is the point known as 'Pareto efficiency', named after a famous economist Vilfredo Pareto.

The main problem with the CBA approach in health care is very obvious, how do we measure or 'convert' benefits from health programmes into monetary values? Well this is a very difficult issue and many health economists would still argue that it is futile to do so. There are, however, two main techniques for the monetary valuation of benefits: the 'human capital' and the 'willingness to pay' approaches. With the human capital approach the benefit of a health programme is measured by how it helps the patient return to or increase his productive output. Productive output can be easily valued using actual or proxy wage rates. Clearly this approach will not always be appropriate, especially in the case of children or the elderly. The willingness to pay approach assumes that the utility an individual gains from an intervention is valued by the maximum amount they would be willing to pay for it (out of their own pocket!). Various research methods have been developed to illicit from individuals their monetary valuation of health benefit. This has proved to be a very successful research area and is developing rapidly. However, it is still difficult to get away from the fact that inevitably willingness to pay is a function of ability to pay and results may be more a reflection of wealth than valuation of benefit.

The final section of this chapter is dedicated to a practical example of a cost–effectiveness analysis. This illustrates some of the methodology outlined above.

ECONOMIC EVALUATION CASE STUDY: THE NOTTINGHAM SAFE AT HOME PROJECT

The Nottingham Safe at Home Project (NSHP) was undertaken to assess the effectiveness and cost–effectiveness of a package of injury prevention interventions. A controlled intervention study was used to test the hypothesis that there was no difference in injury frequency or severity between children aged 3–12 months at entry, who received the primary care based interventions, and those in the control group, who received usual care. The initial study took place in 36 general practices across Nottingham, the final combined study population was 1100 children in the intervention group and 1019 children in the control group. Further details of the trial design and the effectiveness study are reported elsewhere (Kendrick et al 1999), the cost–effectiveness study is reported here.

Interventions

The study intervention consisted of four elements. Parents received a combination of these, based on an assessment of their need for accident prevention education and/or equipment and their willingness to participate.

Safety advice was provided at routine child health surveillance (CHS) discussions. Parents of children aged 6–9 months (315 visits) and 18–24 months (535 visits) received this intervention from health visitors. Parents of children aged 12–15 months (463 visits) received this intervention from practice nurses. Approximately 10 minutes was spent on discussion of safety.

Specific additional home safety checks (HSC) were carried out by health visitors to identify hazards and offer limited advice. This intervention took an average of 1 hour. A total of 235 HSC visits were carried out.

First aid training (FAT) for parents ($n = 152$) was provided at 16 half-day group sessions. Each of these FAT sessions was led by a health visitor. In addition, a free mobile crèche facility was provided (£40 a session).

The safety equipment scheme (SES) provided accident prevention equipment for households in the study. Most received a safety equipment pack consisting of stairgates, fire surrounds, smoke alarms and cupboard locks, depending on their needs and environment. A total of 107 safety equipment packs were provided.

Costs to the NHS of providing CHS, HSC and FAT were calculated on the basis of staff time. The hourly rate for health visitors was taken directly from Netten (1994). This gives a basic figure of £15 per hour; however, based on Dunnel & Dobbs (1982) a client contact multiplier of 1:1.9 is suggested. This means that for each hour of client contact a further 1.9 hours are required in preparation, travel and administration. This produces an overall cost per client contact hour of £44. This figure was used as this study only collected data on client hours, no data was collected on travel or other costs incurred by staff. The same approach was used to cost practice nurse time (£23 per client contact hour).

The average cost per SES pack was £47. A nominal user charge was set at £5 for each stairgate or fire surround, £0.50 for each smoke alarm and £0.20 for each cupboard lock. A total of 143 stairgates, 69 fire surrounds, 96 smoke alarms and 158 cupboard locks were provided.

A total of £25707 was spent on these four interventions targetted at a group of 1100 children. The mean cost of providing the package of interventions is £23.37 per child.

Treatments

For economic evaluation, only NHS costs have been considered. The main items of resource use identified to be associated with the treatment of accidental injuries were treatment at A&E; treatment within primary care; hospital admission; outpatient or GP follow-up consultation.

Treatment at A&E was recorded by type. Many children received multiple treatments. Hospital admissions were measured by length of stay. Outpatient visits were simply counted. Treatment at the GP surgery was also quantified by type. Where a referral from hospital back to the GP was indicated, one additional GP follow-up consultation was assumed. Where a referral from the GP to secondary care was indicated, full service use data was captured in the hospital notes. Injuries involving a fracture were all assumed to require an additional X-ray at the follow-up outpatient visit.

Valuation of these resources employed several methods. A&E treatment costs were estimated by assuming a baseline value (£25), derived from local finance data, for the minimum treatment which consisted of advice only. An increment was then added for other types of treatment based on an estimation of the additional time and materials needed. The same method was used to arrive at unit costs for treatment carried out within primary care, with the anchor point (£15) derived from Netten (1994). Hospital admissions (£120 per day) and outpatient visits (£30) were costed based on local hospital finance data. For injuries involving a fracture an additional cost (£25) was added for a follow-up assessment X-ray.

Treatment costs were observed over a period of 2 years after the initial intervention, a discount rate of 5% per year was applied. Discounted and undiscounted treatment costs are presented.

Results

Effectiveness

The injury rate in the intervention and control groups was found to be very similar. A total of 477 injuries were observed in the group receiving accident prevention interventions and 448 injuries in the control group, receiving no specific health education about accident prevention. Table 10.1 shows the distribution of the number of injuries. There was no statistically significant difference in the number of medically attended injuries between the intervention and control groups.

Table 10.1
Number of medically attended injuries by treatment group

Injuries (no.)	Intervention group[a]	Control group[a]
0	754 (68.6%)	689 (67.6%)
1	248 (22.5%)	231 (22.7%)
2	75 (6.8%)	83 (8.1%)
3	16 (1.5%)	13 (1.3%)
4	4 (0.4%)	3 (0.3%)
5	3 (0.3%)	0 (0%)

$\chi^2 = 2.10$, 3df, $p = 0.55$ (categories 3, 4 and 5 injuries combined)
[a] Number in group given, followed by percentage in parentheses

Simple analysis shows that the mean number of injuries was 0.4336 per child in the intervention group and 0.4396 per child in the control group, a difference of 0.0060 ($P = 0.85$). This represents the incremental gain in effectiveness measured in terms of the number of injuries per child.

Further analysis to account for the clustered nature of these data, calculating the mean injury rate per practice, weighted by the number of children in each practice was carried out. Comparison of matched practice pairs from the intervention and control groups with respect to the proportion of children with at least one medically attended injury found that the weighted mean rate of suffering one or more injuries was 31.4% of children in the intervention group and 32.4% of children in the control group. Thus the difference between the means is 0.93% ($P = 0.77$), which represents the incremental gain in effectiveness measured in terms of risk of an injury.

A further outcome measure was the severity of injuries observed, measured by the abbreviated injury scale (AIS), on a scale of 1 (minor injury) to 6 (fatal injury). Very little difference was found between the two groups. The median, 25th centile and 75th centile values for the AIS for both treatment groups was 1. A mean AIS score was calculated for each child, thereby taking account of injury severity scores in children with repeated injuries. The mean score did not differ significantly between the two groups ($P = 0.87$).

Costs

Injury treatment costs were also found to be similar in the two study groups. Total treatment costs, discounted at a rate of 5%, were calculated at £26 940 for the intervention group and £22 329 for the control group. Thus despite a lower injury rate, the mean overall treatment cost per child was 12% higher in the intervention group (£24.49) compared

to the control group (£21.91). Observed differences between the two groups in total treatment cost were not significant ($P = 0.46$).

Table 10.2 shows a breakdown of mean injury treatment costs per child by cost category, no significant differences were found in any category. In both groups treatment at A&E makes up about half of all treatment resource use. Inpatient and then outpatient treatment account for the next largest proportions of total resource use. The most important difference between the two groups is in the mean costs of treatment at A&E.

Non-parametric tests and log transformations were carried out, to account for the skewness of

Table 10.2
Mean injury treatment costs per child by cost category

Cost category	Statistic	Intervention group cost per child	Control group cost per child	Difference
A&E treatment	Discounted (5%)	£12.58	£11.03	+£1.55 (14.1%)
	Undiscounted	£13.61	£11.93	+£1.68 (14.1%) [95% CI, −£0.47, £3.84]
	% of total	51.3%	50.3%	+1.0%
Primary care treatment	Discounted (5%)	£0.90	£1.09	−£0.19 (17.4%)
	Undiscounted	£0.97	£1.18	−£0.21 (17.8%) [95% CI, −£0.57, £0.16]
	% of total	3.7%	5.0%	−1.3%
Inpatient admission	Discounted (5%)	£6.04	£4.79	+£1.25 (26.1%)
	Undiscounted	£6.55	£5.18	+£1.37 (26.4%) [95% CI, −£4.66, £7.38]
	% of total	24.7%	21.8%	+2.9%
Outpatients (inc. X-rays)	Discounted (5%)	£4.36	£4.61	−£0.25 (5.4%)
	Undiscounted	£4.72	£5.01	−£0.29 (5.8%) [95% CI, −£1.85, £1.28]
	% of total	17.8%	21.1%	−3.3%
GP follow-up	Discounted (5%)	£0.62	£0.39	+£0.23 (59.0%)
	Undiscounted	£0.67	£0.43	+£0.24 (55.8%) [95% CI, −£0.01, £0.49]
	% of total	2.5%	1.8%	+0.7%
Total	Discounted (5%)	£24.49	£21.91	+£2.58 (11.8%)
	Undiscounted	£26.52	£23.72	+£2.80 (11.9%) [95% CI, −£4.61, £10.21]

Stopping the runaway.

Table 10.3
Results of cost–effectiveness analysis

Variable	Discounted (5%)	Undiscounted
Total costs		
Intervention	£52 647	£54 879
Control	£22 329	£24 161
Mean cost per child		
Intervention	£47.86	£49.89
Control	£21.91	£23.71
Incremental cost (I-C)		
Total	£30 318	£30 718
Per child	£25.95	£26.18
Incremental effectiveness (I-C)		
Injury rate		0.0060
Risk of injury		0.93%
Cost-effectiveness ratios		
Cost per injury prevented	£4317	£4355
Cost of 1% reduction in risk of injury	£27.90	£28.14

some cost data. The Mann–Whitney U test found no significant differences between total injury treatment costs in the two groups ($P = 0.9976$). After log transformation of the data, differences in injury treatment costs remained insignificant ($P = 0.968$); this was also the case when zero values were excluded ($P = 0.820$).

Cost–effectiveness

Table 10.3 summarises the results of cost–effectiveness analysis. The combined discounted total of intervention and injury treatment costs for the intervention group is £52 647–£47.86 per child. The total discounted cost for the control group is £22 329–£21.91 per child. Hence the incremental cost associated with the intervention is £25.95 per child. This gives an incremental cost–effectiveness ratio of £4317 per injury prevented and £27.90 for a 1% reduction in risk of injury.

Sensitivity analysis

The cost of the study interventions is dominated by the cost of staff time. Variability in this parame-

ter may therefore alter results. There may be some uncertainty over the most appropriate hourly rate to use for health visitors. One-way sensitivity analysis shows the impact of this change on overall results.

Initially a value of £44 per hour was used for health visitors; if instead a value of £15 is used total intervention cost becomes £11.74 per child. This means that the cost–effectiveness ratios are £2387 per injury prevented and £15.40 for a 1% reduction in risk of injury. Results are sensitive to changes in the hourly rate used for health visitors, but the cost of injury prevention remains considerably higher than observed treatment costs.

Threshold analysis was carried out in order to demonstrate what change is required in the values of key parameters in order to make the study intervention cost-effective. Two parameters are considered here, the reduction in injury rate per child associated with the intervention and the treatment cost per injury (intervention and control).

Table 10.4 shows the three threshold values compared with the undiscounted study values. The

Table 10.4
Threshold analysis (undiscounted treatment costs)

Parameter	Study values	Injury rate threshold value	Cost per injury (intervention group) threshold value	Cost per injury (control group) threshold value
Number of injuries	477	**6**	477	477
Intervention group	448	448	448	448
Control group				
Cost per injury	£61.16	£61.16	**£0.79**	£61.16
Intervention group	£53.93	£53.93	£53.93	**£113.49**
Control group				
Intervention cost per child	£23.37	£23.37	£23.37	£23.37
Reduction in injury rate per child	0.0060	**0.4342**	0.0060	0.0060
Treatment cost per child	£26.52	£0.33	£0.34	£26.52
Intervention group				
Control group	£23.72	£23.71	£23.71	£49.90
Intervention cost per child	£23.37	£23.37	£23.37	£23.37
Cost per injury prevented	£4356	−£0.02	£0.40	−£0.72
Cost–benefit result per child	£26.17	−£0.01	−£0.00	−£0.00

reduction in injury rate required to enable the intervention to generate net cost savings is 0.4342 per child. This would mean that instead of observing 477 injuries in the intervention group, just six would have been observed. This is not a plausible variation in this parameter, since the injury rate within the control group was observed at 0.4396. The threshold value would constitute a 98.8% reduction in the average number of injuries per child. When the cost per injury for intervention group patients reaches a threshold value of £0.79, the intervention generates cost savings.

This is unlikely to be a plausible variation for this parameter given that no variation in injury severity was observed in the study. When the cost per injury for control group patients reaches a threshold value of £113.49, the intervention begins to generate cost savings. This value is some £52.33 higher than that observed in the intervention group, which constitutes a treatment cost difference of 86%. This figure is also more than twice that observed for average treatment costs in the control group. Such a variation would only be plausible if significant difference in injury severity between the two groups was observed.

Conclusion

Thus the conclusion of this economic evaluation is that the package of primary care accident prevention interventions detailed in this study are not a cost–effective means of reducing minor childhood injuries in the home. This is due to very small, insignificant gains in effectiveness associated with the intervention, low cost of treatment for injuries that are avoided relative to intervention costs; and no difference in treatment costs for the intervention group compared to the no intervention group. Future studies are unlikely to demonstrate cost–effectiveness unless they aim to reduce injuries of a greater severity than those assessed in this study. Thus the recommendation for policy-makers would be that these interventions may not in fact be the best use for healthcare resources.

REFERENCES

Drummond M, Stoddart G L, Torrance G W, O'Brien B 1997 Methods for the economic evaluation of health care programmes, 2nd edn. Oxford Medical Publications, Oxford

Dunnell K, Dobbs J 1982 Nurses working in the community. HMSO, London

Kendrick D, Marsh P, Fielding K, Miller P 1999 Preventing injuries in children: cluster randomised controlled trial in primary care. British Medical Journal 318:980–983

Netten A 1994 Unit costs of community care. PSSRU, University of Kent

USEFUL SOURCES OF REFERENCE

BMJ Guidelines for Authors 1996 Guidelines for authors and peer reviewers of economic submissions to the BMJ. British Medical Journal 313:3 August

Economics and Operational Research Division Central Health Monitoring Unit, Statistics Division, Department of Health 1996 Burdens of disease: a discussion document. Department of Health, Wetherby

Economics and Operational Research Division, Department of Health 1994 Register of cost–effectiveness studies. Department of Health, London

Jefferson T, Demicheli V, Mugford M 1996 Elementary economic evaluation in health care. BMJ Books, London

Kobelt G 1996 Health economics: an introduction to economic evaluation. Office of Health Economics, London

Netten A et al 1995 Unit costs of community/care. PSSRU, University of Kent (published annually)

Office of Health Economics 1995 Compendium of health statistics, 9th edn. HMSO, London

WEBSITES

Health Economics Places to Go. Online. Available: http:/www.uni-bayreuth.de/departments/vwliv/hec.html

Health Economics Research Group, Brunel University. Online. Available: http:/http 1.brunel.ac.uk:8080/dept/herg/home.html

Health Economics links. http:/www.york.ac.uk/res/herc resource

11 | A simpleton's guide to management

In draughting the outline to this book, I recklessly put in a chapter on management. It is very much a personal practice essay based upon 25 years' experience as a tight rope walker with vertigo — mainly terrifying, but occasionally exciting. These may be ten pages of personal indulgence or the key to successful practice.

Success in service delivery is dependent not only upon the skills of individuals, but also on the quality of their collaboration and the wider frameworks of the organisation. This short chapter is a personal view, a series of hints for how individual skills blend into a successful organisation. The simpleton is myself (not the reader), who has struggled to balance his roles as manager, individual clinician, team member, advocate, representative, investigator, teacher, servant and friend.

The clinician is often ill-prepared in temperament or knowledge to take on a role in managing a large organisation or a small part of it and training comes far too late, if at all. The following sections discuss some of the major management and team issues that face the clinician. They are not written in management speak. The further reading lists more conventional texts on National Health Service (NHS) management.

MANAGEMENT — A LANGUAGE IN ITSELF

Management has generated a language of its own and this is often not part of the medical curriculum. There can be a conflict of cultures: are managers there to help or control, to impede or facilitate, to make tasks easier or more difficult? Personalities can easily merge into stereotypes of Lancelot Sprat

clinicians and John Clees character managers, with a spot of Mr Bean invading both characters.

Clinical management is described in terms such as consultant episode, untoward event, resource allocation, critical pathway analysis and cost improvement. We may have mastered clinical terms such as multiple idiopathic haemorrhagic sarcomatosis, but management terms and their understanding seem to drive our time away from rather than towards clinical tasks. Yet the paediatrician, whether as a doctor, team leader, clinical director of a speciality service or medical director of a NHS trust, needs to be able to address certain management tasks so that the clinicians can deliver a safe and effective service.

The manager has several key tasks as well as clinical leadership. Just as the general does not simply wave his sabre and shout 'charge' or the conductor just stand up and wave his baton, there are other key tasks that make the battle or the concert a success.

Quality

You need good musicians who can actually play the piece with instruments of quality. The quality of the performance will be reported by the press. In medicine, clinical guidelines will be produced and standards of service capable of being audited will be set. Individuals will require training and updating and their individual performance needs to be reviewed and careers developed. The 25-year-old commando would not be expected or able to carry out the same duties at age 55. Community services often have a 'never mind the quality, feel the width' approach in which contacts are counted, simply adding together severe cerebral palsy and a minor colour vision problem as 1 + 1.

Skill mix and staffing

It's no use having 12 tubas and no violins. In health the mix of professions and grades is more complex than the orchestra. In the army the number of soldiers must meet the needs for combat. An outnumbered army will soon be defeated and a poorly staffed health service will rapidly develop waiting lists with only the most severe cases being seen. This must be provided throughout the year and take account of seasonal variations in demand and supply — school holidays, winter illness peaks. There are also limits to the number of hours that staff can work and there are requirements for rest breaks.

Supplies

The orchestra will require music and programmes, the army will require ammunition and the health service requires medicines and other consumables to be available when needed.

Finance

Soldiers, musicians and health service staff all need to be paid as well as providing for maintenance of their equipment.

Information

The army requires information in terms of intelligence and in terms of its own deployment of troops and their activity. The health service also requires information on morbidity and mortality, the numbers of patients waiting for or enrolled in programmes of care and the outcomes achieved.

Capacity management

Just as the seating in a concert hall is finite, so are the slots for patient appointments. Concert goers may not want to wait 5 years for a ticket and then find they are booked to see a ballet rather than an opera. At the other end of the spectrum the concert hall may be nearly empty with the orchestra outnumbering the audience.

Planning

An orchestra will have a programme of concerts covering the current year with plans for the next 2 or 3 years. In the health service, there is the same need for an annual business plan and a 3-year strategic plan.

Risk management

The army commander wishes to avoid casualties in his own troops and is responsible for individuals being trained for the tasks that they are carrying out and for the battle plan to be superior to that of the enemy. The enemy, may, of course complain if they lose. The health service has just the same requirements to limit risk.

DESCRIBING A SERVICE IN MANAGEMENT TERMS

A service can be divided into individual programmes of care, the delivery of each of which will be covered by a contract or service agreement.

Programmes of care in the community would usually follow the headings given in Box 11.1. A commonly used framework is that of describing structure, process and outcome. *Structure* is the nuts and bolts, including people, required to deliver the service. *Process* is the activities that are carried out as part of the programme and should, where possible, be covered by a clinical guideline based upon the best evidence available. *Outcome* is what is achieved as a result of the programme taking place. Outcomes may be difficult to quantify and are not necessarily described in terms of cure. They may be described in terms of well being, quality of life, support, patient satisfaction. They may also be distant from the programme as is the case in some of the early intervention programmes described in Chapter 23 on health inequalities. Structure, process and outcome may also be the subject of audit.

Established services used to continue for year to year on the basis of the biblical method of assessment — 'He looked at it and saw that it was good'. Nowadays, existing services and especially

---

Box 11.1
Programmes of paediatric care in the community

Services for all children
Child health promotion programme
• Core screening programme

• Accident prevention

• Immunisation

• Health education and promotion

• Dental health
Adolescent health

Services for children in need
Disability
• Developmental paediatrics

• Behaviour

• General paediatrics and chronic illness

Social
• Child protection

• Disadvantage

• Children looked after

• Adoption and fostering

---

requested developments have to stand up to a robust series of questions, which ask more testing questions than in the structure, process, outcome model:

• What unmet need will be addressed by this service?
• Is there existing evidence that the proposed service can meet those needs?
• What are the aims and objectives of the service?
• How will the service be accessed?
• How can equity be ensured?
• Has there been consultation with users and are they supportive of the development?
• What resources are needed to deliver the service?
• What are the costs per case and for the service as a whole?
• What is the process and clinical guidelines to be followed?
• What is the expected capacity of the service in terms of numbers of patients and throughput?

• What collaborative arrangements with other agencies need to be in place? Have they been consulted and are they in favour?
• What outcome measures are expected?
• What performance targets might be set?

These are the sorts of hoops that a manager might have to jump through to set up a new service or justify the continuation of an existing service at its present level.

THE INDIVIDUAL

Balances need to be made between the individual's desire to progress in his career, the needs of the organisation for staffing in each of its specialty areas and the need to ensure a uniformly high and safe standard of practice. This is regulated by a mixture of the supply and demand of the working place and regulation and advice provided by organisations such as Royal Colleges and the General Medical Council.

A system of appraisal is generally in place in which an annual review takes place between an individual paediatrician and his manager. This reviews the previous year's activity in both positive and negative terms, highlighting successes and difficulties. Recommendations can be made in terms of training, professional development or achievements and these are mutually agreed between appraiser and appraisee. The system can be a positive experience that enhances the career progression of the individual, providing protected time for preparation and discussion, with common purpose and harmony between appraiser and appraisee. Training for the role of appriasor is particularly useful. Rarely, it can become a less than symbiotic dreaded encounter.

THE TRAVELLING PAEDIATRICIAN — TIME, PLACE AND TRACKING. PAEDIATRIC 'AIR TRAFFIC CONTROL'. THE DIARY, WATCH AND PHONE

Managing others starts with managing oneself. For the community paediatrician the task can be complex because of the wide range of activities and venues into which he must divide himself. It is important to take control and have a framework into which activities can slot, rather than working in reactive mode, trying to fit in every demand.

A weekly timetable with a fixed number of slots is a good starting point. The slots might be:

- clinics
- home visits
- school visits
- case discussion
- on call
- urgent problems
- staff meetings
- administration
- committees
- teaching
- research
- Continuing Medical Education (CME).

The slots are a sort of paediatric 'Air Traffic Control'.

When the slots are full, no more activities can be fitted in. New work can only be undertaken if a slot becomes available by a task no longer being undertaken, by a task being delegated to another member of staff or if the new task if of such high priority that it displaces another activity.

The overcommitted paediatrician will perform badly, will always have a backlog of work that grows, will be behind time on the daily schedule and constantly under stress. In a team situation, stress is an infectious disease and at the end of the day, the functioning of the whole team becomes poor.

Three key instruments, in addition to clinical 'gear', for the community paediatrician are the diary, the watch and the telephone.

The diary has the overall plan with regular weekly or monthly engagements. It also contains projects, such as planning a new service or writing this book. Each of these projects is assigned a start time and a finish time and the slots in which the work will take place. Without doing this, projects are not completed or indeed never started. How many people serving on a committee rarely or never attend and are represented in the minutes by apologies? The diary also contains the protected time for holidays and leisure activities.

The watch is the more detailed level of organisation to the diary. It is concerned that individual

appointments are of the correct length and timing. There needs to be some flexibility built in to take account of the unexpected. Flexibility also ensures that one is not constantly rushing. There must also be breaks in the working day and continuous activity becomes more and more ineffective.

The telephone is potentially the most dangerous instrument. Mobile phones increase the danger! Communication is clearly a vital function for all doctors. For the community paediatrician, who may visit several different places in the day, communication can be a special challenge. Lodging a weekly timetable and indicating the times when you are available to receive or make telephone calls is a simple means of avoiding unscheduled interruptions which can distort the programme for the rest of the day. Interruptions are particularly unwelcome in clinical consultations when the patient may feel there are competitors for your undivided attention. A pager is often more effective than a telephone as you are in control over when you speak to the caller.

Caseload management

This is a process for being in control of your workload. It means understanding your personal capacity to see and care for patients. If capacity is constant and more new referrals are received than discharged, then you will come under increasing pressure. Knowing the numbers in your caseload, referrals and discharges and trends with time is essential information. A paediatrician should not be a passive recipient of referrals, but must consider whether they are appropriate and take action if they are not. Within a team, cases need to be allocated according to the needs of the patient and the skills of team members.

Case management

This is the overall plan for the care of an individual patient. It prevents drift in the 'follow-up 6 months' syndrome, in which there are no clear plans of what you want to or are able to achieve. Case management increasingly follows local or national clinical guidelines and shared protocols between professions and agencies. The individual is expected to know and adhere to them. An individual care plan, well developed in nursing practice, involves a process of assessment, setting objectives, choosing interventions and their time-scale, identifying the professionals involved, setting outcomes and reviewing progress to achieving them.

WHAT BINDS GOOD CLINICIANS INTO SUCCESSFUL TEAMS?

Even the most unlikely teams can be successful. In the case of the story of the Wizard of Oz, all the team members had a disability: the lion had no courage, the scarecrow had no brain and the tinman had no heart, but their collective effort was successful. The reasons were that they had a common purpose; they had determination; they had confidence in one another; they had leadership; and they had an agreed plan of action. The same criteria could be applied to community paediatric teams. The framework given in Box 11.2 is recommended.

Understanding one another's roles is easier in a team where all members belong to the same pro-

fession. In the multidisciplinary team (a potential clinicians' Tower of Babel), more effort is required to ensure that each profession has a good understanding. It cannot be assumed that this is acquired through initial training. External frameworks, for example legislation or the policy of professional bodies, may constrain (or guide) the freedoms of individual team members.

For most clinicians, the situation is more complicated than that given above in that they belong to several teams, which may include a locality clinical team, one or two subspecialty teams based at district level, a management team and a research team.

SORTING NETWORKS

Community paediatrics is not just about what you know, but who you know. Where there are few services, networks are sparse, but a modern community paediatric service might easily have several hundred contacts. Other organisations and agencies will include: primary health care teams; hospital paediatric services; child and adolescent psychiatry; public health; local education authority;

Box 11.2
Recommended framework for a community paediatric team

- Small, stable teams with a low level of staff turnover (a proxy for job satisfaction)

- Written, clinical evidence based guidelines (wherever possible) for the duties undertaken by the team. Commitment to these guidelines is facilitated by the widest possible consultation and discussion during the process of production or revision. The guidelines would apply to all teams operating within a district, though there is sometimes the need for small local procedural differences to take account of special local circumstances

- Control of workload through case allocation, clear referral and discharge criteria, caseload monitoring (individual caseloads, referrals and discharges) and waiting list monitoring. An estimate needs to be made of the *capacity* of the team to accommodate cases so that any rise in numbers should trigger discussions on staff numbers

- Protected time (preferably weekly) for team meetings to discuss case allocation, to share information and to discuss individual clinical problems

- A designated team leader. This responsibility can rotate

- Effective communication pathways between team members

- Attention to good record keeping, so that team members can pick up the threads of others' cases when ill or on holiday

- To all of these must be added personal respect and commitment to stick to joint decisions. Individual temperament or personality may lead a person to function well in one team, but not in another

A simpleton's guide to management

individual schools; social services; police and voluntary organisations. Each one of these divides into several (or many) other teams, so it is easy to see how large the service network can become.

At one level, we need to know the names, addresses and telephone numbers related to individual service groups. At another level we need to understand their internal structures and hierarchies. In medical practice we would not be confused between a medical student and a consultant, though, in dealing with a social services department, precisely this confusion can be encountered.

Where a programme of care is shared between several teams, for example in monitoring a child protection plan or in the care and education of a child with a disability, a similar set of criteria for effective cooperation arise to those listed above for individual teams. There are, however, several additional considerations to be taken into account.

Local service agreements

These agreements may be required to decide how much time one team will give to another, for example how much school health time will be allocated to an individual team. This, in turn, will depend upon knowledge of the need — in this case pupils with special education and special medical needs, child protection issues, children in need and delivery of the child health promotion programme. Good information systems are required as well as the freedom to share this information for planning purposes.

Sharing costs

Sharing costs can lead to difficult negotiations, especially where both agencies involved have budget deficits. Sometimes there are national guidelines, but usually local agreements need to be made. Lengthy discussions can, in themselves, be costly and hold up the provision of services to an individual child.

Service planning

Joint planning ensures a shared knowledge of what each service provides, prevents duplication and leads to a better level of coordination and most efficient use of resources. The information derived from this process must cascade to all levels.

Service directories

For the general public, bringing together all information about children's services (and keeping it up to date) can be invaluable. Common examples are services for pre-school children or a directory of services for children with special needs.

WELL-RUN PROGRAMMES OF CARE

Individual programmes of care will be covered by a contract or service agreement. At its simplest level, this would consist of a count of contacts. At a more sophisticated level, it might include waiting times, patient satisfaction, uptake, referral pathways and, of course, outcomes and performance targets that might be set locally or nationally. The example in Fig. 11.1 lists some of the information that might be required about a screening programme.

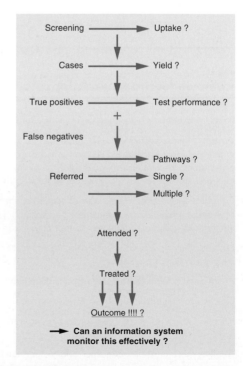

Fig. 11.1 Information that might be required about a screening programme

Where a programme is delivered from several (or many) sites consideration has to be given to access, and the times service is made available.

MEETINGS MATTER

Meetings have been described as 'the practical alternative to work'. They may, in reality be 'the practical alternative to anarchy'. They may vary from corridor discussions to minuted meetings operating under formal procedures. Some may be brainstorming meetings; others involve more detailed planning and many consist of day to day management of business. All can be valuable activities. Effective committees must make decisions and be attended by the majority of its members.

Meetings or committees require:

- A clear remit or purpose.
- A defined place in the organisational structure with pathways for referring questions (setting an agenda), reporting and dissemination of information.
- A record of attendance, discussions, conclusions and recommendations.
- A time period that should not continue beyond the stamina of its members.
- To be chaired in such a way as to facilitate the contributions of all of its members.
- The chairman to keep order and to be able to summarise quite detailed discussions.

MONEY MATTERS

Costs are discussed in Chapter 10 on health economics. Individual managers act as budget holders for their service. In practice there is often very little leeway in spending as most of the budget is used for salaries and fairly fixed costs for consumables, investigations, maintenance, travel and education. However, money can be released for new purposes, for example by better use of skill mix, ensuring that highly skilled and expensive employees are not carrying out tasks that can be accomplished by those working at lower grades. Clinicians should be as comfortable working with accountants as they are with other medical professionals. Accurate costing of service developments is an essential component of management work in the NHS.

SURVIVING OR MANAGING CHANGE

We trained hard — but it seems every time we were starting to form teams — we were reorganised.

I learned later in life that we tend to meet any new situation by reorganising and a wonderful method it can be for creating the illusion of progress while producing confusion, inefficiency and demoralisation.

Petronius Arbiters 210 BC

Public services often seem to be in a constant state of reorganisation. This may consist of building upon present practice or more radical 'knock it down and build it up again' strategies. The keys to surviving this process are:

- Start as early as possible.
- Allocate time even though, inevitably, it will have to be taken away from another activity.
- Import knowledge and experience from the literature or work in other centres.
- Try a small pilot first, before total implementation.
- Ensure open and frequent reporting to all to obtain cooperation, but also to avoid the danger of rumours.

ACCIDENTS DO HAPPEN — MAKING THE BEST OF COMPLAINTS

Every trust will have a local procedure for handling complaints with a short time-scale for investigation and response to the complainants. Small numbers of complaints are inevitable as are, we hope, some compliments. A designated person usually has responsibility for coordinating the management of complaints. Sometimes they can be used in a positive sense to improve the service. They most often arise from some problem with communication or a perceived feeling of offence from a patient. Complaints can usually be resolved by positively addressing the patient's concern rather than adopting defensive approaches.

INFORMATION — FRIEND OR FOE?

Information is needed for both individual medical care, for management, report writing and planning.

Several thousand different forms exist in the public services to feed our appetite for information. Information returns may, at times, appear to have a low priority against the necessities of clinical practice, but may, in the longer term, provide the evidence that supports extra resources being allocated. Information is discussed in Chapter 3 — child public health and Appendices 1 and 2.

The doctor with a management role needs to ensure that information collected is complete and accurate and that information received is critically commented on and its implications thought about. Tables without commentary and interpretation are of little use. Data collections no longer of any use should be pruned, where possible.

Information that might cross a medical manager's desk include the relative proportion of time spent in different activities (e.g. child protection, child development, behaviour management, general paediatrics), and changes in their distribution.

BALANCING FINITE RESOURCES AND UNLIMITED DEMAND

Priorities are the things that are most important or the things that we are told are most important. They are often linked to specific targets, which means we need to have measurements of activity, morbidity or mortality to match each of these targets. They are rarely linked to the permission to stop doing things that are not priorities and new money does not always follow on from new priorities. Demands frequently increase faster than resources.

There is no simple answer to this dilemma until we acquire the ability to turn lead into gold. Suggested approaches include:

- Cap in hand.
- Strict adherence to referral, discharge and capacity principles, which will inevitably lead to a lengthening of waiting lists.
- Pray that the policy will be changed (again).
- A combination of these strategies.

In developing health services (and in research and development programmes) priorities are often set according to the following model:

- Does this fit with national policy guidance? (targets, indicators)
- Is it an important clinical problem? (morbidity, mortality)
- What is its prevalence and variation from locality to locality?
- What are the costs, long and short term, to the NHS and to other bodies such as education, social services, social security?
- Is there evidence for the effectiveness of the planned intervention (and cost effectiveness)?

Aims, objectives, 'to do lists', wish lists, priorities, planning, strategy, policy

Making one's own plans, rather than responding to external pressures or guidance is an alternative or perhaps, more reasonably, parallel approach. There needs to be a broader strategy layered onto the day to day service. A commonly agreed list of two or three joint short- (this year), medium- (2–3 years) and long-term, (5–10 years) goals is about an achievable size. Translating a wish list into an action list requires a list of milestones for the achievement of practical steps to achieve these wishes.

Annual business plan

NHS trusts are required to produce an annual business plan. In essence this outlines the proposals for what the service is to achieve in the next year. It consists of those elements that have been provided in previous years and which need to be continued and service developments. The business plan is costed so that both the cost and expected benefits are available for discussion and publication. Management speak is changing very rapidly with the introduction of primary care trusts in April 2001. Bids for extra funding need to be included in the SaFF (service and financial framework). The 3-year strategic plan addresses longer-term planning and initiatives.

For practical reasons, services need to be measured and described in fairly precise terms.

Volume might mean the number of patient contacts or the number of cases currently managed by a service or team. The capacity of the service is the number of cases that it can manage. New cases can be accepted if some patients are discharged, if the capacity is increased or if the allocation of time to each patient in the system is decreased. There are very delicate balances involved in this process.

Quality standards might be set for the service. This might require meeting targets for structure, process or outcome measures.

Quality may be divided into the following components:

- *Quality policy*: the overall quality intentions and directions of the organisation and this should be formally stated by top management.
- *Quality management*: this will determine and implement the quality policy and must have some control and influence on the planning and distribution of resources.
- *Quality systems*: this is the structure that identifies the service, the standards and the resources needed to ensure quality.
- *Quality control*: these are routine activities aimed at monitoring the service and identifying unsatisfactory performance.
- *Quality assurance*: this is planned systematic action to demonstrate to the management and to the user that the service provided meets the user's requirement.
- *Clinical guidelines* are the agreed professional outlines for clinical practice. They are based upon the best evidence available and the protocols that those working within the service are expected to follow.

Audit is a component of quality assurance. Clinical guidelines need to be subject to audit, a process through which compliance with standards set by clinical guidelines may be monitored. It may result in changes to ensure closer compliance with guidelines or identify areas where guidelines may need to be re-examined or modified.

The value of audit includes the following:

- It is in the children's interests that we should, for the purpose of audit is to raise standards. The risk is that it will merely waste time.

- It is in our interests because it will allow us, if it is effective, to use our time and energy more effectively.
- It is required albeit in a very limited and not too satisfactory a form by the higher professional training bodies which are concerned with the training of consultant staff and therefore might act as a bar to obtaining accreditation.
- It is in itself a valuable educational tool. It allows the introduction of clinical change in a controlled manner. It demonstrates to the established and the learners how to define clinical requirements, how these might be changing, how they might be addressed and which approach is the more effective. The educational value is thought by some to be the main benefit of medical audit.
- It should, linked to financial audit, make all the staff concerned and the 'users', in our situation their families, be aware of the cost of the service and the commitment of the carers.
- Last but not least the government 'invites' us to do it. It may become a required part of any contractual arrangement, though there is no guidance on this at the present.

Audit only makes sense against the background of quality management.

Standards and outcomes

Standards, policy statements, protocols, guidelines, indicators, manuals of practice are all words which are being used in an attempt to set up framework for quality assurance. There are difficulties with such exercises, for even timely statements produced by the most distinguished panels of experts often fail to recognise the complexity of the item of service and settle for what can be measured, which may be a measure of service (short waiting times) or a crude outcome measure like mortality rates which are influenced as much if not more by many factors which are nothing to do with the health provision. It seems probable that there will be much talk in the future about clinical standards, agreed outcome measures and achievable targets.

One aim of this book is to broaden the discussions beyond a narrow review of limited, measurable hospital activities.

A simpleton's guide to management

TIME TO GO HOME — LIVING TO TELL THE TALE!

Medicine can easily overrun every other aspect of human life. The manager needs to ensure for himself and his staff that work does not take over recreation and family life. Without this balance, work does progressively become less productive.

THE LAST STRAW — FORGET THE STIFF UPPER LIP!

It is most important to remember the pressures that all paediatricians are under in terms of stress and workload and recognising what we cannot do — remove poverty, transform poor parenting overnight or double resources. A working environment should be established which provides support to individuals and in which it is both expected and safe to voice personal anxieties, fears and frustrations.

POSTSCRIPT

This is the theory to which we should aspire. In personal terms it is far from the reality. The future climate may prove more favourable for achieving this. Do as I say, not as I do!

FURTHER READING

Drucker P S 1989 The new realities in government and politics, in economy and business, in society, in world view. Heinemann, Oxford

Lessem R 1989 Global management principles. Prentice Hall, New York

Øvretveit, J 1993 Coordinating community care, multidisciplinary teams and care management. Open University Press, Milton Keynes

Rigby M, Ross E M, Begg N 1998 Management for child health services. Chapman & Hall Medical, London

12 | Health services for children

INTRODUCTION

The character and scope of health services for children in the UK have changed progressively during the 50 years since the inception of the National Health Service (NHS) in 1948. The 1990s in particular have seen dramatic changes in the settings in which services are provided, the workforce providing the services and in arrangements to monitor the effectiveness of these services.

Health services in the UK are conventionally classified as primary, secondary or tertiary care (Fig. 12.1) and these are defined below.

Primary care

This describes the services that are available for and are intended to be delivered to all children and to which they may be referred directly. It is based on the primary healthcare team relating to general practitioners and includes child health surveillance and health promotion, which is now largely provided through the primary healthcare team.

Secondary care

This describes the specialist services required by some children, which are based in community and hospital settings within a locality and are accessed by referral from another professional, usually through the primary healthcare team.

Tertiary care

This describes the highly specialist services based in a small number of large centres, and usually accessed by referral from a secondary care team.

Traditionally the health services for children were considered to be either community based or hospital based, the former being provided through the local authority and the latter by the NHS. Following the 1974 NHS Act the local authority services became the responsibility of the district health authority and since that time there has been a gradual blurring of the distinctions between community- and hospital-based services. The first real attempt to reform the anachronistic tripartite system of child health care in Britain was the report in 1976 by Professor Donald Court which achieved little at the time (Court 1976). However his vision was assisted by the development of the concept of a combined child health service, by the British Paediatric Association, bringing together the hospital and community child health services with the aim of integrating them with the services provided through primary healthcare teams (British Paediatric Association 1991). Subsequently a joint working party on medical services for children recommended the creation of a unified career structure in secondary child health by assimilating clinical medical officer and senior clinical medical officer grades into the mainstream medical career structure, and encouraging the creation of more posts with duties in both the hospital and the community (British Medical Association and Department of Health 1992, NHS Management Executive 1993). There is an increasing tendency for both secondary and tertiary paediatric care to be provided both in the hospital setting and in the community, and it is now more helpful to consider children's services simply in terms of primary, secondary and tertiary care, rather than as hospital or community based (British Medical Association and Department of Health 1992).

Health services for children

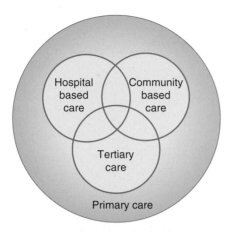

Fig. 12.1 Community, hospital and tertiary care together form a 'combined' child health service, which is 'integrated' with primary care. From British Paediatric Association (1994). Reproduced with permission from the Royal College of Paediatrics & Child Health.

NEW STYLES OF PRACTICE

The 1990s have seen several new initiatives in the way in which health services may be accessed and provided. There has been a tendency for services which traditionally would have been provided in hospital to be provided in a community setting, leading to the development of a variety of ambulatory services for children which are described in detail below. In the UK ambulatory paediatrics is considered to include all non-inpatient services and therefore includes emergency practice as offered in many hospital day-case units.

In 1998 the new Labour government started to introduce NHS Direct, a new nurse-led telephone advice line, which it plans to extend to all parts of England by the end of the year 2000. The service will be provided through approximately 20 major call centres, staffed by approximately 1500 nurses, some of whom will have children's training, and it is likely that 40–50% of calls to NHS Direct will concern children. The introduction of this entirely new service for the public will have significant, but as yet unknown, effects on primary care and on hospital-based emergency services.

Another new government initiative is the introduction of walk-in centres in a variety of settings including shopping malls and stations. While it

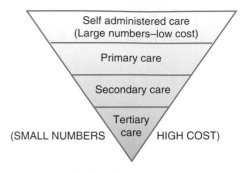

Fig. 12.2 Pyramid of health care

is intended that these centres will offer an emergency service at primary care level the impact on more traditional health service provision is at present uncertain.

PYRAMID OF CARE (Fig. 12.2)

The great majority of clinical care takes place in the community, in other words at home or in school, although it is less visible than the services provided by hospitals. Much of this care is initiated and provided by members of the child's own family, a smaller proportion through primary care services and even less through the secondary and tertiary services. NHS Direct and walk-in centres are both aimed principally at the top layer of the pyramid. Health promotion should largely take place in the home or community as well but responsibility for its coordination lies with the community child health service.

Children who have a disability such as cerebral palsy or Down's syndrome, and their families, have long been cared for primarily in the community and this is increasingly the case for children with chronic illness such as cystic fibrosis or leukaemia, the majority of whose care is now provided in the community with the assistance of outreach teams including children's community nurses.

AVOIDING ADMISSION TO HOSPITAL

National data shows clearly that the number of children admitted to hospital for medical conditions increased steadily during the 1980s and

1990s, although it may now be reaching a plateau (Fig. 12.3).

At the same time the length of stay in hospital has fallen steadily so that the average length of stay in acute paediatric units is commonly less than 2 days (Fig. 12.4). This welcome reduction in the length of time children spend in hospital has been helped by groups such as Action for Sick Children, which has campaigned to improve health services for children and to avoid admission where possible. Reduced

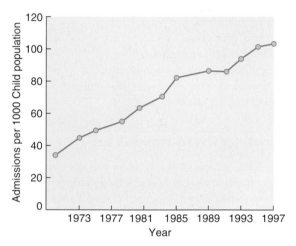

Fig. 12.3 Paediatric admissions per 1000 child population age 0–4 years. After Macfaul and Loerneke.

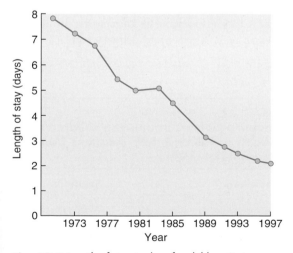

Fig. 12.4 Length of stay in days for children 0–4 years. After Macfaul and Loerneke.

lengths of stay have been achieved by an increased focus on provision of outreach services from hospital, accepting that even quite complex types of care such as nasogastric tube feeding, administration of intravenous antibiotics or subcutaneous infusions can safely be undertaken by parents with appropriate clinical supervision. The development of ambulatory care including children's day units, hospital at home, emergency referral clinics and other new patterns of service provision have all aimed to reduce the need for admission to hospital, while providing a safe and effective service for children.

NEEDS OF THE CHILD AND THE FAMILY

Children's health services must be organised in such a way as to meet the needs of children and families. However often this does not actually happen.

The Audit Commission has pointed out in its report 'Seen but not Heard' that legislation emphasises that people's health and social care needs must be identified and services provided specifically to meet them (Audit Commission 1994).

Social services, the education authority and the health service must assess the overall needs of children and families in their area and develop plans to meet those needs according to agreed priorities. Often this does not happen and the House of Commons Health Committee concluded in 1997 that 'children's health services at present are too often based on traditional custom and practice or indeed on professional self interest. Children's health services must be needs led, not based on historical patterns or the self interest of provider groups', and that 'urgent attention must be given to the present fragmentation of provision within the NHS, in combination with measures to address the fragmentation between the health, social and education services', and 'joint planning and funding between health, social and educational services is required, especially in respect of the care of children who have a chronic health problem or disability.' (House of Commons Health Committee 1997).

The government has made it a statutory requirement that children's service plans should be drawn up and published but this requires a degree of inter-agency cooperation which does not always work effectively at present.

Child health promotion

All children have a need for child health promotion, a generic term which includes:

- A programme of immunisation.
- Child health surveillance, which includes screening tests and developmental assessment.
- Health promotion services which aim to help families in bringing up healthy children through advice and health promotion.
- Access to acute care when required.

These services are defined and detailed in the third edition of 'Health for all Children' (Hall 1996).

Children in need

There is a group of children who are unusually vulnerable and require specialist services. They are often referred to as children in need and include:

- Children who have been abused or are in need of child protection.
- Children with a disability such as spina bifida, cerebral palsy or Down's syndrome.
- Children who are 'looked after' by the local authority and who have often suffered from deprivation or abuse.
- Children with a chronic illness such as cystic fibrosis or leukaemia.

Many of these children have more than one disability. The average number of disabilities experienced by children living in families is 2.6. In severely disabled children under 5 the average number of disabilities was 9.4 per child (Social Services Inspectorate Report 1998). These children and their families therefore have complex needs in terms of health service, education and social service provision. In order to meet these needs there must be joint planning to produce programmes of care ensuring a coordinated approach by professionals and other agencies. Some of these tasks require named paediatric and nursing responsibility from specialised professionals, for example named per-sons for child protection, for immunisation and for children who are 'looked after'.

Key tasks

In order to meet these needs the following key tasks must be undertaken in the community (Royal College of Paediatrics and Child Health 1999):

- A full range of services to children with developmental and physical disability behavioural problems and general paediatrics.
- The full range of educational medicine.
- Adoption and fostering and support of 'looked after' children.
- Child protection.
- Child health surveillance.
- Specialist immunisation advice.
- Audiology and other specialist clinics.
- A public health overview.

Meeting these needs (Table 12.1)

The 1990 reform of the NHS in the UK separated the commissioning of services from their provision. This purchaser/provider split placed a responsibility on health authorities to commission (or purchase) health services from service providers or trusts. The reforms led by the new Labour government from 1997 retained the distinction between commissioners and providers of services and led to the development of primary care groups and primary care trusts which in their fully developed form will be responsible for purchasing certain services as well as providing primary care. The local

Table 12.1 **Major problems in meeting children's health needs and their solutions (Audit Commission 1994)**	
Problems	**Solutions**
Insufficient collaboration	Working together
Ambiguity of roles	Child centred
Support is not needs led	Focus on needs

or district health authorities continue to have a commissioning role and their work is coordinated by the eight regional NHS executive headquarters in England and the Departments of Health in Scotland, Wales and Northern Ireland. From April 2002 Strategic Health Authorities will replace district and regional management. They will be intermediate in size between the two levels they will replace. The service as a whole is directed by the NHS Executive (1998b) (Fig. 12.5).

There has also been a drive to improve quality of care across the health service by setting nationally agreed standards. National Service Frameworks have already been produced for cancer (Calman–Hine) and for paediatric intensive care — 'A Framework for the Future' — and will be followed by frameworks for mental health and coronary heart disease (NHS Executive 1997). These frameworks will help to define the pattern of services and set standards for their provision. Other important national initiatives include the National Specialist Commissioning Advisory Group which is responsible for commissioning highly specialist services such as heart transplantation, paediatric liver services and craniofacial surgery in a small number of specialist centres, and the Clinical Standards Advisory Group which has set national standards for the provision of such services as leukaemia in

children, neonatal intensive care, depression, and outpatient services.

SERVICE PROVIDERS FOR CHILDREN

The principal providers of health services for children are primary care Trusts and acute NHS trusts.

Primary care Trusts are being set up across the UK and in England comprise a collection of primary care services covering a population of approximately 100 000 people. The detailed arrangements differ in Scotland, Wales and Northern Ireland but the basic structure of services is similar. This development will encourage close working relationships between family doctors and others providing primary care and may well lead to the development of more specialist services based in primary care. The role of primary care trusts extends into purchasing secondary services. NHS trusts provide secondary and tertiary services and cover a range of services as follows:

- Acute services.
- Community health services — child and adult.
- Mental health services.
- Teaching hospital or tertiary acute trusts.

The development of primary care trusts together with workforce and financial constraints is leading towards the merger of trusts in many areas and may lead to a reconfiguration of the way in which secondary care services are provided in future.

An integrated child health service

In order to achieve an integrated child health service the primary care and secondary care services must work closely together in order to provide a 'joined up' service. The model shown in Fig. 12.6 has been recommended by the Royal College of Paediatrics and Child Health (1999).

The optimum pattern of service provision is the development of combined paediatric and child health departments, bringing together the acute and community paediatricians and including where practicable child and adolescent mental health.

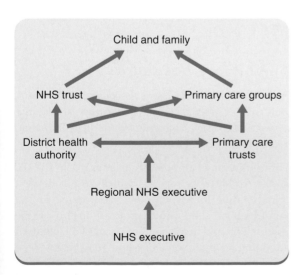

Fig. 12.5 The managerial structure of the NHS in England, from 1998

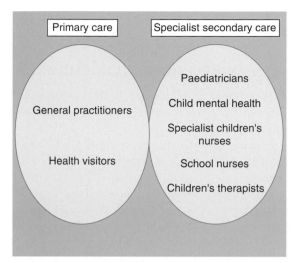

Fig. 12.6 An integrated child health service. From Royal College of Paediatrics and Child Health (1999)

CHANGING PATTERNS OF PRACTICE

The provision of health services and patterns of practice are undergoing progressive change.

Drivers for change

In the UK at present the main drivers for change are:

- The quality agenda and clinical governance.
- Developments in clinical practice.
- Increasing specialisation.
- Changing roles of health authorities and development of primary care trusts.
- Increasing public demands and expectations.
- Changing roles of medical, nursing and other clinical staff.
- Moves towards a consultant provided service.
- Structured training programmes for specialist doctors (Calman training).
- Resource and in particular workforce constraints.

These forces are together encouraging reconfiguration of health services, and this applies in particular to the acute hospital trusts but also affects others including the community child health services.

Reducing admissions

It is clearly in the interests of children and their families for care to be provided without the need for admission to hospital if at all possible. Recognition of this, together with the drivers for change described above, have encouraged attempts to reduce the admission rate of children to hospital and to bring down the length of stay in hospital for those who have to be admitted. This may be achieved through a variety of initiatives:

- Prevention of illness, for example through better immunisation uptake and new immunisation schedules.
- Enhancing the role of the primary care team by improving child health training.
- Providing support to primary care through hospital-based acute assessment units and provision of children's community nursing services.
- Research on different models of service provision including day-case provision.
- Development of community child health services.

If effectively implemented a fall in admission rates for children to hospital and their lengths of stay would be likely to lead to a need for fewer paediatric inpatient units. There would also be effects on the provision of other specialties in acute hospitals, in particular obstetrics and accident and emergency services.

Ambulatory paediatrics

Ambulatory paediatrics is a philosophy of care which aims to avoid hospital admission whenever possible and whenever admission is needed to reduce its duration to a minimum. (RCPCH 1998)

This definition of ambulatory paediatrics in the UK applies to all those services which do not depend on admission to hospital and therefore covers all non-inpatient child health practice including the assessment and treatment of acutely ill children attending hospital, some of whom may be observed for short periods of a few hours (Royal College of Paediatrics and Child Health 1998). The Royal College of Paediatrics and Child Health has commended the development of facilities for specialist assessment of acutely ill children including short stay observation and admission units. A range of different models have been developed which include:

- day assessment units
- emergency referral clinics
- hospital at home services
- paediatric community nursing services.

Day assessment units

Day assessment units have been set up in many hospital children's departments and good examples have been described from the North Middlesex Hospital in London, Wolverhampton and York (Beverley et al 1997, Meates 1997). The aim has been to improve the quality of the children's service but several have described a reduction in admission rates as well. Opening hours vary, some offering a 9 to 5 service, others remaining open through the evening; some for 5 and others up to 7 days a week. Children are usually referred acutely from primary care but in some units elective cases are seen as well. The concept has been extended in Wolverhampton and in Hackney where units are open 24 hours a day but individual children do not stay for longer than a few hours for observation. All these services depend heavily on a well-developed community nursing service which can offer on-going support to the child and family out of hospital.

Emergency referral clinics

Emergency referral clinics have been developed within A&E departments in several large hospitals including those in Leicester, Liverpool and Manchester. They take referrals from primary care and some also from accident and emergency departments and aim to provide a more accessible service and rapid turnover.

Hospital at home

Paediatric inpatient services at Whiston Hospital on Merseyside consist of two inpatient wards, a chil-

dren's day ward and a hospital at-home service for children. Following assessment and observation at the hospital children may be admitted to the hospital at home rather than an inpatient bed if it is considered their clinical care can be managed satisfactorily at home with up to four visits per day by the nursing team. It is staffed by children's trained nurses who rotate from the inpatient wards for a period of 6–9 months in order to maintain their acute nursing skills.

A hub and spoke model

The tendency for acute trusts to amalgamate and their services to reconfigure is likely to lead to the development of hub and spoke models of service with more specialised inpatient services provided in the hub and a range of ambulatory paediatric services in one or more spokes. Examples have been described from Slough (hub) and Heatherwood (spoke), and from Worcester (hub) and Kidderminster (spoke). Worcester and Kidderminster are 18 miles apart and travel time is less than 30 minutes between the two. Acute medical paediatric services were combined in 1996 and a children's day-case centre opened in Kidderminster supported by a full inpatient unit in Worcester, and by a hospital at-home service which covers both districts.

Community paediatric nurses

Most acute paediatric units now employ a number of specialist paediatric nurses who provide outreach to the community usually from a hospital base. They have developed particularly in the fields of oncology, asthma and diabetes and some are now developing generic community children's nursing teams.

Thus practice in the UK in general and community child health, as well as tertiary level paediatrics, is largely ambulatory in nature in that specialist care is delivered where possible in the community.

Ambulatory paediatric practice should offer the following advantages for children and their families:

- Improved management of sick children.
- More accessible and better care for children and families.
- Improved communication and coordination of service between consultants and family doctors.
- A reduction in admission of children to hospital and possibly of accident and emergency attendances.

THE WORKFORCE

Child health services are provided by a wide range of clinical and other professionals including family doctors, consultant paediatricians and supporting staff, child and adolescent psychiatrists, children's therapists, clinical and educational psychologists and a range of nursing staff with a variety of qualifications and skills.

Medical staff

Primary care services including child health surveillance are largely provided through primary care by family doctors, general practitioners who are supported in this work by health visitors. The practice of family doctors is almost entirely generic but it is possible that the advent of primary care trusts serving populations of around 100 000 may lead to a degree of specialisation, particularly in relation to non-acute work such as child health surveillance and child health promotion.

Specialist services for children at secondary level are provided by consultants in community paediatrics or in general paediatrics and these consultants usually have an area of special interest. In community paediatrics for example the special interest may be in child protection, or children who are 'looked after', and in general paediatrics in neonatal care or diabetes. In smaller departments of child health consultants may work both in a hospital setting and in the community and a flexible working arrangement of all clinical staff between the hospital and the community should be an aim of a combined child health service.

Tertiary specialist care is provided by consultant paediatricians or by university clinical staff with specialist training and experience, for example in

paediatric oncology or paediatric nephrology. It is likely that tertiary specialties will develop further in relation to community specialties such as the more difficult areas of child protection and complex disability.

A core training programme for all paediatricians encourages the development of a wide range of skills and experience in general and community paediatrics. This presently takes 4 or 5 years in general professional and higher specialist training before a trainee takes up a particular specialty or subspecialties.

Nursing staff

A variety of staff with different nursing backgrounds are involved in the provision of child health services. They include:

- midwives
- health visitors
- school nurses
- specialist community nurses.

Midwives are responsible for the newborn infant during the early neonatal period. They usually undertake the first examination of the newborn infant for congenital anomalies and are involved in advising and assisting the mother with the establishment of breast feeding.

Health visitors are nurses who have received additional training and play a key part in the provision of child health promotion in the early years. Health visitor services are most often provided through attachment of health visitors to general practices but in some areas they are organised on a patch basis, each health visitor serving a discrete geographical area.

School nurses deliver a service to schools or to groups of schools and are at present likely to cover many different general practices. This arrangement could change with the development of primary care trusts. School nurses now undertake very little routine school medical work and much of their work is with children who have special needs.

Specialist community nurses are usually children's trained nurses who have received additional training in a specialist area of work and most often provide an outreach service from a hospital base.

The House of Commons Health Committee has recently recommended a rationalisation of nursing roles in the community child health services and it is possible that in the future community paediatric nurses may have a more generic training, although a range of specialist skills will still be needed (House of Commons Health Committee 1997).

Professionals allied to medicine

Professionals Allied to Medicine (PAMs) include physiotherapists, speech therapists, occupational therapists and dietitians. There is an increasing trend for those working with children to have specialist training and experience and for their work to be community based. The integration of many children with special educational needs in mainstream schools has increased the complexity of provision of therapy services and their integration with other child health and education services.

Mental health staff

Child and adolescent mental health services are staffed by child and adolescent psychiatrists who work in teams with specialist nurses and social workers and sometimes with clinical psychology support. In addition, approximately 20% of referrals to community paediatricians are primarily for emotional and behavioural problems. It is therefore most important that there are close working relationships between the child and adolescent mental health service and the rest of the child health services.

Education and social services

The need for close liaison between the health services for children and education and social services has been stressed and should be assisted by raising the status of joint children's service plans. At a local level paediatricians usually develop close working relationships with educational psychologists and specialist support teachers.

QUALITY IN THE NHS

The new NHS will have quality at its heart. Without it there is unfairness. Every patient who is treated in the NHS wants to know that they can rely on receiving high quality care when they need it. Every part of the NHS, and everyone who works in it, should take responsibility for working to improve quality

(NHS Executive 1998a p 4)

Quality has been placed at the top of the NHS agenda and is to be implemented through hospitals and primary care trusts. A range of new statutory bodies has been established in order to set, deliver and monitor standards (Fig. 12.7).

The National Institute for Clinical Excellence

The National Institute for Clinical Excellence (NICE) has been established to promote clinical and cost effectiveness through guidance and audit. It will be responsible for appraisal and the production of guidance and its dissemination to the NHS. It will also need to monitor through clinical audit the application of its guidance. NICE represents a new partnership between the government, the NHS and clinical professionals and the government expects the guidance produced by NICE to be implemented consistently across the NHS.

The four established national confidential enquiries, including the Confidential Enquiry into

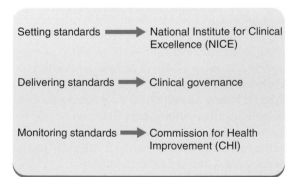

Fig. 12.7 The key elements of 'A first class service — quality in the new NHS'. From: NHS Executive (1998a)

Stillbirths and Deaths in Infancy (CESDI), come under the umbrella of NICE.

A programme of national service frameworks is also planned which will set national standards and define service models for a specific service or care group, support their implementation, and establish performance measures to measure progress.

Delivering standards

The delivery of quality standards is proposed through a programme of professional self-regulation, clinical governance and lifelong learning.

Clinical governance

Clinical governance can be defined as a framework through which NHS organisations are accountable for continuously improving the quality of their services and safeguarding high standards of care by creating an environment in which excellence in clinical care will flourish
(NHS Executive 1998b p 33)

Clinical governance will be part of an overall NHS governance framework and each NHS trust will be responsible for assuring the quality of NHS trust services. The principles of clinical governance apply not only to doctors but also to all those who provide or manage patient care services in the NHS. Trusts will nominate a single person to lead the development of clinical governance and ensure appropriate arrangements are in place.

Lifelong learning

In order to ensure that treatment is up to date and effective and provided by those whose skills have kept pace with new developments, a programme of continuing professional development (CPD) is being introduced into the NHS in order to meet both the learning needs of individual health professionals and to inspire public confidence in their skills. In future an individual's continuing medical education will be tailored to meet the service development needs of the NHS rather than simply the individual's professional needs. It will therefore be overseen and directed by their employer.

Professional self-regulation

Professional self-regulation aims to ensure that the clinical professions are openly accountable for the standards they set and the way that they are enforced. It is likely that the process of professional self-regulation will be open to public scrutiny and will be publicly accountable for professional standards set nationally and action needed to maintain these standards.

Monitoring standards

The government's monitoring programme will be effected through the Commission for Health Improvement (CHI), supported by a national performance framework and a national patient and user survey.

Commission for Health Improvement

The Commission's core functions will be to:

- Provide national leadership to develop and disseminate clinical governance principles.
- Scrutinise local clinical governance arrangements through a rolling programme of local reviews of service providers.
- Monitor national implementation of national service frameworks.
- Help the NHS identify and tackle serious or persistent clinical problems (troubleshooting).

The National Framework for Assessing Performance

The Department of Health has introduced a new performance framework which will focus on six main areas:

- health improvement
- fair access to services
- effective delivery of appropriate health care
- efficiency
- patient and carer experience
- health outcomes of NHS care.

Within these areas a new framework of high level indicators has been established which includes the following which have some application to child health (Box 12.1).

National Survey of Patient and User Experience

A new national survey has been undertaken by the Department of Health and is to be carried out annually. It will attempt to gather systematic evidence to enable the health service to measure itself against the aspirations and experience of its users and to compare performance across the country and to look at trends over time. The results of the first survey have yet to be published.

The government has set a huge quality agenda, the implementation of which will pose a great challenge to all those responsible for providing health services. The particular difficulties of developing evidence-based guidelines in many areas of child health practice must not be underestimated and our present outcome measures are imprecise and often dependent on factors outwith the control of the health service. However clinical guidelines have been produced for several areas of child health practice such as cystic fibrosis, neonatal care and oncology, although implementation of these guidelines has often been difficult.

There are also several examples of good practice guidance produced by professionals working together with voluntary groups. For example Scope (formerly the Spastic Society) assisted paediatricians in developing guidelines for breaking bad news to parents, and Action for Sick Children have produced guidelines for day treatment in children and on the care of young people in hospital, in con-

junction with doctors, nurses and commissioners of health services (Caring for Children in the Health Services 1991, Viner & Keane 1998).

PRIVATE, ALTERNATIVE AND COMPLEMENTARY MEDICINE

These services, which are provided outwith the NHS, have gained increasing prominence in recent years. They include unusual forms of allergy testing, cranial osteopathy as well as more invasive methods of treatment such as hyperbaric oxygen therapy and injection of animal cells as treatments for cerebral palsy and 'brain damage'. The scientific basis of most of these therapies is unclear and most have not undergone controlled evaluation.

The government has indicated its intention to apply its quality agenda and principles to the private sector as well as to the NHS, but it remains to be seen what if any effect these arrangements will have on the provision of alternative and complementary medicine.

OTHER DEPARTMENT OF HEALTH INITIATIVES

A series of important initiatives have been developed by the Department of Health which aim to improve access for the whole population to health promotion and services. These include:

- Inequalities in health which are as prevalent in children and young people as they are in the rest of the population and have been addressed by the 'Independent Enquiry into Inequalities in Health' led by Sir Donald Acheson (see Chapter 23).
- 'Our Healthier Nation' — which aims to improve the health of the population as a whole and to improve the health of those who are worse off in society.
- Health improvement programmes — which will be developed by health authorities, identifying local health needs and setting a programme to meet 'Our Healthier Nation' targets.
- Improving access to health services via NHS Direct and primary care centres (referred to earlier).

Health services for children

These initiatives have been complemented by the setting up of health action zones in England to target health inequalities through a partnership of health organisations with local authorities, community groups, the voluntary sector and local businesses. It is hoped that they will prove to be an effective way of tackling ill health and reducing inequalities in health.

CONCLUSION

The child health service aims to place the needs of children and young people, and their families first. The development of ambulatory styles of practice enables more specialist care to be provided in the community, avoiding unnecessary admission to hospital and reducing lengths of stay. More needs to be done to tackle inequalities, to develop a co-ordinated children's community nursing service, and to encourage joint planning and working with social service and education authorities.

REFERENCES

Audit Commission 1994 Seen But not heard. Co-ordinating community child health and social services for children in need. HMSO, London

Beverley DW, Ball RJ, Smith RA et al 1997 Planning for the future: the experience of implementing a children's day assessment unit in a district general hospital. Archives of Disease in Childhood 77:287–292

British Medical Association and Department of Health 1992 Report of the Joint Working Party on Medical Services for Children. BMA, London

British Paediatric Association 1991 Towards a combined child health service. BPA, London

British Paediatric Association 1994 Purchasing health services for children and young people, vol 1: Summary. RCPCH, London

Caring for Children in the Health Services 1991 Just for the day: children admitted to hospital for day treatment. Action for Sick Children, London

Court S D M 1976 Fit for the future. The report of the Committee on Child Health Services. HMSO, London

Hall D M (ed) 1996 Health for all children — a programme for child health surveillance. Oxford Medical Publications, Oxford

House of Commons Health Committee 1997 Second report. The specific health needs of children and young people, vol 1. The Stationary Office, London

MacFaul R, Werneke U Trends in paediatric hospital utilisation — the problem of "healthy babies" Publication pending

Meates M 1997 Ambulatory paediatrics — making a difference. Archives of Disease in Childhood 76:468–476

NHS Executive 1997 Paediatric intensive care 'a framework for the future'. Department of Health, London

NHS Executive 1998a A first class service. Quality in the New NHS. Department of Health, London

NHS Executive 1998b The New NHS modern — dependable. The Stationery Office, London

NHS Executive 1999 The NHS performance assessment framework. Health service circular HSC 99/078. Department of Health, London

NHS Management Executive 1993 Report of Joint Working Party on Medical Services for Children. NHS ME Executive Letter [93] 28. Department of Health, London

Royal College of Paediatrics and Child Health 1998 Ambulatory paediatric services in the UK. Report of a Working Party. RCPCH, London

Royal College of Paediatrics and Child Health 1999 Paediatric services within the community for the new millennium. RCPCH, London

Social Services Inspectorate Report 1998 Breaking down the barriers in services to disabled children. HMSO, London

Vine R, Keane M 1998 Youth matters: evidence based best practice for the care of young people in hospital. Caring for children in the health services. Action for Sick Children, London

WEBSITES

Up-to-date information on health services in the UK can be found on the Department of Health website: *www.gov.uk/dhhome.htm*.

13 | Child health in primary care

General practice provides the first point of contact with the health service for most people and provides continuity of care for individuals and families. It is estimated that 98% of the population are registered with a general practitioner (GP) (Royal College of General Practitioners 1997a). Patients present with problems that can be physical, psychological or social. GPs need to understand why a patient has come to see them and be able to sort out medical and non-medical problems. There is an increasing focus on preventive care and care of the community, in addition to focusing on individual patients who are ill.

GPs now work as part of a primary healthcare team with administrative, nursing, midwifery, health visiting and therapy staff. The care of children is a significant part of the workload of GPs and some members of the primary healthcare team. Under 15 year olds account for 20% of a GP's average patient list. The majority of children receive all their medical care from a GP, with only 9% requiring referral to secondary care (Royal College of General Practitioners 1996).

CURRENT GENERAL PRACTICE

GP principles are independent contractors, responsible for the care of patients registered with them, for employing staff and for running their practice. Most GPs work full time with only 12% working part time. The proportion of GPs who are female is rising and reached 31% in 1996. The average age of GPs is falling and in 1996, 70% were aged between 30 and 49 years. The size of practices is increasing and in 1995 only 10% of GPs were single handed. The majority of general practices are based in premises owned by GPs and increasingly these are purpose built. In 1997, it was estimated that 92% of practices were computerised (Royal College of General Practitioners 1997b).

From April 1999, the organisation of primary care changed with the advent of primary care groups (PCGs) and the phasing out of GP fundholding. PCGs serve a population of around 100 000 and have responsibility for commissioning care for the locality that they represent. GPs, community nurses, social services and lay people are represented on PCG boards. Key aims of PCGs are; (i) to develop primary care by joint working across practices and (ii) assuring quality of care (Department of Health 1997). Their role in the organisation of community health care will increase over the next few years. PCGs become trusts in April 2001 (see p.181).

HISTORY OF CHILD HEALTH CARE IN GENERAL PRACTICE

Before the introduction of the National Health Service (NHS) in 1948, GPs only provided care for children as private, fee-paying patients. Free health care for the under fives was provided in local authority child health clinics by health visitors and clinic doctors, while children who attended school were cared for by the school health service. The NHS Act made provision for free health care for all. As a result, more children received care from GPs but no change was made to the services provided by local authority child health clinics.

In 1967, the Sheldon Committee recommended that the care provided by child health clinics', for example, child health surveillance, health promotion and immunisations, should be incorporated into the care provided by GPs (Sheldon 1967). As a result, more GPs began to run baby clinics in their practices, and in 1974, there was a change in government policy encouraging health visitors to be attached to general practices rather than being locality based. However, by the time of the Court Report only 15% of GPs were running child health clinics in their practices (Court Report 1976). The Court Report again called for GPs to take over all responsibility for child health. In practicular, it suggested that there should be GP paediatricians with specialist training in child health.

Within the general practice profession major changes have taken place since the introduction of the NHS. In 1952, the College of General Practitioners was set up (now the Royal College of General Practitioners). In 1966, the Family Doctor's Charter introduced fees and reimbursements to encourage GPs to work together in group practices and to employ staff (British Medical Association 1965). In 1982, compulsory 3-year vocational training for general practice began.

In 1982, the Royal College of General Practitioners published guidance on the training and organisation required for providing child health in primary care (Royal College of General Practitioners 1982). There was still great variation in how child health services were organised both in general practice and in child health clinics. Standardising the provision of child health surveillance was of particular concern and successive Hall reports have provided a national framework for improving the quality of child health surveillance (Hall 1989, 1991, 1996).

The 1990 Contract introduced many changes to how GPs work, including targets for immunisations, audit, fundholding, and a new capitation fee for the under fives. This was to be paid for each child under five for whom developmental surveillance was provided. To qualify for this payment, GPs had to be appropriately trained and be registered with their local family health services authority (now their local health authority). The criteria used by different authorities varied greatly (Evans et al 1991).

Before the 1990 Contract, studies showed that between 35% and 55% of practices were providing child health surveillance (Butler 1989, Health Departments of Great Britain 1989). By 1995, 94% of GPs were registered to provide child health surveillance and now, for most children, all aspects of health care are provided by primary care teams in general practice (Department of Health Statistical Bulletin 1995).

GENERAL PRACTITIONER'S TRAINING IN CHILD HEALTH

As part of their vocational training, all GPs spend a year in a training practice and will learn about the care of children. Some will also complete a 6-month paediatric post but this is not compulsory. Surveys have shown that in 1990–91 between 40% and 55% of GPs had completed a paediatric post, either in hospital or in the community (Glickman et al 1994, Brown et al 1998).

Guidelines for the accreditation of GPs in child health surveillance were produced jointly by the Royal College of General Practitioners and the British Paediatric Association in 1989 and updated in 1991 (Royal College of General Practitioners et al 1991). These guidelines should be used by health authorities when GPs apply to be registered for child health surveillance, but they have not been universally implemented. They suggest that GPs should have provided systematic child health surveillance for 3 years or more, have recent experience in community child health, for example held a community paediatric post, or attended a recognised training programme consisting of six theoretical and six practical sessions. Also, a certificate of proficiency in child health surveillance is now a compulsory part of the membership exam of the Royal College of General Practitioners that is taken by many newly qualifying GPs.

CHILD HEALTH WORKLOAD IN GENERAL PRACTICE
Consultation rates

The average number of GP consultations per patient per year is rising and 0–4 year olds have a higher average consultation rate than all other age groups except the over 75s (Office for National Statistics 1997) (Table 13.1).

In 1995, it was estimated that 9% of GP consultations were with 0–4 year olds and 8% were with 5–15 year olds (Office of Health Economics 1997). 0–4 year olds were more likely to have a home visit than other age groups except those over 65 years old (Office for National Statistics 1997) (Table 13.2).

Conditions seen in general practice

The most common illnesses for which children see their GP are respiratory conditions (including asthma), and diseases of the nervous system and sense organs (including ear infections and epilepsy). However, the second most frequent classification for attendance is for reasons other than illness, for example child health surveillance and immunisations (Office of Population Consuses and Surveys 1995) (Table 13.3).

The disease groups for which 0–4 year olds are the most frequent attenders are:

- acute respiratory infections
- otitis media
- other infections, e.g. chicken pox, warts
- asthma
- skin disorders, e.g. atopic eczema.

Prescriptions

Prescribing rates vary greatly between GPs and in different areas but, in general, they are increasing year by year (Jones & Menzies 1999). In 1993, the average number of items prescribed per person was 8.8, but for under 16 year olds it was 4.8. The therapeutic groups for which children under 15 years most frequently received prescriptions in 1994 were:

- Infections (mainly oral antibiotics but also antifungals for thrush and treatments for thread worms).
- Immunology and vaccines (mainly vaccinations).
- Respiratory system, i.e. inhalers and hay fever treatment.
- Central nervous system, e.g. painkillers including paracetamol, and epilepsy drugs.

Table 13.1
Average number of NHS GP consultations per person per year

Patient age (years)	1981	1985	1991	1995
0–4	6	7	7	7
5–15	3	3	3	3
16–44	4	4	4	4
45–64	4	4	4	5
65–74	4	5	6	6
≥75	6	6	6	7
All ages	4	4	5	5

Source: Office for National Statistics 1996

Table 13.2
% Consultations with GPs by type of consultation

Type of Consultation	Patient age (years)					
	0–4	5–15	16–44	45–64	65–74	≥75
Surgery	81	84	89	86	84	59
Home	9	7	4	7	10	35
Telephone	10	9	7	7	5	6

Source: Office for National Statistics 1996

Child health in primary care

Table 13.3
Children consulting their GP by type of condition[a]

Condition	Patient age (years) 0–4	5–15
Diseases of respiratory system, e.g. viral infections and asthma	6 471	3680
Reasons other than illness, e.g. child health surveillance and immunisations	5 313	1140
Diseases of the nervous system and sense organs, e.g. otitis media, otitis externa, epilepsy	4 252	1881
Infectious and parasitic diseases	3 648	1888
Diseases of the skin and subcutaneous tissue	2 715	1418
Ill-defined conditions, e.g. rashes, headache, cough, abdominal pain	2 721	1363
Injury and poisoning	1 293	1375
All conditions	10 221	7234

[a] Rate per 10 000 person-years at risk
Source: Office of Population Censuses and Surveys 1995

- Nutrition and blood, e.g. oral electrolyte replacement, iron and vitamins.

There were at least twice as many prescriptions for under 4 year olds as there were for those aged 5–15 years (Office for National Statistics 1996).

Immunisations

Most children now receive their primary immunisations in general practice and these are usually given by practice nurses. Since the 1990 Contract, GPs have received a payment for reaching immunisation targets and a higher payment is received if 90% of children receive immunisations. In 1994, 91% of GPs were in practices that had achieved the higher target for primary immunisations and 82% were in practices that had received the higher payment for pre-school boosters (Department of Health Statistical Bulletin 1995).

Referrals to secondary care

In 1991/92, on average, 16% of all patients were referred to secondary care and the lowest rate was for the 5–15-year age group (6.7%). The highest referral rates amongst all age groups were to outpatients. Under 5 year olds had a relatively high referral rate to accident and emergency departments and to inpatient beds. Referral rates among adults did not reach the same level until the 65–74 year age group (Office of Population Censuses and Surveys 1991–92).

An example of child health care provided by one GP

To provide a snapshot of child health care as part of the workload of one GP, I analysed my own consultations and home visits in May 1999. Full-time GPs usually provide nine surgeries and have one half day off per week. The traditional working pattern is to do morning surgery followed by home visits, then an evening surgery which on some days might be preceded by an afternoon clinic. I analysed 9 days of consultations and home visits plus one Saturday morning and one baby clinic. This would be the typical workload of a full-time GP during 2 weeks at our practice.

I had 304 face-to-face patient contacts including 229 (75%) patients with booked appointments 49 (16%) emergencies and 26 (9%) home visits. Of the total number of contacts at home or in surgery, 50 (16%) were with under 18 year olds. Of these:

- 30 (60%) were booked appointments in normal surgeries.
- 15 (30%) were emergencies.
- 2 (4%) were home visits.
- 2 (4%) were 6–8 week child health surveillance reviews.
- 1 (2%) was seen at the well baby clinic at the request of the health visitor.

Therefore, under 18 year olds were more likely than older patients to be seen as emergencies.

The 50 contacts with under 18 year olds included four children who I saw more than once. Therefore, during the 2-week period, I saw 46 children. Most children presented with one problem at each consultation, but 9 (20%) children had more than one problem recorded.

The most frequent diagnoses recorded during the 50 face-to-face contacts with under 18 year olds are shown in Table 13.4.

Of the 50 contacts with under 18 year olds, 26 (52%) resulted in a prescription and 7 (14%) resulted in a referral. The most frequent prescriptions were for:

- emollients or low-potency steroid creams
- inhalers
- antibiotics
- the oral contraceptive pill
- antipyretics, i.e. paracetamol and ibuprofen.

The seven referrals included:
- A child where the diagnosis of asthma was uncertain — to a respiratory physician.
- A child with complications following grommet insertion — to ENT.
- A child with a probable distal radius/ulnar fracture — to casualty.
- A baby about whom the Mum and I had concerns about weight gain — to the health visitor for regular weighing and advice.
- A child with possible congenital dysplasia of the hips — to a paediatric orthopaedic surgeon.

Table 13.4
Most frequent diagnoses recorded during 50 face-to-face GP contacts with under 18 year olds

Diagnosis	Contacts (no.)
Upper respiratory tract infection (probably viral)	8
Eczema	7
Asthma	6
Otitis media	3
Oral contraceptive pill advice/ monitoring	3
Tonsillitis	2
Musculoskeletal pain	2
Unsettled/crying baby	2
Urinary tract infection	2
Diarrhoea and vomiting	2
School stress/bullying	2

- A boy with an inguinal hernia — to a paediatric surgeon.
- A child with probable appendicitis — to the on-call paediatric surgeons.

WHO IS INVOLVED IN CHILD HEALTH IN PRIMARY CARE?

The composition of the primary healthcare team can vary from practice to practice. Figure 13.1 shows the staff who generally are agreed to be members of the primary healthcare team and who are usually involved in the care of children.

Practice nurses, practice managers, receptionists and secretaries are usually employed by GPs, whereas the other members of the team have traditionally been employed by a local community NHS trust (previously the local health authority). Some practices may have a team within the primary

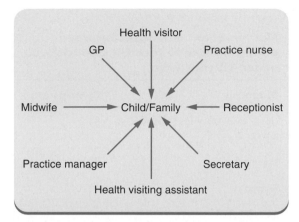

Fig. 13.1 The primary healthcare team usually involved in the care of the child

---

Box 13.2
Most frequent problems referred to GPs by health visitors

- Concern about weight gain
- Acute illness
- Concern about developmental delay
- Possible congenital dysplasia of the hip
- Possible squint
- Hearing problems
- Skin problems
- Problems that require a prescription

From Hampshire et al 1996

Box 13.1
Most frequent aspects of the role of the health visitor mentioned in interviews with health visitors and GPs.

- Advice and reassurance for parents
- Parental support
- Health education
- Child health surveillance reviews
- Referral
- Teamwork

From Hampshire et al 1996

---

healthcare team who have a particular interest in child health and work closely together in providing child health surveillance and baby clinics, for example a health visitor, a GP, a practice nurse and a receptionist.

GPs are involved in the care of well and ill children. The previous section on workload in general practice describes the common reasons why GPs see children. Although most problems are managed in primary care, it is vital that GPs know when and how to refer to secondary care and other services.

They also have an important role in providing continuity of care for children and families, sometimes following children as they grow up and have families of their own.

The role of the health visitor is discussed in Chapter 14. Health visitors mainly work with the under fives and play a key role in child health promotion. Health visitors and GPs in Nottingham were asked about the role of the health visitor, and the aspects they mentioned most frequently are shown in Box 13.1 (Hampshire et al 1996).

GPs and health visitors refer children and families to each other. The most frequent problems they refer are shown in Boxes 13.2 and 13.3 (Hampshire et al 1996).

Practice nurses are usually involved in child health by providing immunisations. A survey of practices in Nottingham found that in 79% of practices, the practice nurse gave primary and pre-school immunisations (Brown et al 1998). They also have a key role in the management of asthma which is common in children (prevalence estimated as over 10%, Crockett 1993) and may also see children for minor injuries.

Midwives are involved in the care of babies during the first month of life, although health visitors usually also visit from 10 to 14 days onwards. Midwives provide a programme of preparation

---

Box 13.3
Most frequent problems referred to health visitors by GPs.

- Feeding/dietary advice
- Sleep problems
- Parenting skills
- Behaviour problems
- Parental concerns/anxiety
- Concern about the mother's health, e.g. postnatal depression
- Child protection issues
- Social problems

From Hampshire et al 1996

---

for parenthood antenatally, provide immediate care of the newborn and advise mothers on infant care (United Kingdom Central Council for Nursing, Midwifery and Health Visiting 1998). They have an important role in monitoring early progress of the baby and helping mothers establish safe feeding.

Practice managers, receptionists and secretaries are all part of the administrative team within general practice. Receptionists are important because they are frequently the first point of contact for families. All are involved in ensuring that families receive the care they need and, increasingly, they are involved in preventive care, for example call-up systems for immunisation.

Teamwork in general practice

For the primary healthcare team to work well there should be:

- Agreed aims or goals.
- Effective communication.
- Individual roles that are defined, understood and valued.
- Mutual respect, trust and confidence.
- Appropriate use of skills.
- Involvement of all in decision-making.
- Commitment to the team.

- Joint audit and review.
- Regular meetings with open and honest discussion.
- Support for innovation (Pearson & Spencer 1997).

It is difficult to achieve effective teamwork with the average size of primary healthcare teams, i.e. 17–18 members. Also, because members are employed by different organisations with differing hierarchies, primary healthcare teams are even less likely to function well. When compared with other teams, primary healthcare teams had particularly low scores for participation, support for innovation and commitment to the team. To improve their effectiveness, there needs to be regular review of the team's goals and how to achieve them, and social support for individual members (Pearson & Spencer 1997).

Concern has been expressed that health visitors and GPs in particular, might not work well together in the care of children (Butler et al 1995). However, when health visitors and GPs in Nottingham were interviewed, only 7% of health visitors and 7% of GPs thought that communication with the other healthcare professional was difficult. Fifty per cent met at least weekly, usually after the practice baby clinic. They thought that teamwork was easier if the health visitor was based in the practice building (Hampshire et al 1996). Nationally, 61% of health visitors are practice based (Health Visitor's Association 1995).

In Nottingham, 82% of GPs had access to health visitor records and all health visitors had access to GP records; 53% of health visitors and 43% of GPs wrote in the records of the other health professional (Hampshire et al 1996). The personal child health record should aid communication between members of the primary healthcare team and with parents. It is almost always available and is well completed (Saffin & Macfarlane 1991, Emond et al 1995). However, not all professionals use the record to its full potential. In Nottingham, we found that 86% of health visitors always or usually wrote in the personal child health record at baby clinics, whereas only 21% of GPs always or usually wrote in it during surgery contacts (Hampshire et al 1996).

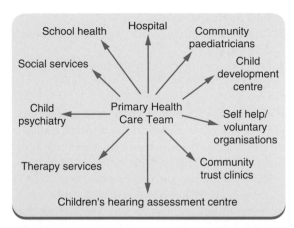

Fig. 13.2 Services to which the primary healthcare team refer children

It is used even less frequently when children attend hospital.

LINKS WITH OTHER SERVICES AND VOLUNTARY ORGANISATIONS

Communication

Most problems that children and families have are managed within the primary healthcare team. When referral is necessary, GPs and health visitors in particular have an important responsibility in accessing appropriate services for the child and family. They need to be aware of all the services that are available, how to refer and also what problems will best be managed by which services (Fig. 13.2). The quality of care that children and families receive from other services is very dependent on the appropriateness of referrals made by the primary care team.

A child needs to be referred with enough information to enable the other service to provide appropriate care. Good communication is very important. Most referrals will be written, usually as a letter but some will be by telephone (e.g. urgent referrals). The quality of communication back from the services to which a child has been referred is also important for maintaining quality of care. This is especially true when a child has complex problems and many people are involved in their care. Regular communication allows the primary care team to support the family and provide care that is com-

plementary to, rather than conflicting with, that being provided by other services. Where the GP is prescribing medication for the child this is vital.

The GP, in particular, provides important continuity for the child and family as the child grows up. Children with a chronic disease or disability will at some point be transferred to adult secondary services. This is a time when the quality of care provided can be severely compromised. GPs should be able to provide support during the transition and ensure that the young adult's health needs continue to be met.

Referrals to paediatricians

When a child needs referral to a paediatrician, in some areas, GPs have a choice of referring to a hospital or community paediatrician. One study that compared referrals from GPs to hospital and community paediatricians showed that GPs were more likely to refer behaviour problems, concerns about nutrition/growth, continence and orthopaedic problems to community paediatricians. Urogenital, cardiovascular, endocrine, respiratory and gastrointestinal problems were more frequently referred to hospital (Blair et al 1997). Another study looking at referrals to hospital outpatients (Ni Bhrolchain 1992), of which 89% were from GPs, found the following to be the most common reasons for referral:

- respiratory, e.g. asthma
- neurological, e.g. epilepsy, syncope and headaches
- cardiovascular, e.g. murmurs
- gastrointestinal, e.g. diarrhoea and vomiting.

In a minority of practices, consultants run outreach clinics. These provide greater accessibility for parents and primary care staff. Such outreach clinics are thought to be particularly useful in deprived areas (Spencer 1992).

Casualty and out of hours care

Children attend A&E services with minor injuries and illness, usually without referral from their GP (Carter & Jones 1993). Nevertheless, a recent study showed that 81% of out-of-hours contacts for 0–4 year olds were dealt with by GPs (Hulland 1997). Out-of-hours care for patients, including children, is changing rapidly with more and more care being provided by GP co-ops and deputising services. Again, communication back to the primary care team about diagnosis and treatment is important to enable continuity of care and to alert the primary care team about children or families with problems.

Child abuse

Identifying a case of child abuse may be a rare event for most GPs (e.g. one child every 5–8 years, Styles 1985). However, GPs and other members of the primary care team can be the first to detect the early warning signs in families where there are problems. They need to communicate their concerns within the team and follow local guidelines regarding referral procedures.

Although the overriding principle is to secure the best interests of the child, it is also important to support the family, to help them meet their child's needs (the Children Act 1989). The GP is likely to have the child, any siblings, their parents and possibly other members of the family registered with them. They have a duty of care to all, and are in the difficult position of needing to maintain a good relationship with the family, as well as notifying social services or any other relevant body of their concerns. Only a small proportion of child abuse investigations result in children being placed on the child protection register (Munro 1998) and all families going through such investigations face a traumatic time whatever the outcome. The primary care team can provide vital support through this process.

Although GPs have been criticised for not attending case conferences, their attendance may not be necessary (Harris 1991). They can provide useful information in the form of a factual written report and read/take action on the minutes of case conferences that they receive. When a child is placed on the 'at-risk register' it is important that all the primary healthcare team are aware and it is good practice for one member of the team to be responsible for ensuring that this occurs (see also Chapter 24).

CARE OF THE CHILD AND THE FAMILY IN GENERAL PRACTICE

A child's health and use of health services is influenced by their family and it also affects the family. The primary healthcare team usually have the advantage of knowing families well and can consider the family situation when caring for a child.

Most children's symptoms are treated at home without contact with the primary healthcare team. Campion & Gabriel showed that under 4 year olds have an average of one new symptom per week but parents consult for only 1 in 12 symptoms (Campion & Gabriel 1985). There are important variations in how children and families use healthcare services and decisions to consult are influenced by a complex mixture of physical, psychological and social factors.

One of the most significant factors is social class, which may be viewed as an indicator of deprivation. Analysis of the 4th National Survey of Morbidity in General Practice showed that the consultation rate of children rose from social class I–II to class IV–V. Children from class IV–V consulted more frequently for illness, for example infections, asthma, injuries and poisonings. However, they had a lower consultation rate for preventive services, for example immunisations and health promotion (Saxena et al 1999). Other studies have also shown that children from deprived families are more likely to consult their GP and use out-of-hours primary care services (Blaxter 1981, Campion & Gabriel 1985, Morrison et al 1991).

There are many possible explanations why there are differences in consultation rates associated with social class. It may be that social class influences uptake of services but social class is also linked with extent of morbidity and with factors that influence the health of children, for example low birthweight, breast feeding, nutrition, growth, housing type, unemployment and smoking (Blaxter 1981).

The 4th National Survey of Morbidity in General Practice also found that children from South Asian families had a higher consultation rate than other children (Office of Population Censuses and Surveys 1995).

Psychological factors may underlie responses to illness and need to be considered in terms of the patient's or, in this case, usually the parent's health belief model (Becker & Maiman 1975). There is conflicting evidence about whether or not children of single parents consult more frequently than those with two parents (Morrison et al 1991, Judge & Benzeval 1993, Office of Population Censuses and Surveys 1995). However, lay referral networks have a major influence on consulting behaviour and those with well-developed social networks consult less frequently (Campbell & Roland 1996). Some families respond to symptoms by attending the doctor more frequently than others and patterns of illness behaviour may also pass from one family generation to the next (Colling 1967, Huygen 1988). Maternal anxiety is associated with higher consultation rates and the perceived threat of an illness to the child is also important (Campion & Gabriel 1985, Kai 1996).

Other factors that are associated with increased consultation rates include the child being under 1 year old, being a first child and the severity of symptoms (Campion & Gabriel 1985, Wyke et al 1990, Morrison et al 1991). Wyke et al also found that children were more likely to consult with respiratory illnesses if there was a smoker in the household.

Another way that the family can influence a child's health is genetically, either through single-gene or multifactorial genetic conditions (Blaxter 1981). They may also influence a child's health through the role model they provide, for example teenagers are more likely to smoke if their parents smoke (Health Education Authority 1989).

It is important to remember that illness in children has an effect on the rest of the family. In particular, children with a disability or chronic illness influence relationships within families and parent's perceptions of their own health (Blaxter 1981).

So far, this section has highlighted the importance of understanding the health of the child in the context of the family. As children mature sometimes conflicts arise between the needs of the child and the needs or wishes of their parents. They start to consult the primary healthcare team on their own, without their parents. One survey of 15 year olds found that 26% had made their own appointment to see a GP and 91% thought that they should be able to see their GP confidentially (Brannen

et al 1994). A common example of this in primary care is when teenage girls consult for contraceptive care and do not wish their parents to be informed. If they have sufficient understanding they can consent to treatment and also have the right to confidentiality (British Medical Association 1993).

ORGANISATION OF CHILD HEALTH CARE WITHIN GENERAL PRACTICE

The organisation of care within practices varies greatly. A few factors that can influence the way that care is provided are practice size, style of premises and the community in which the practice is based, for example inner-city, rural, suburban.

Being child friendly

Ideally, practices should consider the needs of children, teenagers and parents when planning their services and the layout of practice premises. When parents have been asked their views about community and general practice child health clinics the main problems that they have identified are:

- Poor access for prams or push chairs.
- Lack of provision of play areas/toys.
- Premises not sufficiently clean.
- Lack of facilities for private discussion with health visitors in clinics.
- Lack of nappy changing facilities.
- Inconvenient clinic times.

General practice clinics were no worse than community clinics and fewer community clinics were considered to have good standards of cleanliness or provision for private discussion with a health visitor (Boyle & Gillam 1993, Sutton et al 1995).

In Nottingham, we observed child health clinics in 25 general practices (Hampshire et al 1996). The characteristics that were considered are shown in Box 13.4. Almost all the characteristics were achieved by over 80% of general practice clinics. However, 68% of practices had child health leaflets, 56% had a notice board specifically on child health issues and only 16% had a child toilet seat or potty available. There were some particular examples where extra consideration had been given to making the practice child friendly. For example,

Box 13.4
Characteristics of child health clinics observed in 25 practices in Nottingham.

- Generally clean waiting room
- Adequate seating in waiting room
- Toys in examination room
- Appropriate child health records available
- Full set of standard growth charts available
- Tape measure
- Scales suitable for weighing a child
- Suitable temperature of waiting room
- Provision for private discussion with a parent
- Toys in waiting area
- Someone to welcome parents
- Pram park (lockable) or space for prams in waiting room
- Provision for breast feeding in private
- Baby weighing scales (electronic)
- Suitable temperature of examination room
- Measuring mat (standard)
- Relevant child health leaflets freely available
- Notice board on child health issues
- Child toilet seat/potty in toilets

From Hampshire et al 1996

Table 13.5
Return rates of child health surveillance reviews from 28 practices in Nottingham.

Child health surveillance review	Reviews returned
10–14 day	87%
6–8 week	80%
9 month	72%

From Hampshire et al 1996

Another study of all general practices in Nottingham found that 94% provided a child health clinic and only 11% of these did not offer an open access system without appointments (Brown et al 1998).

Child health surveillance

Nottingham practices replying to a postal questionnaire about child health surveillance in 1994 indicated that, 87.5% provided child health surveillance (Brown et al 1998). GPs provided the neonatal and 6–8-week review and health visitors reviewed children at 10–14 days, 6–9 months, 18–24 months and 36–42 months. Some GPs also provided a pre-school review but this is not part of the current recommend pre-school child health surveillance programme (Hall 1996). The content of child health surveillance/child health promotion is discussed more fully in Chapter 20.

When we interviewed health visitors and GPs at 28 practices in Nottingham about child health surveillance (Hampshire et al 1996), a wide variation in how practices organised the call-up and recall of children was found. In general, health visitors were responsible for call-up and recall for the reviews that they provided and practice staff were responsible for call-up and recall for the 6–8-week review. Often GPs were not aware of how health visitors organised 'their' reviews. Having compared health visitor and GP answers per practice, it appeared that there was a call-up system for all reviews in only 21% of practices and a recall system for non-attenders for all reviews in only 29% of practices.

provision of child-size chairs and tables in the waiting area, large wall murals of characters from children's stories or a pet's corner.

General practice child health clinics were held in the late morning or early afternoon so as not to clash with times that parents might have to collect older children from school. All but two of the clinics were open access. A health visitor was always available, and at all but one clinic, a GP was also always available for parents to see. A practice nurse was available at 75% of clinics and immunisations were offered at all but two clinics (Hampshire et al 1996).

All health visitors and GPs recorded child health surveillance in the personal child health record and at least 75% of health visitors and GPs also recorded the reviews in their own professional records. In addition, 43% of GPs recorded child health surveillance reviews on the practice computer.

In Nottingham, we have tried to determine the coverage rate of child health surveillance reviews by collecting copies of the review pages from the personal child health record (Hampshire et al 1996). For 2 years the review pages from the personal child health records returned by health visitors attached to 28 practices were collected. Table 13.5 shows the return rates of child health surveillance reviews per practice. The figures are an underestimate of the coverage rate of child health surveillance reviews because at least 17% of reviews were not returned. Other studies have suggested coverage rates of 84–88% for the 6-week review, 83–90% for the 9-month review and 74–89% for the 18-month review (Colver 1990, Wearmouth et al 1994). In these studies data were collected at a health authority level and again may underestimate actual coverage rates because of low returns.

Immunisations

When uptake rates of immunisations in general practice have been compared with those from child health clinics, they have been found to be higher in general practice whether or not the clinics/practices were in inner-city, rural or suburban areas. Children in general practice clinics also completed their immunisations at a younger age. One of the main reasons for this was thought to be that the children receiving immunisations in general practice were more likely to be called/given appointments for immunisations rather than immunisations being given opportunistically (Li & Taylor 1991). Practices that provided child health surveillance were more likely to achieve higher immunisation rates (Lynch 1995).

Despite general practices being sufficiently well organised to achieve high uptake rates of immunisations, there has been some concern about how well vaccines are stored in general practice, with few practices having minimum/maximum fridge thermometers or thermometers that were checked daily (Haworth et al 1993).

Teenager's needs and primary care

Health issues in teenagers of relevance to primary care staff might include contraception, pregnancy, psychological problems, smoking, alcohol and illicit drug abuse. However, the main concerns that teenagers may wish to discuss with healthcare professionals are:

- sexually transmitted diseases
- contraception
- nutrition
- acne
- weight
- exercise (Epstein et al 1989).

This study also suggested that teenagers were not interested in discussing smoking, alcohol or drugs with health professionals. When asked, almost 90% of teenagers reported attending general practice in the previous 12 months. The most common reasons for attendance were minor injuries, minor illnesses and travel immunisations (Balding 1996). Others have also found that teenagers often attend for upper respiratory tract infections, injuries, asthma, gastrointestinal problems, skin problems, general check-ups and immunisations (Macfarlane et al 1987, Kramer et al 1997). A more recent study in Nottingham showed that in the previous 12 months, 72% of teenagers had been seen at their general practice. In comparison, 29% had been to hospital outpatients and 26% had been to casualty. Only 5% had been to a family planning clinic and 4% had been to a teenage clinic (Churchill et al 1997). This suggests that teenagers are most likely to be seen in primary care.

Unfortunately, teenagers may have difficulties with seeing their GP. The most commonly reported reasons in one study were embarrassment and difficulty in booking a quick appointment (Kari et al 1997). By far the most important aspect of primary health care for teenagers is being sure of confidentiality either with the doctor, practice nurse or receptionists (McPherson 1996). Other aspects of care that were also thought to be important were:

- Friendliness of reception staff.
- Being able to phone for advice.
- Notices and magazines for young people in the waiting room.
- Good written information on contraception.
- Having a clinic specially for young people.

If primary care staff are to improve their services for teenagers, then these concerns and priorities need to be considered. In particular, young people need reassurance about the confidentiality of their contacts with the primary healthcare team.

Payments for child health services in primary care

GPs are independent contractors but are paid by their local health authority. Most GPs do not receive a salary and payments are received for many different aspects of the care they provide. Usually, payments are received quarterly from the health authority. In relation to children, GPs receive a payment for each patient registered with them, which includes each child. GPs also receive an extra payment for each child under five for whom they provide child health surveillance, if they have been accepted onto the child health surveillance list of the local health authority. In addition, GPs receive a payment for immunisations if they achieve a coverage rate of 70% and a higher payment if they achieve 90% coverage. There are two separate payments: one for primary immunisations completed by the time children are 2 years old and another for pre-school boosters.

THE FUTURE

Primary care groups (PCGs) have great potential to change the way child health care is provided in the community. With community nurses and social services being represented on PCG boards, hopefully there will be closer working between all services involved in the care of children. As PCGs become established, they will take on greater responsibility for commissioning care and will hold the budget for care provided in their locality. This may, at last, end the traditional division between community trusts and general practices in the provision of child health care. The aim of PCGs to assess local needs and provide appropriate services may mean a redeployment of staff and services into more deprived areas which should help to improve the provision of child-care services in these areas. Other government initiatives such as health action zones may also improve services and child health in deprived areas.

The government is set on improving the quality of health care (Department of Health 1998). There will be national standard setting and monitoring of services as well as local quality assurance through PCGs. This will include health services for children. However, appropriate standards and outcome measures for child health in primary care have yet to be determined. Also, the means of collecting accurate data to assess the quality of service provision needs to be developed.

Recently, the General Medical Council and the Royal College of General Practitioners decided that a system of demonstrating that GPs continue to be fit to practice should be organised (General Medical Council's Revalidation Steering Group 1999, Pringle 1999). This is likely to include;

- reflection on practice, e.g. audit
- keeping up to date
- communication skills
- professional values
- performance indicators

As child health is an important part of general practice care, it should be included in the revalidation process.

Hopefully, all these changes will promote the continuing improvement of child health services in primary care. For many years, child health care has been an integral part of general practice. This has been strengthened in the last decade with primary healthcare teams taking responsibility for child health surveillance and closer teamwork between GPs, health visitors, practice nurses, midwives and GP administrative staff. In the future, child health will continue to be a very important part of general practice.

Child health in primary care

REFERENCES

Balding J 1996 Young people in 1995. Schools Health Education Unit, Exeter

Becker M, Maiman L 1975 Socio-behavioural determinants of compliance with health and medical care recommendations. Medical Care 13:10–24

Blair M, Horn N, Polnay L 1997 General practitioner's use of hospital and community based paediatric out-patient services in Nottingham. Public Health 111:97–100

Blaxter M 1981 The health of the children. Heinemann, London

Boyle G, Gillam S 1993 Parents' views of child health surveillance. Health Education Journal 52:42–44

Brannen B, Dodd K Oakley A, Storey P 1994 Young people, health and family. Open University Press, Milton Keynes

British Medical Association 1965 A charter for the family doctor service. British Medical Journal Supplement 1:89–91

British Medical Association 1993 Medical ethics today. BMA, London

Brown K, Hampshire A, Groom L 1998 Changes in the role of general practitioners in child health surveillance. Public Health 112:399–403

Butler J 1989 Child health surveillance in primary care. HMSO, London

Butler J, Freidenfeld K, Relton J 1995 Child health surveillance in the new NHS. Centre for Health Services Studies, University of Kent

Campbell S, Roland M 1996 Why do people consult the doctor? Family Practice 13:75–83

Campion P, Gabriel J 1985 Illness behaviour in mothers with young children. Social Science in Medicine 20:325–330

Carter Y, Jones P 1993 Accidents among children under five years old: a general practice based study in north Staffordshire. British Journal of General Practice 43:159–163

Churchill R, Allen J, Denman S et al 1997 Final report: factors influencing the use of general practice based health services by teenagers. Division of General Practice, University of Nottingham

Colling A 1967 The sick family. Journal of the Royal College of General Practitioners 14:181–186

Colver A 1990 Health surveillance of preschool children: four years' experience. British Medical Journal 300:1246–1248

Court Report 1976 Fit for the future. A report of the Committee on Child Health Services. HMSO, London

Crockett A 1993 Management of asthma in primary care. Blackwell Scientific Publications, Oxford

Department of Health 1997 The new NHS. HMSO, London

Department of Health 1998 A first class service. Quality in the new NHS. Department of Health, London

Department of Health Statistical Bulletin 1995 Statistics for general medical practitioners in England: 1984–1994. HMSO, London

Emond A, Howat P, Evans J 1995 Reliability of parent held child health records. Health Visitor 68:322–323

Epstein R, Rice P Wallace P 1989 Teenagers' health concerns: implications for primary health care professionals. Journal of the Royal College of General Practitioners 39:247–249

Evans A, Maskery N, Nolan P 1991 Admission to child health surveillance lists: the views of FHSA general managers and general practitioners. British Medical Journal 303:229–232

General Medical Council's Revalidation Steering Group 1999 Report of the revalidation steering group. GMC, London

Glickman M, Gillam S, Boyle G, Woodroffe C 1994 What makes general practitioners do child health surveillance? Archives of Disease in Childhood 70:47–50

Hall D 1989 Health for all children. Oxford University Press, Oxford

Hall D 1991 Health for all children, 2nd edn. Oxford University Press, Oxford

Hall D 1996 Health for all children — Report of the third joint working party on child health surveillance. Oxford University Press, Oxford

Hampshire A, Blair M, Crown, N et al 1996 An audit of pre-school child health surveillance in Nottingham 1993–1996: final report to the Department of Health. Division of General Practice, University of Nottingham

Harris A 1991 General practitioners and child protection case conferences. British Medical Journal 302:1354

Haworth E, Booy R, Stirzaker L, Wilkes S, Battersby A 1993 Is the cold chain for vaccines maintained in general practice? British Medical Journal 307:242–244

Health Departments of Great Britain 1989 General Practice in the National Health Service. The 1990 Contract. The Health Departments of Great Britain, London

Health Education Authority 1989 Tomorrow's young adults. Health Education Authority, London

Health Visitor's Association 1995 Membership survey. Health Visitor's Association, London

Hulland J 1997 Use of out of hours primary health care services on behalf of children aged under five years old: a descriptive study. BMedSci thesis, Division of Public Health Medicine, University of Nottingham

Huygen F 1988 Longitudinal studies of family units. Journal of the Royal College of General Practitioners 38:168–179

Jones R, Menzies S 1999 General practice: essential facts. Radcliffe Medical Press, Abingdon

Judge K, Benzeval M 1993 Health inequalities: new concerns about the children of single mothers. British Medical Journal 306:677–680

Kai J 1996 What worries parents when their preschool children are acutely ill and why: a qualitative study. BMJ 313:983–986

Kari J, Donovan C, Li J, Taylor B 1997 Adolescents' attitudes to general practice in North London. British Journal of General Practice 47:109–110

Kramer T, Iliffe S, Murray E, Waterman S 1997 Which adolescents attend the GP? British Journal of General Practice 47:327

Li J, Taylor B 1991 Comparison of immunisation rates in general practice and child health clinics. British Medical Journal 303:1035–1038

Lynch M 1995 Effect of practice and patient population characteristics on the uptake of childhood immunisations. British Journal of General Practice 45:205–208

Macfarlane A, McPherson A, McPherson K, Ahmed L 1987 Teenagers and their health. Archives of Disease in Childhood 62:1125–1129

McPherson A 1996 Primary health care and adolescence. In: McFarlane A (ed) Adolescent health. Royal College of Physicians, London, pp 33–41

Morrison J, Gilmour H, Sullivan F 1991 Children seen frequently out of hours in one general practice. British Medical Journal 303:1111–1114

Munro E 1998 Changing the response of professionals to child abuse. British Journal of General Practice 48:1609–1611

Ni Bhrolchain C 1992 A district survey of paediatric outpatient referrals. Public Health 106:429–436

Office for National Statistics 1996 Key health statistics from general practice. The Stationary Office, London

Office for National Statistics 1997 Living in Britain; results from the 1995 General Household Survey. The Stationary Office, London

Office of Health Economics 1997 10th Compendium of Health Statistics. Office of Health Economics, London

Office of Population Censuses and Surveys 1995 Morbidity statistics from general practice. Fourth national survey 1991–1992. HMSO, London

Pearson P, Spencer J 1997 Promoting teamwork in primary care. Arnold, London

Pringle M 1999 Revalidation. British Journal of General Practice 49:259

Royal College of General Practitioners 1982 Healthier children — thinking prevention. RCGP, London

Royal College of General Practitioners 1996 Information Sheet 13: children in general practice. RCGP, London

Royal College of General Practitioners 1997a Information Sheet 1: profile of UK general practitioners. RCGP, London

Royal College of General Practitioners 1997b Information Sheet 2: profile of UK practices. RCGP, London

Royal College of General Practitioners, British Paediatric Association, GMSC, JCPTGP 1991 Training and accreditation of general practitioners in child health surveillance. RCGP, London

Saffin K, Macfarlane A 1991 How well are parent held records kept and completed? British Journal of General Practice 41:249–251

Saxena S, Majeed A, Jones M 1999 Socio-economic differences in childhood consultation rates in general practice in England and Wales: prospective cohort study. British Medical Journal 318:642–646

Sheldon W 1967 Child welfare centres. A report of the sub-committee of the Standing Medical Advisory Committee. HMSO, London

Spencer N 1992 Consultant paediatric outreach clinics — a practical step in integration. Archives of Disease in Childhood 68:496–500

Styles W 1985 Caring for children in general practice. In: Harvey D, Kovar I (eds) Child health: a textbook for the DCH. Churchill Livingstone, Edinburgh, pp 41–58

Sutton J, Jagger C, Smith L 1995 Parents' views of health surveillance. Archives of Disease in Childhood 73:57–61

United Kingdom Central Council for Nursing, Midwifery and Health Visiting 1998 The midwives code of practice. UKCC, London

Wearmouth E, Lambert P, Morland R 1994 Quality assurance in preschool surveillance. Archives of Disease in Childhood 70:505–511

Working together under the Children Act 1989 A guide to arrangements for interagency co-operation for the protection of children from abuse 1991. HMSO, London

Wyke S, Hewison J, Russell I 1990 Respiratory illness in children: what makes parents decide to consult? British Journal of General Practice 40:226–229

14 | Community nursing

HEALTH VISITING

Introduction

The health visiting service is unique within the nursing professions because of its contact with the well population and its ability to act on its own initiative. Its practice is based on philosophies of partnership and empowerment and is influenced by social, environmental and economic factors.

The health visiting service offers preventive health care to individuals, children and their families and groups in local community settings, where it also seeks to influence health agendas. As the role of the primary healthcare team has developed and expanded, the majority of health visitors working in the community have integrated their work within the primary care team, recognising the value of coordinated team working as a powerful means of influencing health agendas both locally and nationally.

Health visitor practitioners also work within more specialist health settings, either in the community or hospitals, where their skills in holistic health assessment, communication, facilitation and empowerment contribute to those teams who provide more complex services to families with young children. Health visitors' knowledge of primary care and local community facilities and services ensure an integrated approach to health care for children and families in these circumstances.

At an individual level the service enables and supports people and families to take more control over their lives and manage their responsibilities including that of parenting and caring for children.

At a group level health visiting seeks to initiate and collaborate in healthy alliances, stimulating and promoting choices in healthy lifestyles which will bring improvements in health and well being.

Within local communities and populations health visiting encourages wider social responsibility for health, seeking to redress inequalities in health. Health visiting recognises the effectiveness of community participation and the need to enable and facilitate the participation of groups who are marginalised or families who are living in poverty.

The health visitor

Background

Health visitors are registered nurses holding an additional postgraduate qualification in health visiting. They are part of a live register of nurses and are regulated through the United Kingdom Central Council for Nursing, Midwifery and Health Visiting.

Health visitors began to be trained in 1892. A range of people were involved from backgrounds including sanitary inspectors, doctors and nurses who were selected for their characters and who had an interest in fighting disease. Their roles at that time seemed to be connected to cleanliness and godliness and had a missionary aspect, with the notion of disease and bad health being ascribed to bad smells.

A recognised course of training was established in 1919 through the new Ministry of Health and Board of Education, with access arrangements for qualified nurses and later to include midwifery qualifications.

In 1929 the Local Government Act provided statutory rules and orders setting out qualifications

Community nursing

of health visitors. Their role continued to be based on responses to public health needs and focused on teaching and helping activities within local communities, where poverty and its consequences were having serious effects on child health and welfare and where child death rates were high. Activities were centred on home visiting of families with children, teaching and facilitating improvements in basic household and personal hygiene, diet and the welfare of children.

During the 1930s the profession joined forces with doctors working in the public health sector.

A number of other major changes continued to influence the development of the profession, the NHS Act 1946, the Children Act' 1948, the Health Visiting and Social Work (Training) Act 1962. A new syllabus of training was agreed in 1965 which established the current aims and principles of health visiting.

During the last 30 years the profession has grown and developed with significant roles continuing to emerge and develop with the children, young people and their families in the community. Changes in legislation, most notably the Children Act 1989, set out principles which have influenced the development of health visiting practice, together with particular working together arrangements which feature the primary healthcare and interagency team working contribution of health visiting. In supporting the rights of the child, this legislation has given new impetus to the principles of health visiting, though its clear focus on the needs of the child within the changing face of the family today and in its purpose of seeking to ensure each child has the right to a reasonable, healthy and safe childhood.

The principles

The ultimate aim of health visiting is encompassed by four principles:

- The search for health needs.
- The stimulation of awareness of health needs.
- The influence on policies affecting health.
- The facilitation of health-enhancing activities — applicable at individual, family and community level.

The role

Health visitors work as members of multidisciplinary health teams, both primary and specialist, and within interagency teams. Their work is largely within community settings. At an individual family level much of the work continues to be face to face within family homes.

Primary healthcare teams and community paediatric teams will have health visitors as core members of their teams. The health visitor is typically based with the primary healthcare team in the local health centre or general practice surgery and will work within a geographical area, linking into and liaising with the local paediatric child health team, the child psychology team and the child and adolescent mental health team. Strong links and routine liaison arrangements will also be in place with the local midwifery team, the school health team and the local paediatric departments of hospitals. The health visitor role within these teams will focus on primary and secondary prevention of ill health.

Most health visitors within primary healthcare teams will have developed a specialist area of interest or expertise, for example, stress management, childhood immunisation, management of a Care Of the Next Infant scheme. These particular programmes will be offered within the local population and may be offered more widely across a district, based on level of need and local resources.

Some health visitors will perform a part-time or full-time specialist role. These health visitors will be part of a specialist clinical team, for example a child development centre team will usually have a specialist health visitor for childhood disability. A multiagency homeless team will have a health visitor who specialises in work with homeless families and/or travellers. Health visitors working in these teams will focus on tertiary prevention and crisis interventions.

In addition, health visitors based in hospital paediatric units provide an essential liaison role acting as a professional networking and liaison service between paediatric accident and emergency centres, paediatric wards and clinics, the primary healthcare teams, school health service and community paediatric teams. Where resources allow these health visitors provide a full range of health visiting services to parents and children within the ward setting.

The health visitor, as part of primary health work, is often drawn in to the interagency team where core teamwork involves work with families with children in need or where there are child protection issues. Health visitors give priority to this work which can range across the whole spectrum of primary, secondary and tertiary preventative work, but, in the initial stages, will usually focus on crisis interventions.

Partnerships are developed by the health visitor within the wider community where the health visitor will operate across organisational boundaries, local authorities, voluntary and community groups. Health visitors will often be the cornerstone of these partnership arrangements which are valuable in seeking to gain knowledge or to raise interest and support in local health issues or national health agendas and campaigns. They provide the basis of information about need and the help and support available to families locally. Agencies and groups will respond to local need through these collaborative working arrangements.

Skills and knowledge

These are based on:

- health promotion
- health assessment
- health surveillance
- epidemiology
- community development
- knowledge of health and in particular child health
- risk assessment and management
- change management
- models of health — social and public.

Core elements which underpin activities

These are described as:

- management of systems and caseloads
- prioritisation of caseloads and workloads
- research and evidence-based practice
- partnership working based on models which are enabling and empowering

- team working, both interdisciplinary and interagency
- liaison and formal communication
- professional development and reflective practice.

Priority areas of work

Target groups are identified through census data and primary health profiling of local communities. In relation to children's health these groups are commonly:

- Families, parents/carers where children are under 5 years.
- Community groups including young people.
- Antenatal women.

Particular emphasis would be placed on those groups where there was disadvantage and/or minority issues affecting health. Criteria include:

- A population of between 7000 and 10000 per full-time health visitor.
- Areas of disadvantage, using census and profiling information:
  — identifiable communities: social and geographical identities
  — identifiable assessed health needs
  — identifiable outcome measures.

Models

Models of service delivery in health visiting vary across the country and vary locally in response to the needs of communities. Each model will at least expect to reflect the aim and principles of health visiting and will have an agreed philosophy which will reflect measurable standards of care (e.g. team working, client involvement in care planning, honesty and confidentiality, evidence-based practice).

In practice most health visiting activity follows a systems model, focusing on the groupings described below.

Individual case management

Client-related activities are recorded against the client record. The parent-held child health record, for example, is used routinely for this purpose.

Assessment

A range of qualitative and quantitative measures are utilised. Tools will be validated and will include percentile charts, sleep diaries, diet diaries, Edinburgh postnatal depression score. Health visitors use their professional judgement through listening and observing, considering social/vulnerability factors and client perceptions, utilising attitude scales and process of change information.

Health education/health promotion

This is linked to health of the nation targets and local health improvement programmes and child health promotion programmes. A range of activities carried out within the primary healthcare team led by or involving the health visitor would include raising awareness, dealing with resistance, providing information, programmes of education and public campaigns and screening programmes.

Programme of child surveillance of individual health and development with associated health promotion through parents

Within the primary healthcare team the health visitor will plan collaborative activities with the team to ensure delivery of this programme locally for all children under 5 years. Any deviation from the norm and any observation or concern by the parent is considered and acted on. Factors which are particularly significant, such as attitude and health of parent/carer, housing, safety measures, local facilities and access, are considered. The health visitor may facilitate a group support link for the parent and child, or make a referral to other agencies. Where paediatric advice or a second medical opinion is required the health visitor, in discussion with the GP, will liaise with, or refer to the local community paediatric team, or in agreement with the paediatric team, refer directly to other specialist community teams, for example the child development team or child and adolescent mental health team.

Protection of children/families at risk

Health visitors remain alert to the needs of children and act in a child's best interests where there was a question of need or a risk of significant harm. Typically figures from a local social services office would demonstrate upwards of 70% of all referrals of children under 5 years as coming from health visitors.

Health visitors contribute to an initial and full assessment of need or risk and would routinely be involved in child protection case conferences. Where there were children under 5 years the health visitor routinely forms part of the core group who will plan and work with the family/carers.

Health visitors frequently provide a valuable contribution to family proceedings or directions hearings where orders are being sought in court to settle a child's arrangements.

Interventions based on programmes of care

Health visitors make interventions available based on assessed need which will be negotiated and agreed with parents/carers. A variety of programmes focusing on children's health will be planned and provided individually or within groups. The health visitor will work alone or as part of a team arrangement. Any programme undertaken will seek to ensure active listening, empowering through raising of self-awareness and encouragement and will include active monitoring. Examples of programmes would include toddler behaviour management, nutritional guidance, play, support programmes including bereavement and management of a diagnosed problem.

Public health function

Health visitors initiate or work collaboratively towards organised efforts to protect and promote health and well being, prolong life and prevent illness within local communities. The Royal College of Nursing publication (1994) 'Public Health: Nurses Rise to the Challenge', identified six key areas of work in nursing. These key areas are reflected in examples of health visiting activity:

- Assess the health needs of local populations through the compilation of health profiles.
- Support people to participate in the life of their community to influence factors that affect their health.

- Increase health resources in communities by establishing local networks.
- Build healthy alliances and a supportive infra-structure to provide information, resources and practical help for community initiatives.
- Engage with local statutory and voluntary groups to work towards health-related policies and actions.
- Increase uptake of services by ensuring they are accessible, offered appropriately and effectively targeted.

Successes in health visiting

There is evidence available to support the effec-tiveness of health visiting in various areas of health promotion and public health summarised in a Community Practitioner Health Visitor Associa-tion briefing paper (CPHVA 1989). This evidence includes demonstration of impacts on the health and well being of children and young people. Examples of areas where this has been effective are given below.

The child development programme
(Barker & Anderson 1992)
This programme brought about highly significant changes in almost every home environmental vari-able, as well as children's development levels, com-pared with controls.

The positive parenting programme
(Angeli 1994), **parent support initiatives** (Sutton 1995, Brown 1997), **parenting health education** (Kerr et al 1997)
This range of health visiting programmes, initia-tives and health education programmes, the posi-tive parenting programme in particular according with the spirit of the Children Act, demonstrated positive benefits for parents and children. Support was offered for example in toddler behaviour man-agement, infant and child sleep disturbances, hyperactivity in children, child injury both acci-dental and physical abuse.

Child health promotion
The report of the joint working party on child health surveillance 'Health for all Children' (Hall 1996) recognises that health visitors are closely identified with child health promotion and take lead responsibility in primary healthcare teams for an under fives child surveillance programme.

Child accident prevention
A systematic review on preventing unintentional injuries carried out by the University of York (NHS Centre for Reviews and Dissemination 1997a) iden-tified good evidence that the use of safety devices, targeting households at risk and provision of home visits and education make the most impact.

Clover et al (1982) concluded that health visitors are particularly well placed for a role in accident prevention. Health visiting interventions can reduce the incidence of children presenting at accident and emergency with head injuries (Walsh 1995).

Other initiatives have provided positive outcomes.

Infant nutrition
Research has shown that health visitors can influ-ence both initial choice of infant feeding method and factors influencing the duration of breast feeding (Dracup & Sanderson 1994). A survey of weaning practices of first-time mothers shows that the health visitor is the most used and useful source of advice. (Walker 1995). A Bristol study found that health visitors working as a part of a multidiscipli-nary team were able to bring about improvements (Griffiths et al 1995).

Sun safe education
A health visitor-led sun education programme for 11 and 12 year olds in Derbyshire (Syson-Nibbs 1996), showed that sun safe educational interven-tion can improve knowledge and attitudes in this age group.

Services for children with special needs and chronic conditions
A study has shown that health visitors make a range of contributions to the work of child devel-

Community nursing

opment teams and continuing care of children and their families. The study looked at the work of 12 district child development teams (Yerbury & Thomas 1994). Specialist knowledge of disability, specialist skills in direct care, liaison with local colleagues and face to face support in the home were valued by parents.

Mental health promotion

A recent systematic review of mental health promotion by the NHS Centre for Reviews and Dissemination (1997b) identified that it is possible to identify vulnerable groups and that there are several interventions that can help promote mental health and prevent health problems. High-quality pre-school education and support visits for new parents have been shown to improve the mental health of children and parents in disadvantaged communities. Mental health problems in children of separating parents can be reduced. Health visitors may take a lead within primary healthcare teams in applying the Edinburgh postnatal depression scale and have demonstrated satisfactory responses from active listening or non-directive counselling (Holden et al 1989).

Studies have shown that these interventions have demonstrated significant reductions in child behaviour problems (Seeley et al 1996).

Care Of the Next Infant (CONI) programme

This programme was developed by the Foundation for the Study of Infant Deaths (1997), as a possible means of reducing cot deaths. Health visitors are involved as key professionals in making this programme widely available. The CONI programme provides a framework of care offered to parents who have suffered a child death, particularly where the death has been unexpected.

A report on 5000 babies using the CONI programme demonstrates:

- A high take-up and wide acceptance of all aspects of the programme.
- The programme was really valued by parents, who particularly appreciated the involvement of their health visitor.

- Some evidence to suggest the scheme may be preventing further deaths (CONI National Organiser 1998).

Future direction

The future direction of health visiting continues to be the subject of healthy debate, investigation and review. The Community Practitioner Health Visitor Association and the Office of Public Management published a report, 'Leading the Future' (CPHVA 1999), which provides a challenging agenda focused on a family-centred public health role. Recent debate and information available suggests success for children and young people and their families, where the core health visiting elements of partnership, non-directive approaches and collaborative interagency working are visible.

A recent government publication, 'Saving Lives: Our Healthier Nation' (Department of Health 1999a), has identified health visitors as leaders of public health practice and encourages them to develop a family-centred public health role, working with individuals, families and communities to improve health and tackle inequalities.

As a result of this modernised role and supported by government initiatives, for example 'Surestart' (Department for Education and Employment 1999a), these publications identify that:

- Parents will receive improved support.
- Individuals and families will have a tailored family health plan.
- Health needs of families will be met by a team led by a health visitor.
- Health visitors will initiate and develop programmes based on models such as Homestart, NEWPIN and PIPPIN as summarised in 'Surestart: A guide to evidenced based practice' (Department for Education and Employment 1998).
- Neighbourhoods or special groups such as homeless people will have their health needs identified by health visitors.

The Surestart programme proposes that health visitors will provide a range of health improvement activities including:

- Child health programmes.
- Parenting, support and education.
- Development of support networks in communities.
- Support and advice for breast-feeding mothers.
- Advice on family relationships and support to vulnerable children and their families.

These proposals, plans and initiatives will ensure that health visiting continues to play a central, pioneering role in preventing disadvantage and social exclusion for children and their families.

SCHOOL NURSING

To give a full and comprehensive account of the role and remit of school nurses and the school nursing service is a task that is beyond the scope of these few pages. However what can be done is to give the reader a flavour of what is currently occurring within the field under the subject areas:

- The range of school nursing activity.
- The philosophy and process of school nursing.
- School community profiles.
- Future school nurse development.

The range of school nursing activity

School nurses work with a client group that is in a period of physical, psychological and emotional transition. Their remit is the care of school age children and young people who range in age from the 'rising fives' to young people at the brink of young adulthood. It also encompasses the period of adolescence with all its varied and turbulent connotations. It is a client group that will challenge accepted adult norms and contains much risk-taking behaviour. School nurses regularly encounter and are expected to deal with such issues as sexual health problems, teenage pregnancies, substance misuse, behavioural problems, mental health issues and eating disorders to name but a few.

School nurses also have some of society's most vulnerable children and young people in their care, such as the abused and neglected, children who are 'looked after' or those with profound and complex physical and/or mental health needs. In its broadest sense it is a dynamic and challenging client group that requires a high degree of adaptability and specialist expertise on the part of the school nurse to manage successfully.

The school nursing service is as varied as its client group. It has evolved throughout the UK as a disparate service with many different service models in current operation, with even neighbouring trusts offering widely differing services. The Amalgamated School Nurses' Association (Fletcher & Balding 1992) produced data to this effect when it undertook a national survey of its members in 1990 which looked at trends in school nursing practice. The Community Practitioners' and Health Visitors' Association (Health Visitors' Association 1996), then known as the Health Visitors' Association, undertook a similar process in 1996 which again highlighted the variation in practice of its school nursing members across the UK. This disparity in service provision was exacerbated during the 1990s as many trusts disinvested in their school nursing services. A survey published by the Queen's Nursing Institute (Bagnall & Dilloway 1996a) also noted some of the managerial differences in service provision. The survey indicated that many trusts were operating without appropriate service level agreements for school nursing in place and that significant numbers of trusts were in contravention of the Court Report's (Department of Health 1976) recommendation of a minimum of one full-time school nurse per 2500 pupils. In one unfortunate case the survey found that the ratio was one school nurse per 12 973 pupils.

As service provision has varied so has the role of the school nurse, although a Royal College of Nursing (1992) survey found that school nursing activities undertaken in the UK could be generally placed within six broad categories which were:

- Health promotion.
- Health surveillance and screening.
- Liasing with professional colleagues and parents.
- Clinical activities.
- Teaching and research.
- Clerical/administrative activities.

However these categories and the emphasis placed on each will be affected by various factors, one of

Community nursing

which is caseload composition. The role of the school nurse and what she is able to effectively undertake will also be considerably affected by the numerical size of the caseload especially if the numbers are based on historical precedent rather than need. The type of client will also influence the activities undertaken. For example the school nurse may work solely with children with profound physical and/or mental health needs, or specialise in a particular area such as 'children looked after'. The range, emphasis and quality of service that school nurses are able to offer to the children and young people in their care will also vary according to the commissioning contract under which their trust is currently operating.

A philosophy for school nursing

Despite the wide variation in current school nursing provision it is the author's considered belief that there is an underpinning philosophy within the school nursing service that is rarely articulated but in reality has a profound influence on the process of school nursing. It is a philosophy of:

- *Advocacy* — Which speaks out for, and promotes the interests of, children and young people in their care.
- *Empowerment* — Which encourages and desires children and young people to begin to learn to take control and to be proactively involved in their own health.
- *Protection* — To be actively involved in the protection of children and young people from abuse and harm.
- *Partnership* — That children and young people are given respect and dignity and are involved in, and listened to when any decisions or actions are taken that affect them.
- *Equity* — That all children and young people of school age have open access to the service without stigma or prejudice.

It is a clear understanding and articulation of this philosophy that will allow school nurses to create the collective 'thread' that can be used to link all their extensive and myriad range of activities regardless of where or how these services are being provided.

The process of school nursing

A clearly articulated philosophy for school nursing also helps to clarify and define the processes by which school nursing activities are undertaken and carried out. Although the format of school nursing service provision may well vary from area to area according to need the processes will, to a large extent, remain the same. If the philosophical tenets underpinning the service are that of advocacy, empowerment, protection, partnership and equity, then it is the authors' considered belief that the processes by which school nursing activities are carried out to comply with this philosophy can be considered in terms of:

- *Informing* — By being a giver of information either through health education/promotion on a one-to-one basis with children and young people or through input into school personal health and social education (PHSE) programmes, etc. School nurses also act as a source of information to parents and carers and the wider school community.
- *Listening* — By being a 'listener' and hearing what children and young people are saying either as a counsellor when it is required or acting as an advocate on their behalf when they are vulnerable and their voices are not heard.
- *Supporting* — By actively supporting children and young people through the life events, often traumatic, they may experience in their transition to young adulthood such as bereavement, parental divorce, pregnancy, mental health problems, behavioural problems, etc.
- *Providing* — By providing the care required by children and young people with specific needs such as those with profound and complex medical and/or physical problems either in mainstream or special schools. By providing services such as 'drop-in' clinics providing contraceptive advice, etc. to nurse-led enuresis and soiling clinics.
- *Facilitating* — By being a facilitator and providing the 'glue' which seamlessly joins all the many disciplines and professionals that may be involved in the care of one particular child or young person such as paediatricians, social workers, school staff, parents, clinical psychol-

ogy, etc. to allow a coherent care programme to emerge.

- *Consulting* — By consulting with children and young people to ascertain what services they require from school nursing and in what format and by actively involving them in any decisions that will involve or affect them when care or services are offered.
- *Profiling* — By developing ongoing and dynamic school community profiles to assess need and appropriately target school nursing resources.

School community profiles

A vital and important element of the school nurse's role is the ability to undertake a needs assessment of her caseload in order to provide the appropriate care and input required and to target the use of available school nursing resources efficiently. A thorough health needs assessment of a caseload will also provide the evidence base from which to develop individual service level agreements with schools within that caseload. Efficient and effective health needs assessments can also provide an accurate source of information that can be used to influence the commissioning process. In addition it can be used to lobby for additional resources to ensure that school nursing service provision matches the needs of the children and young people within that caseload (Bagnall & Dilloway 1996b).

However the production of an effective and detailed school community profile is a time-consuming exercise requiring commitment and skill (Billings 1996). It is therefore important that school nurses acquire the necessary public health skills that will enable them to undertake such a process. It is equally necessary to ensure that sufficient time is negotiated and appropriate resources are put in place to allow the school nurse to undertake and complete the process adequately.

One effective way for school nurses to undertake a health needs assessment is to use a school community profile School community profiling is an ongoing and dynamic process that if done well provides a sound basis from which to develop school health plans that are proactive in promoting health. It is also a collaborative process that seeks out the views and opinions of its key stakeholders both

within the school and wider community. School community profiling can also identify school nurse training issues that will require addressing if specific needs identified in the profile are to be met, for example an increased expertise in dealing with children and young people involved in substance misuse. The frequency with which they are undertaken should also reflect the specific needs and circumstances of the school involved.

Future school nurse development

Despite the 1990s being a period when many school nursing services were being reduced and disinvestment was common, the late 1990s began to see an increasing interest in discovering how the service was being provided and how it might be developed. For example Lightfoot & Bines (1997) in their research on the role of school nursing in keeping children healthy identified four key roles:

- Safeguarding the health and welfare of children.
- A confidante for children and young people.
- Health promotion.
- Family support.

DeBell & Everett (1997) undertook an extensive mapping process of the roles and responsibilities of school nurses' within three trusts (commissioned by East Norfolk Health) to try and assess the effectiveness of current school nursing service provision. Subsequent recommendations made in the report included a proposed model for school nursing provision. This model proposed the idea that skill mix teams led by a 'school health advisor' (i.e. a school nurse) might be a more effective method of delivering the service to specified groups of schools. It also recommended that the school nursing service has a professional lead, distinct from operational management, who would be a specialist practitioner in school nursing responsible for interagency liaison at policy and strategy level. The professional lead would also have a strong research and development remit. DeBell & Everett's (1997) recommendations are similarly being echoed by development work on a 'service framework' for school nursing which is currently being undertaken jointly by The Royal College of Nurses, the Community Practitioner and Health Visitor Association

Community nursing

and the Queens' Nursing Institute. It is anticipated that the definitive document on the framework will be produced in summer 2000.

The influence and importance of the role of school nursing was again highlighted in the White Paper 'Excellence in Schools' (Department of Health 1997). This document identified education as providing a lifeline to many disadvantaged children and young people who receive little systematic health input and cite the school as a vital means of providing this input. It also stated that schools could not be proactive in the development of health policies without the support and cooperation of the relevant health professionals. The National Healthy School Standard (Department for Education and Employment 1999b) also discussed the school nurse as a key professional in jointly developing health education and health promotion initiatives within schools to promote the healthy school programme.

The publication of two White Papers at the very end of the 1990s, 'Making a Difference' (Department of Health 1999b) and 'Saving Lives' (Department of Health 1999a), is also beginning to have a profound influence on how future school nursing services will be developed and configured. In 'Making a Difference' (Department of Health 1999b), the strategy document for strengthening the nursing, midwifery and health visiting contribution to health and health care, the government's expectations of the school nursing role were, for the first time, clearly addressed:

- Assess the health needs of children and school communities and to agree individual and school health plans.
- Deliver these plans through multidisciplinary partnerships.
- Play a key role in immunisation and vaccination programmes.
- Contribute to personal health and social education and to citizenship training.
- Work with parents to promote positive parenting.
- Offer support and counselling, promoting positive mental health in young people.
- Advise and coordinate health care to children with medical needs.

(Department of Health 1999b p 62)

In 'Saving Lives: Our Healthier Nation' (Department of Health 1999a) which was published later in the same year the government further expanded their expectations of the school nursing role. School nurses would be expected to lead school nursing teams that would assess the health needs of individuals and school communities and agree individual and school health plans. They were also charged with the development of effective multiagency partnerships in order to deliver the agreed plans. The school nursing team would also be expected to provide a range of health improvement activities, which included:

- Immunisation and vaccination programmes.
- Support and advice to teachers and staff and other school staff on a range of child health issues.
- Support to children with medical needs.
- Support and counselling to promote positive mental health in young people.
- Personal and social education programmes and citizenship training.
- Identification of social care needs, including the need for protection from abuse.
- Providing advice on relationships and sex education by building on their clinical experience and pastoral role.
- Aiding liaison between, for example, schools, primary care trusts, and special services in meeting the health and social care needs of children.
- Contribute to the identification of children's special educational needs.
- Working with parents and young people to promote parenting.

(Department of Health, 1999a pp 134–135)

The mid to late 1990s also saw the training needs of school nurses being addressed as specialist school nurse degree courses started to be developed across the country to give school nurse training parity with other specialist community practitioners. School nurses were now becoming better equipped with the skills necessary to develop, audit and critically examine their practice. The need for school nursing to become a research-based profession was also high on the agenda and school nursing services were being actively encouraged to have professional leads whose remit was heavily biased towards research and development. There was also an increasing realisation that the service should move away from the idea of a 'school-based' service to that of a 'school-aged' one and that the needs of those children and young people who are outside of the school system must also be addressed. At the beginning of the twenty first century school nursing is being considered as a potent public health resource and a major contributor in ensuring that children and young people maintain their optimum health. The potential development of school nursing to meet these expectations will be an exciting and challenging enterprise.

REFERENCES

Angeli N 1994 Facilitating parenting skills in vulnerable families. Health Visitor 67:130–132

Bagnall P, Dilloway M 1996a In search of a blueprint: a survey of school health services. Queen's Nursing Institute, London

Bagnall P, Dilloway M 1996b In a different light: school nurses and their role in meeting the needs of school-age children. Queen's Nursing Institute, London

Barker W, Anderson R 1992 The child development programme; an evaluation of process and outcomes. Early Child Development Unit, University of Bristol

Billings J 1996 Profiling for health: the process and practice. Health Visitors' Association, London

Brown I 1997 A skill mix parent support initiative in health visiting; an evaluation study. Health Visitor 70:339–343

Clover A F, Hutchinson P J, Judson E C 1982 Promoting children's home safety. British Medical Journal 285:1177–1180

CONI National Organiser 1998 CONI (Care of Next Infant), Report. Division of Child Health, University of Sheffield

CPHVA 1989 (Briefing paper) Making a difference: evidence of the effectiveness of health visiting. Health Watch, London

CPHVA 1999 Leading the future report. Office for Public Management, London

DeBell D, Everett G 1997 In a class apart: a study of school nursing. City College Norwich, Norwich

Department for Education and Employment 1997 Excellence in schools. Stationery Office, London

Department for Education and Employment 1998 Surestart: a guide to evidence based practice. DfEE, London

Department for Education and Employment 1999a Surestart, making a difference for children and families. DfEE, London

Department for Education and Employment 1999b National Healthy School Standard. Stationery Office, London

Department of Health 1976 Fit for the future; report on the committee for child healthcare services (The Court Report). HMSO, London

Department of Health 1999a Saving lives: our healthier nation. Cm 4386. Stationery Office, London

Department of Health 1999b Making a difference: strengthening the nursing, midwifery and health visiting contribution to health and healthcare. Stationery Office, London

Dracup C, Sanderson E 1994 Health visitors' perceptions of breast feeding mothers. Health Visitor 67:158–160

Fletcher K, Balding J 1992 School nurses do it in schools!: trends in school nursing practice. Amalgamated School Nurses' Association, London

Foundation for the Study of Infant Deaths 1997 Cot death — facts, figures and definitions, fact file 1. FSID, London

Griffiths B, Poynor M, O'Connell K 1995 Health education and iron intake of weaning children. Health Visitor 68:418–419

Hall D M B (ed) 1996 Health for all children. Oxford University Press, Oxford

Health Visitors' Association 1996 School nursing: here today for tomorrow. Health Visitors' Association, London

Holden J M, Sagovsky R, Cox J L 1989 Counselling in a general practice setting; a controlled study of health visitor intervention in the treatment of post natal depression. British Medical Journal 298:223–226

Kerr S, Jowett S, Smith L 1997 Education to help prevent sleep problems in infants. Health Visitor 70:224–225

Lightfoot J, Bines W 1997 Keeping children healthy: the role of school nursing. Social Policy Research Unit, University of York

NHS Centre for Reviews and Dissemination, University of York 1997a Preventing unintentional injuries in children and young adolescents. Churchill Livingstone, Edinburgh

NHS Centre for Reviews and Dissemination, University of York 1997b Mental health promotion in high risk groups. Churchill Livingstone, Edinburgh

Royal College of Nursing 1992 Survey of school nursing. Royal College of Nursing, London

Royal College of Nursing 1994 Public health: nurses rise to the challenge. Royal College of Nursing, London

Seely S, Murray L, Cooper P J 1996 The outcomes for mothers and babies of health visitor intervention. Health Visitor 69:135–138

Sutton C 1995 Educating parents to cope with difficult children. Health Visitor 68:284–285

Syson-Nibbs L 1996 Measuring the effectiveness of sun safety messages. Health Visitor 69:274–277

The Children Act 1989 HMSO, London

Walker C 1995 When to wean, whose advice do mothers find helpful? Health Visitor 68:109–111

Walsh D 1995 Preventing childhood accidents. Primary Health Care Journal 5:18–20

Yerbury M, Thomas J 1994 Health visitor role in services for children with disabilities. Health Visitor 64:86–87

15 | Education services

Education shares the characteristics of all complex systems. It is guided by legislation and policy; it has many interlinked parts; it has a 'language' of its own; and it is accompanied by a set of belief systems, which may be different according to the people holding them or the era. In addition it is high profile, constantly evolving, and people have high expectations for what it can and should do.

The complexity of the system and its evolving nature have a major impact on all children, but particularly when those with significant education and health needs are considered.

WHAT ARE EDUCATION SERVICES

Nationally education is governed by legislation. (Most of this chapter refers to arrangements in England and Wales. There are different requirements and legislation in Scotland and Northern Ireland, and in Wales there are some differences, e.g. National Curriculum.) There have been around 40 Acts directly concerning education since 1944. Some of the key Acts are listed in Box 15.1.

The Department for Education and Skills (DfES) administers education throughout the country, headed by the Secretary of State for Education and Employment. The DfES ensures that legislation is carried out at local level, issues policy and guidance, oversees a variety of other bodies and commissions research into various aspects of education.

Locally, education is administered by elected councils with a department, the local education authority (LEA), which employs officers to carry out the functions. Most councils have an education committee, but this is likely to alter under radical changes to be made by the government. However, exact arrangements have yet to be determined.

Funding for the LEA comes from two main sources — local funding raised by local taxation and central government via the DfES. The latter is increasingly allocated in grant form with clear guidelines from the DfES on how it should be spent.

An LEA delivers its service at two levels — school level, with schools having a measure of independence but also being overseen by the LEA and DfES, and at a central administrative level, which includes a variety of central and support services.

Over the last decade legislation has moved the balance of responsibilities away from being predominantly with the LEA towards a tripartite model, where power and responsibility is shared between the DfEE, LEA and schools. The increasing role of school governing bodies is one aspect of this. An example of the work of DfES, LEA and schools is the setting of targets.

All schools have to teach the National Curriculum, which is set down in detail by the DfES. It includes programmes of study (what pupils should be taught) and attainment targets (what they should have learned at each stage). Pupils are tested at key points of their education by standard assessment tasks (SATs).

The structure of education is illustrated on the following pages (Figs 15.1, 15.2).

Box 15.1
Some key legislation

Education Act 1944
The 'Principal Act' which is the foundation of the current education system. Consolidated into the Education Act 1996.

Education (Handicapped Children) Act 1970
Discontinued the classification of handicapped children as unsuitable for education at school. Consolidated into the Education Act 1996.

Education Act 1981
To make provision for children with special educational needs. Consolidated into the Education Act 1996.

Education Reform Act 1988
Amending the law, mostly consolidated into the Education Act 1996.

Education (Schools Act) 1992
Making provision for inspections of schools and with respect to information about schools and their pupils. Consolidated into the School Inspections Act 1996.

Education Act 1996
Overarching and consolidating Act, which covers a wide variety of educational legislation including the statutory system of education, functions and funding, LEA-maintained schools, special educational needs, the curriculum, schools admissions and attendance, independent schools, etc.

Education Act 1997
Includes school discipline, admissions, baseline assessments and pupils' performance, inspections of LEAs and schools.

Schools Standards and Framework Act 1998
Includes measures to raise standards of school education and nursery education.

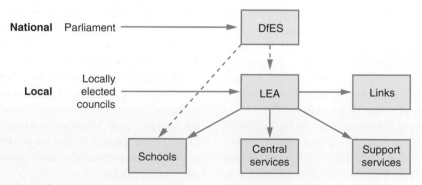

Fig. 15.1 Relationships of structure of education at national and local government levels

SOME KEY PRINCIPLES (Table 15.1)

Several key principles guide the way education is evolving. They are part of the total picture, but can be described separately to help clarify some of the many expectations and requirements that face those working in education services.

Raising standards of achievement for all children and all schools

Successive governments have placed a high emphasis on raising standards. A variety of approaches is used, including:

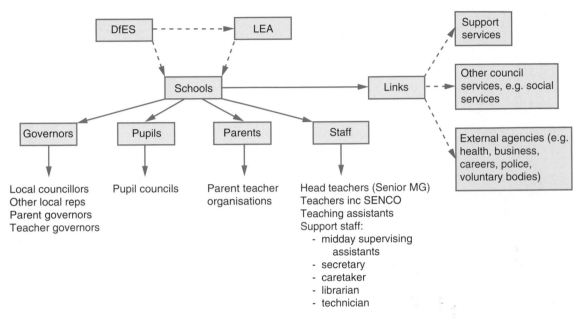

Fig. 15.2 Structure of education at schools level

- Independent inspections of schools through the Office for Standards in Education (OFSTED), now extended to include inspections of LEAs.
- The setting of targets (e.g. the standard of reading which should be achieved by 80% of all 11 year olds by 2002).
- The publication of test results, commonly known as 'league tables'.
- The requirement that LEAs will support schools who are not achieving and help them improve.
- The 'naming and shaming' of failing schools, and ultimately requirements for them to be closed if they do not improve.

Increasingly, the government is not only determining *what* should be taught, but is telling schools and LEAs *how* it should be taught. The National Literacy Strategy, described as a framework for teaching, sets out the DfES requirements for the teaching of literacy skills in reading, comprehension, spelling and writing. The strategy prescribes the practical arrangements that should be put in place, via a literacy hour of teaching in all schools, with detailed information about how that hour should be organised and taught. Similarly, schools have to follow the National Numeracy Strategy for the teaching of mathematics.

Inclusion of pupils with special educational needs

Although there is still a wide range of views about where children with special educational needs should be educated, the overall trend of the last decade has been towards inclusion. The concept means different things to different people.

The DfES regards inclusion as a 'process, not a fixed state'. Ultimately it means there should be a place for every child at his local mainstream school, and that they should be totally accepted and their needs met. In other words, it is about 'belonging' and not experiencing segregation or discrimination.

It is important to be clear about the different meanings of 'inclusion' and 'integration'. Inclusion is about accepting children as they are and adapting schools' curricula and ways of working so that they are accessible to young people, while integration is generally regarded as trying to support a young person with aids or personal assistance so that they can access the unchanged school.

Children with even the most complex needs are now being educated in the local mainstream school, and there is less use of more segregated options such as special schools and units. The DfES requires

Education services

Table 15.1
Education phases

Phase	Age (years)	'Year'	National Curriculum	Compulsory education[a]	Establishment	'Run by' tests/exams	Assessment
Foundation Stage (nursery and reception)	3–5	–	Not applicable (but there are Early Learning Goals [ELGs])	No	Nursery schools	LEA	ELGs
					School nursery units (separate building in the school grounds)	LEA	
					School nursery classes (classroom within the school)	LEA	
					Playgroups Family centres Private nurseries	Pre-school learning alliance Voluntary organisations Social services Private owners	
Primary	5–7	Y1 Y2	Key stage 1	Yes	Primary schools or	LEA (diocese for denominational schools)	National Curriculum (NC) Standard Assessment Tasks (SATs)
	7–11	Y3 Y4 Y5 Y6	Key stage 2	Yes	separate infant schools and junior schools In some areas: First schools Middle schools Upper schools		
Secondary	11–14	Y7 Y8 Y9	Key stage 3	Yes	Secondary schools In many areas, fully comprehensive, but some parts of England and Wales still retain grammar schools and selection Names vary, e.g. some call themselves community colleges	LEA (Diocese)	NC SATs
	14–16	Y10 Y11	Key stage 4	Yes			GCSEs
Sixth Form	16–18/19	–	Not applicable	No	Sixth forms in schools Sixth form colleges	LEA College and FEFC[b]	'A' levels National Vocational Qualifications (NVQs)
Tertiary					Further education colleges	College and FEFC[b]	
Higher	18+	–	–	No	University	University	Degrees

[a] The law does not dictate that children must attend school to receive their education, simply that they must receive an education. Some parents elect to provide this themselves for their children at home. This arrangement is generally known as 'education otherwise'
[b] Further Education Funding Council: the government have made some early moves on reviewing post-16 education, and have indicated their wish to move towards a unified funding system for post-16 education that takes place in FE colleges, and that which takes place in schools

Partnerships

Promoting partnership is a keystone of the government's approach to improving educational attainment. It expects a partnership approach in a variety of ways: between parents and schools; between LEAs and various agencies; by formal agreements or groups and through less formal arrangements. There are many forms of partnerships, depending on the focus and local interpretation. Some examples are given below.

Home school agreements

The DfEE expects all schools to have written home-school agreements, drawn up in consultation with parents. These are intended to explain the school's aims and values to parents, spell out the responsibilities of school and parents, clarify what is expected of pupils, and provide information on topics such as homework and behaviour.

Parents are expected to sign the agreement to show that they understand and accept it.

Parent partnership schemes (Box 15.4)

All LEAs are expected to have a scheme for the parents of pupils with special educational needs (SEN). The aim is to provide parents with independent information and advice about SEN procedures, school-based provision, support available for their child, and additional sources of help and information. As with many initiatives, there are differences in local operation of such schemes. Some are based within the LEA using LEA officers, others are distanced as in the next example.

that all initiatives should involve children with special educational needs, including the National Curriculum, the literacy hour, target setting and the rest.

Compare the example given in Box 15.2 with little more than a generation ago, when children with severe learning difficulties (at that time described as severely subnormal) were not entitled to education, being labelled 'ineducable'. Others with less learning difficulties but other specific disabilities were put into special schools or even 'sent away' to residential schools without their parents having any say, and without considering the feelings or rights of the child (Box 15.3).

Today parents and children, and young people themselves, are expected to be properly consulted about their wishes. Schools themselves appreciate the benefits of inclusion. More enlightened schools recognise that having pupils with special needs is an enriching experience for the school as a whole, and gives all students the opportunity to benefit from being part of a varied and inclusive community.

Box 15.4
The Nottingham and Nottinghamshire Parent Partnership Project

The project is run independently, although it is jointly funded by the two LEAs, and is located in the voluntary sector. It provides support for parents of children with SEN, through telephone and personal advice and the provision of independent parental supporters (formerly called named persons). The project produces a variety of information leaflets for parents and professionals, it organises and delivers workshops and training for volunteers, parents and professionals.

Partnerships between NHS and local authorities

There are no formal arrangements in place at the moment, but health, social services and education generally have good working liaison. The DfES plans to develop a more integrated local planning framework for all children's services, including those for children with special educational needs. They are also considering therapy needs, especially for speech and language therapy, where difficulties in securing services are felt to result partly from the different statutory responsibilities and priorities of health authorities and LEAs, but also from lack of clarity over funding. The DfES Programme of Action plans for new powers to enable more flexible funding between NHS and local authorities.

Early years development and child care partnerships

These are groups of people from statutory, private and voluntary organisations with a brief to plan for education in the early years (mainly 3 and 4 year olds), and child care for children from 0 to 14. Among the targets for these partnerships are to strengthen provision for the early years, to increase opportunities for child care, and to ensure maximum choice and high standards for parents and their children.

WHAT PEOPLE IN THE EDUCATION SERVICES DO

Local education authorities

The LEA is responsible for the planning and delivery of education policy and practical arrangements. It must ensure that DfES requirements are carried out and develop its own policies. Some examples of what is expected of LEAs are given below:

- An education development plan, which must set out targets for improving pupils' achievement, for improving school attendance and reducing exclusions. The plan must say what the LEA intends to do to help schools achieve these targets.
- A behaviour support plan, which should describe current provision and future plans for development to support those pupils whose behaviour in schools causes concern.
- Information on their policy for the inclusion of pupils with special educational needs.
- Early years and child care development plan, which should include arrangements for the education of children under five and child care arrangements for day care of young and older children.

All policies and plans have to go through a consultation and reviewing process, and be integrated into the local authority planning system.

In addition, the LEA takes decisions on pupils with special educational needs: whether to carry out a statutory assessment; whether to issue a formal statement of those needs; and on school placements and arrangements. In all of this, they have to follow DfES requirements to involve parents and, in the case of statutory assessments, to meet set timelines.

Most LEAs employ expert advisory staff on specific difficulties such as autism and dyslexia. They also arrange and provide a variety of training, including for teachers, support staff and governors.

Schools

The head teacher is responsible for the day to day running of the school, including making decisions, planning and allocating the school resources of finance and personnel, and being responsible for the education of the pupils. He or she is responsi-

---

Box 15.5
The role of a special educational needs coordinator (SENCO) in a primary school

Mrs Brooks is the SENCO for a primary school. She has a class of her own which she teaches on 4½ days of the week. She has half a day[a] to carry out her SENCO role. This will typically involve her in most of the following activities:

- Writing and taking responsibility for the school's own policy for SEN.
- Being aware of the requirements of the Code of Practice and of any developments in the field of SEN.
- Maintaining and overviewing the school's SEN register.
- Supporting her colleagues in meeting the needs of children with SEN in the school.
- Having an overview of individual education plans (IEPs) for the children at the relevant stages of the Code of Practice.
- Organising and monitoring any additional support provided for those children.
- Liaising with and informing the parents of the children with SEN.
- Liaising with support services and agencies, such as outreach/learning support teachers, educational psychologists, speech and language and other therapists, school and community doctors, social services.
- Planning and attending review meetings on children at relevant stages of the Code of Practice.

[a] This is an example. The time given to a SENCO varies according to the school and is decided by the head teacher and governors in liaison with that person.

---

ble in turn to the governing body of the school. Governors, locally elected or appointed and unpaid, have major responsibilities and powers. Among the teachers, the role of the special needs coordinator (SENCO) is a relatively recent and increasingly important one (Box 15.5).

Apart from teachers, there is a wide range of people working in schools who have an important role to play, ranging from the kitchen and midday supervisory staff to caretaker, librarian or technician. Some who work more directly in classrooms and with the pupils are those who support learning, especially for children with special educational needs (Box 15.6). These are teaching assistants who may have a variety of titles, including learning support assistants or welfare assistants, and who will mostly be qualified in child care and development, play and early learning.

Support services

A characteristic of LEA support services is that they are not usually based in or employed by schools.

Box 15.6
The role of a support assistant in a mainstream primary school

Mrs Jones is a support assistant in a mainstream primary school. She has the National Nursery Examination Board (NNEB) qualification and 5 years' experience working in a school nursery. She is employed for 10 hours a week to provide teaching support for a boy with Down's syndrome. Mrs Jones has taken a Makaton course provided by the speech and language therapy department, and helps to support the boy's language development using Makaton, and following a programme provided by the therapist.

Mrs Jones is responsible to the class teacher, and supports the boy during in-class activities. He is able to carry out many class activities on his own, and she is helping to encourage his independence. The 10 hours' support was allocated by the LEA, who review it on a regular basis.

> ### Box 15.7
> ### The role of an early years worker
>
> Mrs Brown is a qualified and very experienced nursery nurse who is part of a team of early years workers and teachers. She has high level teaching skills, with an in-depth knowledge of child development and learning. She visits a number of children under five on a regular basis, usually once a fortnight. She starts by completing a baseline assessment, focusing on what the child *can* do. Then, in liaison with the parents, she plans activities to enable the child to learn new skills through play and at the child's own pace. The basis of the early years teaching service is recognition that parents and carers are the main educators of the child. The focus is on the parent helping the child's learning through an informal but structured approach, leading the child through the relevant developmental stages and attainments. Mrs Brown works closely with other professionals from education, health and social services, and she links with nurseries and schools.

Employed by the LEA, they visit schools and/or children regularly to help support children's learning, or to support schools in their own development and in meeting DfES requirements.

Specialist support teaching staff

Early years staff work with children aged 0–5 who have a range of special needs (Box 15.7). They usually provide home teaching, often following a Portage model, supporting parents and carers in their role as the child's first educators. They also liaise with nurseries, other professionals and with schools.

Special needs teachers (sometimes called outreach staff) will visit schools to assess and monitor pupils with learning difficulties, and to advise staff on teaching approaches.

Sensory teachers are those qualified to teach deaf or visually impaired children. They will be involved in supporting and teaching children under five and in supporting older children in schools, through regular monitoring and advising staff.

Emotional and behavioural difficulties (EBD) services, or sometimes called behaviour support teachers, work to help support children with particular behaviour difficulties, working sometimes directly with the pupils, but mainly advising staff. They are 'outreach' staff, and are often based in pupil referral units (PRUs), which are units for pupils with severe behavioural difficulties where plans are for the pupil to return to full-time mainstream schooling.

Advisory and inspection services (often now called school effectiveness and improvement services) are committed to support schools in raising standards. They advise on curriculum and practice and school development.

Educational psychology services provide advice on children's learning and development, including emotional and behavioural difficulties. Each school within an LEA usually has a named educational psychologist who provides a service within the area for children aged 0–19.

The main focus of work for the *education welfare service* is with those pupils who do not attend school regularly. They work with and for these pupils in a number of ways, including individual counselling and support, support for parents/carers, liaison with other services and agencies, and negotiating packages of alternative provision. Some LEAs employ education welfare officers especially for pupils who are 'Looked after', since they are a very vulnerable group of pupils.

PERSPECTIVES

The medical and the educational perspectives on children with disabilities are different.

Understanding the differences in the types of questions asked about disability and the kind of interventions made is of more than philosophical interest: it is crucial to any effective partnership between school health personnel and staff in the teaching profession. It has only been within the last 20 years that the educational perspective on disability has been clearly articulated. Previous to this, teachers responsible for the education of disabled children borrowed heavily from the medical model of disability to make sense of their practice. Thus children diagnosed as 'educationally subnormal' (ESN) were seen as requiring 'special educational treatment' by specialised 'remedial' staff. Such terms are now rarely if ever used within educational thinking, and an understanding of the edu-

Education services

Box 15.8
Questions asked about disabled children from a medical perspective

Diagnostic questions:
How are the typical features of the disability best described?
What are the common features across individual cases?
How do these features interrelate?
How does the overall picture differ from that seen in other conditions and disabilities?

Epidemiological questions:
Who is affected by this disability?
What is its prevalence?
Is this increasing or decreasing?

Aetiological questions:
What is the cause of this condition?
What is the influence of pre-, peri- and postnatal factors?
What weight should we give environmental versus genetic factors?

Prognostic questions:
What is the likely course of this condition?
What are the likely outcomes?
Can normal functioning be restored?

Therapeutic questions:
What treatment or combination of treatments is likely to be most effective in restoring normal functioning or limiting further deterioration?
Where is this treatment available?

---

skills, attitudes and resources of the individual teacher, as well as the overall organisation and ethos of that school itself. Thus what may be viewed as a special need or difficulty in one teaching situation may not be apparent, or be much less apparent, in another differently organised situation. It is for these reasons that such questions as: 'What is this child's handicap?'; 'What is his IQ?'; 'What are the correct treatments for his condition?' do not figure amongst the prime concerns of an educational venture. *Schools are not treatment centres* (if they were they would be organised quite differently). They are social institutions responsible for delivering a curriculum, a range of learning experiences, to their pupils regardless of their disability.

Because of these fundamental differences in the questions asked by each approach to disability, and the differences in the overall aims, there are as a result important differences in the way a child with a disability is viewed from each perspective (Box 15.10).

It is clear from the list of differences in emphasis shown in Box 15.10 that the outcomes for disabled pupils in terms of type of provision likely to be made are also likely to differ. Broadly, a medical perspective will tend to highlight a need for segregated or special education, and an educational perspective will tend to give rise to education being provided in an integrated setting.

Despite these differences in aims and outcomes, an understanding of the medical perspective on an individual pupil is important to the work of teachers. A knowledge of the child from this perspective is likely to provide helpful pointers to those areas of curricular planning likely to need particular attention to ensure access to learning experiences for that pupil. This will be most obviously true for pupils with visual and auditory impairments, where a medical profile of deficit will be essential to enable appropriate teaching arrangements. It will also be true for pupils with less objectively definable disabilities such as 'autism' — for a teacher to know that a child is viewed as 'autistic' from a medical perspective is very likely to mean that those aspects of the curriculum concerned with interaction and relationships will figure highly in the child's overall timetable.

cational model that has replaced them is needed by the health service personnel working with schools. One useful way of clarifying the differences between the medical and educational approaches to disability is to consider the typical questions asked from within each perspective (Box 15.8).

In clear contrast, to understand a disability from an educational perspective leads us to ask a quite different set of questions about the individual child (Box 15.9).

The primary concerns of a teacher are to look at the individual child and his unique educational needs. Those needs will be seen as essentially *relative* and only capable of being understood in the context of the learning situation the child is in. This situation crucially includes such factors as the

---

Box 15.9
Questions asked about disabled children from an educational perspective

---

Profiling questions:
What are this child's strengths and weaknesses?
What observations will the teachers need to make, and in what settings, to ensure a full profile is achieved?

Questions about learning history and style of learning:
In what situations does the child appear to learn most effectively?
How has the child learned the skills already achieved?

Questions about a child's overall needs:
What development has taken place in the child's self-help skills, personal and social development?
Emotional and behavioural needs and independence are of interest, along with academic and language skills.

Questions about curricular priorities:
What aspects of this child's present approach to learning are acting as barriers to future learning?
What types of learning experiences are priorities for this child?

Questions about curricular access:
What teaching conditions/resources/styles will need to be provided in order to maximise this child's access to the
    National Curriculum?
What must the teacher plan to ensure that the curriculum offered has breadth, balance and provides learning
    experiences which are age appropriate and relevant to this child's particular situation?

Questions about future learning:
What are the next steps in development?
What teaching plans can be made?
What learning targets can be set?

However, knowing the diagnostic label that has been assigned to a child does not change the fundamental nature of the teacher's task, which is to ensure maximum access to the curriculum. This is the teacher's task, *whatever their pupils' difficulties*, and it is essentially an individualised exercise that will need to be gone through for each child in turn. It will be based on a detailed understanding of that child's particular strengths and weaknesses in learning. From an educational perspective there is no 'one size fits all' treatment for any child's difficulties. However, the aims of education are the same for all.

SOME OF THE TENSIONS

Inevitably in such a complex system there are bound to be tensions. The demands do not always sit comfortably with the expectations. On the one hand, there is the desire, pressure and indeed requirement that children and young people with special educational needs should be included in their local mainstream school. On the other hand, the raising of standards is a dominating theme that may overshadow all others. Thus the issue of inclusion may be in tension with the raising of standards. However, schools which are successful at being inclusive are also successful at other things as well, usually having high standards and raising achievement for all. This is because the same underlying characteristics — good leadership, good planning, good monitoring and review — are common to both enterprises.

With the large number of people who are involved in education, there is a variety of views. Not all teachers are totally supportive of inclusion or of the approach to the teaching of literacy. Most parents are happy to work in partnership with schools and teachers, but there are some who would rather hand over total responsibility, despite a desire for their children to succeed. Many therapists believe that whatever they can deliver is best delivered in a special school. Some doctors maintain that 'labels' are the answer, that a 'within-child' explanation is

---

Box 15.10
Different views of a child's disability from medical and educational perspectives

Medical perspective:
- Child is described in terms of his deficits and divergence from the norm. These deficits exist exclusively within the pupil

- Child is categorised by diagnostic label

- School placement by categorical label

- Exceptionality defined by comparison with the norm
- Specialist staff and specialised resources characterise remediative approaches
- Curriculum for disabled pupils is specialised and different from regular curriculum

- The exceptional needs of disabled pupils are highlighted

Educational perspective:
- Child is described by unique individual profile of strengths and weaknesses. Needs and difficulties seen as *relative* to variety of environmental factors. Difficulties arise as a result of interaction between pupil and environment

- Child is categorised by curricular needs and support required to meet those needs

- School placement determined by availability of resources needed for curricular access

- Individual assessment identifies teaching priorities

- All teachers have a role and contribute to curriculum delivery

- Curriculum is same for all, but modified in level, rate and methods of delivery for disabled pupils (i.e. the curriculum is 'differentiated')

- Needs in common of all pupils emphasised

---

the way, rather than acknowledge an interactionist perspective which recognises that children's difficulties are caused by a combination of factors, including external ones such as the demands of the curriculum or the setting of the class.

Yet everyone wants the best for their children, for all children. Everyone wants quality schools and quality education services. The challenge is to work together to achieve this.

FURTHER READING

Department for Education and Skills (DfES) publications
Code of practice on the identification and assessment of special educational needs (1994) — a revised version is due to be published in 2002

Meeting special educational needs: a programme of action (1998)
The National Literacy Strategy — framework for teaching (1998)
Supporting pupils with special medical Needs (1996)

Local publications
Most LEAs will have written information about their policies, development plans and support services. Support services themselves will have leaflets describing their work. It is helpful to approach your area LEA for relevant local information
Schools Achieving Success, White Paper. DfES 2001 Updated information is on the DfES website: *www.dfes.gov.uk*.

16 | Social services

INTRODUCTION

Personal social services help children and young people, elderly people, disabled people, people with mental illness or learning disabilities, their families and carers. At any one time up to 1.5 million people rely on help from social services. Everyone is likely to need their help at some point in their lifecycle, and very often at a point of crisis.

Personal social services are administered by local authorities but central government is responsible for establishing national policies, issuing guidance and overseeing standards, through the Department of Health (DH) and the Social Services Inspectorate (SSI). Joint finance and planning between health and local authorities aims to prevent overlapping of services and to encourage the development of community services.

The statutory services are provided by local government social services departments (SSDs) in England and Wales, social work departments in Scotland, and health and social services boards in Northern Ireland. Alongside these providers are the many and varied contributions made by independent private and voluntary services.

This chapter outlines the range of social services responsibilities for vulnerable people, but with a focus on their specific functions as regards to children and young people.

HISTORICAL CONTEXT AND CURRENT STRUCTURE

The Second World War precipitated major reforms in health and social care. The Beveridge Report, published in 1942, recommended extensive changes, including the extension of health, social security and personal social services. Two years later the government published their first plan for a comprehensive national health service, later embodied in the National Health Service Act 1946. The NHS came into operation in July 1948, providing a complete general practitioner and hospital service for all.

In the same year the 1948 National Assistance Act finally brought to an end the Poor Law, while introducing a national social security system and an expanded role for local authorities in delivering personal social services to adults. The 1948 Children Act for the first time also placed a clear duty on local authorities to provide a comprehensive service for the care of children deprived of the benefits of a normal life. Later legislation significantly increased the responsibilities of social care in helping those with mental health needs or physical disabilities to lead independent lives in the community.

Social work as an activity, and social workers as a professional group, become more powerful during the 1950s to early 1970s, indeed, they owed their very existence and status as 'experts' to the power of the state.

By the 1960s it had become apparent that many families required services from more than one local authority department and so the 1965 Seebohm Committee recommended the structural changes, many of which were implemented by the 1970 Local Authority Social Services Act. This brought together a number of services which had previously been run separately to form generic social services departments. The intention was, as far as possible, to ensure that families or individuals in need of care or protection would be served by a single social worker from a single department.

Social services

It was the 1988 Griffiths Report on community care (Griffiths 1988), and the NHS and Community Care Act 1990, however, which were to have the most radical implications for the shape and activities of SSDs. Griffiths endorsed the philosophy and values of social services, not the primacy of social work, in delivering community-based services. Many SSDs in the 1990s split their organisation and operation between children's and adult services, propelled by the Griffiths report and subsequent adult (community care) legislation, and by the quite separate 1989 Children Act.

Services for adults include residential care homes for elderly and other vulnerable people, day care for elderly people and those with physical or learning difficulties, alcohol and drug misuse services, community care assessments of vulnerable service users and family carers, care management, inspection and complaints work and direct service provision for care in the community, for example home help and home care services, meals on wheels, etc. The legislative context for much of this work is provided by the NHS and Community Care Act 1990 (finally implemented in 1993), the Carers (Recognition and Services) Act 1995 (implemented in 1996) and other pieces of legislation concerning the needs of elderly or disabled people, those with mental health problems and other vulnerable groups. Services for adults account for about three-quarters of all social services spending, the majority of which is spent specifically on services for elderly people.

The split between adult services and children's services within SSDs has not only widened social services remit, but has also required departments to move away from being direct providers of services, to arrangers and purchasers of services supplied by voluntary and independent (private) agencies. Moreover, there has been a resurgence of old problems, including a lack of coordination between adult and children's services (characteristic of the immediate postwar period), a move away from a 'whole person' approach, and increased difficulties with joint working between social services and other agencies, including the health service.

Table 16.1
The main groups in all social care sectors

Group	Social care workers (no.)
Home care services	169 000
Day services for adults	26 000
Residential services for adults	416 000
Occupational therapists	2 000
Social workers, care managers and assistants	55 000
Day services for children	156 000
Residential services for children (includes foster carers)	37 000
Managerial and administrative staff	186 000
Total	**1 047 000**

SOCIAL CARE

Today, approximately one million people work full or part time in providing social care in England — as many as the number employed in the NHS (Table 16.1). About 30% of these staff work for local authorities in SSDs. Over half of all social care staff (about 562 000) are employed by the private sector and about 172 000 staff are employed by the voluntary sector (Fig. 16.1).

The majority of staff employed in social care, both in the independent sector and within social services departments, have no or few formal qualifications. Most staff therefore rely on the training provided by their employers to undertake increasingly complex tasks. A new General Social Care Council will set and enforce standards of conduct and practice for all those who work in social care. This should put social care on to a proper professional footing on a similar basis to other caring professions.

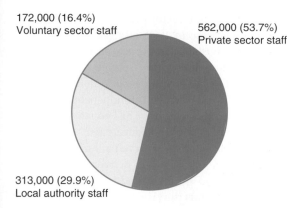

172,000 (16.4%)
Voluntary sector staff

562,000 (53.7%)
Private sector staff

313,000 (29.9%)
Local authority staff

Fig. 16.1 Size of social care workforce: 1996. Source DH 1998a

LOCAL AUTHORITY SOCIAL SERVICES DEPARTMENTS

Local authority SSDs exist to keep vulnerable people safe and to promote independence. These departments are now regarded widely as the 'fourth arm' of the welfare state, alongside the health service, social security and education. Around one-third of a million people are employed in SSDs in England.

There are about 150 local authorities with social services responsibilities in England which relate to 100 health authorities and over 500 NHS trusts. Only 34 health authorities have the same boundaries as SSDs. Over time the number of health authorities will be reduced as primary care groups develop. This means that the number and complexity of relationships will increase.

Each year the government decides what it believes local authorities need to spend on social services, provision for which is made through the Revenue Support Grant (RSG) and special or specific grants. Authorities may spend more or less in the light of local priorities and circumstances. The RSG is distributed on the basis of standard spending assessments (SSAs) for each local government service, which take account of measures of relative need (e.g. the age profile of the local population, the number of children of lone parents, etc.). The resource allocation formulae are reviewed each year. Special and specific grants are distributed in a variety of ways. Some use a combination of the SSA formulae, others are distributed by competitive

bidding or on the basis of the number of local service users.

SSDs account for about 13% of all local authority staffing and about 10% of all local authority spending. Expenditure on SSDs nationally was about £9.5 billion in 1997–98. This expenditure has increased tenfold over the last 25 years, although it is still less than one-tenth of what is spent on the social security system. Over the 10 years from 1986–87, gross expenditure on social services trebled in cash terms, from about £3 billion. Over the same period, gross expenditure on social services has increased by 89% in real terms.

Most social services provision is provided within a statutory framework. So, for example, the Chronically Sick and Disabled Persons Act 1970 is a primary piece of legislation to enable and encourage disabled people to live reasonably independent lives in their own homes; the Children Act 1989 recasts the legislative framework for children's services, care and protection into a single coherent structure; while the NHS and Community Care Act 1990 provides the framework for the provision and delivery of health and social care services to adults, including those with mental health problems, physical disabilities, learning difficulties, elderly people and those who misuse alcohol or drugs.

While local authority SSDs have to implement central government policies and legislation in the fields of child care and adult services, they still have considerable power to determine their own local priorities based on their own local profile of needs. Priorities and policies are determined by local politicians; implementation is through paid officers — professionals such as social workers, care managers, home helps and so on. However, professional judgements influence local political decisions, and vice versa.

TYPES OF SERVICE PROVIDED, ARRANGED OR FUNDED BY SOCIAL SERVICES DEPARTMENTS

Residential care

Many vulnerable people, including those with physical or mental impairments, elderly people, children and others, may not be able to live at home on their own, or with family, because they are frail, need care or protection, need control or have no one else available to care for them. SSDs provide or fund residential care for such groups, including residential care homes and children's homes.

- There were 17800 staffed residential care homes providing about 371000 places for vulnerable adults in 1997. The majority of places (about 75%) were in homes for elderly people. In addition, there are around 6700 small homes with fewer than four places and around 4000 independent sector nursing homes. Local authorities are no longer the main providers of residential accommodation; by 1997 local authorities provided only 18% of the total provision compared to 45% in 1987. While the number of people in local authority homes has reduced, the percentage placed in the independent sector rose from 20% in 1993 to 66% in 1997 and an increasing proportion were supported in independent nursing homes.
- The number of children in children's homes has declined from about 18000 in 1984 to 7000 in 1996.
- About 66000 people work in social services residential care establishments. In 1997, 44% of all full-time equivalent posts were filled by part-time staff. Only a small minority of residential staff are professionally qualified.

Day centres

There were about 632000 day centre (whole-day equivalent) places available for local authority clients during 1997, 24% more than in 1992. The majority (78%) continue to be provided in local authorities' own day centres, although independent sector provision increased from 10% of the total in 1992 to 19%.

Home care and meals on wheels

About half a million households receive some home help or home care. About 2.64 million contact hours of home help or home care was purchased or provided by local authorities each week in 1997. One-quarter of all social services staff are involved in home care.

The independent sector provided 2% of publicly funded home care in 1992, rising to 44% by 1997. One of the most noticeable effects of the growth of independent home care services has been an increase in flexible care at evenings and weekends.

About one-quarter of a million people a week receive meals on wheels. This equates to about three-quarters of a million meals per week delivered to people's homes or served at luncheon clubs. Most meals (about 85%) are delivered to people's own homes, and the independent sector provides almost half of this service (41%). Around 9% of meals are provided at weekends, with two-thirds of this service being provided directly by local authorities.

Welfare rights services

Many SSDs now employ specialist welfare rights advisers to advise local people, and other SSD staff, about benefits and other welfare entitlements (services in kind as well as cash), and help them to secure their rights. Welfare rights workers will be involved in individual casework with vulnerable clients to maximise their incomes, and with larger campaigns to help groups of claimants.

Field social work

Only 13% of SSD staff, around 35000 people, are field social workers. Most field social workers have a professional qualification gained from a university course accredited to the Central Council for the Education and Training of Social Workers. Social work practice is largely governed by a framework of legislation — social workers fulfil statutory requirements under children and adult legislation. However, despite the legal framework much practice is discretionary, based upon professional judgments and assessments.

Social workers provide help and support to, and also social control of, many different groups of people defined as in need of care or protection. So, for example, social workers will be involved in assessing and responding to cases of child abuse and neglect, compulsory detention of people with mental health problems where they are a danger to themselves or others, arranging fostering and adoption services for children in need, counselling people with trauma, and many other activities.

SOCIAL SERVICES SPECIFICALLY FOR CHILDREN

Work with children and families includes child protection, children looked after, children in need, children's homes, secure units, fostering and adoption (substitute family care), family work, youth offender teams, work with disabled children, guardian ad litem work, etc. Much of this activity, and many of these services, are provided within the legislative context of the 1989 Children Act and consequent guidance. Services for children account for about one-quarter of all personal social services spending.

Local authorities must safeguard the welfare of any child in need, and promote the upbringing of such children by their families, by providing a range and level of services appropriate to those children's needs. These services can include advice, guidance, counselling, help in the home, or family centres, and can be provided for the family of the child in need or any member of the family if this will safeguard the child's welfare. Local authorities can provide these services directly or arrange for them to be provided by, for example, a voluntary or private organisation. They are also required to publicise the help available to families in need.

In England and Wales a child may be brought before a family proceedings court if he is neglected or ill treated, exposed to moral danger, beyond the control of parents or not attending school. The court can commit children to the care of a local authority. Certain pre-conditions have to be satisfied to justify a care order. These are that the children are suffering or are likely to suffer significant harm because of a lack of reasonable parental care or because they are beyond parental control. An order is made only if the court is also satisfied that this will contribute positively to the children's well being and be in their best interests. In court proceedings children are entitled to separate legal representation and the right to have a guardian to protect their interests. All courts have to treat the welfare of children as the paramount consideration when reaching any decision about their upbringing. The law requires

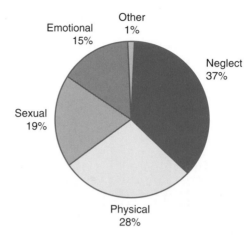

Fig. 16.2 Percentage of children on child protection registers 1998, by category of abuse. Source DH 1998b

that wherever possible children should remain at home with their families.

Since 1996 it has been mandatory for local authorities to assess the level of need for children's services in their area and draw up a Children's Service Plan, prepared by the SSD in liaison with the health and education authorities, certain voluntary organisations, the police, probation service and other relevant bodies. The plan should reflect the medium-term strategic planning process by projecting ahead 3 years, being reviewed regularly in the interim.

Children on child protection registers

Children and young people are placed on a child protection register if abuse has already taken place or if they are considered to be at risk of abuse or neglect, and if they require an interagency plan to protect them. Since 1993 the numbers on child protection registers in England have stabilised at about 32 000 (Fig. 16.2). This represents about 28 children on the register for every 10 000 children. However, there are significant local variations, with some authorities having around eight children on the register in every 10 000, and others with as many as 78 per 10 000.

Younger children have higher rates of registration than older children, and boys have similar rates

Social services

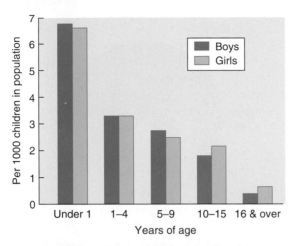

Fig. 16.3 Registrations to child protection registers during 1997, by age group and sex. Source DH 1998a

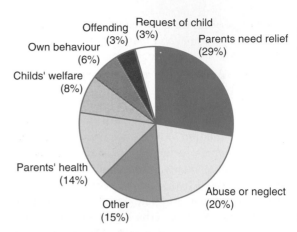

Fig. 16.4 Reasons why children are looked after: 1996. Source DH 1998a

to girls up to the age of ten, but after this the rates for girls are higher (Fig. 16.3).

Children looked after by the local authority

Children looked after by local authorities are those children and young persons for whom local authorities, primarily through their SSDs, provide accommodation and care. Children can be looked after by local authorities for a number of reasons (Fig. 16.4). Their own families may be unable to care for them because of illness or death, or because of disability or mental health needs, or respite care may be needed in the case of families of children with disabilities. Other families may have failed to provide proper care, putting children at risk of abuse or neglect, or the children may have been accused or found guilty of a criminal offence. Most children looked after come from low-income and disadvantaged families. Some children are accommodated under a voluntary agreement, others are subject to court orders. The Children Act 1989 puts emphasis on partnership with parents and on the principle that generally court orders should only be made if in the best interests of the child.

Local authorities are responsible as corporate parents for the welfare of looked after children. They are required to support children and their

families and, where possible, take measures to prevent the necessity arising for children to leave home.

Through the 1980s and until 1994 the number of children looked after by the local authority reduced significantly each year. In 1986, the total number of children looked after was about 67 000. Since 1994 it has stablised at around 50 000 children. This represents about 47 children looked after per 10 000 children under 18.

Children looked after can be placed in a number of different settings. The majority (about two-thirds) are placed in foster care. The number placed in children's homes reduced significantly from 15 000 in 1986 to 6000 in 1996. Some (about 5000 in 1996) were placed with their own family, often as a step towards a permanent return home.

Much public concern has been expressed in recent years over the treatment of children looked after by local authorities. This concern has focused chiefly on allegations of physical and sexual abuse, or SSI concerns about poor practice and management. In 1996 the Prime Minister established a review of safeguards for children living away from home, conducted by Sir William Utting. The Utting report, 'People Like Us', was published in November 1997 and presents a woeful tale of failure at all levels to provide a secure and decent childhood for some of the most vulnerable children in society. It shows that in far too many cases children were harmed in care rather than helped. Failings were not just the fault of individuals but also of the whole system.

The House of Commons Health Committee (1998a) also examined the experiences of and outcomes for children looked after and reported that it was gravely concerned about policy and practice in this area. Inspections of planning and decision-making for children looked after, and of the safety of children looked after (Social Services Inspectrate 1998), reveal a catalogue of concerns about how important decisions are made and the arrangements to ensure that children are safe. There was evidence of good and bad practice in most authorities but no authority could be fully confident about the services it provided. While all departments had developed a range of planning, policy and procedural documents, these were not always followed by staff. Managers did not have the systems to check that workers complied with procedures and guidance. This led to inconsistency in practice, service delivery and placement of children.

The government's response to the children's safeguard review was published in November 1998 and was linked to the establishment of the 'Quality Protects' programme, a major initiative to improve social services policy and practice with children in need, and children looked after in particular. Quality Protects is discussed in more detail later in the chapter.

Children's homes

In 1997 there were about 1200 homes in England accommodating children, these were either run by local authorities or were registered with them or with the Department of Health. Two-thirds are local authority maintained or controlled community homes, approximately one-sixth were private registered homes and the remaining sixth were either care homes registered under the 1984 Registered Homes Act, registered voluntary children's homes, assisted community homes or dual-registered schools. The maximum number of places available in these homes is around 11 000 in total, although only about half the places were in use at any one time in 1996.

Day care for young children

Playgroups

These are run by trained playgroup leaders and the playgroup movement is represented by the Pre-school Playgroups Association. Playgroups need to be approved and registered with the local authority. Attendance may be from one to five mornings a week. They provide an opportunity for children to meet, play and socialise and for parents to meet too. Playgroups may be held in church halls, community centres, private premises or attached to schools, health centres or various social work agencies.

Childminders

Childminders have to be legally approved and registered with SSDs. In spite of this requirement much illegal and unsatisfactory childminding still takes place, characterised often by overcrowding, inadequate space, lack of toys or inadequate stimulation. The provision of training courses for childminders and appropriate support services can ensure a higher level of care. The child who is quiet and withdrawn is perhaps particularly vulnerable in the childminding setting. Between 1991 and 1996, places with childminders increased by 61%, from 233 000 to 367 000 nationally.

Day nurseries

These are generally run by social service, but others are run privately or by various voluntary organisations (Fig. 16.5). They all have to obtain registration and approval by the local authority SSD. Day nurseries are staffed by nursery nurses (who have undergone a 2-year training) and have an experienced matron and deputy in charge. Places in day nurseries increased by 68% from 106 000 in 1991 to 178 000 in 1996.

Family centres

The family centre is essentially a day-care setting in which parents attend as well as their children and in which a number of programmes are established to teach parenting skills and to increase the confidence and self-esteem of parents.

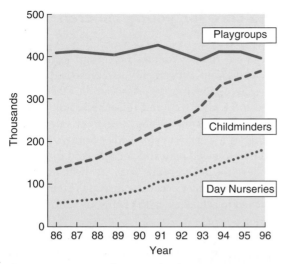

Fig. 16.5 Day care places, England: 1986–96. Source: DH 1998a

Children placed for adoption

Local authority SSDs are required by law to provide an adoption service, either directly or by arrangement with approved voluntary adoption societies, and many SSDs also provide a postadoption service for children and adults. It is illegal to receive an unrelated child for adoption through an unapproved third party. The registrars-general keep confidential registers of adopted children. Adopted people may be given details of their original birth record on reaching the age of 18 (or 16 if adopted in Scotland), and counselling is provided to help them understand the circumstances of their adoption. An Adoption Contact Register enables adopted adults and their birth parents to be given a safe and confidential way of making contact if that is the wish of both parties. A person's details are entered only if they wish to be contacted.

The number of adoption orders peaked at 25 000 in 1968 and fell to about 6000 in 1996 (3000 boys, 3000 girls). Of these, about half are adopted by one legal parent and a new partner, following marriage or remarriage. The average age at which children were adopted in 1996 was $5\frac{1}{2}$ years. As the number of placements reduces, fewer social work staff have experience and confidence in adoption work.

Children in need

In addition to children looked after and those on child protection registers, there are about 300 000 more children in need at any one time, of whom about 50 000 are disabled children. Many 'young carers' (see Chapter 23) could also be considered to be children in need.

QUALITY PROTECTS

On 21 September 1998 the government launched Quality Protects, a 3-year programme to transform the delivery and management of children's services. The initiative comprised the publication of a set of government objectives for children's services, a framework for the preparation of new Quality Protects Action Plans by local authorities and guidance for local councillors. In addition, the government committed about £350 million additional resources over 3 years to social services, in the form of a special grant for children's services.

Quality Protects will have a strong concentration on better outcomes, for which targets will be set. The key changes are:

- The reform and renewal of the public care system.
- Improving the education of looked after children.
- Increasing the choice of placements for looked after children.
- Improving services for care leavers.
- Radical improvements to procedures to prevent dangerous people from working with children.
- Stronger emphasis on interagency working and the corporate responsibility of local authorities.
- Better safeguards for children and young people in all settings away from home.

The Quality Protects programme sets out eight national objectives, each of which is accompanied by a list of subobjectives. The objectives are intended to be clear, affordable and enforceable. SSDs will be required to develop effective systems to measure their performance in achieving them. While the government is particularly concerned with service provision to children looked after, its objectives are intended to cover all those children and families who receive help of any kind which is funded or part funded by SSDs.

The objectives of Quality Protects are:

- To ensure that children are securely attached to carers capable of providing safe and effective care for the duration of childhood.
- To ensure that children are protected from emotional, physical, sexual abuse and neglect.
- To ensure that children in need generally, and children looked after in particular, gain maximum life chances from educational opportunities, health care and social care.
- To ensure that young people leaving care, as they enter adulthood, are not isolated and participate socially and economically as citizens.
- To ensure that referral and assessment processes discriminate effectively between types and levels of need and produce a timely service response.
- To ensure that children with specific social needs arising out of disability or a health condition are living in families or other appropriate settings in the community where their assessed needs are adequately met and reviewed.
- To ensure that resources are planned and provided at levels which represent best value for money, allow for choice and different responses for different needs and circumstances.

All local authorities had to submit their first Quality Protects Action Plan to the DoH by the end of January 1999. These plans set out how the authority proposes to address 20 key tasks that are identified in the government's framework document, and which they will be expected to have achieved by March 2002 at the latest. Central to these key tasks is the need to develop local management strategies in line with the government's national objectives, which can be demonstrated to lead to clear and identifiable benefits for children. The key tasks place a particular emphasis on the development of plans which expand the range of placement choices available to children entering care; which improve the management of adoption services; and which enhance support for care leavers up to the age of 21. Specific provision is also made for ensuring that appropriate mechanisms are in place to listen to the views of children and young people about the services they receive. Many of the key tasks are concerned with the development of effective management strategies and systems to ensure that the government's objectives for children's services are effectively and efficiently met.

The government expects local authorities, as corporate parents, to recognise that they have a parenting role which is additional to the responsibility simply to provide basic care. These parenting responsibilities include:

- To provide a mixture of care and firmness to support the child's development, and be the tolerant, dependable and available partner in the adult–child relationship even in the face of disagreements.
- To protect and educate the child against the perils and risks of life by encouraging constructive and appropriate friendships, and discouraging destructive and harmful relationships.
- To celebrate and share the child's achievements, supporting them when they are down.
- To be ambitious for them and encourage and support their efforts to get on and reach their potential, whether through education, training or employment.
- To provide occasional financial support, and to remember birthdays and Christmas or annual celebrations within the individual child's religion and culture.

FUTURE CHANGES
Social services white paper

November 1998 saw the publication of the government's white paper, 'Modernising social services' (Department of Health 1998f). The white paper identifies six main problems with the current system of social services:

- *Protection*: Vulnerable children and adults have been exposed to abuse and neglect by their supposed carers.
- *Coordination*: Elderly people are left in hospital, blocking beds, while authorities argue over who should pay for their further care.

Social services

- *Inflexibility*: Services are often what suits the provider, not the client.
- *Clarity of role*: There is no clear understanding of what services should be provided and to what standard.
- *Consistency*: Huge differences persist in service standards, levels, allocation criteria and charging rules, leading to a feeling of unfairness.
- *Inefficiency*: Running costs of services can vary widely, suggesting poor value for money from much of the money spent on social services.

The most radical change proposed in the white paper is to inspection arrangements. Local authorities will lose the inspectorial function and new independent bodies will be established. Eight commissions for care standards, based on NHS regions in England, will regulate not just residential and nursing homes but, for the first time, local authority run services including domiciliary care. They will also regulate independent home care agencies, independent fostering agencies, family centres, maintained boarding schools and small residential homes. The commission will be independent of both local and health authorities. Children's rights officers will be appointed by each commission.

The white paper also proposes to introduce: national standards and rules for care services; a General Social Care Council to regulate and train staff; performance-linked funding; requirements for greater compatibility on eligibility criteria and on charging policies. It may take up to 4 years before these proposals are fully implemented.

Assessing children: a new framework

Systematic gathering and evaluation of information has an important part to play in child protection and family support, since the quality of initial assessments is known to relate directly to the quality of outcomes for children and their families. The DH has initiated work on developing a new framework for needs-led assessments of children and their families. This will focus on children in need (rather than just on children in need of protection), and reflects an holistic approach to addressing children's needs, including the need for protection, within a broad context rather than focusing mainly on incidents of abuse. The framework requires the collection and evaluation of information on the child's needs and development, on parental capacity and external factors such as income, housing, etc. (DH 2000). Social services will need to help improve the capacity of parents to meet the needs of their children. Adult and children's services will need to provide an integrated service to parents to ensure children's welfare is safeguarded. This is particularly important where adult mental health, substance misuse and domestic violence problems result in impairment of the health and development of children, or in their neglect or abuse. The new framework was introduced early in the new millennium and should restructure the whole assessment process for children and families. At the same time the DH has published new guidance for health, social services and other agencies, about how best to work together. The guidance provides details of the roles and responsibilities of the different sectors and agencies with regards to interagency working to safeguard children in need of care and protection (DH 1999).

REFERENCES AND FURTHER READING

Becker S 1997 Responding to poverty: the politics of cash and care. Longman, London

Department of Health 1998a Social services facing the future. The seventh annual report of the chief inspector, social services inspectorate 1997/98. The Stationery Office, London

Department of Health 1998b Health and personal social services statistics for England, 1998 edn. The Stationery Office, London

Department of Health 1998c The government's response to the children's safeguards review. The Stationery Office, London

Department of Health 1998d Quality protects. Framework for action. The Stationery Office, London

Department of Health 1998e The government's expenditure plans 1998–1999. Departmental report, The Stationery Office, London

Department of Health 1998f Modernising social services. The Stationery Office, London

Department of Health 2000. Framework for the Assessment of Children in Need and their Families. The Stationery Office, London

Department of Health 1999. Working Together to Safegaurd Children. The Stationery Office, London

Griffiths R 1988 Community care: an agenda for action. A report to the Secretary for State for Social Services. HMSO, London

House of Commons Health Committee 1998a Children looked after by local authorities, vol 1, Report and proceedings of the committee. The Stationery Office, London

House of Commons Health Committee 1998b The relationship between health and social services, vol 1, Report and proceedings of the committee. The Stationery Office, London

Howe D 1997 Patterns of adoption. Blackwell Science, Oxford

Social Services Inspectorate 1998 Someone else's children. Inspections of planning and decision making for children looked after and the safety of children looked after. The Stationery Office, London

Utting W 1997 People like us: the report of the review of the safeguards for children living away from home. The Stationery Office, London

17 | Benefits

The link between financial deprivation, ill health and social exclusion is one which has been regularly cited in many recent surveys on poverty. Whilst disability can occur throughout all sections of society, not having sufficient money to cope with the additional cost of having a disability places parents and carers at a considerable disadvantage. A civilised and caring society is often judged by the way that it supports its more disadvantaged members, and how it provides help where and when it is needed.

There is a growing number of children and young people living in the community who need high levels of support — partly because more of these children are surviving infancy and partly because there is no longer an assumption that disabled people should be cared for in hospitals or institutions. There are nearly 400 000 disabled children in England and Wales and more than 100 000 who are severely disabled having at least two different sorts of significant impairment (Department of Health 2000). There are also over 7500 families who are caring for more than one severely disabled child.

The degree to which these children and their carers are catered for is governed by many factors: economic, political, social, personal. Governments will always cite the difficult balancing act between funding the resources to meet this need, and setting up reasonable criteria to allow an equitable access to these resources. Many carers would argue that in the past too much emphasis has been placed upon establishing a very restrictive framework of entitlement, which, once satisfied, leads to an insufficient level of assistance.

This is probably the reason why families with disabled children identify money as their biggest unmet need. It costs on average three times more to bring up a child with significant impairments than a non-disabled child — about £100 a week extra. However, parents of disabled children have lower incomes than other parents, because the demands of caring mean they are less likely to be able to get and keep a full-time job. Consequently a large number of these families are dependent upon benefits. Unfortunately, surveys have identified that many families do not get all the benefits to which they are entitled to and even when they do, these benefits would have to be increased by between 20% and 50% to meet the actual cost of a such a family's minimum budget (Dobson & Middleton 1998).

The inadequacies of the benefit system were identified by Dobson & Middleton (1998) in their report for the Joseph Rowntree Foundation 'Paying to care: the cost of childhood disability'. They surveyed 300 families with a child with severe disabilities, reached an agreed minimum essential budget for three different conditions and compared these to the maximum level of benefit income. The calculations assumed that the family was in receipt of their maximum level of Disability Living Allowance and Income Support. Their findings (Table 17.1) were that even if the child and family were receiving their maximum entitlement, benefits would need to be increased by between £30 and £80 per week in order to meet the minimum essential costs identified by parents.

To a certain extent recent changes introduced by the Disability Income Guarantee are intended to rectify the shortfall between the actual cost of disability and benefit provision. However, whilst these changes are helpful, they have done little to address the other main complaint that parents and carers have about the benefits system, namely the level of complexity.

Benefits

Table 17.1 **Budget standards and benefit income.**[a] **From Dobsen & Middleten (1998)**						
Age group (yr)	Mobility disability	Maximum benefit income[b]	Sensory impairment	Maximum benefit income[c]	Traumatic intermittent conditions	Maximum benefit income[c]
0–5	£170.68	£87.35	£143.20	£70.95	£134.45	£70.95
6–10	£151.08	£121.95	£131.23	£84.10	£117.95	£84.10
11–16	£169.61	£129.80	£126.63	£91.95	£128.01	£91.95

[a] The benefit rates included in the table are for 1997/98 when the budget standards were constructed, for comparability
[b] Assumes the highest rate of Disability Living Allowance. Children less than 5 years of age were not eligible for the Mobility Component in 1997/98. It is assumed that those in the older age groups receive the higher rate of the Mobility Component
[c] This assumes the middle rate of Disability Living Allowance. Children less than 5 years of age are not eligible for the Mobility Component. It is assumed that those in the older age groups receive the lower rate of the Mobility Component

The Government have yet to arrive at a simplified system of entitlement, and although this chapter does much to stress the increases brought in by the Disability Income Guarantee, the level of detail and lengthy descriptions of the interrelationships between benefits serves only to highlight how bewildering the current system must appear to the average parent and carer.

The range of benefits, their conditions of entitlement and the ever-changing nature of the social security system causes much confusion in the minds of the parent and carer. As health professionals are very often amongst the first people to confirm the extra needs of a disabled child, they are often best placed to provide the parent and carer with some initial advice about the benefits to which the child and their carer might be entitled. By passing on a general outline of what benefits are available, the health professional will be doing much to ensure that as well as providing medical support, they are also ensuring that the child and the family are obtaining the maximum level of financial support.

Therefore to assist health professionals in fulfilling this role, the remainder of this chapter will look at the benefits that can be claimed in the UK for children with disabilities and their carers. Table 17.2 provides a basic guide to the benefits that can be claimed from birth through to 16. Each of the

major benefits is then examined in turn with reference made to the general rules of entitlement, the way in which they relate to other benefits and how they can be affected by spells in hospital. Finally a case example is included in Box 17.1 later in this chapter. This example has been designed to show how, by claiming all of the benefits available, parents and carers will achieve their full level of entitlement and thereby ensure that they are receiving their maximum statutory entitlement.

CHILD BENEFIT

This is a non-contributory benefit which is paid for all children from birth and continues, without further claim until the age of 19 for children remaining in full-time education. It has an almost 100% uptake which is probably a result of the ease with which it is obtained and it being perceived as free from the unfavourable stigma that many people associate with claiming benefits. The child does not have to be a blood relative but in most cases must be living with the claimant.

Receipt of Child Benefit is generally accepted by other benefits as being an indication of the carer having responsibility for the disabled child. It should therefore trigger dependent child additions payable with these benefits.

Table 17.2 **Claiming benefits from birth to 16 years**	
Age	**(Child benefit)**
Birth	Health benefits, e.g. prescriptions A working parent or carer can claim Working Families Tax Credit A non-working parent or carer can claim extra Income Support, income-based Jobseekers' Allowance, Housing and Council Tax Benefit for a dependent child
3 months	Disability Living Allowance Care Component Invalid Care Allowance for the carer if the disabled child receives either the High or Middle rate of the DLA Care Component A working parent or carer can claim extra Working Families Tax Credit or Disabled Persons Tax Credit, Housing and Council Tax Benefit for a disabled child A non-working parent or carer can claim extra Income Support, income-based Jobseekers' Allowance, Housing and Council Tax Benefit for a disabled child. From April 2001 children on the High rate of the Disability Living Allowance Care Component will qualify for an Enhanced Disabled Child's Premium Assistance from Family Fund Trust
2 years	Vaccine Damage Payments
3 years	From April 2001 children with severe physical disabilities or with a severe mental impairment which causes profound behaviour problems, will be able to claim the High rate of the Mobility Component from their third birthday
5 years	Disability Living Allowance Mobility Component. From April 2001 claims from the age of 5 will usually involve claims for the Lower rate of the Mobility Component
16 years	A young person can claim for Social Security benefits in their own right, e.g. Severe Disablement Allowance. From April 2001 this is being abolished and replaced by a non-contributory based version of Incapacity Benefit Income Support For young people who are able to work for over 16 hours a week they can claim Disabled Persons Tax Credit

DISABILITY LIVING ALLOWANCE

The major disability benefit was introduced in April 1992 and replaced the Attendance Allowance (AA) and the Mobility Allowance (Mob All). The Disability Living Allowance (DLA) is available to anybody under 65. It is not means tested and is tax free.

The Disability Living Allowance is divided into two parts, a Care Component (which replaced the Attendance Allowance) and a Mobility Component (which replaced the Mobility Allowance). The rules governing the Disability Living Allowance are similar to the rules of the old benefits, but it has extended the scope of these benefits to allow new rates to be paid to claimants with less severe disabilities.

To be eligible the claimant must have been needing the help for the last 3 months and must remain likely to require the help for a further 6 months. The claimant must have been resident in Great Britain for 26 weeks out of the last 52 (13 out of the last 52 weeks for children under 1 year). For children under 16 they have to show that their need for personal care is 'substantially' higher than that of a 'non-disabled' child of the same age.

The Care Component

The Care Component of DLA is for people who need help with their personal care, for example help with bodily needs, supervision and watching over because of their disability. The rate at which it is

Box 17.1
Case example: a young unemployed family with a disabled daughter

Mr & Mrs Jones are a young, unemployed, married couple, who 3 months ago had a little baby girl with Downs syndrome called Sally. They live in a council house and have no other children and no savings.

Sally is now showing some signs of developmental delay, in addition to the physical problems which she has had since birth, such as poor muscle tone, severe respiratory problems (especially at night), sinus problems, ear infections, dry skin, poor sleeping patterns and severe feeding difficulties.

Mr Jones is 'signing on' as available for work, and claiming income-based Jobseekers' Allowance for the whole family. The family has successfully applied for a maternity grant from the Social Fund. They are now asking for advice about what other benefits are available.

When assessing Sally's case the following benefits should be considered:

1. **Disability Living Allowance.** The DLA Care component should be claimed from when Sally was 3 months old. A DLA 1 should be used and returned to the appropriate regional disability benefit centre for the area. In addition to the form a covering letter could be sent providing an accurate description of all the 'extra' personal care that Sally requires during the day and at night, when compared to that needed by a non-disabled baby of the same age and sex. Special emphasis should be made of the serious nature of Sally's breathing problems at night. The claim may take about 4–6 weeks to come through.

2. **Income Support.** This should be claimed instead of Jobseekers' Allowance on the grounds that the Jones's are having to look after a child who is ill and because they are waiting for the outcome of a claim for Disability Living Allowance. Their entitlement to Income Support should be checked to make sure that the Jones have been awarded the extra premiums that they are now entitled to, e.g. the Family premium and a dependent child addition for Sally and Milk tokens. This should have happened if Mr and Mrs Jones have claimed Child Benefit.

After 4 weeks the DLA Care Component is awarded at the High rate. The couple also tell you that their washing machine has broken down and that they have run out of bedding. Mr and Mrs Jones should be advised to do the following:

1. **Income Support.** As a result of the award of the DLA Care Component Mr Jones should be advised to contact his local benefits agency office, to ask them to add the Disabled Child's Premium. This should be awarded from the date on which the DLA Care Component was awarded. The award of the High rate of the DLA Care component will also mean that the Jones's will qualify for an Enhanced Disabled Child's Premium.

2. **Invalid Care Allowance.** Now that the High rate of the DLA Care component has been awarded either Mr Jones or Mrs Jones should claim the Invalid Care Allowance. Who they decide to claim ICA, should then become the Income Support claimant. Their entitlement to ICA will be deducted from their entitlement to Income Support, but it will mean that the Carer's Premium will be awarded.

3. **Social Fund.** An award of the DLA Care Component will have the effect of confirming the severity of Sally's condition, this will mean that a claim to the Social Fund for a Community Care Grant for bedding may be more likely to succeed.

4. **Family Fund Trust.** The Jones's could apply for help from the Family Fund Trust for a new washing machine.

Mr & Mrs Jones' benefit entitlement given in financial terms using 2001/02 benefit rates

The amount of entitlement before the claim for the Disability Living Allowance,

Income-based Jobseekers' Allowance:

£ 83.25	Personal Allowance for a couple
£ 14.50	Family Premium
£ 31.45	Dependent Child Addition for under 16
£ 129.20	Total entitlement to Jobseekers Allowance

Total family income of £129.20 which includes £15.50 child benefit

Box 17.1
Continued

Mr & Mrs Jones's entitlement to benefits after the Disability Living Allowance Care Component at the Higher rate, a claim for Income Support and for Invalid Care allowance

Income Support:

£ 83.25	Personal allowance for a couple
£ 14.50	Family Premium
£ 31.45	Dependent Child Addition for under 16
£ 30.90	**Disabled Child's Premium**
£ 11.05	**Enhanced Disability Premium**
£ 24.40	**Carer's Premium**
£195.55	Total entitlement to Income Support
+ £55.30	Disability Living Allowance Care Component at the High rate

Total family income is £250.85 which includes Child Benefit of £15.50 and Invalid Care Allowance worth £41.75

paid depends on the amount of care and/or supervision required:

- The High rate is awarded if the baby or young child requires help and/or supervision for both day AND night.
- The Middle rate is awarded if the baby or young child requires help and/or supervision either for JUST during the day or the night.
- The Lower rate is awarded if a baby or young child needs a small amount of help with their personal needs amounting to over 1 hour per day. This rate is also payable if a person aged over 16 requires help to prepare and cook a main meal.

Special rules for the terminally ill

Babies and children who are terminally ill may be able to qualify for the highest rate of the care component without the usual requirement of a 3-month qualifying period. To claim under the special rules the child's death must be likely to occur within the next 6 months, and this has to be confirmed by a doctor or consultant on form DS 1500.

The Mobility Component

The Mobility Component is available to children over 3 years and adults claiming before their 65th birthday. It is to help people who have severe mobility problems or who need guidance and supervision whilst out walking in unfamiliar areas. The Mobility Component is paid at two rates.

The high rate of the Mobility Component

The High rate is awarded to a child over 3 or young person who:

- Is unable to walk.
- Is virtually unable to walk.
- Because of the exertion required to walk, danger is caused to the child's/person's health.
- Has had both legs amputated at or above the ankle or was born without legs or feet.
- Is both deaf and blind.
- Is severely mentally impaired with severe behavioural problems.

To qualify under all but the last category the child's walking difficulties must be caused by a physical condition. To qualify under the last category the child must have a 'severe mental impairment' and 'severe behavioural problems' for which they need continual control and restraint whilst out walking. To use this last condition the child or young person must also be entitled to the DLA Care Component at the High rate.

Extra help due to receiving the High rate of the Mobility Component

Receipt of the Mobility Component at the High rate can also allow the following forms of assistance: help to lease a car through the Motability scheme; enhanced parking rights under the Blue Badge Scheme (this replaced the Orange Badge scheme in April 2000) and exemption from Road Tax.

The Low rate of the Mobility Component

The Low rate is awarded if the child or young person can walk, but due to a physical or mental disability needs someone with them to ensure that they are safe or to help them find their way around in unfamiliar areas.

It is anticipated that most young children with severe learning disabilities will qualify for this level of the Mobility Component from the age of 5. Children who need guidance due to impaired vision or severe hearing impairment may also qualify for this help. Children have to show that the need for guidance and supervision is 'substantially' in excess of that which would be given to a child without special needs.

How to claim the Disability Living Allowance

One of the major changes introduced by the Disability Living Allowance scheme is the use of a very long self-assessment form. The claim form is called DLA 1 for children under 16 and it is a very long questionnaire assessing the baby's or young child's care needs and their walking difficulties. (Claim forms can be ordered from the Benefits Enquiry Line on 0800 882200.)

The parent or carer has to complete this form, and claim the benefit on the child's behalf. It is also their responsibility to notify the Disability Living Allowance of any change in the child's condition and circumstances.

These forms have replaced the doctor's visits that were a regular part of claiming under the earlier scheme. The forms also ask for the names and addresses of professionals who know the child well. For children with a special or rare condition, it is sensible to nominate the professional who is the most familiar with the child and his diagnosis. This is because it is likely that this professional will be contacted by the Disability Living Allowance Unit to provide confirmation of the child's diagnosis and degree of disability.

Initial claims should be sent to the regional Disability Benefit Centre that is local to the parent's or carer's address. Once a decision has been made and issued, the case is sent to the Disability Living Allowance Unit in Blackpool, to be stored on file.

The Disability Living Allowance Unit uses similar forms to the initial claim form to revise and renew the child's entitlement. These forms should be completed as carefully as the original claim form.

The decision-making process

After requesting a claim form, the parent or carer has 6 weeks in which to return the completed claim form. If the parent or carer is aware that they will not be able to return the main section of the form within this period, they can return just section 1 of the claim form with a letter of explanation about the delay.

Once the Disability Benefits Centre has received all of the completed form, the case will be determined by a Decision Maker. This will be a lay person with no specialist medical knowledge. Therefore to assist the Decision Maker with their deliberations, the Benefit Agency have provided several sources of information. The Decision Maker will have access to the Disability Handbook. This gives guidance to the Decision Maker about the care needs of children, both generally and in relation to specific disabilities.

When claiming for a child, the need for care and supervision has to be substantially in excess of what is normally required by a child of the same age. When deciding this in relation to the principle concerns of the Disability Living Allowance Care Component, the main point for consideration is the practical effect of the disability in terms of the child's need for personal care, supervision and watching over. In short the child's needs must be substantially more than what is normally required, they must be outside the range of attention or supervision that would be normally be required by the 'average' child.

For very young babies the guidance rests on the incidence of non-standard interventions or actions which the baby requires because of this disability. Babies that are likely to qualify under this guidance are those who are severely hearing or vision impaired; babies with severe multiple disabilities; frequent loss of consciousness; seizures; babies with renal failure; cerebral palsy or who are extremely premature.

The Disability Handbook contains whole chapters of guidance on the care and mobility needs caused by specific conditions. The existence of such guidance highlights the considerable advantage that children with a clear diagnosis have over children whose condition has yet to be diagnosed.

Revisions and appeals

Since 1999 the Benefits Agency has introduced changes to the rules on how claims can be revised or reconsidered at an appeal. These changes to the decision and appeals regulations have reduced the amount of time that claimants have in order to ask for a reconsideration following their receipt of a decision.

The details for challenging a decision under the new system are given in the Benefits Agency leaflet GL24 'If you think our decision is wrong'. This leaflet also contains an application slip that can be used to register an appeal.

In brief, following the claimant's receipt of the decision, they have 1 month to request that the decision is looked at again. As long as this request is made within a month, the Disability Living Allowance Unit will look at the decision again and will either revise or uphold it from the date of claim.

A parent or carer may also request a reconsideration on the grounds that the child's condition has changed or deteriorated. If the Disability Living Allowance Unit accepts that the change has lead to an increase in the child's care or mobility needs then they can replace the old decision, either from the date when the child's condition changed, or from the date that their carer applied for a reconsideration.

If the claimant disagrees with the outcome of the reconsideration, they can ask for an appeal. Once again this must be done within 1 month of getting the decision. This appeal will be handled by the Tribunal Appeal Service. This agency will deal with the administration of the appeal and they have powers to dismiss appeals on the grounds that they will not succeed, or because the claimant fails to provide further information or if they fail to respond to letters.

Appeals will be heard by tribunals, and these will comprise either three, two or one person(s), according to which benefit is being reconsidered. It is expected that Disability Living Allowance appeals will be heard by a three-person tribunal. The claimant can also choose to have the appeal dealt with as a paper hearing or to attend in person. Professionals can accompany the claimant to an appeal. With complex cases it is also a good idea for the claimant to seek someone to represent them.

How is the Disability Living Allowance paid

The Disability Living Allowance is paid to the carer on behalf of the child. The Disability Living Allowance Unit can use a variety of methods. Both components can be paid on a monthly order book issued by the Disability Living Allowance Unit in Blackpool, or they can be paid directly into the carer's bank account.

The Disability Living Allowance and other benefits

The Disability Living Allowance is a very important disability benefit, because if a baby or young child receives the Care Component at either the High or Middle rate, their carer may qualify for Invalid Care Allowance.

For parents and carers on benefit or low incomes, Disability Living Allowance is ignored by all means-tested benefits such as Income Support, means-tested Jobseekers' Allowance, Housing Benefit and Council Tax Benefit. It is also ignored by Working Family Tax Credit and Disabled Person's Tax Credit. Indeed, if the child is entitled to any level of the Disability Living Allowance, the parent and carer will qualify for extra help on this benefits known as the Disabled Child's Premium or Disabled Child's Tax Credit.

Benefits

From April 2001 if the child is allowed the High rate of the Disability Living Allowance Care Component their parent or carer will qualify to have an Enhanced Disabled Child's Premium added to their entitlement to their means-tested benefit on top of the usual Disabled Child's Premium.

Parents and carers should therefore be encouraged to contact the office responsible for administering their benefit entitlement, as this will result in extra assistance.

The Disability Living Allowance and going into hospital care

Children under the age of 16 who go into hospital will have both the Care Component and the Mobility Component withdrawn after 12 weeks of consecutive or 'linked' care. (Separate periods in hospital can be linked together only if they are separated by less than 28 days in the claimant's normal home.)

After 16 the claimant's entitlement to Care and Mobility Components will be withdrawn after 4 weeks of consecutive or linked care.

INVALID CARE ALLOWANCE

Invalid Care Allowance (ICA) is a weekly benefit paid to people of working age who look after someone with a disability receiving the Attendance Allowance or the Disability Living Allowance Care Component at either the High or Middle rates. ICA can be claimed by men and women, married or single, who are of working age and who meet the basic qualifying conditions. It does not matter whether the disabled person and their carer are related, nor whether they live in the same household.

Qualifying conditions

To qualify the claimant must meet all of the following conditions:

- Looking after the person at least 35 hours per week.
- Between 16 and 65 for women and men.
- Living in Great Britain. They must have been resident for 28 weeks out of the last 12 months.

- Not in full-time education.
- Not earning more that £72.50 p per week. Earnings are gross earnings minus National Insurance contributions, trade unions subscriptions, the cost of looking after another member of the household, e.g. childminding fees, the cost of getting a uniform or work clothes cleaned and the cost of travel whilst at work.

How much is it?

Invalid Care Allowance comprises a payment for the carer and then extra payments for a partner and for any dependent children subject to certain conditions.

Invalid Care Allowance and other benefits

Invalid Care Allowance will be considered in full by Income Support, income-based Jobseekers Allowance, Housing Benefit and Council Tax Benefit. It is still useful to claim Invalid Care Allowance because it helps to confirm the carer's status so that they don't have to be available for work, and it qualifies the claimant for a Carer's Premium to be added to their benefit entitlement.

The claimant will not be allowed Invalid Care Allowance if they receive such National Insurance-based benefits as contributory-based Jobseeker's Allowance, Incapacity Benefit and Retirement Pension A dependent adult addition on these benefits would also be lost if the dependent adult claimed Invalid Care Allowance in their own right.

How to claim

Claims should be made on a Invalid Care Allowance claim pack DS 700. All claims will be dealt with by the Invalid Care Allowance Unit at Palatine House, Lancaster Road, Preston, PR1 1NS.

Backdating

Invalid Care Allowance can be backdated for a maximum of 3 months, just as long as the claimant can prove that they could have satisfied the qualifying conditions for the whole of the 3 months.

Invalid Care Allowance and going into care

If the baby or young child goes into care and has their DLA Care Component stopped, then the carer's Invalid Care Allowance will stop. For children under 16 going into hospital this will usually mean that the Invalid Care Allowance will stop after 12 weeks of consecutive or linked hospital care.

A carer can be in hospital and away from the disabled child and keep Invalid Care Allowance for a maximum period of 12 weeks.

INCOME SUPPORT

Income Support was introduced in April 1988. It is a means-tested benefit which is to help people who don't have to be available for work, or who work for less than 16 hours per week. It is intended to bring an individual or family's income up to the minimum level which the government says they need to live on. If the money which the claimant has coming in is less than this set level, a claim for Income Support will 'top up' their money, raising the claimant's income to their Income Support 'applicable' amount.

Income Support is made up of a basic Personal Allowance, which is awarded in accordance with the claimant's age and marital/partnership status. In addition any claimant who cares for a baby or young child who receives either or both the Care Component and Mobility Component of the Disability Living Allowance will automatically qualify for a Disabled Child's Premium. From April 2001 children on the high rate of the Disability Living Allowance Care component will qualify for an Enhanced Disabled Child's Premium on top of the normal Disabled Child's Premium.

If the baby or young child is entitled to either the High or Middle rate of the Disabled Living Allowance Care component and their carer receives the Invalid Care Allowance, then the carer will have the Carer's Premium added to their Income Support.

As well as these premiums connected to disability, the claimant can also receive a Family Premium if they have one or more dependent children. To qualify for Income Support most people have to be over 18, although special conditions exist which mean that most 16/17 year olds with severe learning disabilities can claim Income Support, even if they stay on in first-time 'specialist' education.

The claimant must also have less than £8000 in savings, and they must be exempt from having to be available for work. If they work part time it must be for less than 16 hours per week.

How to claim for Income Support

Claims for Income Support should be made direct to the local Benefit Agency office. Along with the Income Support application form, there are forms to enable the claimant to receive assistance with their rent and council tax under schemes that are administered by the claimant's local authority.

When the person claims for help with rent or the council tax, if they are awarded Income Support, they will receive the maximum levels of help, for example 100% rent rebate and 100% council tax rebate.

Other housing costs

Help with mortgage interest can also be included as part of a person's entitlement to Income Support. Income Support may also meet the interest payments on a loan used to adapt the home for the special needs of the disabled child.

Other sources of help due to getting Income Support

Income Support acts on an 'automatic passport' to a number of welfare benefits. Anyone receiving Income Support is entitled to free subscriptions, dental treatment and vouchers for NHS glasses. A person on Income Support can also make a claim to the Social Fund.

Income Support and going into hospital care

When a dependent child goes into hospital their carer's entitlement to benefits such as Income

Benefits

Support and Child Benefit will be unaffected for the first 12 weeks. After 12 weeks of consecutive or linked care their carer's Income Support will be reduced to a set amount. If the carer receives Housing Benefit or Council Tax benefit, this will **not** be reduced. Child Benefit can remain in payment just as long as the carer can show that the Child Benefit is being spent in the dependent child's interests.

JOBSEEKERS' ALLOWANCE

For carers who choose to be available for work, or who are 'signing on', they can claim income-based Jobseekers' Allowance, which is calculated in much the same way as Income Support and can be claimed from the local employment office or benefits agency.

THE SOCIAL FUND

If the parent or carer is entitled to Income Support, they may be able to get payments from the DSS Social Fund. A payment may be a grant or a loan. If they have savings of more than £500 (£1000 for people over the age of 60) these will affect the size of the payment and may stop the claimant from getting a payment altogether. The DSS have a budget for each month, which they must stick to.

The Social Fund is made up of two parts, one part is known as the Statutory Social Fund and deals with such statutory payments as Maternity grants, Funeral grants, and Budgeting loans for specific items in specific circumstances. The other part is known as the Discretionary Social Fund, which means that grants are awarded at the discretion of the Social Fund officers and on their view of the urgency of the claimant's need and their circumstances.

There are two sorts of discretionary payments from the second part of the Social Fund: the Crisis Loan, which has to be paid back, and the Community Care Grant (CCG). Grants do not have to be paid back and should be the type of payment awarded to a family who are trying to cope with the extra stress and expense caused by caring for a child with disabilities.

Community Care Grants

CCGs are lump sum payments that can be made to:
- help families under stress
- help people at risk of going into some sort of institutional care
- help people who are leaving some sort of institutional care
- help people with some travel expenses.

Most families on Income Support and looking after a child with a disability will come under the first criteria — 'families under stress'. They may be able to qualify for such items as clothing, bedding, laundry equipment, redecoration, and furnishing if damaged by a child's behaviour problems.

How to claim help from the Social Fund

To claim a Social Fund payment from the Community Care Grant, claimants must use form SF 300 for the DSS office that is paying their benefit. A claim can be made at any time, but claims stand a better chance of succeeding if they are submitted at the beginning of the month.

The Social Fund is cash limited, so even though the family making the claim may be in serious and genuine need, if there is limited money in the budget, then they may receive little or no help. The other problem is that 'family under stress' has a low priority, and in order to overcome this problem extra emphasis has to be made of the child's disabilities and the extra expense that it causes:

WORKING FAMILIES TAX CREDIT

Working Families Tax Credit is a means-tested benefit for working families who have children. Awards normally last for 26 weeks. To qualify either the claimant or their partner must be working for 16 hours a week or more. They must have less than £8000 in savings. The amount of Working Families Tax Credit paid depends on the number of children the claimant has, their ages and how much income the family has.

Disability Living Allowance is not treated as an income by Working Families Tax credit, and any child with a DLA entitlement will qualify the claimant for a Disabled Child's Tax Credit. From more information and a claim form telephone 0845 609 5000.

DISABLED PERSON'S TAX CREDIT

Disabled Person's Tax Credit is a means-tested tax benefit that tops up income for people in work, whose disabilities put them at a disadvantage in getting a job. It can be claimed from the age of 16. The claimant must be working for 16 hours or more and must have less than £16 000 in savings. In order to qualify the claimant must be receiving a disability benefit such as Disability Living Allowance or Incapacity Benefit.

The amount of benefit awarded will depend on the amount of income coming into the household, any savings between £3000 and £16 000, how many hours the claimant works, any child care costs, whether the claimant has any dependent children and whether any of the children are disabled.

An award of Disabled Person's Tax Credit usually last for 26 weeks. For more information and a claim form telephone 0845 605 5858.

HOUSING BENEFIT

Housing Benefit is a means-tested benefit which provides assistance with a claimant's rent. A claimant can apply for Housing Benefit even still in work, but he must have less than £16 000 in savings.

Carers on Income Support or income-based Job-seekers' Allowance qualify for full Housing Benefit. Carers on a low income will have their income assessed against a set figure. This set figure can include a Disabled Child's Premium, the Enhanced Disabled Child's Premium and the Carer's Premium.

For more information about Housing Benefit and to claim it, the parent or carer should contact their local council.

COUNCIL TAX BENEFIT

Parents or carers who are responsible for their household council tax bill can claim assistance with

paying it. Once again it does not matter whether the claimant is in work, but they must have less than £16 000 in savings.

Carers on Income Support or income-based Job-seekers' Allowance will qualify for full Council Tax Benefit. Carers on a low income will have their income assessed against a set figure. This set figure can include a Disabled Child's Premium, the Enhanced Disabled Child's Premium and the Carer's Premium.

For more information about Council Tax Benefit and to claim it, the parent or carer should contact their local council.

A parent or carer may be able to get a further reduction in their Council Tax if the child they care for uses a wheelchair indoors or needs an extra room because of their disability. This help is not means tested and it is not affected by any savings. If a carer thinks that their house might qualify, due to any aids or adaptations that have been carried out for their disabled child, they should contact their local Council Tax department and ask for information about The Council Tax Disability Reduction Scheme.

THE FAMILY FUND TRUST

The Family Fund Trust is a fund set up to help families caring for a child with a severe disability, by providing goods, or services or by giving grants of money. Any family with a child who is severely disabled can apply for help, so long as the child is under 16 and lives in the UK. In most instances the child should be receiving the Disability Living Allowance.

The fund can provide help that will relieve stress arising out of the day to day care of the child. In the past it has helped families by providing hire cars, taxi fares and driving lessons to enable a family to go on outings, washing machines and dryers to help with laundry problems, clothes, bedding and furniture, family holidays. To apply parents or carers should write to: The Family Fund Trust, PO Box 50, York YO1 2ZX.

After an application has been made the family will be visited by a representative of the fund who will discuss the best ways in which they can help.

Benefits

The fund has to take the family circumstances into account, and limits offers of help to families with an annual income of less than £18 500. Claimants may have to go through a means test as part of their application.

FARES TO HOSPITAL

If a parent or carer is on Income Support, income-based Job Seekers Allowance, and in some cases Working Family Tax Credit or Disabled Person's Tax Credit they will be entitled to help with travel costs to and from hospital in order to receive NHS treatment. These costs are for either the parent or carer or their child if they require treatment.

If the parent or carer is not getting these benefits but is on a low income, they may still be able to get help. They should apply for help under the low income scheme by using claim form AGI, available from the hospital or their local benefits agency (DSS) office.

Payment can made at the hospital each time the child has to go for treatment. Normal public transport fares or the estimated amount of petrol used if travel is by private care will be paid (whichever is the less). Payment will only be made if the person takes proof of their entitlement to the appropriate benefits or of their entitlement to help under the low income scheme. Fares should be paid for the disabled child and the accompanying parent or carer.

HELP TOWARDS THE COST OF VISITING A CHILD IN HOSPITAL

If a parent or carer is visiting a child in hospital and they are on Income Support or income-based Job Seekers' Allowance, they may be able to get help with fares and related expenses from the Social Fund.

For more information about help with travel costs to hospital, ask for leaflets GL 12 'Going into Hospital' and HC 11 'Help with health costs'.

HEALTH WARNING FOR THIS CHAPTER

Whilst every effort has been made to ensure that the details given in this chapter are as accurate as possible at the time of writing, readers should be aware that payment levels change, regulations are amended and some benefits completely abolished — Severe Disablement Allowance for new claimants from April 2001 for example. It is therefore strongly recommended that in addition to passing this information on to parents and carers, health professionals should also suggest that parents and carers make contact with some of the excellent statutory and voluntary bodies that exist to provide benefit information. A list of these bodies can be found in Appendix b of the edition. As well as the traditional ways of accessing the information that these groups can provide, an increasing number are now offering support and up-to-date benefit information on the Internet.

The following sites are strongly recommend as a way as ensuring the accuracy of this chapter:

- http://www.dss.gov.uk/index.htm — Benefits Agency site which offers direct access to basic benefit information, and lists of useful leaflets and publications.
- http://www.mencap.org.uk. — Mencap site, offering information about the largest charity working on behalf of children and adults with learning disabilities.
- http://www.nacab.org.uk — Citizens Advice Bureaux site provides list of local CAB offices which can offer free confidential advice on a wide range of subjects including benefits and debt.
- http://www.after16.org.uk. — excellent site offering up-to-date information on benefits for young people with disabilities.
- http://www.cpag.org.uk — provides information about the services and information that the Child Poverty Action Group can provide to individuals and groups concerned about child poverty.

REFERENCES

Department of Health 2000, Quality protects: disabled children numbers and categories and families. DoH, London
Dobson B, Middleton S 1998 Paying to care: the cost of childhood disability. York Publishing Services, York

18 | Legal framework

Practitioners whose responsibilities concern children need to be aware not only of the general principles of law relating to the delivery of medical services but also those that specifically apply to children and reflect their vulnerability and inability to protect their own interests. It is also important to understand the framework on which co-operation and joint working, essential for the effective provision of services, depends. This chapter addresses the law as it is applied in England and Wales. Elsewhere in the United Kingdom, while the principles may be similar, the sources of those principles may be different.

The Children Act 1989 ('the Act') provides a framework of law, determines the jurisdiction of and the approach to decision making about children's welfare by the courts, and establishes the responsibilities of public agencies to deliver services in order to safeguard and protect children from abuse and neglect and promote their welfare.

STATUTORY FRAMEWORK FOR SAFEGUARDING AND PROMOTING CHILDREN'S WELFARE

The statutory scheme for the protection of vulnerable children and the promotion of their welfare places with the local authority in each local government administrative area the responsibility to carry out enquiries and take action. The responsible local authority is that carrying out the functions of a local social services authority and the practical exercise of these functions is delegated to social work staff.

When social services are informed that a child who lives, or is found, in their area has been subject to emergency action by social services or the police because of concerns with regard to his welfare or they otherwise 'have reasonable cause to suspect that a child . . . is suffering, or is likely to suffer, significant harm', they have a duty to 'make or cause to be made such enquiries as they consider necessary to enable them to decide whether they should take any action to safeguard or promote the child's welfare' (Section 47(1)).

Local authority action under these provisions has become widely referred to as 'Section 47 enquiries.' It is important to recognise that the reason for concern may arise from suspicion of significant harm but the enquiries must be sufficiently thorough and extensive to enable social services officers to decide whether they should take *any* action to safeguard and promote the child's welfare.

In particular, but not exclusively, the enquiries must be directed towards establishing whether the authority should make any court application, exercise any other powers under the Act or apply for a child safety order with respect to the child (Section 47(3)). Amendments to this section made by the Crime and Disorder Act 1998 reflect the government's determination to bring young children who are involved in anti-social or criminalised behaviour within the scope of welfare provisions.

Under Section 17 of the Act, social services have a duty to:

'(a) safeguard and promote the welfare of children within their area who are in need; and
(b) so far as is consistent with that duty, to promote the upbringing of such children by their families, by providing a range and level of services appropriate to those children's needs.'

Box 18.1
Glossary of abbreviations

DFEE — Department for Education and Employment (from 2001 Department for Education and Skills).

LAC — Local authority circular, followed by the year issued and the number in sequence from the beginning of the year.

FLR — Family Law Reports — Series of law reports, preceded by year of publication and volume for the year, and followed by the page on which the report appears in the volume.

FCR — Family Court Reporter — Series of law reports, preceded by year of publication and volume for the year, and followed by the page on which the report appears in the volume.

SI — Statutory Instrument (subordinate legislation), followed by the year made and the number in sequence from the beginning of the year.

A child is to be taken to be in need if:

'(a) he is unlikely to achieve or maintain, or have the opportunity of achieving or maintaining, a reasonable standard of health or development . . .'

or

'(b) his health or development is likely to be significantly impaired, or further impaired,'

without the provision of services by a local authority or:

'(c) he is disabled' (Section 17(10)).

A child is disabled if blind, deaf or dumb or suffers from mental disorder of any kind, or is substantially and permanently handicapped by illness, injury or congenital deformity or such other disability as may be prescribed (Section 17(11)).

Part III and Schedule 2 of the Act provide further duties and powers regarding the services to be provided in fulfilment of this duty. A local authority in meeting a child's assessed needs, has a discretion to provide assistance in kind, or in exceptional circumstances, cash, and may provide services to members of a child's family, including persons with parental responsibility or any other person with whom the child has been living but may not be compelled to do so (Section 17(3), (6), (10)).

Clearly, social services are unable to carry out these important statutory responsibilities without access to information and expertise held and services delivered by staff working in other agencies. The Act empowers social services to call upon other agencies to assist them with the delivery of these functions.

If so requested in connection with enquiries under Section 47 an agency may only refuse if it would be unreasonable in all the circumstances of the case (Section 47(9), (10)). If requested, to assist, either in an individual case or for strategic planning of services, in relation to duties under Part III of the Act, an agency is obliged to comply if it is compatible with its statutory or other duties and obligations and does not unduly prejudice the exercise of any of its functions (Section 27(2)).

The agencies that may be required to assist social services include:

- any health authority
- any special health authority
- any national health service trust
- any primary care trust.

INTER-AGENCY WORKING

The Secretary of State has powers under Section 7 Local Authority Social Services Act 1970 to require local authorities in the exercise of their social services functions to act under his general guidance. Such guidance, although it does not have the full force of statute, must be complied with unless local circumstances indicate exceptional reasons justifying a variation.

This power is used to issue guidance that requires social services to establish and lead inter-agency working to ensure that statutory welfare and protection functions are effectively carried out. Recent guidance issued under this section has included Working Together to Safeguard Children (TSO 1999), Framework for Assessment of Children in Need and their Families (TSO 2000) and Safeguarding Children Involved in Prostitution (TSO 2000).

Social services are required by the guidance to exercise their powers, in particular those under Sections 47 and 27, to require other agencies to co-operate with the application locally of this national guidance. The interaction of these statutory provisions underpins inter-agency co-operation and the establishment and working of Area Child Protection Committees.

It also requires agencies to establish child protection procedures and working protocols and ensure that these are applied and followed by their staff, and to include negotiated expectations for the delivery of services within contract specifications between commissioners and providers of health services. It requires the appointment of designated professionals by health authorities and named doctors and nurses or midwives by trusts to lead on inter-agency working in child protection (see in particular paragraphs 3.18 to 3.53 Working Together 1999).

The Secretary of State has also exercised powers under the Children Act to make regulations that have statutory force. These place further duties and responsibilities on social services regarding the manner in which they shall carry out their functions under Part III of the Act in relation to particular categories of vulnerable children, including those looked after by the local authority in foster or residential homes. These regulations have been supplemented by further guidance issued under section 7 of the 1970 Act published by the Department of Health in a series of ten volumes (The Children Act 1989 Guidance and Regulations. Volumes 1–10).

The duties owed to vulnerable children established by these provisions cannot be met without significant co-operation from health personnel in the planning and delivery of services. For example, the Children and Young Persons Review of Children's Cases Regulations 1991 (SI 1991 No. 895) require local authorities regularly to review and plan cases of children whom they look after and for whom they provide accommodation. The schedules to the regulations set out the information social services must acquire when reviewing such cases and this includes under Schedule 3:

1. The child's state of health.
2. The child's health history.
3. The effect of the child's health and health history on his development.
4. Existing arrangements for the child's medical and dental care and treatment and health and dental surveillance.
5. The possible need for an appropriate course of action which should be identified to assist necessary change of such care, treatment, or surveillance.
6. The possible need for preventive measures, such as vaccination and immunisation, screening for vision and hearing.'

Before placing a child, or as soon as practicable thereafter, social services must arrange for a medical examination. Once placed arrangements must be made for medical examination by a registered medical practitioner every six months before the second birthday and thereafter every year. The practitioner is required to provide a written assessment of the state of health of the child and the need for health care (Review of Children's Cases Regulations 1991, reg.6).

In respect to every child it is looking after, a local authority must ensure that he is provided with health care services, including dental and medical treatment (Children and Young Persons Arrangements for the Placement of Children (General) Regulations 1991, S.I. 1991/890 reg.7(2)).

The statutory mechanism by which the co-operation of health personnel is expected, both for the strategic planning of services and on individual cases, is through the provisions of Section 27 of the Act.

The failure in the past to ensure effective co-ordination of services for vulnerable children and the poor outcomes particularly for those looked after by local authorities led to the government's initiative, Quality Protects (LAC 1998/28). This programme sets standards and inspection targets and makes increased funding conditional on improvements, which are unlikely to occur unless the statutory provisions, in particular those requiring liaison and co-operation across agencies, are carried out.

TAKING HISTORIES IN CHILD PROTECTION CASES

Care must be taken when taking histories from adults or children about events that have led to the need for medical or nursing intervention. Suggestion and comment should be avoided and recording should carefully set down the source of historical explanations. Later discrepancies can then be identified and the danger of stated facts being interpreted as the practitioner's opinion of what has occurred will be avoided. Local protocols agreed with local authorities and police may give guidance on these issues.

Particular care must be taken when speaking to a child in order to avoid contaminating potential evidence from that child by inappropriate or leading questions, or encouraging explanations by voice or gesture. Courts have been critical of professionals in cases involving possible sexual abuse for failing to read the full Cleveland Report published in 1987 and in particular for failing to heed the guidance set out in Chapter 12 of the Report concerning interviewing children (Re E (1991) 1 FLR 420).

Evidential and practice issues are particularly complex when it is suspected that carers of a child may be inducing or fabricating illness in a child. A Department of Health circular is to be issued as Supplementary Guidance to Working Together to Safeguard Children to address inter-agency co-operation and practice in such cases.

SPECIAL EDUCATIONAL NEEDS

The Education Act 1996 codifies previous statutory provisions concerned with education functions. Section 321 requires local education authorities (LEAs) to identify if children over the age of two years and under compulsory school leaving age have special educational needs and if necessary determine the provision which their learning difficulty may call for. A child has special educational needs if he has a learning difficulty that calls for special educational provision.

LEAs must give notice to parents of children whom they propose to assess for special educational needs and are expected to involve them fully in the process which leads to the preparation of a Statement of Special Educational Needs setting out the extent of the needs and how they will be met. Special Educational Needs Tribunals have jurisdiction to determine disputes.

While not all children with medical conditions will have special educational needs, many will and medical and nursing services will often be required to identify and assess needs and assist in the planning and delivery of provision.

Essential inter-agency co-operation is encouraged by Section 322, which provides that if it appears to the LEA that any Health Authority, Primary Care Trust or local authority could by taking any specified action help in the exercise of any functions concerned with special educational needs, it may request the help specifying the action necessary. A health service so requested has a duty to comply unless it considers it not to be necessary or having regard to its resources it would be unreasonable.

Local authorities must comply unless the request is not compatible with their own statutory functions and obligations or would unduly prejudice the discharge of any of their functions.

The extent and level of the services expected to be provided should be negotiated through the Children's Services Planning process. To assist practice in this sensitive area, Codes of Practice on the Identification and Assessment of Special Educational Needs are published by the government from time to time, the most recent revision of which is expected to be placed before Parliament and implemented with effect from 1 January 2002.

Assessments for special educational needs may be carried out at the same time as any assessment of need under the Children Act, legislation concerned with meeting the needs of disabled persons or their carers or any other enactment (Paragraph 3 Schedule 2 Education Act 1996).

SCHOOL MEDICAL SERVICES

For pupils in schools maintained by LEAs the Secretary of State has a duty to arrange for their medical inspection and treatment at appropriate intervals and to the extent he considers necessary to meet all their reasonable requirements for dental inspection, treatment and education in dental health (Section 5(1) (1A) National Health Services Act 1977). LEAs are required to make arrangements for encouraging and assisting pupils to 'take advantage of the provision for medical and dental inspection and treatment in the National Health Service' (Section 520 Education Act 1996).

If a parent objects to a pupil using the services, that pupil is not to be encouraged or assisted to do so. However, it is not necessary for parents to positively consent — an objecting parent must make known opposition — and a pupil who is competent to give necessary consents may take advantage of the services offered even if the education authorities are prevented from encouraging or assisting involvement.

It is expected careful planning will ensure that children who have medical needs will have these needs catered for within the school environment. The DFEE Circular 14/96 Supporting Pupils with Medical Needs in Schools published jointly with the Department of Health in October 1996 gives guidance on how this should be achieved.

PARENTAL RESPONSIBILITY

The Children Act replaced previous principles concerned with parental rights and duties in relation to children with the concept of 'parental responsibility' which is defined as

'. . . all the rights, duties, powers, responsibilities and authority which by law a parent of a child has in relation to the child and his property'

(Section 3(1)).

It therefore includes responsibility for important decisions relating to a child's welfare and life opportunities when that child is not able to exercise that responsibility. It is important therefore when delivering services to a child to know whether that child has the capacity to determine such issues and, if not, which adult(s) have parental responsibility in relation to that child. Adults with parental responsibility have a duty to exercise that responsibility in the interests of the welfare of the child.

Mothers have parental responsibility from the time of the birth of a child and may only lose that responsibility on the making of an adoption order.

Fathers who are married to the mother at the

time of the birth acquire parental responsibility at that time, and fathers who subsequently marry the mother acquire parental responsibility from the date of the marriage.

Fathers not married to the mother may acquire parental responsibility by agreement with the mother through a formal process involving registration or may be granted parental responsibility by an order of the court, otherwise they do not have parental responsibility.

A provision in proposed legislation, if enacted, will in due course provide for unmarried fathers to acquire parental responsibility if they enter their name on the birth certificate at the time of the registration of the birth of a child (clause 91 Adoption and Children Bill 2001).

Adults without parental responsibility may, by the court making a residence order in their favour under Section 8 of the Act, acquire parental responsibility, which they lose on the subsequent discharge of the order.

Several adults may hold parental responsibility at one time and may exercise it independently. They may not give it up but may arrange for others to exercise all or some of responsibilities on their behalf. It is reasonable for a professional dealing with a child to insist on evidence of these arrangements having been made.

Adults with the care of a child but not parental responsibility may do what is reasonable to safeguard and promote the welfare of the child — this may include arranging for urgent medical care.

The courts have powers to determine the exercise of parental responsibility by those who have it. It is particularly important in circumstances in which a child is living apart from a parent to understand whether either parent's ability to exercise parental responsibility has been limited to any extent.

When a child is by order of a court committed to the care of a local authority, that authority acquires parental responsibility and the power to determine the extent to which parents with parental responsibility may exercise their parental responsibility (Section 33(3) (b) Children Act 1989). It is important to ascertain from a responsible care authority what arrangements have been made for the exercise of this power and to whom a practitioner should relate on issues that arise with respect to the child.

Local authorities that are looking after a child under section 20 of the Act but in respect of whom there has been no care order made, do not acquire parental responsibility and must reach agreement with those who have it concerning the exercise of the responsibility. Children in such circumstances are particularly vulnerable if adequate arrangements are not made or professionals involved with the child and family are unclear of those arrangements.

Although parental responsibility continues until the end of childhood at 18 years of age, a child acquires an increasing ability to influence matters that affect his or her welfare since so far as the parent is concerned it is:

'a dwindling right which the courts will hesitate to enforce against the wishes of the child, the older he is. It starts with the right to control and ends with little more than advice'

(Gillick v West Norfolk and Wisbech Health
Authority and Another (1986) 1 FLR 224).

CONSENT TO MEDICAL TREATMENT

As with an adult, medical treatment in the absence of lawful authority may amount to trespass to the person and an assault. Failure to consider the issue appropriately may also lay the ground for a negligence claim. The principles apply to treatment, examination, assessment, or disclosure of information.

A child who has attained the age of 16 years is capable of giving effective consent (Family Law Reform Act 1969 Section 8(1)) unless lacking capacity applying the same principles that apply to adults.

If under 16 years, a child may give effective consent if, in the judgment of the practitioner, the child is of sufficient understanding to comprehend the consequences of consent or refusal or to be capable of making up his or her own mind on the matter requiring decision. The judgment may differ according to the matter at issue for the same child and may involve different ages for different children on similar issues (Gillick v West Norfolk and Wisbech Health Authority and Another (1986) 1 FLR 224).

However, the right of determination and the right of consent are different. The right to determine whether to have medical treatment may be made by the competent child or otherwise by a person with parental responsibility if he or she is not. Consent to the treatment can be given by the competent child, or the parent, whether or not the child is competent, or by some other competent authority including the court. Therefore a child may consent against the wishes of a parent, but may not be able to prevent treatment if a parent or some other competent authority provides the lawful source of consent (Re R (1992) 1 FLR 190).

Practical issues may however affect the ability to carry out treatment in such circumstances.

A person with parental responsibility is a possible source of lawful consent until the child reaches the age of 18 years.

Where a number of adults have parental responsibility, it is unnecessary to secure the agreement of all those adults — each may independently be a source of lawful consent, even where it is known that one may oppose the proposal. However, if it is known that a person with parental responsibility opposes the treatment, unless delay or involvement will expose the child to risk, it would be wise to allow a reasonable time for the person opposing the steps to make an application to the court.

Disputes or concern over potential damage to a child that may result from a failure to secure appropriate treatment may be resolved by the court. This may involve applying for a specific issues order under Section 8 of the Act or for the exercise of powers in the wardship jurisdiction. The court will consider carefully parental views but will resolve the matter by applying the principle of what is in the best interests of the child.

In appropriate cases it may be necessary for child protection procedures to be followed and for the local authority to acquire parental responsibility by invoking public law proceedings, seeking the making of a care order so that the local authority may give any necessary consents. The appropriateness of particular action in an individual case should be agreed through inter-agency strategy discussions as envisaged in Working Together to Safeguard Children (TSO 1999).

When local authorities are involve with determining the placement of a child, regulations require them to have clear policies and procedures in relation to the consent to the medical examination and treatment of children placed by them, and to make these known to the health authority and the child's carers (Arrangements for Placement of Children (General) Regulations 1991, S.I. 1991/890, reg.7).

CONFIDENTIALITY

The important statutory duties in relation to vulnerable children cannot be met without effective and appropriate sharing of relevant information, some of which may usually be regarded as confidential between a practitioner and patient or client.

Confidentiality should not be confused with secrecy. Patients and others are entitled to have confidence in their relationships with professionals and that information will only be shared for proper purposes. Such information may be shared in order to comply with a statutory obligation or if it is in the public interest.

The statutory obligations arising from the Children Act are set out above and it is clearly in the public interest that the carefully constructed legislative framework and government guidance designed to provide services for the most vulnerable children operates effectively.

Provisions of the Crime and Disorder Act 1998 encourage effective sharing of material in the interests of reducing crime and disorder and complement the public interest obligation for public agencies to co-operate with the detection and prevention of serious crime.

It is important, however, that disclosure of information takes place according to principles of good practice and on a need to know basis. Those seeking disclosure should be clear about the reasons information is required and the purposes for which it is likely to be used.

It should be remembered that only the receiver of information is in a position to fully understand its relevance. In child protection cases in particular, 'often, it is only when information from a number of sources has been shared and is then put together that it becomes clear that a child is at risk of or is suffering significant harm' (Paragraph 7.27 Working Together to Safeguard Children, (TSO 1999)).

The Data Protection Act 1998 and the Human Rights Act 1998 encourage the adoption of sound decision making in this area and the need to be able to justify the course adopted. While encouraging good practice, however, their provisions are not intended to inhibit the proper protection and safeguarding of the welfare of the most vulnerable.

The establishment of protocols between agencies will reassure professionals and members of the public that high standards of practice will be applied to these issues.

Concerns over inconsistencies within the health service in the treatment of sensitive personal health information led to the government establishing the Caldicott Committeee which reported with recommendations in December 1997. A key recommendation of the Report was that a network of Caldicott Guardians of patient information should be established throughout the NHS. Government circular required each Health Authority, Special Health Authority, NHS Trust and Primary Care Group to make appointments by 31 March 1999.

The appointments are intended to assist work to improve confidentiality and security and guardians will oversee access to patient-identifiable information as a new framework for handling patient information in the NHS is developed. This will include the development of local protocols governing disclosure to other organisations, restrict access by enforcing strict need to know principles, establish reviews and improve organisational performance (HSC 1999/012: Caldicott Guardians).

CARE PROCEEDINGS

Prior to the implementation of the Children Act, provisions by which children could be compulsorily committed to the care of a local authority were to be found in a range of statutes. The grounds to be satisfied varied according to the statute and the court before which the matter was being considered.

The Act repealed these statutes and provided that the only route by which a child may now be committed to care or placed under supervision following an application by a local authority or the NSPCC is under Section 31. The processes are termed 'public law proceedings' to distinguish them from issues concerning private individuals. The grounds that must be satisfied before magistrates sitting in a Family Proceedings Court, or judges sitting in a County or High Court, may consider making a care or supervision order are:

(a) that the child concerned is suffering, or is likely to suffer, significant harm; and

(b) that the harm, or likelihood of harm, is attributable to:

  (i) the care given to the child, or likely to be given to him if an order were not to be made, not being what it would be reasonable to expect a parent to give him; or

  (ii) the child's being beyond parental control (Section 31 (2)).

These grounds have become known as 'the threshold criteria' and must be satisfied on evidence established to the required standard of proof, which is the balance of probability. However, since serious events occur less frequently than more serious events, the courts insist that the more serious the allegations, the more cogent must the evidence before a fact is proven. Unproven facts are treated as not having occurred (Re H and R (1995) 1 FLR 643).

'Likely' means that there is a real possibility, one that cannot sensibly be ignored (Re H and R (1995) ibid.).

'Significant' is not defined in the Act and means, according to ordinary usage, noteworthy or important (Oxford English Dictionary). It does not mean serious. Presenting circumstances may be significant because they are indeed serious or because they give rise to particular implications.

The Act defines the following terms:

- 'harm' means ill-treatment or the impairment of health or development;
- 'development' means physical, intellectual, emotional, social or behavioural development;
- 'health' means physical or mental health; and
- 'ill-treatment' includes sexual abuse and forms of ill-treatment which are not physical.

If satisfied that the threshold criteria is met, the court, after considering the 'welfare checklist' of issues relevant to the upbringing of a child set out in Section 1 (3) of the Act, will decide whether an order should be made. The principle that the welfare of the child shall be the court's paramount consideration is applied (Section 1 (1)).

In specified public law proceedings, a guardian ad litem will be appointed by the court from the Children and Family Court Advisory and Support Service (CAFCASS) to enquire into the circumstances in the interests of the child, instruct a solicitor on his behalf and prepare a report for the court.

The Crime and Disorder Act 1998 Section 11 introduced the Child Safety Order to address the problems of children under ten years of age who commit criminal acts or anti-social behaviour. If provisions of the order are breached a local authority may apply to the court under Section 31 of the Act for a care order. In these circumstances the order may be made without the court being satisfied that the threshold criteria are met but in all other respects the matter will proceed as for other applications under Section 31.

APPEARANCE IN COURT

Medical and nursing personnel may be required to appear to give evidence in public or private law proceedings, when the future welfare of a child is at issue, or in criminal proceedings. The obligation of a professional witness is to assist the court to reach an appropriate decision by ensuring that it has all the relevant information and benefit of relevant expertise.

Appropriately qualified and experienced professionals are regarded as experts and are privileged in that they may within the scope of their expertise give evidence of opinion and inferences based on factual material. It is important to consider all material facts, properly research and identify any data not available. Experts must be objective and non-partisan in the presentation of material and opinions. The court must not be misled by omission and if only a provisional view is being expressed, this must be made clear (Re J (1991) FCR 193).

Opinions expressed should be within the scope of a competent body of professional opinion, be logical and within the scope of judicial functioning on the issue.

Where appropriate it is important to be firm when expressing opinions and not to be drawn into making concessions that distort the evidence.

Arrangements may be made for experts with differing opinions to discuss the areas of difference before court appearances in order to reduce or clearly identify the scope of disagreement.

When giving evidence and during the processes that may precede court proceedings, care must be taken to ensure that medical terms and phrases are correctly understood and interpreted by those to whom they are addressed. In particular, members of other professions may need considerable assistance in drawing appropriate inferences from the material.

REACHING SOUND JUDGMENTS

It is helpful to consider the means by which the soundness of judgments and conclusions are challenged and undermined in proceedings before the courts. To be sound the approach must be demonstrably reasonable in the sense that it has been properly reasoned. Table 18.1 sets out the issues commonly explored and against which the forming of judgments or making of diagnoses may be measured. If integrated into practice, these principles will raise the quality of judgments and expose them less to successful challenge.

HUMAN RIGHTS

The Human Rights Act 1998 was implemented for most purposes with effect from 2 October 2000. From this date it is unlawful for public authorities to carry out their functions incompatibly with the European Convention for Human Rights and Fundamental Freedoms, the relevant provisions of which are set out in the First Schedule to the Act.

The Act does not create new statutory functions — it determines how existing functions should be exercised. In particular, consideration of the Convention Rights should not inhibit action necessary for the protection of vulnerable children. They should be seen as encouragement for good standards of practice — 'the expectation is that best practice in the services already respects the Convention' (LAC (2000) 17).

Working Together to Safeguard Children 1999 and the Framework for the Assessment of Children in Need and their Families 2000 were written taking account of the Convention. Application of the processes and expectations within those documents will therefore reflect the principles of the Convention.

Table 18.1 **Reaching sound judgments**	
Demonstrate proper reasoning	*Consider human rights implications*
Take account of all relevant factors	Consider any relevant guidance
Give each factor appropriate weight	Consult appropriately
Consider all the options or alternatives	Acknowledge lack of expertise and its impact
Keep an open mind until it is appropriate to close it	Acknowledge lack of information and its impact
Know and act in accordance with the law	If the position is provisional identify what required to make final
Know and apply procedures or know why deviated	Ensure full and accurate recording of these issues

Everyone, in particular the vulnerable child, is entitled to the protection of the Convention Rights and practice should therefore consider the impact of the delivery of services on all those likely to be affected and not simply the most obvious recipients. There is an obligation to actively promote the freedoms set out in the Convention and not simply avoid their infringement. In this way the standards of practice should be enhanced and delivered on a basis that respects individual needs.

Article 2, which prohibits intentional ending of life, Article 3 which provides for protection against torture and inhuman and degrading treatment or punishment and Article 8, concerned with respect for private and family life, home and correspondence, are clearly relevant to the delivery of services to the most vulnerable.

The Court of Appeal has emphasised the focus of Article 8 in the following way:

'The family life for which Article 8 requires respect is not a proprietary right vested in either parent or child: it is as much an interest of society as of individual family members, and its principal purpose, at least where there are children, must be the safety and welfare of the child. It needs to be remembered that the tabulated right is not to family life as such but to respect for it. The purpose . . . is to assure within proper limits the entitlement of individuals to the benefit of what is benign and positive in family life. It is not to allow other individuals, however closely related and well intentioned, to create or perpetuate situations which jeopardise their welfare' (Re F (2000) 2 FLR 512)).

REFERENCES AND FURTHER READING

The Challenge of Partnership in Child Protection Practice Guide. 1995 HMSO, London

The Children Act 1989 Guidance and Regulations Volume 1 Court Orders. 1991 HMSO, London

The Children Act 1989 Guidance and Regulations Volume 3 Family Placements. 1991 HMSO, London

The Children Act 1989 Guidance and Regulations Volume 4 Residential Care. 1991 HMSO, London

The Children Act 1989 Guidance and Regulations Volume 7 Children with Disabilities. 1991 HMSO, London

Child Protection: Medical responsibilities. 1994 HMSO, London

Child Protection: Clarification of Arrangements between the NHS and other Agencies. 1995. HMSO, London

Child Protection: Guidance for Senior Nurses, Health Visitors and Midwives and their Managers. 1997. HMSO, London

Darbyshire, P 2001 The English Legal System in a Nutshell (5th edition). Sweet and Maxwell, London

Department of Health 2001 www.doh.uk/consent Reference guide to consent for examination or treatment.

Department of Health 2001 12 key points on consent: the law in England. www.doh.uk/consent

Department of Health 2001. Safeguarding Children in whom Illness is Induced or Fabricated by Carers with Parental Responsibilities: Supplementary Guidance to Working Together to Safeguard Children. Consultation Document. The Stationery Office, London

Department of Health 1999 Working Together to Safeguard Children. The Stationery Office, London

Department of Health 1996 Children's Services Planning Order and Guidance. The Stationery Office, London

DFEE 1996 Supporting Pupils with Medical Needs in School. DFEE Circular 1996/14

DFEE 1994 The Organisation of Special Needs Provision. DFEE Circular 1994/6

Framework for the Assessment of Children in Need and their Families. 2000 The Stationery Office, London

GMC 2000 Confidentiality: Protecting and Providing Information

HSC 1999 Caldicott Guardians. 1999/012

An Introduction to the Children's Act 1989. 1990. HMSO, London

NHS Executive 1996 Child Health in the Community: A Guide to Good Practice. HMSO, London

Quality Protects Programme: Transforming Children's Services. 1998. LAC 1998/28

Reporting to Court under the Children Act. 1996 HMSO, London

Report of the Inquiry into Child Abuse in Cleveland 1987. HMSO, London

19 | Voluntary organisations

INTRODUCTION

This chapter aims to map the voluntary sector in Britain today, its variety, role and functions, and to provide paediatricians with some signposts for contacting and working with voluntary organisations.

Voluntary organisations have for many years been a central source of support for children and families. They operate in almost every sphere of life, care and welfare, in most areas of work covered by this book, and in a wide variety of different guises. This chapter attempts to describe the variety and diversity of organisations, their links to other sectors of society and their strengths and limitations.

BACKGROUND

The close connection between voluntary and charitable organisations and the mainstream services is usually forgotten. Many statutory services and institutions began as voluntary, charitable and community initiatives, whether they be local hospitals and trusts now absorbed into the health service, or large areas of social services which grew out of voluntary and philanthropic effort.

At the same time, the boundaries of statutory provision change constantly through rationing which leaves lower-priority recipients seeking help in the voluntary or private sectors, 'contracting out' of directly provided services to voluntary organisations, and the assimilation of new areas of work (e.g. alternative therapies) into mainstream services. Now the division of the health service into yet more self-governing trusts, and the development of new kinds of non-profit charities, companies and so on, blurs the boundaries between

definitions of voluntary, statutory and private still further. In reality the boundary between voluntary and statutory is always changing.

WHAT IS A VOLUNTARY ORGANISATION?

There have been a number of attempts to answer the question 'What is a voluntary organisation?' and to classify different types of organisation. A good basic definition is:

Voluntary organisations are not-for-profit organisations, set up and run by voluntary, unpaid Management Committees. As such the voluntary sector differs from the private sector which is run for profit; from the statutory sector which is set up by statute; and voluntary organisations differ from not-for-profit organisations which are run by paid staff rather than voluntary Management Committees. [Some] voluntary organisations do employ paid staff as well as involving volunteers in the work of the organisation. Some but not all, voluntary organisations are charitable in the sense of being registered charities or having charitable objectives
(National Council of Voluntary Organisations 1990).

While most larger organisations do employ staff, there is a tension in the voluntary sector between professionalism and 'pure' voluntarism. On the one hand there are doubts about the reliability of volunteers and on the other about the cost, remoteness and bureaucracy of organisations employing staff. The 'pro-professional' view can be explained simply in terms of statutory bureaucracies identifying most easily with similar organisations, as well as a mistrust of 'amateurism'. However, this is to ignore both the autonomy of voluntary organisations as well as the expertise and value associated with voluntary commitment. From all perspectives, however, the key issue is an organisation's reliability in what it sets out to do.

QUALITY AND VOLUNTARISM

Concerns about quality and accountability are now commonplace in monitoring and evaluating the work of even the smallest of voluntary organisations. The issue of trustworthiness is not primarily a question of whether an organisation delivers services through volunteers or through paid workers, but relates to issues such as image, training and adherence to standards and guidelines. A simple prejudice against volunteers ignores the often excellent professional services they can deliver, but it is also true to say that in the voluntary sector there is a tendency over time for organisations to supplement or replace volunteers with paid workers as services become more complex or demanding, and as the safeguards required by society increase.

Questions of liability are more urgent because people are more ready to make legal challenges to inadequate services. Also although accidents or active wrongdoing may not be frequent or common, isolated cases are highly publicised in the voluntary sector as in others, and lead to demands for more checks and balances. The idea of public accountability can seem uncomfortable to voluntary groups which developed from notions of independence, trust and the basic good intentions of philanthropy.

However, the idea that voluntary organisations owe a duty of care, or are accountable to, the wider community, to government or to public agencies has strengthened alongside the growth of formal 'standards in public life'. We have realised that charitable funding, in a different but equally clear way to funding from the public purse, uses public money and demands public accountability. The historic, stuffy image of charities is being replaced by expectations of openness and clarity, and the arrival of the National Lottery has intensified the feeling that charitable funds are in a real sense public funds.

> **Box 19.1**
> **Self-help**
>
> The term *self-help* acquired politically contrasting meanings in the last 20 years, on the one hand reflecting Conservative notions of self-reliance, individual responsibility and active citizenship (Johnson 1990). On the other hand the sense in which it is used in the voluntary sector, while it is less focused on helping others than on mutual aid within a group, is fundamentally different from this stress on the *individual*: it relates instead to the *collective* support available through a group of people acting cooperatively.

WHAT VOLUNTARY ORGANISATIONS DO

There are different ways of analysing voluntary organisations' activities. Handy (1988) includes four commonly used categories apart from clubs set up for mutual self-interest and benefit of members (sports, travel, theatrical and so on):

- *Service*: Providing something for individual people other than members.
- *Advocacy and campaigning*: A range of activities including individual support and joint action to promote a particular viewpoint or policy.
- *Support*: Supporting other voluntary organisations or groups, providing advice and services for them as distinct from providing them to individuals.
- *self-help*: (See Box 19.1).

These categories are not mutually exclusive. Indeed, the nature of the voluntary sector is such that many organisations combine two or more of these functions.

Self-help groups (Box 19.2)

The self-help category is separate in origin, in that members come together entirely for their own benefit: they do not initially aim to offer a service to non-members. But of course, self-help groups are often strong campaigners or advocates on behalf of their members and may easily develop into service-

Voluntary organisations

Box 19.2
Example of a self-help support service

Self Help Nottingham is a registered charity based in Nottingham. It enables people concerned with their own health, disability and social issues to develop support systems through self-help groups and mutual aid networks. Self Help Nottingham offers support and development to self-help groups and also advocates, through training, research, development of services and dialogue, the benefits of self help in society. Its services primarily relate to self-help groups in Nottingham and surrounding areas, but it also has many national and international contacts. Self Help Nottingham's website at www.selfhelp.org.uk offers information on how self-help groups can help individuals and professionals, on publications, training and research relating to self help, and on how to contact groups. It also invites users to become involved in discussions about the development of self-help groups.

Box 19.3
Example of voluntary organisation supporting families

Home-Start is a national voluntary organisation supporting local autonomous Home-Start schemes in which volunteers offer support to families in their own homes who have children under the age of five. Volunteers offer support, friendship and practical help, preventing family breakdown or crisis. Families are often referred to Home-Start by their health visitor or social worker but anyone can contact them to ask for help.

Home-Start supports families for many reasons. These include: new mothers, multiple births, single parents, mothers with postnatal depression, families who are isolated, families where either or both parents or children have health problems, families who are experiencing financial problems, housing or relationship problems, and other things which make life stressful.

Volunteers are carefully matched to a family and then visit regularly. They often help by listening and offering companionship, helping with trips to the doctor, hospital or clinics, playing with the children, or just providing an extra pair of hands.

Home-Start offers a confidential service: information will not be shared outside the organisation except when a child needs protection. Home-Start volunteers are all parents themselves and understand the stresses and strains in bringing up a young family. All volunteers are police checked, and trained.

providing organisations in a wider sense. It is common for self-help groups to oppose medical orthodoxy, but if antagonism is avoided there are many examples of productive partnership between health professionals and self-help groups.

Organisations of service users
(Box 19.3)

Another distinction is between organisations *of* service users or patients (and/or their carers or parents) on the one hand, and other voluntary organisations on the other. The definition of *user* itself, in the context of community care, needs separate examination, but organisations run (managed and staffed) by people who are themselves service users, carers or parents have become stronger and more assertive during the late twentieth century.

One issue is who represents the service user or patient in consultation, planning and other partnerships with statutory agencies: this is especially problematical in the field of services for children and their families. Very often in the past it was assumed that voluntary organisations generally

could convey the user's (and/or carer's) perspective. However, government policy now leans firmly towards partnership with and involvement of service users, carers and parents. The complexity and the dilemma involved in this area is well summarised in 'Building Bridges' (National Institute for Social Work, 1993 p 9):

Consulting voluntary organisations is very different from consulting people who use services. Debates about representativeness can be a mechanism for devaluing contributions from people who get services. Some groups . . . are often accused of being unrepresentative when they are angry, articulate or assertive. This can be a way for others to avoid hearing what someone has to say.

> **Box 19.4**
> **Example of a group of relevance to people of Africo-Caribbean origin**
>
> *The Sickle Cell Society* was first set up as a registered charity in 1979. It was formed by a group of patients, parents and health professionals who were all concerned about the lack of understanding and the inadequacy of treatment for sufferers of sickle cell disorders. The website of the Sickle Cell Society www.sicklecellsociety.org is a comprehensive source of information on Sickle Cell disorders which affect people of African-Caribbean origin. In addition to practical advice about day-to-day care of children, it has information for health professionals and a directory of over 50 locally based support groups nationwide, some based in NHS trusts and others elsewhere.

> **Box 19.5**
> **Example of a voluntary organisation of disabled people**
>
> *Nottingham Young Disabled People* (NYDP) describes itself as 'an advocacy project run by disabled people for disabled people'. 'Young' in this context means between 16 and 65 years old. 'Young' disabled people can find out about their rights, express their concerns and discover ways of changing things for themselves. They meet together in small groups, initially facilitated by the project's development worker, to discuss everyday experiences and issues. NYDP supports and encourages young disabled people to speak for themselves and to find support through contacts with other disabled people.

Children's voices

In the case of children as service users, there is a long history of expecting others to speak for them, and legal issues arise if it is suggested that they have a direct say in their own treatment or care. However, children's rights are now more prominent and there is at least a commitment in rhetoric to children having a voice. In practice most interagency plans have found it more difficult to make this a reality, but there are examples of good practice.

Black and ethnic minority groups (Box 19.4)

A special category of user group is the organisation of black people. Such groups sometimes cover a whole range of 'ethnic minorities' (e.g. Afro-Caribbean communities, or Asian) but more often reflect a specific religious/cultural/national origin and identity (Indian, Bangladeshi, Muslim, Pakistani, Vietnamese and so on). Sometimes groups form within these areas — Muslim women, black mental health for example.

Black and ethnic minority voluntary organisations reflect different cultural identity, but they also exist because of the widespread, longstanding neglect of the different needs and cultures of these groups in mainstream services, combined with the racism experienced by people in black and ethnic minority communities in our society. In the area of family policy and services such organisations can be valuable sources of information about culturally appropriate services.

Geography and voluntary organisations (Boxes 19.5–19.7)

Voluntary organisations can also be defined according to their geography. Geography relates not just to the physical area covered by their services and/or membership: it is also to do with the way in which they are managed. Essentially, an organisation providing services in a defined area can either be set up for and confined to that area alone, or it can act as a local arm of an organisation set up to cover a wider area. This is important for two reasons.

On the one hand some people attach importance to local management: in other words, they believe that the essential voluntary element of the organisation, its management committee, should be drawn from the community it serves. On the other hand, there is a concern that services should provided uniformly in different areas. But while rational planning and provision is a longstanding

> Box 19.6
> **Example of a charity providing early help for children with emotional and behavioural difficulties**
>
> *Think Children*, based at Newark in Nottinghamshire, aims to prevent a young child's emerging emotional and behavioural difficulties from becoming a pathway to educational marginalisation, social disaffection and violence or self-harm. Their experience, based on research, is that very early help is vital, and they work with children from 5 to 11 years old, targetting the most vulnerable children and their parents.
>
> The charity's methods include focused playwork for the child, using the safety of the imaginary world to clarify and confront issues in the real one. They also offer person-centred counselling to parents. The charity stresses the necessity of partnership with primary schools. This is a unique organisation which began in one corner of Nottinghamshire and which is gradually developing its work across neighbouring areas as resources grow.

> Box 19.7
> **Example of a voluntary organisation providing a community-based resource for disabled children and their families**
>
> *A Place To Call Our Own* (APTCOO) is a voluntary organisation offering an accessible, community-based resource to disabled children, their carers and families in North Nottinghamshire. Formed in 1991 by a group of carers, APTCOO aims to support disabled children and young people and their families through offering a range of services and facilities. APTCOO offers an information services (including website: www.proweb.co.uk/~aptcoo/), a telephone helpline for carers and families of disabled children, one-to-one support, support groups including A Time To Call Our Own (for carers), a Dad's Group, Bereavement Support and a Sibling Group.
>
> It has a fully equipped community sensory room for children, for stimulation and development, or relaxation in a safe and specialised environment. The room uses sight, sound and touch to encourage and stimulate the development of the child: 'This magical "Moon in the Sky Room" helps to calm, reduce frustrations and promote a feeling of well being'. Equipment includes bubble tubes, optic fibres, star carpet, infinity tunnel, projector, light board, waterbed and soft music. The sensory room facility is free to individuals and families and may be booked by groups.
>
> In partnership with Mansfield Play Forum, APTCOO offers an integrated toy library with toys and specialist play equipment for children of all abilities.

aspiration of statutory agencies, it has never been a strong feature of voluntary sector operation.

The three main geographical 'types' operating locally are:

- National organisations managed nationally (e.g. NSPCC, Barnardos, NCH Action for Children, Childline).
- National organisations operating through affiliated autonomous locally managed organisations (e.g. HomeStart, Mencap, Councils for Voluntary Service).
- Local organisations (which naturally vary from locality to locality).

THE VALUE OF VOLUNTARY ORGANISATIONS

For busy professionals, the question is obviously 'Why work with voluntary organisations?' To summarise, they may offer:

- Complementary services to those provided by statutory agencies.
- Expertise and knowledge based on direct experience and involvement.
- Greater approachability for those suspicious of officialdom and statutory agencies.
- Alternative perspectives and therapies.

CONTACTING AND WORKING WITH VOLUNTARY ORGANISATIONS

Once a paediatrician or any other professional is aware that voluntary organisations may offer some additional support to patients, the question will then be how to find out what is available. Usually the enquiry will start by trying to identify locally accessible groups, and with support available by telephone, post or the internet. In the case of, for example, uncommon and specific illnesses, conditions or disabilities the enquiry will need to take account of national and even international specialist groups. The assumption should be that 'there is an organisation somewhere' which has the appropriate knowledge or support to offer.

In most localities in the UK there are 'intermediary' or 'umbrella' organisations which act as signposts to all the voluntary organisations in their area. In England these are usually know as Councils for Voluntary Service (CVS): they can usually be found in the Yellow Pages under 'Charitable & Voluntary Organisations' along with a large number of more specific local voluntary groups. The CVS usually publishes some kind of directory of local organisations.

At a national level the list of support organisations at the end of this volume (Appendix 1) is an obvious first source of contact details of key national voluntary organisations. The annual voluntary agencies directory (National Council of Voluntary Organisations, 2000) is the main source for information on groups of all sizes and kinds. The 2000 edition includes details of 57 organisations under 'Children: health', 36 under 'Disability: children . . .' and nearly 100 under 'Children: childcare'. The directory usually includes references to websites. Internet directories to voluntary organisations are less certain but search facilities and specialist sites are developing very fast (a recent search for pages on 'dyspraxia' for example produced 2618 entries!).

SUMMARY

The voluntary sector is diverse in purpose and expertise, but it offers access to a rich mixture of experience and services which complement those offered by statutory health services. In the past professionals have shown mistrust of such resources, but experience of joint work between voluntary organisations and statutory services shows that it is worth moving beyond these barriers. The growing culture of partnership and the pressure for greater user involvement in service planning and delivery at the beginning of the twenty-first century offer powerful encouragement to health professionals and voluntary and self-help groups to find areas of common ground, whether in answering the needs of individual children and their families, or in developing even better health care for children.

REFERENCES AND FURTHER READING

Handy C 1988 Understanding voluntary organisations. Penguin, Harmondsworth

Johnson N 1990 Reconstructing the welfare state: a decade of change, 1980–1990. Harvester Wheatsheaf, Hemel Hempstead

National Council of Voluntary Organisations 1990 Nathan report. NCVO, London

National Council of Voluntary Organisations 2000 The Voluntary Agencies Directory 2000 [annual publication]. NCVO, London

National Institute for Social Work 1993 Building bridges. Building bridges between people who use and people who provide services. National Institute for Social Work, London

Wilson J 1995 How to work with self-help groups: guidelines for professionals. Arena, Aldershot

20 | Child health surveillance and promotion programme

INTRODUCTION

The last century has seen the emergence of 'surveillance medicine' where normal/healthy populations have become the areas of concern rather than the sick. The focus has largely been on early identification of children with problems and knowledge of the normal child and child care to promote better parenting. The latter is at least in theory an exercise in primary prevention. There have long been concerns however about the value of many of the surveillance activities, particularly in the context of evidenced-based health provision. The emphasis of surveillance programmes has shifted away from screening towards more health promotional activity. The benefit of these activities is also extremely difficult to evaluate. The shift towards partnerships with families and away from surveillance methods in which they may be more or less passive recipients of tests lends itself to less formalised approaches. At the same time as refocusing the universal programme, the service is able to provide a graduated response according to need.

The current UK population is diverse and health care and promotion needs to be designed to reflect these differences. The changing nature of the population imposes new demands on the health service which must adapt its delivery to reflect this new morbidity (Box 20.1). The focus has moved from individual checks to a broader public health approach with a holistic view of the child and his family and environment. Checklists and testing have often led to a pass–fail attitude to a child's development and not necessarily taken into account the natural variations in children's development and may undermine the parents' own superior knowledge of the child.

The UK programme published as Health for all Children (Hall 1996) and the new edition (2001 www.health-for-all-children.co.uk) address these issues with a smaller core 'surveillance programme' in comparison to previous years and greater emphasis on targetted more intensive support to those in greatest need. This will alter the role of school nursing services where more effort can be directed at those children requiring additional support. This should also pave the way for innovative health promotion programmes which are already being instigated in some schools, for example in sexual/reproductive health.

Child health surveillance

The current policy places less emphasis on secondary prevention (identification of children with problems) and more on primary prevention (health promotion). It rests upon the assumption and evidence that many problems which earlier programmes might have sought to identify through surveillance of all children, would present through parental self-referral, or opportunistic observation by informed individuals. It also stresses the danger of false reassurance provided by 'tests' with poor sensitivity and specificity.

Primary prevention acts by decreasing the incidence (number of new cases) by advice or education, for example accident prevention, nutritional advice, immunisation, Back to Sleep programme. **Secondary prevention** decreases the prevalence by early detection, shortening the duration and reducing the impact. **Tertiary prevention** is referring to minimising disability once a condition is established (Box 20.2). (see 'Screening' in Chapter 2).

There are a number of key issues around the surveillance of children for health and developmental

Box 20.1
Composition of UK population

- 20% of children live in lone-parent families
- 24% of children will experience parental divorce before the age of 16
- 30% of births take place outside of marriage
- 75% of married women and 50% of lone parents of preschool children work
- >8% of children under 16 are from ethnic minorities
- 25% of all children are growing up in poverty
- 200 000 are homeless
- 8% of births are to teenage mothers
- 4% of children live in housing unfit for use

From Woodroffe et al 1993

Box 20.2
Division of preventative health care for children

Primary prevention: activities include dental prophylaxis, immunisation, accident prevention, prevention of child abuse, health education for the child, education, advice and support to parents and health promotion

Secondary prevention: individual screening activities, tests and examinations, and non-specific oversight of health, e.g. screening for CDH, hearing impairment

Tertiary prevention: for the child with recognised special needs

From Butler 1989

Box 20.3
Principles of child health surveillance

- Child health surveillance is carried out in partnership with parents. The programme acknowledges the parents as the most important and effective identifiers of health, developmental and behavioural problems in their children

- The process of child health surveillance is a learning experience for parents, for children and for the health professionals. It involves an exchange of information and provides opportunities for guidance on important child health issues such as behaviour, nutrition, accident prevention, immunisation and the use of services for children

- Child health surveillance should be a positive experience with opportunities to reassure, build confidence, relieve anxiety and promote good health

- The process should be continuous and flexible, taking advantage of every consultation on an opportunistic basis as well as the fixed age components of the programme

- History taking and observation are the main tools for child health surveillance, complemented by clinical examination and screening tests

- A high standard of child health surveillance depends upon team work and good communication between all those involved. This includes education and social services as well as the health services

- The provision of the programme is a form of shared care between the primary health care teams and the child health services provided by community paediatricians

- The health visitor is the major health professional engaged in child health surveillance for pre-school children with close working links with the rest of the primary health care team and the district child health services. Child health surveillance by the health visitor is part of a wider family health assessment

- The school nurse is the key person for children of school age

problems. The principles described in Box 20.3 should be applied to any programme being implemented.

The current core programme is indeed much smaller than previous protocols because only those 'tests' of proven effectiveness are considered. The screening tests need to be considered as any other screening test. This means that not only will the test identify the child in need of help, with few false positives and false negatives, but also that there are interventions that will improve outcomes (Box 20.4). These programmes are expensive and need therefore to be planned with evidence-based knowledge of outcomes and effectiveness.

Problems with surveillance checks are illustrated in Boxes 20.5, 20.6, and fall into the following categories:

- Professional versus parental judgement — devalues the parental view.
- Initial impressions may be wrong.
- Failure to make allowance for prematurity.

- Developmental testing is not the best means of detecting developmental delay.
- Differing social context.
- Language and cultural context.
- Uncooperative child.

One of the major pitfalls of screening tests for development is illustrated in Fig. 20.1, with similar outcomes for two children who had very different testing results at age 1–2 years.

Child health promotion

Child health promotion reflects the move towards a more holistic care and partnerships with parents (Box 20.7). Child health promotion programmes differ in detail or emphasis between different health authorities and primary care trusts, however the

---

Box 20.4
Criteria for a 'Good' screening test

The condition:
- Should be important
- Natural history and epidemiology known

The test:
- Cost-effective test available
- Test has to be acceptable to patient and family
- High number of true positives (high sensitivity)
- Low number of false negatives (high specificity)
- Agreed policy of further diagnostic evaluation

The treatment:
- Identified pathway and services available
- Effective intervention available agreed and evidence based
- Early intervention shown to improve outcome

The screening programme:
- Evidence from randomised controlled trials that the programme is effective in reducing mortality and morbidity
- Programme acceptable to community
- Should be economically balanced in relationship to expenditure on medical care as a whole
- Agreed plan for management and quality assurance

Box 20.5
Does early detection matter?

- Parents value early diagnosis
- Improved outcome, e.g. phenylketonuria, congenital hypothyroidism
- Improved quality of life for child and family, e.g. physiotherapy in cerebral palsy
- Access to educational and social services — health authority has legal obligation to notify LEA when a child with special needs is recognised

---

Box 20.6
Pitfalls of screening

- Anxiety
- Subjected to unnecessary referrals and procedures
- Litigation in missed cases
- Unclear referral pathways
- Insufficient secondary services

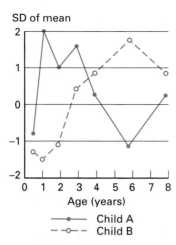

Fig. 20.1 Developmental quotients of individual children can vary markedly at different ages. (Adapted from Largo et al 1990)

Box 20.7
Child health promotion versus child health surveillance

- Central role of parents
- Parental empowerment
- Emphasis on primary prevention
- Use of parent-held record

---

core child health programme offers the opportunity for issues to be addressed with individuals and their families. Specific groups may need programmes tailored to their needs, for example travellers. There is also the opportunity for a more robust public health approach to be used within the school health system, for example sex education programmes, drug education programmes, etc.

Changing trends

Opportunistic screening and health promotion

It is recognised that many of the children most at risk of behavioural and developmental problems are in fact missing out on routine surveillance pro-

---

Box 20.8
Children most at risk of behavioural and developmental problems

- Mobile and homeless
- Poor parenting
- Maternal mental health problems
- Premature
- Children in need

---

grammes (Box 20.8). This is evidence of the inverse care law, where those in most need are not receiving services (Tudor Hart 1971, Webb 1998). Opportunistic surveillance and health promotion including immunisation is recommended for those children at risk (e.g. travellers and homeless), as these children usually present for other reasons (e.g. accidents, infections, etc.).

Our healthier nation

The 'Saving Lives: Our Healthier Nation' (OHN) White Paper (Department of Health 1999) is a comprehensive government-wide public health strategy for England. It was published as a White Paper in July 1999 with twin goals:

- to improve health
- to reduce the health gap (health inequalities).

The strategy aims to prevent up to 300 000 untimely and unnecessary deaths by the year 2010.

'Our Healthier Nation' seeks to encourage and support action being taken to address a wide range of influences (or determinants) on health. To do this it supports the setting of both national and local priorities and targets.

One of the problems with national strategies is that they can often fail to take account of local level variability. To overcome this, the 'Our Healthy Nation' health strategy has identified a limited number of key national priorities which each area must address while allowing local flexibility to set additional priorities based on local assessments of need.

Nationally the four main priorities identified are:

- **Cancer.** To reduce the death rate from cancer in people under 75 years by at least a fifth by 2010, saving up to 100 000 lives in total by tackling factors which cause them such as diet, smoking or the environment.
- **Coronary heart disease and stroke.** To reduce the death rate from coronary heart disease and stroke and related diseases in people under 75 years by at least two-fifths by 2010, saving up to 200 000 lives in total.
- **Accidents.** To reduce the death rates from accidents by at least one-fifth and to reduce the rate of serious injury from accidents by at least one-tenth by 2010, saving up to 12 000 lives in total.
- **Mental health.** To reduce the death rate from suicide and undetermined injury by at least a fifth by 2010, saving up to 4000 lives in total.

Government initiatives

Health Action Zones
Health Action Zones (HAZ) have been part of a government initiative to try to improve health in areas of deprivation with high morbidity (Box 20.9). There have also been a number of other initiatives such as Education Action Zones (EAZ; see below) to improve educational attainments. In many areas HAZs and EAZs coexist.

Sure Start
This programme is for under fours in deprived areas and has been funded to £452 million nation-

ally (Sure Start 2001). The main short-term aim is that a greater number of children are 'ready for school'. This involves the concept of school readiness and includes the following facets of a child's development:

- language
- motor
- emotional
- behavioural
- social interaction.

The long-term aim is an improved educational outcome at 16 years.
Other targets include:

- general health
- child abuse and neglect
- postnatal depression.

Methods used include:

- health promotion
- teaching parenting skills
- encouraging parents to help/stimulate their children
- joint working between social services, education, voluntary agencies, e.g. provision of day care, crèche.

Sure Start particularly emphasises the recognition of and support for socially excluded families in a local community framework.

Other examples of Government initiatives
Connexions is a government strategy aimed at facilitating the transition between adolescence and adulthood. The Connexions strategy has four main themes:

- Flexible curriculum that enables young people to seek alternative qualifications and work-related learning.
- High quality provision of education in school sixth forms, colleges of further education and work-based learning.
- Targetting financial support for those in learning, e.g. youth card for discounted travel and leisure.
- Outreach, information, advice and support (this includes anti-truancy and anti-exclusion measures).

Box 20.9
Examples of areas targetted in Health Action Zones

↓ Homelessness

↓ Accidents

↓ Child abuse and neglect

↓ Pregnancy in under 16s

↓ Unemployment in deprived areas

Delay first use of alcohol and drugs in young people

Education Action Zones are part of a government initiative to ensure that children from deprived urban and rural areas have an equal chance to succeed in school. There are currently 99 zones identified and more are planned. Applications are made within these zones to fund particular local initiatives.

Recognition of the importance of partnerships with others assists in targeting high-risk groups, for example **Youth Offending Teams** which are part of a government initiative to reduce youth crime. They involve a multidisciplinary approach to youth and include participation by police, mental health, social services, health and voluntary organisations.

PROFESSIONALS INVOLVED

The primary healthcare team (see Chapter 13; Table 20.1)

For the purposes of Child Health Promotion the primary healthcare team consists of:

- general practitioners
- health visitors
- midwife
- practice nurse
- practice manager
- receptionists.

Who does what

Agencies and roles in child health promotion

Promoting children's health is not solely the role of health services. As shown in Fig. 20.2, it can be seen that parents and family play a major role in child health promotion. They are supported primarily by health services but also by the local education authority, department of social services and national government.

The **primary healthcare team** has the responsibility for ensuring all children take part in the programme, i.e. scheduled checks, immunisation and health promotion advice for pre-school-aged children. The lead professional is the **health visitor**. The **school health service** has a similar respon-

Table 20.1 **Role of members of the primary health-care team in the first 2 years of life**					
	Birth visit	10–14 day visit	6–8 week check	6–9 month review	2 year review
GP	✓		✓		
HV		✓		✓	✓
MW	✓				

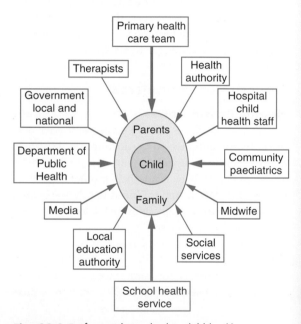

Fig. 20.2 Professionals involved in child health surveillance and promotion

sibility for school-aged children. School nurses carry out these activities.

The **community paediatrician** becomes involved after referral, for example advising on the treatment of iron deficiency anaemia or when assessing a child for developmental delay. Health promotion should always be an integral part of any consultation with a paediatrician.

The **hospital child health staff** also play an important role, with most newborn reviews being carried out by senior house officers. An ideal opportunity for health promotion arises in the accident and emergency department after injuries, for example head injuries, poisonings.

The **midwife** has responsibility for promoting breastfeeding, ensuring vitamin K is given where appropriate and promoting maternal health.

Therapists, for example speech therapists, occupational therapists, help children to overcome or adjust to their disability.

The **Department of Public Health** advise on immunisation and infectious disease control and on accident prevention.

The **health authority** is responsible for implementing national policy on a local level and for collating data returns (e.g. COVER statistics — Cover of Vaccination Evaluated Rapidly (Begg et al 1989); Public Health Laboratory Service and Communicable Disease surveillance Centre (Department of Health 2000).

The **local education authority** must provide adequate resources for children with special needs in school and can provide free school meals to those on a low income or provide a special diet for children whose conditions dictate this.

The **government** through the Department of Health sets national guidelines and targets for child health promotion.

The **media** may have both a positive and a negative role in child health promotion. Local newspapers, radio and television are useful tools in promoting new immunisation campaigns but at the same time vaccine safety issues may be overexaggerated by the media with disastrous effects.

Clinic set-up

There are a number of requirements for the set-up of an appropriate child health promotion clinic, and these are outlined in Boxes 20.10 and 20.11.

Personal child health record (Red Book)

The Personal Child Health Record (PCHR or Red Book) should be regarded as the main health record for pre-school children in the UK (Fig. 20.3). Many countries have similar child health record books with local emphasis. Ideally it should be given to

---

Box 20.10
Facilities needed in buildings of a primary care practice

Waiting room:
- Child-friendly layout
- Pram/buggy park available
- Well heated
- Privacy for breast feeding
- Children's toilet

Examination room:
- Private
- Child friendly
- Well heated

Box 20.11
Equipment required in the waiting and examinations rooms of a primary care practice

Waiting room:
- Age-appropriate toys
- Health promotion literature
- Changing mat
- Electronic scales
- Rollameter measuring mat or similar
- Lassoo tape measure
- Growth centile charts
- Safety measures e.g. plug covers, protect against sharp corners

Examination room:
- Changing mat
- Age-appropriate toys
- Equipment for developmental assessment
- Ophthalmoscope
- Lassoo tape measure
- Growth centile charts
- Safety measures as above

Child health surveillance and promotion

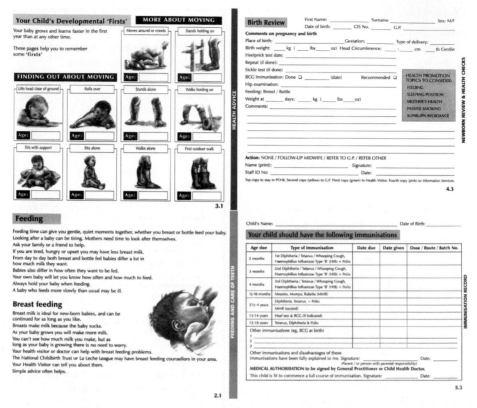

Fig. 20.3 Examples of pages from the Parent Held Child Health Record. (Reproduced with permission from RCPCH)

parents antenatally by either the health visitor or the midwife, in order that parents are able to read through it before the birth of their child. If this is not possible the Red Book should be given as soon as possible after birth.

The Red Book typically contains:

• Feeding and weaning advice.
• Health promotion topics, e.g. accident prevention, dental advice, management of common illnesses.
• Record of health checks carried out.
• Advice regarding developmental milestones.
• Immunisation record and advice.
• 1990 growth centile charts.

The Personal Child Health Record should be seen as a two-way sharing of information between parents and health professionals with empowerment of both, particularly parents. Parents should be made aware that some pieces of information from the Red Book, for example results of developmental checks, are entered onto the child health computer system. This information is treated with the strictest confidence but may then be available to other professionals working with the child or the local health authority. Parents have the right under the Data Protection Act to see the information held about their child on the computer or in written records.

The Personal Child Health Record also offers an opportunity for providing an explanation to parents as to the nature and pitfalls of screening tests in general, in order to minimise misconceptions about screening tests and hopefully reduce litigation from missed cases. New guidelines suggest the Red Book should:

• Be given prior to birth by health visitor or midwife.

Box 20.12
Examples of items that are included in the essential core data set

NHS number	6-week check
NHS number of mother	8-month check
Date of birth	2-year review
Sex	Primary school entry review
Postcode	Secondary school entry review
GP practice code	Secondary school 16+ review
Ethnic group	Significant conditions
Mother's educational status	Disability status at 2 years
Birth order	Disability status at 5 years
Birthweight	Immunisation status
Place of birth	Status on Child Protection Register
Gestational age	Care status
Breastfeeding status	Stage of Educational Code of Practice
Admission to neonatal intensive care	Accidents
Neonatal screening — PKU result	A&E attendance
Neonatal screening — hypothyroidism result	Hospital admission
Neonatal screening — sickle cell result	Hospital outpatient attendance
Neonatal screening hearing	Date of death
Neonatal examination	Cause of death

- Be standard across the UK.
- Contain space for parents to make notes.
- Ideally run from birth to 18 years.
- Be cross referenced to the Health Education Authority* book 'Birth to five'.

Essential core data set

Data collection now forms an important part of the child health promotion process with information coming from parent-held record returns, primary care and community child health computer systems (Box 20.12).

The formulation of a core data set for child health has the following advantages (Blair 2000):

* Note that the Health Education Authority became the Health Development Agency (HDA) in April 2000.

- Allows the assessment of the health needs of a population.
- Data is collected in a standardised way such that it may be compared nationally.
- Allows evaluation of screening programmes.
- Facilitates the development of outcome measures.
- Supports clinical audit and research.

The Child Health Informatics Consortium has proposed a key set of indicators for monitoring child health services and the identification of health needs in the child population. This has resulted in the development of the proposed essential core data set (Child Health Informatics Consortium 2000). The current core set will evolve as requirements change. Information about this can be accessed on the website *http://www.chiconsortium.org.uk*.

THE CHILD HEALTH PROMOTION PROGRAMME

The Child Health Promotion (CHP) programme has been under intensive review using evidence-based criteria and is undergoing many changes, particularly in the way the school health system is utilised.

It is generally agreed that any child health package should include both universal and targetted care. The universal package should include:

- Antenatal care and screening processes.
- Information, advice and support.
- Agreed and recommended programmes of screening and immunisation.
- Health promotion for all children (pre-school and school aged).
- Access to school health service.

Targetted care involves programmes to support individuals and communities with specialised needs. These groups might include traveller families, those in homeless accommodation, asylum seekers and deprived areas. Children 'looked after' and those placed for adoption form a special group. Other groups that are also identified as having special requirements are those with parental mental health needs (Box 20.13), children with disability or child protection needs. Many of these services are statutory, particularly for child protection and special educational needs. A number of programmes are in place to provide this type of targetted service (Box 20.14).

The interrelationship of all these services and child and adolescent mental health services is complex, and ideally the child should have access to any of these services via a 'one-stop shop'. The complexities of a seamless service to provide this are profound and better working arrangements or partnerships need to be forged to optimise accessibility.

The recommended child health promotion programme

Each child health promotion consultation should take the following form:

- Review of records and immunisation status.

Box 20.13

Example of high-risk group and reasons for targetted intervention: maternal depression

- Non-psychotic-postnatal depression in around 10%
- Depressive symptoms in up to 40% of mothers in low-income deprived populations
- Impaired mother–infant interaction
- Boys affected more than girls
- Lower cognitive scores at 18 months
- Poorer concentration
- More behaviour problems, e.g. sleeping, eating, temper tantrums
- Insecure attachments
- Suggestion that difficulties may persist when depression has resolved

Murray et al 1996

Box 20.14

Programmes in place to target care at individuals and communities with specialised needs

- Sure Start and related parental support programmes
- Voluntary sector groups both local and national
- Specific medical, nursing, therapeutic educational and social services
- Child protection services

- Examination/developmental assessment/screening procedure.
- Health promotion.
- Listening/counselling.

Preschool
Screening programme

This should be dictated by an evidence base and by the criteria above. Screening programmes may differ between different populations and countries depending on numerous factors, including prevalence (e.g. haemoglobinopathy screening).

Immunisation programme
The Department of Health prescribes the current programme (see Chapter 21).

Health promotion
Health promotional activities in the pre-school period should include:

- Nutrition — information about breast feeding and support for breastfeeding mothers. The WHO's Baby Friendly Initiatives may provide support for this. Information should also been provided on vitamin K policy, formula feeding, weaning, vitamins and iron (screening for iron deficiency is not recommended), dental care, failure to thrive and obesity.
- Reducing the risk of sudden infant death syndrome (SIDS), through recommended programmes such as 'Back to Sleep'.
- Identification of maternal depression.
- Reducing the risk of abuse and neglect through community awareness and supporting families at risk, e.g. domestic violence.
- Accident prevention — this occurs at a community and individual level. Many would argue that individual support particularly at times of stress can reduce the incidence of accidents.
- Behavioural and emotional development — general information about normal child development and how to recognise problems will help most parents. Information about where to access further information will benefit families not involved in programmes such as Sure Start.

School-aged child
Screening of school-aged children has been dramatically reduced but it is important that an opportunity exists to ensure that all children have had access to pre-school care including immunisations.

There has been a consistent move away from routine medical examination in school. The community paediatrician's role has changed from this routine screening role to a secondary or tertiary role with referrals from school nurses where concerns

> **Box 20.15**
> ## Definition of special needs
>
> A child has special needs if he has significantly greater difficulties with learning than the majority of children of the same age

arise. Importantly each school has a named nurse and doctor; however, their roles and functions have changed.

Twenty per cent of the population have special needs (Box 20.15) at some point in their school career and with the social policies of inclusion extending to the education system, the numbers of these children within mainstream education is likely to increase. Currently only 1.8% of children are educated within the special school system and this figure is dropping.

The roles of the school health system will involve supporting these children identified as having special needs and in the screening and health promotional activities as recommended.

In recent years Woodroffe et al (1993) have demonstrated that the epidemiology of disability within school-aged children has changed from an illness model to the larger proportion of disability involving emotional and behavioural disorders.

Risk behaviours for future disease include smoking, alcohol misuse, drug taking, lack of physical activity, unhealthy eating, unsafe sex. Social factors implicated in future disease include poverty, unemployment, single parenthood. Therefore targeting specific programmes to groups at high risk makes sense in terms of long-term health. This may take place in the form of:

- Class-based education, e.g. sex education.
- Accident prevention programmes, e.g. cycle helmet use.
- Mental health initiatives.
- Clinic-based activity, e.g. drop-in clinics.
- Health promoting schools.

The Health Promoting School Programme has grown out of the World Health Organization's

Health for All initiative and adopted by the UK in 1993 as part of the Health of the Nation strategy. This involves the general philosophy of the school and includes school ethos, health-related policies, physical environment, curriculum, support systems, role models and links (Health Education Authority 1999). The effectiveness of this initiative is being evaluated by WHO (Health Development Agency 2001, WHO 2001).

Examples of current programmes

Sex education (see Chapter 8)

School sex education is likely to be seen as the most sensitive of topics within health education and it has a special position with regard to legal requirements.

Legal position

All schools must have an up-to-date sex education policy which is available to parents. Sex education for pupils provided with primary education is discretionary. The Department of Health recommends that programmes in primary school should ensure that children know about puberty and how a baby is born. Every pupil receiving secondary education must receive sex education, including education about the acquired immune deficiency syndrome (AIDS), human immunodeficiency virus (HIV) and other sexually transmitted diseases. The programme should also include education about relationship, esteem and safe sex. However, parents have the right to ask for their children to be wholly or partly excluded from sex education (except where it is taught as part of the science National Curriculum). Governing bodies are required to maintain a separate written statement of their policy for the provision of sex education and make copies available for inspection by parents at all reasonable times.

Further guidance on sex education is contained in the Department for Education and Employment (DfEE) Circular 0116/20 (2000). This circular outlines the position and the responsibilities of governors, school head teachers and the local education authority (LEA). A number of LEAs have produced guidelines on health and/or sex education in schools. Members of the school medical service should be familiar with any relevant LEA policies.

Planning and organisation

While the legal requirements of school sex education give it a unique status, approaches to its planning, organisation and teaching have much in common with any other area of health education.

Pupils with moderate learning difficulties may have special needs in relation to the way in which sex education is given, but the content should be very similar to that offered to any child. For a comprehensive sex education programme for older pupils with learning difficulties, Craft and members of the Nottinghamshire Sex Education for Students with Severe Learning Difficulties Project (Craft et al 1991) have produced material for students with severe learning difficulties, and this offers a useful overall plan and a wealth of teaching strategies.

Parental involvement

Under the 1986 Education Act parents were given opportunities for a larger say in school sex education. The number of parent governors was increased and any parent can make representations on sex education to the governors and head teacher. In addition, any parent can raise matters concerning the operation of the school at the annual parents' meeting called specifically for that purpose. Parents have the legal right to withdraw their child from school sex education, except where it forms part of the statutory National Curriculum.

All this means that schools have to pay careful attention to the way in which parents are informed about and involved in classroom sex education. One widely used approach is to invite parents to come along to look at the teaching resources the school plans to use. If the school nurse is involved in the programme her presence is important, signalling clearly that a cooperative, team approach has been adopted. Such meetings can serve several purposes — besides putting parents in a position to be able to answer a child's questions in relation to, for example, a teaching video, the occasion can allow group or individual discussion of parental anxieties (for other approaches see Coombes &

Craft 1987, Craft & Cromby 1991). The school nurse or doctor can have a special role to play in offering individual advice to parents.

DARE (Drug Abuse Resistance Education)

DARE is part of an international family, currently operating in 50 countries around the world. The established DARE curriculum's are taught in schools around the world. In the UK each year, over 400 schools and 20 000 youngsters receive the programme. The curriculum involves education and peer support, usually under supervision of local officers, often the police.

The aim of the programme is to ensure that children are able to deal with issues relating to drugs and violence that they will inevitably face during their lives. The life skills based programme encourages young people to achieve their best in life (DARE 2001).

A number of other initiatives and programmes exist and can be referred to for:

- Skin cancer:
  http://www.doh.gov.uk/sunknowhow/ index.htm
  http://www.sunsmart.com.au/
- Accident prevention:
  http://www.patient.co.uk/health.htm#acc
  (Child Accident Prevention Trust)

Core programme

Antenatal screening and health promotion

Initially contact is via primary care, and health promotion around folic acid supplementation, alcohol consumption, cigarette smoking and a healthy diet during pregnancy should ideally take place when a couple is planning a pregnancy. Conditions routinely screened for antenatally are:

- neural tube defect
- Down's syndrome
- infectious disease, e.g. rubella, hepatitis B.

These are performed by the GP and midwifery services.

Part of the Core programme for Child Health also takes place prior to birth. The objective of this early visit is to ensure the parent is familiar with the health visitor service, ensure access to breast feeding support, and to identify those that may need extra support, for example those with learning disability or mental health problems. This may be done by health visitor or midwifery services.

Newborn

The midwife should perform a general inspection immediately after birth with the more formal examination to be performed within 48–72 hours (Box 20.16). At this time there is the opportunity to review issues identified antenatally and to discuss immunisations, vitamin K and feeding issues. The midwife will usually visit the family on several occasions in the first 10 days to review progress and support breast feeding.

Neonatal screening

At 7 days blood spots for screening are collected by midwives on the Guthrie screening card. This Guthrie (heel prick) test currently screens for:

- congenital hypothyroidism
- phenylketonuria
- cystic fibrosis (now recommended to become universal)
- haemoglobinopathy (in some geographical areas).

Universal hearing screening should also take place at this time by trained professionals (see below). This is currently (2001) being piloted in 20 centres with others offering neonatal screening to those at high risk.

Vigilance is required by primary health care providers in the first weeks of life to identify problems that present after the first 48 hours, for example congenital cardiac defects and feeding problems. If required there should be prompt access to paediatric services as many of these conditions can deteriorate rapidly.

New birth review

A new birth review by the health visitor is also recommended primarily for pragmatic reasons. At this visit the health visitor reviews parental concerns and the newborn's progress, explains the

---

Box 20.16
Newborn review: this should be carried out within 48 hours after birth

Review	**Examination**	**Health promotion**
Pregnancy complications	Tone	Breast feeding
Birth complications	Dysmorphic features	Sleeping position
Risk factors for hearing loss	Jaundice	Vitamin K
Risk factors for DDH	Red reflexes/cataracts	Car safety
Passage of meconium	Palate	Dangers of shaking
Feeding	Heart and pulses	Need for BCG, hepatitis B vaccine
	Organomegaly	Passive smoking
	Genitalia	
	Hernias	
	Hips	
	Spine	
	Weight	
	Head circumference	

---

child health surveillance and immunisation programmes, and plans further visits as required.

6–8-week review

The 6–8-week review is generally performed by the GP (Box 20.17). The aim is to identify important conditions that have not been previously detected, for example cataracts, congenital dislocation of the hip, undescended testes. All babies should be reviewed *by 8 weeks* of age. There is some concern that if the examination is brought forward to 4–6 weeks as some have suggested to identify congenital dislocation of the hips and cataracts earlier, then uptake rates for the 8-week immunisation will fall.

2-, 3- and 4-month review

The primary care team performs these at the time of the primary immunisations. Weight should also be followed at this time. There is also the potential to identify other difficulties such as postnatal depression.

8-month, 2-year, 3–4-year reviews

These are an opportunity to review all children, but the formal screening that took place in the 1996 programme is no longer is required. In general there are two aims; one to ensure that the parents have no concerns, the baby is growing normally, in good health and development and behaviour are normal for age. The second is to provide an opportunity to complete the PCHR for the core dataset. The approach is flexible. In those that are known to have any disability that might require extra services, i.e. special educational needs, review may be needed; in those whose records do not reveal recent information this acts as a reminder to the team for the child to be reviewed. Preschool booster immunisation by primary care team is also carried out at this stage.

4–5 years

Orthoptists perform vision screening to identify refractive errors and amblyopia. At this stage there is a review of the records to determine via the GP whether the child is healthy, whether there is long-

---

Box 20.17
6–8-week review

Review	**Examination**	**Health promotion**
Feeding	As newborn check	Immunisation
Weight gain	Weight	Recognition of illness
Visual behaviour	Length	Feeding and weaning advice
Socialisation	Head circumference	Accident prevention
Hearing concerns		Maternal health (postnatal depression)
Risk factors for DDH		
Other parental concern		

---

term illness or disability and whether there is any information needed by school. This can be done by the primary care team, usually the health visitor, by reviewing records and seeing child if necessary. Information should be passed on to the school nurse with parental permission. PCHR forms should also be completed for core dataset.

School entry

The school nurse or technician to performs height and weight measurement. Currently a hearing testing also occurs at this stage but the evidence to support this as a screening procedure is variable and this is under review.

11 years

Vision testing for myopia occurs at this stage but the value of this is currently also being debated.

Specific areas: sensory impairment and hip dysplasia

Hearing impairment (see Chapter 34)

Hearing impairment in childhood may be either conductive or sensorineural in nature or a mixture of both types. Conductive loss is by far the most commonly occurring, usually secondary to otitis media with effusion. It is thought that up to 50% of children suffer from otitis media with effusion at some time in their lives with the peak incidence being in the first 2 years.

Sensorineural hearing impairment is much less frequent, approximately 1.1 per 1000 births. It is congenital (or acquired for example after meningitis) and may be either unilateral or bilateral. There is now good evidence to show that children with congenital hearing impairment who are diagnosed before 6 months of age have improved language development with the possibility of improved educational attainment, compared to children whose hearing impairment is diagnosed later in infancy or childhood (Yoshingaga-Itano et al 1998).

Risk factors for sensorineural hearing impairment are:

- Family history of permanent hearing impairment in childhood.
- Admission to a neonatal intensive care unit for greater than 48 hours.
- Administration of ototoxic drugs.
- Congenital cranio facial abnormalities.
- Congenital infection.
- Meningitis.

Hearing testing in the first year
(see Chapter 34)

Despite widespread awareness of the above risk factors, selective screening of high-risk groups in the neonatal period only identifies approximately 50% of babies born with permanent congenital hearing impairment. A further small proportion of children will be detected by the infant distraction hearing test, although this test has a poor specificity and sensitivity for detecting congenital hearing impairment.

The above factors have led to the preparation for and introduction of universal neonatal hearing screening in several countries in Europe and the USA.

The screen is a two-stage process. Initial screening is performed using otoacoustic emissions (OAE), whereby low-intensity sounds emitted from the hair cells of the cochlea in response to a click, are picked up by a microphone on a probe placed in the ear. The screening threshold should be 45–50 dB.

Babies who fail this stage of the test should then have automated auditory brainstem response (AABR) testing, whereby electrical response to auditory stimuli is recorded on scalp electrodes. The sensitivity and specificity of both these methods are high. For OAE sensitivity is 100% and specificity is 82–87%. For AABR sensitivity is 89% and specificity 82–87% (Report of Children's Subgroup of the National Screening Committee June 2000).

Further research is required, looking at issues of parental anxiety arising from screening failures.

Evidence from the Wessex Study in the UK and from several studies in the USA show that universal neonatal screening is achievable with coverage rates of 90–95% of births (Wessex Universal Hearing Screening Trial Group 1998). Implementation of a programme for the detection of bilateral congenital hearing impairment commenced in the UK in 2000 in centres with adequate audiological facilities, with a view to this becoming a nationwide programme with the phasing out of the infant distraction test. A set of 'Family Friendly Hearing Service' standards have been produced for centres starting a screening programme (Hall & Davis 2000). Universal neonatal screening also compares very favourably with the infant distraction test on economic grounds. The cost per case detected for universal neonatal hearing screening is approximately £20000 compared with up to £84000 for distraction testing.

For areas where universal neonatal screening is not yet feasible the infant distraction hearing test is the standard assessment tool. As outlined above, distraction testing is a relatively costly procedure and quality is dependent on the person who performs the test. It has a high failure rate, usually due to intercurrent upper respiratory infection, and a sensitivity as low as 20%.

It is important to remember that parents are often the best screeners of their children and parental anxieties should always be taken seriously. Most parents find additional information about hearing loss, for example 'Can your baby hear you?', to be useful. (See Fig. 34.8; McCormick 2000)

Hearing screening in school-age children (ref to OME)

Most cases of hearing impairment are identified before school entry. However there may be a small number of children whose impairment has not yet been diagnosed because either their hearing loss is progressive and was not present at birth or because they have not had access to preventative health services due to poor social circumstances. In addition some children will have otitis media with effusion severe enough to cause significant disability.

Screening for hearing impairment at school entry using pure tone audiometry is recommended as a screening procedure although case definition is not always clear cut. No further routine hearing screens are recommended for school-age children.

Vision screening
Vision screening in the newborn period

Visual examination in the newborn period is primarily to exclude the presence of cataracts. This is a treatable condition occurring in 2–3 per 10000 births in the UK. Other abnormalities such as colobomata should also be looked for.

A separate screening programme for retinopathy of prematurity exists for at-risk babies.

Vision screening in the pre-school period

There has been much debate about the necessity of vision screening in the pre-school period. The main concerns are around the detection and prevention of amblyopia usually occurring as a result of a squint or refractive error which leads to poor vision in one eye and impaired stereoscopic vision. Many ophthalmologists and orthoptists argue that amblyopia should be diagnosed and treated by 3½ years of age to prevent permanent visual impairment. However screening for visual acuity in each eye of children in this age group has many problems associated with it and needs to be carried out by a professional with expertise in this field, that is an orthoptist. The present recommendation for the UK is that all children should be reviewed by an orthoptist before school entry at 4–5 years of age via school eye clinics (Report of the Children's Subgroup of the National Screening Committee 2000).

It is recommended that professionals other than orthoptists do not test pre-school children's vision in the community but that they should have a low threshold for referral of parents' concerns even when no abnormality is seen.

Vision screening after school entry

Screening in this age group is primarily for refractive errors. Myopia occurs in approximately 15% of 15 year olds. Current guidelines suggest that this should not be regarded as a screening test and there is debate (related to the lack of evidence) about the value of routine vision testing at ages 11 and 14. Vision screening will be retained however at 11 and 14 until better evidence is available. The majority of children in this age group will be seen by local optometrists for vision testing.

Colour vision defects

Colour vision defects affect approximately 8% of boys and 0.4% of girls. The Ishihara plates are the standard assessment tool. Although common, this test has little educational significance but may affect career choice (e.g. armed forces). There is little rationale therefore for routine testing of colour vision in schools. Alternatively information could be made available to teenagers regarding colour vision defects and career choices and the colour vision testing be carried out by optometrists.

Screening for developmental dysplasia of the hip

The term developmental dysplasia of the hip (DDH) incorporates congenital dislocation of the hip (CDH) and other developmental hip abnormalities. It occurs in 1.2 per 1000 births. If established

CDH is left untreated it results in a limp and pain and osteoarthritis in later life. It is generally accepted that early diagnosis and treatment reduces the need for surgical intervention and minimises long-term disability.

Screening for hip problems in the first 2 months

Screening for DDH begins in the first week of life. Risk factors for DDH are:

- breech birth
- family history of hip problems as a child
- first-born females
- babies with postural foot deformities.

Hip screening is a two stage process:

1. All babies should have a clinical examination by an experienced clinician in the first week of life using the Ortolani and Barlow test and by checking for leg-length discrepancy and major skin crease asymmetry (Figs 20.4, 20.5).
2. Ultrasound examination. Those with abnormal physical signs, i.e. hip instability, limited abduction in flexion, leg-length discrepancy or asymmetry of major creases, e.g. inguinal or buttock, should be referred for ultrasound examination. In addition babies born by breech or those with a positive family history should also be scanned.

The identical screening process should be carried out for all babies at 6 weeks of age. Some centres also recommend an additional hip examination at 10–14 days of age. There is insufficient evidence at present to recommend universal ultrasound screening.

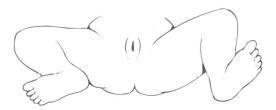

Fig. 20.4 Limited abduction of left hip due to DDH. (Adapted from Department of Health and Social Security 1986 Guidelines: 'Screening for the Detection of Congenital Dislocation of the Hip')

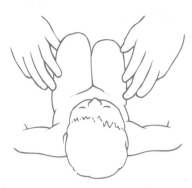

Fig. 20.5 Shortening of the right femur due to DDH. Adapted from 1986 Department of Health and Social Security Guidelines: 'Screening for the detection of Congenital Dislocation of the Hip')

Screening for hip problems after 2 months of age

There is much less evidence to suggest that routine screening for hip dislocation after 6–8 weeks of age is a worthwhile procedure and this is not now recommended as part of the Child Health Promotion Programme (www.health-for-all-children.co.uk). However a further hip check is still recommended by some orthopaedic surgeons and paediatricians at 3–5 months of age in order to detect those who present late. Nevertheless parents' concerns about their children's hips or their child's gait should always be taken seriously and clinical examination performed where there are concerns. In children much older than 6–8 weeks it is not possible to perform the Ortolani and Barlow tests; instead the hips should be examined for limited abduction in flexion, leg-length discrepancy and skin crease anomalies. Abnormalities of gait should also be observed in the walking child.

For the child less than 5 months of age ultrasound is the examination of choice for suspected DDH. In children over 5 months of age X-rays should be performed. These children should be referred to appropriate orthopaedic surgeons experienced in dealing with CDH. For details of treatment options for DDH the reader should refer to orthopaedic texts.

REFERENCES

Begg N T, Gill O N, White J M 1989 COVER (Cover of Vaccination Evaluated Rapidly): description of the England & Wales scheme. Public Health; 103:81–89

Blair M E 2000 Taking a population perspective on child health. Archives of Disease in Childhood 83:7–9

Butler J 1989 Child health surveillance in primary care. HMSO, London

Child Health Informatics Consortium 2000 Monitoring the Health of the Nation's Children. Child Health Informatics Consortium and Royal College of Paediatrics and Child Health, London. Online. Available: http://www.chiconsortium.org.uk March 2001

Coombes G, Craft A 1989 Special health: a professional development programme in health education for teachers of pupils with mild or moderate learning difficulties. Health Education Authority, London

Craft A, Cromby J 1991 Parental involvement in the sex education of students with severe learning difficulties: a handbook. Department of Mental Handicap, Nottingham University Medical School

Craft A and members of the Nottinghamshire Sex education for Students with Severe Learning Difficulties Project 1991 Living your life: a sex education and personal development programme for students with severe learning difficulties. LDA, Cambridge

DARE 2001 Drug awareness and resistance programme UK. Online. Available: http://www.dare.uk.com Jan 2001

Department for Education and Employment 2000 Sex and relationship guidance for DfEE circular 0116/2000. The Stationery Office, London. Online. Available: http://www.dfee.gov.uk/sreguidance/sexeducation.pdf 2000

Department of Health 1999 Saving lives: our healthier nation. The Stationery Office, London. Online. Available: http://www.ohn.gov.uk/ohn/ohn.htm Feb 2001

Department of Health 2000 NHS Immunisation statistics, England: 1999–2000. Government Statistical Service Bulletin 2000/26. The Stationery Office, London

Department of Health 2001 Immunisation statistics. Online. Available: http://www.doh.gov.uk/public/sb0026.htm Feb 2001

Department of Health and Social Security Guidelines 1986 Screening for the detection of congenital dislocation of the hip. Department of Health, London

Hall D M B 1996 Health for all children, 3rd edn. Oxford University Press, Oxford

Hall D, Davis A 2000 Neonatal screening for hearing impairment [commentary]. Archives Disease in Childhood 83:382–383

Health Development Agency UK 2001 Online. Available: http://www.hea.org.uk Jan 2001

Health Education Authority 1999 Whole school — healthy school: an essential guide to the health promoting school. Health Education Authority and NFER, London

Largo R H, Graf S, Kundu S, Hunziker U, Molinari L 1990 Predicting developmental outcome at school age from infant tests of normal, at risk and retarded infants. Developmental Medicine and Child Neurology 32:30–45

McCormick B 2000 Can your baby hear you? In: Personal child health record 2000, 3.5. Harlow Printing, Newcastle

Murray L, Fiori-Cowley A, Hooper R, Cooper P J 1996 The impact of postnatal depression and associated adversity on early mother–infant interactions and later infant outcome. Child Development 67:2512–2526

Report of Children's Subgroup of the National Screening Committee 2000

Stewart Brown S 1998 New approaches to school health. In: Spencer N (ed) Progress in community child health, vol 2. Churchill Livingstone, Edinburgh, pp 137–157

Sure Start UK 2001 Online. Available: http://www.surestart.gov.uk Feb 2001

Tudor Hart J 1971 The inverse care law. Lancet i (7696):405–412

Webb E 1998 Children and the inverse care law. British Medical Journal 316:1588–1591

Wessex Universal Neonatal Hearing Screening Trial Group 1998 Controlled trial of universal neonatal screening for early identification of permanent childhood hearing impairment. Lancet 352:1957–1964

WHO 2001 Healthy Schools. Online. Available: http://www.who.int/hpr/gshi/docs/index.html Jan 2001

Woodroffe C, Glickman M, Barker M, Power C 1993 Children, teenagers and health: the key data. Open University Press, Buckingham

Yoshinaga-Itano C, Sedey A L, Coulter D K, Mehl A L 1998 Language of early- and later-identified children with hearing loss. Pediatrics 102:1161–1171

FURTHER READING

British Paediatric Association 1995 Health needs of school aged children. Report of a joint working party. British Paediatric Association, London

Hall D M B 1996 Health for all children, 3rd edn. Oxford University Press, Oxford

Health Education Authority 1999 Whole school — Healthy School: an essential guide to the health promoting school. Health Education Authority and NFER, London

Murray L, Cooper P J 1997 Post partum depression and child development. The Guilford Press, New York

http://www.doh.gov.uk/dhhome.htm Department of Health Feb 2001

http://www.doh.gov.uk/sunknowhow/index.htm Sun Know How programme UK

http://www.health-for-all-children.co.uk

http://www.nacro.org.uk NACRO-Crime reduction UK Jan 2001

http://www.patient.co.uk/health.htm#acc (health promotion including accident prevention and antismoking programmes)

http://www.standards.dfee.gov.uk/eaz Education Action Zones Feb 2001

http://www.sunsmart.com.au/ Anti Cancer Council of Victoria Australia, Sunsmart programme

http://www.who.int World Health Organisation Homepage Feb 2001

http://www.wiredforhealth.gov.uk Health information for teachers Feb 2001 (includes information on a wide range of issues and programmes for healthy schools)

http://www.youth-justice-board.gov.uk Youth Justice Board UK Jan 2001

21 | Avoiding infection

Infectious diseases are still a major cause of illness throughout the world. Although falling mortality rates in the western world have taken much of the fear out of childhood infections, it would be a mistake to become complacent. If one assumes that most of those designated on the death certificate as 'respiratory' are due to infections, then in the UK infections are still the commonest cause of death in the post-neonatal period. In much of the rest of the world, pneumonia, gastroenteritis, tuberculosis, HIV/AIDS, measles, malaria, tetanus, pertussis and diphtheria, remain collectively by far the most important causes of death in all age groups. According to the latest WHO health report of 10.4 million deaths in children under 5 years, 99% occurred in developing countries and over 70% were due to these major infections. Poor nutrition and lack of adequate facilities for treatment are important contributory factors. In the UK, infections are the commonest reason for children of all ages being seen by family doctors and admitted to hospital. Children under the age of 9 years can be expected to have between six and eight upper respiratory tract infections each year, of which three will be accompanied by constitutional symptoms.

Recording infection

Information on infection is often inaccurate or incomplete. There is a great variation in response between individual hosts and microbes — a case of measles in a malnourished African infant is often fatal whereas a healthy 7 year old in the UK may not be taken to the doctor. Many clinical syndromes such as gastroenteritis or sore throat may be caused by a wide range of microbes which cannot be distinguished without microbiological investigation,

so the cause of death will be uncertain. Statutory notification of some infectious diseases, although a legal responsibility of doctors, is also an incomplete exercise (Box 21.1). Until recently a fee of only 25 pence was payable for each notification; this has now been increased to £3. Nevertheless the data do provide a basis for local and national monitoring. The Communicable Disease Report from the PHLS Communicable Disease Surveillance Centre at Colindale provides regular information on notified diseases and laboratory reports of infections.

The Royal College of General Practitioners produces weekly data from a sample of practices (sentinel practices); this is particularly helpful for following infections like chickenpox and influenza, which are not notifiable and would not otherwise be recorded. A recent survey of acute infectious diarrhoea in England and Wales coordinated by the PHLS showed the magnitude of underreporting of gastroenteritis. There are probably 1600 times as many cases of viral infection due to rotavirus and small round structured viruses, seven times as many campylobacter and three times the number of salmonella as are reported to the public health officials.

Susceptibility to infection

Children are not all equally susceptible to infection. Although a certain element of infection is 'bad luck', such as being in the wrong place at the wrong time, other factors can be identified.

Genetic

Certain children are more prone to infection; for instance, children with Down's syndrome are more likely to develop upper respiratory tract infections.

Avoiding infection

Box 21.1
Notifiable infectious diseases, UK

Acute encephalitis	Measles	Scarlet fever
Acute poliomyelitis	Meningitis	Smallpox
Anthrax	Meningococcal septicaemia	Tetanus
Cholera	Mumps	Tuberculosis
Diphtheria	Ophthalmia neonatorum	Typhoid fever
Dysentery	Paratyphoid fever	Typhus fever
Food poisoning	Plague	Viral haemorrhagic fever
Leprosy	Rabies	Viral hepatitis
Leptospirosis	Rubella	Whooping cough
Malaria	Relapsing fever	Yellow fever

Mild and severe immune deficiency states run in families and complement deficiency increases significantly the risk of meningococcal disease.

Environmental

Environmental factors are important with respect to the spread of infection. Good housing, clean water supplies and adequate sanitation contribute enormously to the control of infectious diseases such as tuberculosis. Likewise, poor environment as well as poverty is a factor in the continual high prevalence of infectious disease in inner city areas.

Age

The number and severity of certain infectious diseases relates strongly to age. Thus the prevalence and mortality rate of whooping cough and bronchiolitis are greatest in very young infant whilst tuberculosis peaks in the pre-school child and in adolescence and early adult life. Mumps and chickenpox tend to be more severe in adults.

Geographical

Many infectious diseases are largely confined to certain climates or areas of the world depending on conditions for the survival of insect vectors. However rapid international travel means that children can travel far in the incubation period.

Background nutrition

This is of paramount importance in the susceptibility and reaction to infection. In the malnourished the death rate due to measles or whooping cough can be very high. Children with any chronic illness are also more susceptible to infection, particularly if the disorder or its treatment results in undernutrition or immunosuppression.

Immunisation history

Immunisation history is of obvious importance in determining individual susceptibility to particular infections. Also when new infections are introduced into communities where there is little herd immunity the effects can be devasting. This was seen most markedly when measles and influenza were introduced by explorers and colonists into many island communities.

DIAGNOSIS AND MANAGEMENT OF INFECTION

This account cannot give complete details of all childhood infections and the reader is referred to textbooks and reviews in paediatrics, microbiology or infectious diseases. However, all health professionals working in domiciliary practice see children with infection so frequently that they need to be

Prevention
Government policy
Family doctor
Health visitor
Child Health Service

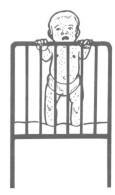

Control
Public health physician
Environmental Health Officer
Microbiologists
Public health laboratories
Isolation units

Fig. 21.1 Agencies involved in controlling infection

aware of the basic principles (Fig. 21.1). It is seldom necessary to take specimens for microbiological investigation from most cases of respiratory infection, and as the majority of these are due to viruses with no specific therapy the benefit to the patient is minimal. When there is suspicion of an outbreak or when illness is severe or there are unusual features, it is advisable to take samples from some of the subjects with the acute illness. One important lesson is to instruct when and how to investigate. Too frequently laboratories receive rock hard stools from an episode of diarrhea and throat swabs when the child is in convalescence. There are sound epidemiological grounds for asking for laboratory help in the investigation of an outbreak or incident and in determining vaccine efficacy (see below).

However convinced a clinician may be about the diagnosis of a rash, without laboratory confirmation the issue is in doubt. Following the widespread coverage with MMR vaccine the Public Health Laboratory Service (PHLS) have been trying to get saliva antibody tests from children notified as measles, mumps or rubella. In almost every case in

the past 3 years the clinical diagnosis has not been confirmed.

The crucial questions in the management of an acute infection are: Does the child need admitting to hospital? Does the child require antibiotic or other specific therapy? Is there a need for isolation from others or exclusion from school?

Prevention of infection

Improving the conditions under which people live, for example by ensuring clean water supplies, adequate sanitation, adequate food supplies and storage, has a major impact on the incidence, spread and severity of infectious disease. Improved housing with adequate light, heating, ventilation and abolition of overcrowding had been shown to reduce the incidence and spread of infection.

The main means to prevent infection that are under the control of a health professional are shown in Box 21.2.

The traditional way to deal with many infectious diseases was isolation. Many children used to be incarcerated for many weeks in remote hospitals with chickenpox or scarlet fever — diseases now considered sufficiently trivial that children are now sometimes sent back to school contagious. There is no doubt that strict exclusion from other susceptible people is an excellent way to stop the spread of an infectious disease; however, it is seldom justified because of the resources involved and the harm it can do to those isolated. Nevertheless, there are good reasons to use isolation wards for those with open pulmonary tuberculosis before effective antimicrobials have been given. Excluding children from school is a more contentious issue and the decision needs to be taken on the basis of local and national guidelines, often with consultation with the consultant in communicable disease control (CCDC) or other public health doctor. In March 1999 the Departments of Health (DH) and Education and Employment issued guidance with the PHLS on infection control in schools and nurseries. Table 21.1 shows a shortened version of the poster which is available for all schools from the DH.

Day nurseries and infant schools have a constant dilemma when they have an outbreak of diarrhoea

---

Box 21.2
Main means of preventing infection

Isolation/exclusion

Treat cases/contacts

Personal hygiene

Health education

Immunisation

---

which can spread rapidly in this environment. Sometimes it is necessary to close the nursery for a short time, especially if the cause has been shown to be *Escherichia coli* O157. When the outbreak is self-limiting and due to a virus, a balance needs to be struck between what can be achieved to prevent further cases against the disruption to the lives of the children and their families and carers. Outbreaks of diarrhoea should be reported to the CCDC and environmental health officer who will investigate the cause.

Table 21.1
Exclusion from schools or nurseries

Condition	Days away (after well)	Comments
Chickenpox	5 from onset	Care with pregnant staff, special care with immunosuppressed
Hand, foot and mouth	None	Mild disease due to enterovirus
Impetigo	Until lesions dry	Earlier if lesions covered
Measles	5 from onset	Check vaccination status
Rubella	5 from onset	Care with pregnant staff
Scabies	Until treated	Outbreaks may occur
Slapped cheek	None	Also known as fifth disease (parvovirus)
Diarrhoea/vomiting	1–2	Unless due to *E. coli* O157
Tuberculosis	Ask chest physician	Most children not infectious
Whooping cough	5 after treatment started	Cough persists for weeks
Glandular fever	None	
Head lice	None	Treat family actively if live lice
Hepatitis A	5 after onset	Only necessary if poor hygiene
Meningococcal	Ask CCDC	Contacts may attend school
Mumps	5 after onset	Check immunity of contacts
Hepatitis B/C	None	Clean spillages, use universal precautions
HIV	None	Not infectious by social contact

There is good evidence that antibiotics have revolutionised childhood infections. Scarlatina was a feared disease before penicillin was available and although meningitis is still a cause for anxiety the outcome is usually good, provided therapy is started quickly. One major benefit of antibiotics which is not always mentioned is in preventing further cases by quickly making cases non-infectious. For example it is thought that usually 24 hours of penicillin is sufficient to remove streptococci from the throat of a child with tonsillitis. Another advantage which is used in disease control is chemoprophylaxis. Close contacts of a case who may be harbouring the causative organism are given a short course of antibiotic to eradicate carriage. The best example is in the management of a case of meningococcal disease in which rifampicin or sometimes ciprofloxacin is given to the household, family and other close, prolonged contacts.

The effect of good personal hygiene on reducing infection cannot be overemphasied. Children need to be taught the importance of handwashing, food hygiene and the importance of a clean environment. Some of this may be done by formal education as part of the national curriculum, but there is a need for this subject to be included in parenting classes for young mothers.

Health education has an important part to play in the prevention of all infectious diseases where it can lead to change in behaviour. It is particularly important in the prevention of the blood-borne virus infections such as hepatitis B and HIV. Their association with unprotected sexual activity and drug abuse are important messages for adolescents to understand, but education needs to start earlier.

Immunisation has had a dramatic effect on diseases like smallpox, diphtheria and poliomyelitis; smallpox has been eradicated, indigenous polio is now not seen in many countries, and diphtheria is rare.

IMMUNISATION

The aim of immunisation is to produce a specific resistance to infection without significant risks to the recipient. The first recorded evidence of immunisation was in the sixth century BC in China when dried smallpox crusts were introduced intranasally. Modern developments in immunisations start with Jenner who in 1796 demonstrated experimentally the protective effect of cowpox extracts against smallpox.

Theoretical basis of immunity

During an infection there is both a humoral antibody (B-cell) and T-cell lymphocyte response. Antibodies which are produced specifically against the organism may neutralise toxin (antitoxin) or enhance phagocytosis (opsonic activity). T cells previously exposed to the specific antigen are mobilised to release chemical mediators (cytokines) which invoke a local inflammatory reaction and recruit other cells to attack the organism and cells harbouring the microbe (Fig. 21.2). This specific memory is usually lifelong but wanes with age, especially if the host has not encountered the infection for some time. Few vaccines can produce a degree of immunity to match a natural infection but the aim is to achieve high efficacy with few of the unpleasant features of the natural illness. This may be achieved by using attenuated live organisms (e.g. oral polio, BCG), killed organisms or parts of them (e.g. pertussis, typhoid) or modified toxins (e.g. diphtheria, tetanus). With live vaccines the very low grade infection from a single dose provides a prolonged stimulus and long-lasting protection. With killed vaccines or toxins the stimulus is usually short lived and more than one dose needs to be given to give satisfactory immunity unless the person has been in contact with the organism before, in which case the antigen administered boosts the response. Some vaccines are made by recombinant DNA technology which has the potential to produce a very wide range of vaccines. Temporary protection can be given by passive immunisation. Immunoglobulins must be given by injection, usually intramuscular. They may be given as pooled human immunoglobulin which contains a mixture of antibodies against the infections prevalent in blood donors, or specific immunoglobulin prepared from blood taken from patients in the convalescent phase after a natural infection or immunisation. Varicella/zoster (VZ) immunoglobulin is used to give temporary protection to immunosuppressed people after contact with chickenpox (Box 21.3).

Avoiding infection

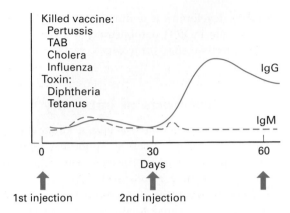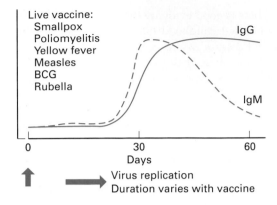

Fig. 21.2 Reaction to vaccination

Effectiveness and safety

In the laboratory the likely potency of vaccine may be assessed by a variety of methods such as calculating the number of live organisms in a dose, assay of antibody responses to the vaccine in healthy volunteers, inoculation of animals before exposure to the infection and measuring the degree of protection.

The effectiveness of a vaccine within a population can be calculated by the following equation:

$$\frac{\text{Attack rate in unvaccinated} - \text{Attack rate in vaccinated}}{\text{Attack rate in unvaccinated}} \times 100\%$$

Assessment of safety may be made by injection of large doses of the vaccine into laboratory animals and observing for signs of toxicity. In the field, trials

of a new vaccine will estimate safety prior to general use. Continuing monitoring of safety is provided in the UK by the mechanism of reporting reactions to the Committee on Safety of Medicines by the 'Yellow Card' system. There have been many concerns in the UK about the safety of many vaccines which have been in widespread use for many years such as MMR. This has been fuelled by single reports of an alleged association with autism and inflammatory bowel disease (mainly Crohn's). These findings have been widely publicised by the media, of which certain sections are interested in magnifying any scare story. This is in the interests of the antivaccine lobby who are always keen to further hype the issue, making the job of the immunisation teams extremely difficult. Coverage for MMR has fallen by nearly 10% in some districts; this in turn leaves a sufficiently large number of susceptibiles to restart measles outbreaks.

Uptake and herd immunity

It is not always necessary to immunise all individuals in order to protect the total population. In some situations, such as tetanus, all individuals need immunisation because of the ubiquitous nature of the organism. For other infections such as polio where infection spreads directly from one person to another and where the vaccine is highly effective, high levels of uptake in the community (probably >90%) will prevent epidemics. This provides protection for unimmunised people and has lead to eradication of the organism in many parts of the world. Immunising one group of people can protect another group; ensuring a high immunisation rate in older children against whooping cough reduces the spread of infection and thereby protects very young children prior to completing their immunisations. The issue of vaccine uptake and herd immunity is important in the design of immunisation programmes.

Immunisation programmes (Table 21.2, Box 21.4)

The decision to initiate an immunisation programme, the practical aspects of running such a programme and its final success depend on many factors.

Political

At national level it is politicians rather than doctors who decide on national programmes and campaigns. They are influenced by health professionals but also by individual pressure groups and publicity. Politicians may also affect people's responses to immunisation programmes, either by support, by casting doubts about effectiveness or by emphasising side-effects. Whether they are well or ill informed, what they say is reported in the press. Moral issues will also influence political discussion; introduction of a vaccine against HIV will probably be surrounded by controversy.

Economic

The budget available for health care is not unlimited; one group of priorities must be weighed

Table 21.2 Recommended immunisation programme for UK: 2000		
Age	**Immunisation**	**Comments**
Neonatal	BCG Hep B	High-risk infants
2 months	Diphtheria Pertussis Tetanus Hib MenC Oral polio	1st dose primary course DPT/Hib
3 months	DTP/Hib Polio MenC	2nd dose primary course
4 months	DTP/Hib Polio MenC	3rd dose primary course
12–18 months	Measles mumps rubella (MMR)	
4–5 years	Diphtheria Tetanus aP (acellular pertussis) MMR Polio	Booster
10–14 years	BCG	If Heaf negative
14–16 years	Tetanus/diphtheria (Td) Polio	Booster (school leaving)

Avoiding infection

Box 21.4
Administration of immunisation programmes

I   Register of susceptible individuals

II   Explanation of benefits — appropriate literature

III Obtain consent

IV   Call and recall system (manual or computer)

V   Immunisation clinic:
     appropriate clerical, medical, nursing staff arrangements for transport and storage of vaccines maintaining the cold chain

VI   Record of attendance and uptake of vaccine

VII System for identifying and immunising non-attenders (opportunistic or home immunisation)

VIII Monitoring uptake

---

against another. In the case of an immunisation programme the benefit of prevention must be weighed against the cost of treatment. For instance, the falling rate of tuberculosis in the UK led to consideration of giving up routine immunisation of adolescents, because it might no longer be economically justified; some health authorities in the UK have already decided this and stopped. Against the cost of developing a vaccine programme must be weighed the lives saved and the long-term burden of disability. There are also many indirect costs such as the hours lost by parents from work and consequent fall in productivity caused by the disease, and less tangible factors such as the distress and unhappiness caused by the disease. Common respiratory infections must be very expensive in these terms.

Medical

The medical task is to assess the trends in morbidity and mortality from the infection, and assess the possible influence of an immunisation programme. Once a programme is established, it is not easy to determine what would be the effects of its withdrawal. Where there are no recorded cases of polio

in the country, the presence of a reservoir of infection abroad, combined with the severity of the disorder, would seem to warrant continued whole-population immunisation. Obviously the benefits of the programme for the whole community must outweigh the risks to individuals.

Public motivation

This may range from complete antipathy to demands for instant immunisation depending on fear when there has been adverse publicity to panic when an outbreak occurs. When the dire consequences of the illness are not within the experience of the community the general public is usually apathetic. All these reactions have been seen over a short period of time with pertussis immunisation and MMR. Changes in public attitude can only occur with positive messages through health education and by presentation of accurate, clear information to public figures and journalists. At the individual level this is best achieved by health visitors and primary care teams counselling parents and carers.

Immunisation schedules

Schedules should not be rigidly interpreted. Primary courses can be commenced at any age after the first 2 months, though clearly the immunisation schedule is designed to protect against infectious disease as early as possible and at the ages of particular risk. The intervals between immunisations are the minimum required. If the intervals between immunisations in the primary course are longer than those indicated in the schedule, there is no need to restart the course but simply to carry on where the course was interrupted. This is most important with tetanus where the risk of reaction increases the greater the number of doses given.

Immunisation uptake (Table 21.3)

Factors affecting uptake can be divided into two broad categories: professional knowledge/attitudes and administrative problems. Many studies on uptake rates have identified inappropriate advice received by parents of unimmunised children. This may be inaccurate or outdated advice on

Table 21.3
Uptake of immunisations by 2 yeras of age[†] (%), England and Wales

Year of birth	Measles	Diphtheria	Pertussis	Tetanus	Polio
1970	34	80	79	81	79
1975	48	77	39	77	77
1980	58	84	53	84	84
1985	76	87	73	87	87
1990/91*	84	89	78	89	89
1995/96	92	96	94	96	96
1999/00	88	95	94	95	95

[†] Primary course completed by 2 years of age
* Recording changed from calendar to financial year
Data for England and Wales from PHLS

contraindications (e.g. asthma as a contraindication for measles vaccine). Inconsistent advice from different professionals is quoted by parents as a reason for avoiding immunisation. There have been many changes in the field of immunisation in recent years and this will continue with new vaccines becoming available and more information on vaccines currently in use. All those involved (administrative and clerical as well as medical and nursing staff) need to have regular updating of their knowledge.

Another consistent feature of studies is that the uptake rate recorded is inaccurate; children who are recorded as having no immunisations or partial immunisation are found to have been fully immunised. This may be because they have been immunised in another clinic, or have moved into the area following immunisation. Other problems arise when reliable recall systems are not in place and appointments are not sent. Children may have failed to attend appointments, but when they turn up to a clinic for some other reason the information on missed immunisations is not available so the opportunity is missed. Good information systems, either manual or on computer, should identify children due immunisations. This information can then be used to encourage attendance at appointments or to tag the records (perhaps of the whole family)

in order to enable immunisations to be given opportunistically. Some groups may need a specially tailored system, such as immunisations taken into the home.

POLIO

There are three distinct strains of poliovirus — types 1, 2 and 3 — and there is very little antigenic overlap. Type 1 has been associated with most of the major epidemics and shows the greatest propensity to cause paralytic forms of the disease (Fig. 21.3).

Vaccine

Oral poliovirus vaccine (OPV, Sabin vaccine) is a mixture of live attenuated strains of virus types 1, 2 and 3, grown in monkey kidney or human cell cultures. This vaccine is given orally on three separate occasions during which both local gut and systemic immunity are established. This may not occur to all three strains on the first occasion, so the dose needs to be repeated in order to ensure immunity to all three types. Inactivated poliovirus vaccine (IPV, Salk vaccine) is an inactivated vaccine containing all three strains given by injection. Although it

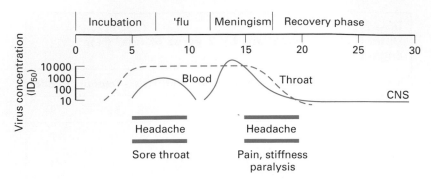

Fig. 21.3 The clinical course of poliomyelitis

provides satisfactory systemic immunity and will prevent poliomyelitis, it does not provide local gut immunity so that the virus can still replicate in the gut and be transmitted to other people.

Effectiveness

Introduction of the two forms of vaccine has led to the elimination of indigenous polio in the UK and much of the world. Unfortunately the WHO target of eradication by the year 2000 has not been achieved. It is hoped that it may be eliminated worldwide soon depending on delivering vaccine to areas of conflict. With OPV the attenuated virus is excreted in the faeces and may spread to other members of the family and immunise them as well. However there is a slightly increased risk of reversion to a more virulent form in this situation, so it is preferable to immunise susceptible carers at the same time as the child. In the UK and the USA the benefits of herd immunity from OPV, the acceptability of an oral vaccine and the lower cost are thought to outweigh the rare complication of vaccine-associated polio. Other countries such as Holland, which had an outbreak of polio in a group opposed to immunisation, use IPV.

Contraindications

Polio vaccine is contraindicated in pregnancy unless at very high risk of the disease. It is also contraindicated in those with immune deficiency; close contacts of those with immune deficiency should receive IPV because of the risk of transmission of the vaccine virus.

Reactions

Vaccine-associated polio resulting from reversion to a more virulent form in the gut occurs in recipients of OPV in about one case per 4–5 million doses and in unvaccinated contacts in one case per 2–3 million doses given.

MEASLES

The maculopapular rash of measles appears first behind the ears and on the face, spreading downwards to form a confluent blotchy appearance. Encephalitis affects 1 in 5000 children who have measles; 15% of these will die and 25% will suffer cerebral damage. In developing countries in the presence of malnutrition, the severity and mortality of measles is much higher than in the UK (Fig. 21.4). Uncomplicated measles requires only rest, fluids and an antipyretic. Prophylactic antibiotics are not indicated. Where secondary infection does occur this is likely to be a mixed bacterial infection and a broad-spectrum antibiotic is required. The patient is infectious from a few days before to 7 days after the onset of the rash (Fig. 21.5). In parts of the world where measles has been nearly eradicated it is important to attempt to confirm every suspicious case: this can be easily done by using a swab taken from the gingival margins and asking the laboratory to look for specific antibody. IgM is

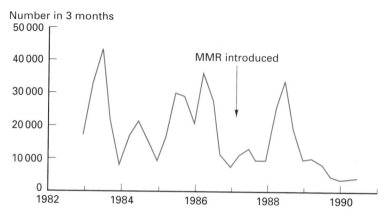

Fig. 21.4 Measles notification

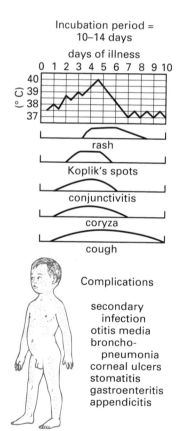

Fig. 21.5 Measles

indicative of recent infection whereas IgG is suggestive of past infection or immunisation.

The vaccine is a freeze-dried aqueous suspension of live attenuated measles virus grown on fibroblast tissue derived from chick embryos. It is given at 12–18 months of age with mumps and rubella as MMR. It can be given safely even if the child is thought to have had measles infection or during the incubation period. If the vaccine is given from 12 to 15 months of age, it is highly effective. Under the age of 1 year a significant number of children fail to seroconvert because of the presence of maternal antibodies to measles. A new vaccine (Edmonston–Zagreb) that is effective in the presence of maternal antibodies is being investigated in developing countries because of the high risk of measles illness under 1 year in these countries. Studies of single-dose MMR immunisation have shown that the efficacy of the measles component is around 95% and that when the uptake is below this figure the numbers of susceptibles in the population is sufficient to allow small outbreaks to occur. The duration of immunity of the early vaccines has also been questioned. These factors lead in the UK to the mass school measles immunisation as MR in 1994 and the introduction of a two-dose schedule of MMR in 1997.

Contraindications

Live vaccines should not be given to children with any immune deficiency. Severe allergy (anaphylaxis) to eggs may be a contraindication because the vaccine is grown on chick embryo fibroblasts and there is a theoretical risk of cross-reaction. However, immunisation can probably be safely carried out under controlled conditions and many children labelled as egg allergic are not hypersensitive to the minute quantities of egg protein found in a dose of vaccine. The vaccine may contain small amounts of various antibiotics (e.g. polymyxin, neomycin) and should not be given to those known to be allergic to the particular antibiotic in the vaccine being used. If there is a history of febrile convulsions it is important to stress antipyretic measures.

Reactions

It is not uncommon for children to develop a fever, mild irritability and even a measles-like rash 5–10 days after the immunisation. There is a small increase in the risk of a convulsion during this time (1 per 1000). Because it is a live vaccine, any of the complications of measles illness can occur but much less frequently than with the illness.

Passive immunisation

Suppression of measles can be achieved by giving human normal immunoglobulin and may be indicated at certain times in exposed unimmunised children with chronic heart, lung or malignant disease.

MUMPS

The distinguishing feature of mumps is the enlargement of the salivary glands, usually the parotids. There may be a prodromal illness with fever, headache and malaise lasting for 1–2 days. Aseptic meningitis occurs in about 1 in a 1000 cases though a mild form may be much commoner. Sensorineural deafness, usually unilateral, can occur and mumps is thought to be the commonest cause of this. Orchitis affects 20% of postpubertal males but sterility following this is rare.

Vaccine

This is a live attenuated virus grown on chick embryo tissue culture. It is given combined with measles and rubella at 12–15 months.

Effectiveness

It is a highly effective vaccine. Since its introduction in the UK in 1988, there has been a noticeable fall in mumps illness.

Contraindications

As for measles.

Reactions

A mild mumps illness occurs in about 1 in 100 children about 3 weeks after immunisation. Aseptic meningitis may occur but is less frequent than in the mumps illness. It is usually mild and then recovery is complete.

RUBELLA

Rubella is a mild illness with a maculopapular rash, occipital lymphadenopathy and mild fever. Arthritis and thrombocytopenia are occasional complications. Its importance lies in the effects on the fetus, which can be devastating. Diagnosis of congenital rubella relies on a combination of the clinical features, antibody levels and isolation of virus from the urine. High specific IgM titres indicate a recent infection, whereas IgG levels may be positive indefinitely. The easiest way to detect antibody is to use a gingival swab rather than a serum sample. Virus may remain in the urine for up to a year following congenital infection (Fig. 21.6).

Vaccine

This is a freeze-dried suspension of live attenuated virus grown in human tissue culture cells. It is given in combination with measles and mumps vaccines at the age of 12–18 months. Until 1988 in the UK, rubella immunisation was only given to girls at the age of 11–13 years and to susceptible

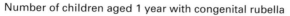

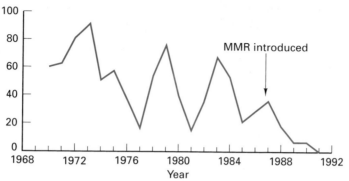

Fig. 21.6 Rubella notifications

women in the childbearing years. This policy helped to reduce the incidence of congenital rubella, but there were still affected children born each year and terminations for possibly affected pregnancies. By 1987/88 the national immunisation rate for 14 year olds was 86%, leaving a potential 14% susceptible girls with epidemics of rubella still occurring regularly. In 1988 the policy was changed to universal immunisation at 12–18 months, in order to try and get herd immunity and stop epidemics. The programme to immunise older girls continued until it was realised that susceptible men were keeping the infection circulating in the community. The mass school campaign with MR and the introduction of the second MMR as a pre-school booster has lead to the virtual eradication of rubella in the UK. The vaccine is still offered to all seronegative women of childbearing age.

Effectiveness

After the initial rise antibody levels slowly decrease over the subsequent years, though after 30 years there is still normally adequate immunity serologically. Reinfection is known to occur and though this does not normally affect the fetus, it may do so.

Contraindications

Rubella vaccine, as with all live virus vaccines, is contraindicated in pregnancy, though there have been no cases of congenital rubella caused by the current vaccines. Accidental immunisation during pregnancy would therefore not be a reason for termination of pregnancy. Other contraindications for live virus vaccines also apply. If children have arthritis, it would be wise to discuss immunisation timing because of the association of rubella illness with exacerbations of arthritis.

Reactions

Mild fever, rash and lymphadenopathy are sometimes seen. Arthritis and arthropathy are rare complications.

WHOOPING COUGH

Pertussis is caused by the bacterium *Bordetella pertussis*, though milder infection may occur with *Bordetella parapertussis* or *Bordetella bronchiseptica*. A variety of viruses can also cause illnesses with symptoms indistinguishable from whooping cough. Adults and older children who have been inadequately immunised may get a milder form of the disease yet remain infectious to susceptible infants. The incubation period is 7–14 days, the catarrhal phase 7–14 days, the paroxysmal phase 4–6 weeks and recovery usually takes a further 2–6 weeks. Complications include bronchopneumonia, convulsions, apnoeic spells, and rarely now bronchiectasis. The child may remain infectious from 7 days after exposure to 21 days after the onset of the paroxysmal cough.

Avoiding infection

Erythromycin given in the catarrhal phase may attenuate the infection and it may be helpful if given as prophylaxis amongst infant contacts. Otherwise treatment depends on good nursing care, which may include oxygen, suction and tube feeding, plus the treatment of complications as they occur.

Prognosis is much worst under 1 year of age. There was a case fatality rate of 0.9–2.6/1000 notifications in the 1977–79 epidemic, and large numbers required hospital admission. There may be an association between whooping cough and cot death as epidemiologically there are parallels.

Vaccine

This is made from killed organisms of several serotypes of *B. pertussis*. It is usually combined with diphtheria and tetanus vaccines in 3 doses in early infancy, but can be given at any age. It is particularly important that children with chronic illness or handicap are immunised since they will be at particular risk from whooping cough. Acellular vaccines are widely used in some countries and are available in the UK for those known to or likely to have a reaction to the whole cell type. These comprise the main antigens without the rest of the bacterium which greatly reduces its reactogenicity without loss of efficacy.

Effectiveness

Protection rates of 85–90% are achieved after standard primary immunisation, and if the illness does affect immunised children it is likely to be milder.

Reactions

Mild reactions are common. These may consist of local pain and swelling or a transient irritability, pyrexia and fretfulness. These are not contraindications to further doses. A few children have a more severe reaction with marked swelling and redness of the injection site or severe systemic upset. These children are likely to recover fully. Immunisation against pertussis became the subject of considerable controversy in the UK in the mid 1970s, following well-publicised reports of neurological damage associated with reactions to pertussis vaccine. The frequency of such reactions and the incidence of pertussis illness and its complications were not known and varying figures were reported. The debate led to a considerable fall in the immunisation rate to about 31% in 1978, and as a consequence there was a bad epidemic of whooping cough in 1978–80. It became clear that pertussis was still a serious disease especially in infants. There were at least 30 deaths in England and Wales. At the same time the efficacy of the vaccine was clearly demonstrated. Attempts have been made to establish the risk of encephalopathy following pertussis vaccine, but there is no conclusive evidence of a link. On the other hand the risks from pertussis illness are well established. Immunisation rates have risen again in recent years with a resulting fall in the number of cases.

Contraindications

A severe reaction to a preceding dose is a contraindication to any vaccine. In the case of combined DTP (diphtheria, tetanus, pertussis) vaccine there is a problem because the cause of the reaction could be any of the components. All three may be omitted, or pertussis alone may be omitted with the rationale that this is the most frequently associated with reactions. The definition of a severe reaction is set out in the Department of Health Guidelines which are regularly updated. There are other children with 'problem histories' such as an increased risk of fits or those thought at higher risk of having a neurological problem. In these children care must be taken to counsel the parents fully on the small risk of fits following the immunisation but also on the increased risk of severe problems of the illness. This is best done by referral to a community paediatrician with a specialist interest in immunisation. Most of these children can be safely immunised.

TUBERCULOSIS

Although tuberculosis has declined in incidence it remains an important disorder in the UK and has been declared a worldwide emergency by WHO because of the sharp increase in the number of deaths, especially in people with concomitant HIV infection. The incidence has remained static, with an increase in the number of notifications in families originating in the Indian subcontinent. In other countries there has been an increase in incidence attributed to the rise in HIV-infected people who are particularly susceptible to reactivation of tuberculosis. Although deaths from tuberculosis are unusual in children compared with the toll exacted in adult life, most infants are highly susceptible to infection. In developing countries tuberculosis kills about 100 000 children compared with approximately 3 million adults per year. Many of those infections would have been acquired in childhood by droplet spread from an adult with open TB who may be an elderly relative or, in the case of school children, someone with undetected illness working in the school (Fig. 21.7).

Presentation of tuberculosis

The diagnosis of tuberculosis cannot be made simply and quickly on clinical grounds alone and requires laboratory confirmation which may take several weeks as the causative bacilli are slow growing.

Asymptomatic subjects
Tuberculosis may be identified by tuberculin testing of contacts of known cases or by routine testing

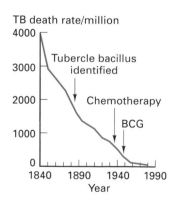

TB death rate/million

Fig. 21.7 Immunity is more than vaccination

prior to BCG immunisation. It may also be identified in people having routine chest X-rays. If a contact has a negative tuberculin test it should be repeated after a further 6 weeks because the test may not become positive in the incubation period of the illness.

Sensitivity reactions
Where primary infection has been recent, children may present with a febrile illness, erythema nodosum or phlyctenular conjunctivitis.

Vague ill health
Children may present with primary tuberculosis with very ill-defined symptoms. There may be complaints of lethargy, tiredness and poor growth. There may be signs of lymphoreticular involvement with an enlarged liver, spleen or neck glands.

Pulmonary tuberculosis
This may present as: (a) pleural effusion, the onset often being with acute breathlessness, pyrexia, pain and occasional cough; (b) caseation and cavitation — the child has a cough, is constitutionally ill and has a pyrexia. If the cavity connects with the main bronchi, the bacilli may be found in the sputum or gastric washings; (c) bronchial obstruction due to lymph node enlargement. This may cause either collapse or hyperinflation of part of the lung.

Miliary tuberculosis
This may be acute or slow in onset. The features are again non-specific with fever, weight loss and lethargy. The liver and spleen may be enlarged and choroidal tubercles may be seen as yellow dots along the retinal vessels.

Tuberculous meningitis
This is another feature of haematogenous spread and presents with a slowly developing lymphocytic meningitis, low CSF sugar and bacilli visible on microscopy of the fluid.

Bone or joint involvement
This may present as synovitis or osteitis which may affect the spine, hip, knee, ankle, elbow, wrist, hands or feet.

Avoiding infection

Primary tonsillar infection with cervical lymphadenopathy

This was more commonly seen as the main presentation of bovine TB from unpasteurised milk.

Abdominal tuberculosis

This is a very rare presentation in the UK and is also caused by bovine infection. It presents with abdominal pain and the findings of a doughy mass in the abdomen. If the mesenteric lymph nodes rupture, tuberculous peritonitis will occur.

Diagnosis

The diagnosis is not always easy. The various forms of tuberculin testing to be described below probably provide for the easiest approach. Radiology is sensitive but non-specific, sputum microscopy is specific but very insensitive, and culture is slow.

Mantoux test

An intradermal injection of 10 units of PPD (purified protein derivative) in 0.1 ml is made on the flexor surface of the left forearm. If active tuberculosis is suspected a lower starting dose of 1 unit should be used. The date, time, position of injection and strength of solution are recorded and the site inspected 72 hours later. An area of induration of 5 mm or more is regarded as a positive reaction. This is not generally used for routine screening because of the difficulty of intradermal injections.

Heaf test

A Heaf gun with disposable single-use heads is now recommended. If you are using a re-usable Heaf gun, it should be set to penetrate the skin at 2 mm, except for children under 2 years when it is set at 1 mm. The gun is sterilised by immersion in spirit and followed by flaming. The gun must be allowed to cool before use. Purified protein derivative equivalent to 100 000 units per ml is applied to the skin over the flexor surface of the left forearm. Sites containing superficial veins should be avoided. The result is read between 3 and 10 days later. Grade I and Grade II reactions may be due to avian tuberculosis or to previous BCG. All children

with Grade III or IV reactions require X-ray and follow-up. False-negative results may be obtained from using materials that have deteriorated, if the material is injected too deeply, if the test is read too soon or too late, or if the test was performed near an inflamed site so that rapid removal of tuberculin occurred. False-positive results may be obtained by a burn from the Heaf gun, local infection or a rupture of small blood vessels.

BCG (Bacillus Calmette–Guerin)

BCG is a freeze-dried live attenuated bovine strain of *Mycobacterium tuberculosis*. It is derived from the original bacillus grown by Calmette and Guerin in 1921. The vaccine is given by intradermal injection of 0.1 ml into the skin at the insertion of the deltoid (Fig. 21.8). Most Health Authorities in the UK offer BCG to all tuberculin-negative children at 10–14 years. It is also given to newborn babies of high-risk families (certain ethnic groups and families with a close relative with recent tuberculosis) in a dose of 0.05 ml. Immunisation results in a small papule appearing 7–10 days later which enlarges over a

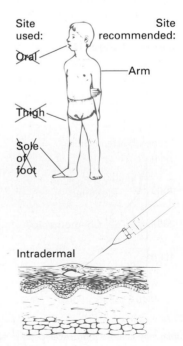

Fig. 21.8 BCG

few weeks and often ulcerates. Peeling occurs in 6–8 weeks with a residual scar forming. Mantoux conversion occurs within 3–4 weeks of immunisation, though this is slower in babies. Abnormal reactions to BCG are often the result of a faulty injection technique. If given subcutaneously there is much more likely to be abscess formation. Ulcers that are slow to heal are best treated with simple dressing and with antimicrobial ointment if secondary infection has occurred. If an abscess or lymphadenopathy develops, this may need treatment with antituberculous drugs and should be dealt with at a specialist clinic.

Effectiveness

Immunity seems long lasting with an 80% protective effect after 15 years. TB can occur after BCG immunisation but it effectively prevents the development of miliary TB or TB meningitis.

The decision to immunise against tuberculosis at birth depends upon the incidence of the disease. The World Health Organization recommended that where 5% of children aged 10–14 years have been infected, BCG should be given at birth. Where the rate is more than 2% but less than 5% it should be given on school entry, and in places with less than 2% affected BCG should be given at 12–13 years. Where tuberculosis does occur in people who have already received BCG the diagnosis may be delayed.

Chemoprophylaxis

This may be given in several circumstances. If the mother of a newborn baby is infected with active pulmonary tuberculosis the baby may be given isoniazid by mouth and isoniazid-resistant BCG. Secondary chemoprophylaxis is given to those with asymptomatic disease. This will include children with strong tuberculin reactions on routine testing, children who are contacts of patients with tuberculosis whose tuberculin test converts, and any tuberculin reactor under the age of 5 years. Chemoprophylaxis currently recommended is isoniazid for 6 months or isoniazid and rifampicin for 3 months. A local chest physician or consultant in communicable diseases will normally coordinate this.

TETANUS

Tetanus is caused by a Gram-positive anaerobic spore-bearing organism, *Clostridium tetani*, found universally in the soil. The disease is caused by the neurotoxin produced by the organism. After an incubation period of 5–14 days there are progressive intermittent muscle spasms, often triggered by stimuli such as noise or touch. Tetanus is now rare in this country because of immunisation. When the disease occurs it still carries a high mortality.

Vaccine

This is a formol-inactivated toxoid given in conjunction with an adjuvant by intramuscular or deep subcutaneous injection often combined with diphtheria and pertussis vaccines. After a primary course of three injections in infancy and the boosters at school entry and leaving, this may be sufficient for lifelong protection. If a contaminated wound occurs a single booster dose only is required. Too frequent reinforcing doses, as may occur in children who have frequent accidents, are unnecessary and can provoke severe hypersensitivity reactions. Human tetanus immunoglobulin may be given to unimmunised people suffering from major wounds with a high degree of contamination.

DIPHTHERIA

Diphtheria is rare in the developed world and caused by strains of *Corynebacterium diphtheriae*. The infection may be caught from infected individuals or healthy carriers. The incubation period is 2–7 days, after which the toxin causes destruction of the superficial epithelium of the respiratory tract producing obstruction by formation of a membrane. It can also infect the skin in abrasions. This may give rise to protective antibody naturally. The toxin can also produce a myocarditis and lower motor neurone symptoms.

Vaccine

This is a formol-inactivated toxoid adsorbed to an adjuvant. An adult form (more dilute) should be used for children over 10 years, because of the small

Avoiding infection

possibility of the child already being immune to diphtheria and therefore having a severe reaction to the standard dose. In the routine schedule it is given with tetanus (Td) at school leaving.

HAEMOPHILUS INFLUENZAE TYPE B (HIB)

Most strains of *Haemophilus influenzae* found in the respiratory tract are uncapsulated but it is the encapsulated type b (Hib) organism that almost always causes invasive disease. This organism was one of the main causes of meningitis in young children. There is a high morbidity with 10–15% of children developing severe neurological sequelac such as profound deafness, cerebral palsy and epilepsy and the mortality rate is 3–4%. Hib is the predominant organism causing epiglottitis and can cause other invasive diseases.

Vaccine

The polysaccharide capsule of the organism is conjugated with a protein. The vaccine is only effective against type b infection. This vaccine was introduced in the UK in 1992 and is given at 2, 3 and 4 months, at the same time as DPT. Booster doses are not needed. It is a highly effective vaccine with a low incidence of side effects. The introduction and success of this programme in virtually eliminating haemophilus invasive disease within 2 years paved the way for the mass immunisation of the UK population under 18 years with the conjugate meningococcal C vaccine in 1999–2000.

MENINGOCOCCAL DISEASE

Neisseria meningitidis has become the most important bacterial infection in children between the ages of 1 and 5 in the UK, causing as much disability as accidents and more deaths. There has also been a noticeable increase in cases in adolescents and university students especially due to group C. Like the haemophilus, meningococci have a polysaccharide capsule which determines the serotype. Simple polysaccharide vaccines against group A and C have been available for a number of years. These have been suitable for foreign travel but because of

poor efficacy in the young and short duration of immunity (usually about 3 years) they have not been widely used for the prevention of meningococcal disease except in outbreaks. The development of protein conjugate vaccines for group C (called menC) has lead to the possibility of eradicating another cause of meningitis. Unfortunately, group B meningococcal infection is more common than group C in infants and vaccines against this are still in development.

Vaccine

At present menC is only available as a single preparation and is given separately in the opposite arm to the primary immunisations. In time it will be combined with them and given as part of the routine course. Children up to age 18 in the UK have been vaccinated in a single dose 'catch-up' programme. The conjugate proteins used in the vaccines are the same as in Hib. There are very few contraindications and the reporting of adverse events has been low.

HEPATITIS

Hepatitis A is the commonest cause of jaundice in older children and has an incubation period of 15–20 days or sometimes longer. Outbreaks sometimes occur in schools or institutions where the level of hygiene is in question. In children the illness is normally mild. The period of infectivity is from 1–2 weeks before to 1 week after the onset of symptoms. Good hygiene remains the main method of control.

Vaccine: hepatitis A

Passive immunisation with immunoglobulin used to be the main method for family and close contacts and for those travelling in high-risk areas, but the introduction of hepatitis A vaccine has completely changed the approach to prevention. Concerns about the safety of human serum derived products such as immunoglobulin has spurred the use of the genetically engineerred vaccine. Recent studies have also indicated that this vaccine is valuable in the control of outbreaks of hepatitis in closed communities as well as in travellers to endemic areas.

Hepatitis B is transmitted largely by the parenteral or sexual route. This means that it is only likely to be acquired in special circumstances in children, i.e. contamination by blood, blood products or other body fluids. Once the virus is acquired it may cause a fulminating hepatitis, chronic hepatitis or be asymptomatic. Many people who acquire the virus in early life become carriers, unaffected themselves but at risk of transmitting it to others. Children are most likely to become infected with hepatitis B virus by vertical transmission before or during birth from an infected mother. In the past, transfusion or injection of blood products was a source of infection, but many countries including the UK, now test blood products. Close contact with body fluids is another source of infection, as may happen in institutions for children with severe learning difficulties who may bite and scratch. In adolescence sexual intercourse and drug addicts sharing needles need to be considered.

Vaccine: hepatitis B

The current vaccine is surface antigen produced by a recombinant DNA technique. Three doses are given at 0, 1 and 6 months. Serological testing should be carried out following this and if unsatisfactory immunity is demonstrated a further dose should be given. The vaccine is not offered routinely to all people in the UK, but is recommended in certain high-risk groups, such as health workers, emergency workers, infants of infected mothers. All pregnant women should be screened antenatally and if appropriate the infant can be immunised at birth and given specific immunoglobulin. In many countries it is included in the routine immunisation programme and is recommended by WHO. The effect on reduction of liver cancer has been demonstrated in China.

Hepatitis C is more commonly found in the UK than hepatitis B. Most cases are related to drug injecting or other parenteral routes. More cases are asymptomatic and about 70% appear to become long-term carriers. So far the prevalence in children is low except for drug users.

OTHER VACCINES

Influenza vaccine is available and can provide 60–70% protection from the illness, but only for a few months. The components of the vaccine are changed annually to keep up with the shift in virus strains circulating throughout the world. It is recommended for certain high-risk groups, particularly the elderly, but also children at risk with chronic heart or lung disorders and the immunocompromised and severely disabled.

Pneumococcal vaccine is of value in certain high-risk children, particularly those with absence of the spleen. Children with sickle cell disease often have a non-functioning spleen and may be at risk. It is only effective in children over 2 years of age at present until the protein-conjugate vaccine is available.

Varicella/zoster vaccine is licensed in many countries but at present is not available in the UK.

Future developments will include vaccines against rotavirus, RSV and the bacterial causes of diarrhoea.

TRAVEL ABROAD

The most important factors in preventing infection while travelling are those involved with good hygiene, care in what is eaten and drunk, and physical protection against bites. Routine immunisations should be up to date. Depending on the country to be visited, some additional immunisations may be recommended, for example typhoid, yellow fever, hepatitis A. Some countries require certificates of vaccination before allowing entry. Up-to-date advice on this and other recommendations can be obtained from the Department of Health leaflets and website, from local travel clinics or from the London School of Hygiene and Tropical Medicine.

FURTHER READING

Department of Health. Online. Available: http://www.doh.gov.uk
DH Immunisation. Online. Available: http://www.immunisation.org.uk

Avoiding infection

Greenwood D, Slack R, Peutherer J 1997 Medical
microbiology. 15th edn., Churchill Livingstone,
Edinburgh
Health advice to travellers 1995. HMSO, London
Immunisation against infectious disease 1996. HMSO,
London
Long S, Pickering L K, Prober C G 1997 Principles and
practice of paediatric infectious diseases. Churchill
Livingstone, New York

Public Health Laboratory/CDSC. Online. Available:
http://www.phls.nhs.uk
Scottish Centre for Infection. Online. Available:
http://www.scieh.co.uk
US Centers for Disease Control. Online. Available:
http://www.cdc.gov

All of the Websites above have links to other sites
which may provide more detailed information.

22 | **Unintentional injuries**

The World Health Organization (WHO) has defined an accident as:

An unpremeditated event, or sequence of events, that results, or could result in recognisable injury.
(World Health Organization 1957)

Over recent years the term unintentional injury has increasingly been used, as 'accident' implies an element of randomness, unpredictability and therefore a lack of preventability. Epidemiological studies have shown that most 'accidents' are indeed predictable, with identifiable at-risk groups. This chapter will therefore use the term unintentional injury. It is clear, however, that accident is not synonymous with injury. A child can fall down stairs and not be injured, but an accident has still occurred. It is therefore important when we consider how to prevent injuries that both the events leading to the injury and the actual injury are considered.

THE SIZE AND NATURE OF THE PROBLEM OF UNINTENTIONAL INJURIES

Death resulting from injury

Above the age of 1 year, unintentional injuries are the leading cause of death in childhood (Office for National Statistics 1996) (Fig. 22.1). Sixty years ago the mortality rate for injuries was similar to that for diseases such as tuberculosis, whooping cough, measles and pneumonia. The death rate from infectious diseases has fallen sharply since then, whereas the injury mortality rate has fallen much more slowly, at about 6% per year (DiGuiseppi & Roberts 1997). Death from injury has been the major threat

to the life of children in the UK for the last 50 years, and continues to be the greatest challenge to child health today. In 1994, 549 children aged under 15 died from an unintentional injury and a further 65 died from an injury of undetermined intent (Office for National Statistics 1996).

The number of deaths by type of injury is shown in Table 22.1. Under the age of 1 year, inhalation of a foreign body or suffocation causes most deaths. Between 1 and 4 years, death occurs most commonly by fire and flames, usually in house fires, with drowning as the second most frequent cause. In older children, road traffic injuries account for the majority of deaths. The types of fatal road traffic injury vary with age; as children become more exposed to traffic as pedestrians and cyclists, more deaths result from these activities. By school age, pedestrian injuries make up almost two-thirds of the fatalities on the roads (Fig. 22.2). The risk of pedestrian injury is related to exposure to traffic. Children living in families without a car are more likely to walk, spend more time walking and cross more streets on average than children from families with two cars, and are therefore more likely to suffer a pedestrian injury (Roberts et al 1997). Children now walk fewer miles per year than 10 years ago, which may largely account for the reduction in pedestrian deaths over the same period of time, but which may cause concern because of higher levels of inactivity.

Ill health resulting from injury

Deaths represent only the tip of the iceberg of injury-related ill health. They are a major cause of hospital admission, A&E department attendances and attendances in primary care as shown in Fig.

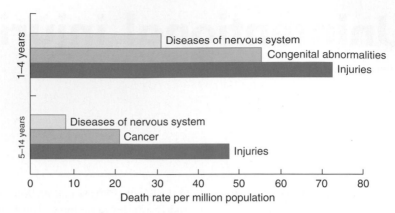

Fig. 22.1 Unintentional injury mortality rate by age: 1994. Source: Office for National Statistics 1996

Table 22.1 **Mechanisms of fatal injuries in children aged 0–14 years: 1994**	
Injury mechanism	**Deaths (no.)**
All injuries	614
Unintentional injuries	549
Non-transport injuries	272
Fire and flames	40
Drowning	37
Suffocation by inhalation or ingestion	33
Mechanical suffocation	27
Falls	22
Poisoning	13
Electrocution	5
Other injuries	95
Transport injuries	277
Pedestrian	140
Vehicle occupant injuries	65
Pedal cyclist injuries	34
Motor cyclist	5
Other transport injuries	33

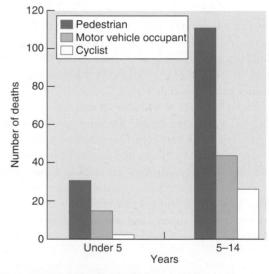

Fig. 22.2 Road traffic deaths by age: 1994. Source: Office for National Statistics 1996

22.3. In addition, many minor injuries occur which are treated at home, as do many 'near misses', where a child does something which could have resulted in an injury, but fortunately no injury occurred, for example a fall which did not result in an injury. A recent study from Nottingham found that over a 2-week period 56% of children aged between 3 and 12 months experienced a near miss and 44% experienced a minor injury which did not require medical attention (Marsh & Kendrick 2000). Overall each year, as a result of injury, 1 in 5 children will attend an A&E department, 1 in 10 to 1 in 20 will attend a GP surgery and between 1 and 2 in 100 will be admitted to hospital. Falls are the most common mechanism of injury at all ages in childhood, but poisonings, foreign bodies and burns and scalds are more common under 5 years, whilst being struck by an object and cutting or piercing are more common over 5 years (Depart-

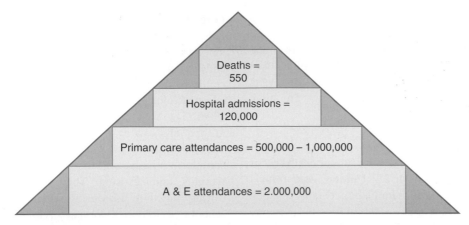

Fig. 22.3 The 'iceberg' of injury-related mortality and morbidity in childhood

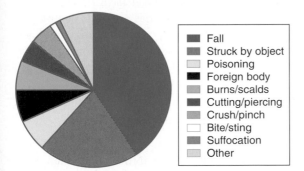

Fig. 22.4 Mechanisms of injury in children aged under 5 years attending the A&E department. Department of Trade and Industry 1998

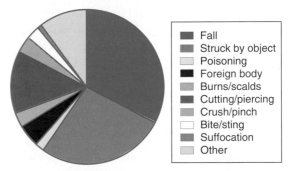

Fig. 22.5 Mechanisms of injury in children aged 5–14 years attending the A&E department. Department of Trade and Industry 1998

ment of Trade and Industry 1998) (Figs 22.4, 22.5). Forty five per cent of children admitted to hospital will have at least a moderately severe injury, whilst one-quarter of admitted children will have a severe injury.

Injury-related ill health does not end with the hospital episode. WHO has estimated that 15% of all disability across all ages is caused by injury (World Health Organisation 1982). Most children who have attended an A&E department leave with some limitation to their activities as a result of their injury. One study found approximately one in three children suffered a short-term disability immediately following the injury, most often limitations in toiletting, dressing, bathing and running. Six months following the injury, 12% of children were still experiencing limitations in running and 8% in walking (Gofin & Adler 1997). Psychological mor-

bidity following injury is also common but research suggests many children suffering an injury receive little or no emotional support from the health service (Heptinstall 1996).

Where and when do injuries happen?

Home injuries

Under the age of five most fatal and non-fatal injuries occur in the home. In 1994, 83 children aged under five and 28 children aged 5–14 years died following an injury at home (Office for National Statistics 1996). More than 550 000 children under five attend an A&E department each year as a result of a home injury (Department of Trade and Industry 1998). These most commonly occur in the living room (19%), the bedroom (9%) and the kitchen

(8%). Six per cent of all non-fatal injuries in children under five involve stairs (Department of Trade and Industry 1998). Home injuries are less common amongst school-age children, but they still account for more than 400 000 A&E attendances each year. Injuries such as falls and poisonings are more common in summer months.

Transport injuries

Over the age of five, most injury and deaths occur on the roads. In 1994, 277 children died from a transport injury (Office for National Statistics 1996). In addition, more than 43 000 children in 1995 were involved in non-fatal road traffic injuries in England and Wales, of which 16% (6983) were classified as being seriously injured (Department of Transport 1996). Road traffic injuries are more common between spring and autumn, in the early morning, late afternoon and evening, corresponding to school journeys and playing after school. Children are most likely to be killed or seriously injured as pedestrians. Injury severity is closely linked to the speed at which a vehicle is travelling; at 40 mph 80% of pedestrians will be killed, at 30 mph 50% will be killed and at 20 mph 20% will be killed. Pedestrian injuries most commonly occur in urban areas on residential streets, close to the child's home, and happen whilst the child is crossing a road. In 1995, 1250 children were killed or seriously injured as pedal cyclists. Most injuries occur when children lose control of the bicycle they are riding. Only about 10% occur in collision with a motor vehicle, but serious injury is much more likely to result from such collisions and also at greater cycle speeds. Cycle helmets are effective in reducing the risk of head injury (Thompson et al 1989). Serious injury and death occurring as a passenger accounted for 1600 casualties in 1995. Seat belts and child restraints are highly effective in reducing injury and death (Towner et al 1996); but there is evidence that older children are less likely to use seat belts; one study found only 60% of children aged 10–13 restrained in cars (Transport Research Laboratory 1992). Other transport injuries occurring on railways and water transport are very uncommon causes of death.

Leisure injuries

Leisure injuries are very common, especially amongst school-age children. More than 170 000 children aged under 5 and more than one million children aged 5–14 years attend A&E following a leisure injury each year (Department of Transport 1996). The vast majority of injuries in both age groups are caused by falls, followed by being struck by an object. The resulting injuries most commonly involve soft tissues, bones, joints, open wounds and bruising. They occur most often during play, but also during sporting activities in school-age children. Sports involving balls, wheels, sticks and winter sports most frequently result in injury. These are most likely to occur on urban roads, sports or recreational facilities and school playgrounds. Sports injuries are most common at the start and end of sporting seasons; drowning and horse riding injuries are most common in the summer.

Injuries are expensive

Childhood injuries are estimated to cost the National Health Service (NHS) more than £200 million per year. This does not include the cost of providing long-term care for severely injured children, or the cost to the child and the family of the suffering and distress and the parental costs of caring for an injured child (Child Accident Prevention Trust 1992). As unintentional injuries disproportionately affect the young, they account for 8.3% of all potential years of life lost under 75 years of age (Department of Health 1993). This represents a huge burden to society in terms of the costs of lost production. The estimated value of preventing road traffic injuries is £784 090 for a fatal injury, £70 910 for a serious injury and £6930 for a slight injury. The cost of lost output is estimated at more than a quarter of a million pounds for each fatal injury. Similar figures have been produced for home injuries; £28 830 for serious injury, £3920 for slight injury treated by the hospital and £120 for slight injury treated by the GP. The total annual cost to the community for childhood injury is estimated to be more than £10 000 million pounds (Roberts et al 1998).

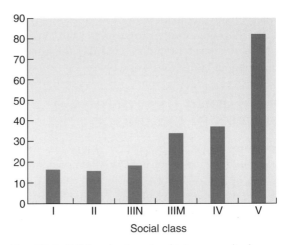

Fig. 22.6 Childhood unintentional injury mortality by social class: 1989–92. From Roberts & Power 1996

Which children are at greatest risk of unintentional injury? (Box 22.1)

The risk of injury is not static over a child's life, but changes as the child develops, as he experiences new and more complex environments and becomes more independent. The mortality rate from road traffic and leisure injuries increases with increasing age, whereas that of home injuries decreases. Injuries, both fatal and non-fatal, are one and a half times more common in boys than girls above the age of 1 year. The gradient across the social classes is steeper for childhood injuries than for any other cause of death in childhood. The standardised mortality ratio for injury and poisoning in children from social classes IV and V is five times that for children in social classes I and II (Roberts & Power 1996) (Fig. 22.6). These children are exposed to more hazards at home, their families possess fewer items of safety equipment and they are exposed to greater risk of injury as pedestrians. Although these families perceive the risks faced by their children, barriers such as low income may reduce their ability to respond to that risk, for example by purchasing safety equipment (Kendrick 1994a). Similarly, families renting accommodation or living in temporary accommodation may have little control over the structure of the environment in which they reside.

Children living in stepfamilies or single-parent families are twice as likely to be admitted to hospital following injury during the first 5 years of life (Wadsworth et al 1983), and the proportion of children experiencing an injury increases as maternal age decreases (Taylor et al 1983). Family stress is associated with childhood poisonings (Sibert 1975, Erikkson et al 1979, Beautrais et al 1981). One study found maternal use of tranquillisers or antidepressants was the single most important predictor of poisoning. Children with sensory deficits are at greater risk of pedestrian injury (Roberts & Norton 1995), children with epilepsy are at an increased risk of drowning injuries and children with a learning disability have a doubling of the injury rate compared to children without a learning disability. Several studies have assessed the contribution of ethnicity to injury risk; all have concluded that factors other than ethnicity, such as social disadvantage are more important in determining injury occurrence (Learmouth 1979, Alwash & McCarthy 1988, Lawson & Edwards 1991). Finally children who suffer an injury are at greater risk of future injury. Children suffering three or more injuries in the first 5 years of life are six times more likely to have three or more injuries in the next 5 years of life (Bijur et al 1988). Children admitted to hospital at least once under the age of 5 are 2.5 times more likely to be admitted during the next 5 years (Bijur et al 1988). A study from Nottingham found children who attend an A&E department are twice as likely to be admitted to hospital than children who have never attended an A&E department following an injury (Kendrick 1993).

PREVENTING UNINTENTIONAL INJURIES IN CHILDHOOD

The importance of preventing injury has been recognised by the choice of unintentional injury as one of the areas for action in the white paper 'Saving Lives: Our Healthier Nation' (The Stationery Office 1999). A national target for reducing injuries has been set.

> **Target:** to reduce the death rates from accidents by at least one-fifth and to reduce the rate of serious injury from accidents by at least one-tenth by 2010

Levels and approaches to injury prevention

There are three levels at which injuries can be prevented:

- primary prevention
- secondary prevention
- tertiary prevention.

Primary prevention aims to prevent the events that cause injuries, for example the use of a stair gate to prevent a fall down stairs, the storage of medicines in a locked cupboard or cycle lanes which separate cyclists from motor vehicles. Secondary prevention aims to prevent or reduce the severity of an injury occurring during the event. Wearing a cycle helmet will not prevent a fall from a bicycle, but will significantly reduce the risk of head and brain injury. Having a smoke detector may not prevent a house fire, but by alerting the occupants to the fire will allow more time for them to escape. Tertiary prevention aims to reduce the consequences of an injury that has already occurred, such as providing appropriate first aid at the scene of an injury.

Within these three levels of prevention three different approaches can be used:

- education
- engineering
- enforcement.

Educational approaches are often conceptualised in terms of trying to achieve behavioural change at the level of the individual parent or child, for example mass media campaigns such as the 'Kill Your Speed' campaign, or the Home Office campaign to increase smoke alarm ownership. Many educational programmes are based on the preventive model of health education. Here information and advice is provided for parents and children, and it is assumed that everybody has an equal opportunity to act on the information. However, barriers prevent or hinder parents from taking action, such as poverty, limited control over rented accommodation, insufficient support with child care, lack of amenities such as safe play areas or inadequate public transport. Providing information without attempting to address these barriers is unlikely to be effective. The empowerment model of health education attempts to increase the control that individuals have over their environment by increasing self-esteem and facilitating the development of the skills required to achieve greater control. Many community development projects use this approach, for example the work in Corkerhill, a deprived housing estate in Glasgow where parent's identified hazards in the environment in which they lived and made suggestions for change to policy-makers (Roberts et al 1995). The third model is the radical model that is aimed at changing society rather than changing the individual, for example lobbying for an improved public transport system to reduce road traffic injuries. Education is also important in bringing about a culture whereby other approaches to injury prevention are accepted. It may be needed to influence policy-makers and the general public prior to legislation, as in the Australian educational campaigns prior to the introduction of cycle helmet legislation. The education of health professionals is also important. Several studies have clearly shown the injury prevention training needs of members of the primary healthcare team are not being met (Kendrick et al 1995, Marsh et al 1995, Morgan & Carter 1996).

The engineering approach to injury prevention involves the design, manufacture and use of safe products and safe environments. The re-design of pen caps to reduce the risk of suffocation if they are inhaled, the design and implementation of area wide traffic calming schemes to reduce the speed and volume of traffic in residential areas and the design and use of safety equipment such as stair gates, fire-guards, child-resistant containers or cupboard locks, are all examples of the engineering approach.

The enforcement approach involves the use of standards, regulations or legislation to enforce safe behaviour, safe products or safe environments. Seat belt legislation is aimed at enforcing safe behaviour, the use of the British Safety Standard on a wide range of products ensures their manufacture to particular specifications and building regulations are aimed at ensuring the safety of the environment, for example by the use of safety glass in newly built homes.

Active versus passive prevention

Active injury prevention is that which requires some action on the part of a parent or child. For example, preventing poisoning by storing medicines in a cupboard too high for the child to reach requires the parent to always put the medicine in the same place. Passive prevention does not require any action on the part of the parent or child, for example fitting a thermostat to the hot water supply in newly built homes would prevent hot water scalds without the parents having to take any action at all. Passive injury prevention measures are often more effective than active measures.

The effectiveness of injury prevention

The effectiveness of the three approaches to injury prevention is outlined below. There is some evidence that combining approaches may be more beneficial than using individual approaches (Towner et al 1996).

Education and parental support

Some educational interventions have been demonstrated to be effective in increasing knowledge,

improving safe behaviour or reducing hazards. Very few have demonstrated reductions in injury frequency or severity (Pless 1993, Towner et al 1996). Many educational interventions have been inadequately evaluated, including interventions using models of health education other then the preventive model. Two systematic reviews have now demonstrated that home visiting programmes providing a range of activities aimed at supporting parents can reduce unintentional injuries in childhood (Roberts et al 1996, Elkan et al 2000) (Table 22.2).

Engineering interventions

Engineering interventions have achieved more success in terms of hazard reduction and reduction in injury frequency than educational interventions (Pless 1993, Towner et al 1996) (Table 22.3).

Enforcement interventions

In several areas legislation, regulations and standards have been found to be extremely effective in reducing unintentional injury mortality and morbidity in childhood (Pless 1993, Towner et al 1996) (Table 22.4).

OPPORTUNITIES FOR INJURY PREVENTION

Working with families (Box 22.2)

Community paediatricians and members of the primary healthcare team have many opportunities for injury prevention as part of their routine work (Kendrick 1994b). The child health surveillance programme provides repeated contacts with children and their parents, at home, in clinics and in surgeries. It also provides contacts at the ages at which childhood injuries are most common, and the ages at which parents have expressed the greatest need for injury prevention (Coombes 1991). It is important that within the child health surveillance programme attention is paid to providing interventions that have been demonstrated to be effective. Providing safety advice will reduce hazards in the home, and providing low-cost safety equipment will help reduce inequalities in health by increasing

Unintentional injuries

Table 22.2
Effective educational and parental support interventions

Intervention	Effect
Home visiting programmes	Reduced unintentional injury rates
GP safety advice and low-cost equipment	Increased safety equipment use and other safety behaviours
Health visitor home visits and safety advice	Reduced home hazards, increased use of safety equipment
Paediatrician safety education	Increased parental safety knowledge, reduction in home hazards, increased smoke alarm use
Community and individual education and free window guards	Reduction in window falls and mortality from window falls
Nurse counselling	Increased safe tap water temperature
Educational campaigns and subsidised cycle helmet schemes	Increased rates of cycle helmet use
Road safety education	Increased knowledge and safer behaviour
Infant car seat/restraint campaigns and loan schemes	Increased correct restraint use
Teaching older children to swim	Reductions in risk of drowning

Table 22.3
Effective engineering interventions

Intervention	Effect
Child-resistant containers for analgesics	Reduction in poisoning from analgesics
Paraffin container distribution scheme	Reduction in paraffin ingestions
Barriers for domestic swimming pools	Reductions in deaths from drowning
Cycle helmets	Reduction in head injury, brain injury and death
Area wide traffic calming schemes	Reduction in pedestrian injuries
Product re-design	Reduced injuries from coffee makers, vacuum cleaners and washing machines

access for those at greatest need (Clamp & Kendrick 1998). Barriers that prevent parents from acting on safety advice need to be examined as part of the child health surveillance programme. Health professionals will need to develop lobbying or advocacy roles to address barriers such as unsafe local authority housing, lack of safe play areas and dangerous local roads. The parent-held child health

Table 22.4
Effective enforcement interventions

Intervention	Effect
Smoke detector legislation	Reductions in fire-related injuries
Child car seat restraint legislation	Reductions in motor vehicle occupant injuries
Seat belt legislation	Reductions in motor vehicle occupant injuries
Cycle helmet legislation	Reductions in cyclist head injuries
Lifeguards on beaches and public pools	Reductions in drowning deaths

Box 22.2
Opportunities for prevention — working with families

- Age-specific advice at child health surveillance
- Opportunistic advice at other consultations, especially at injury consultations
- Identifying hazards on home visits
- First aid advice during consultations for acute injury
- Access to low-cost safety equipment, equipment loan schemes, second-hand equipment and information on financial help available for the purchase of equipment
- Educating parent groups about injury prevention and first aid
- Continued support of families where children have suffered injury including the provision of educational and engineering measures to prevent future injury
- Advice regarding the safe storage of medicines and disposal of unwanted medicine at the time of prescription and dispensing

record can be used as a tool for providing injury prevention and first aid information, and also for recording injury occurrence (Boxes 22.3, 22.4).

In addition to safety advice through the child health surveillance programme, consultations can be used opportunistically for injury prevention. Hazards can be identified on home visits; consultations for acute injury can be used to explore sensitively how similar injuries could be prevented in the future. The parent's first aid actions can be

explored with positive reinforcement of correct actions and information about action to take in case of future injury. Many parents feel guilty following an injury to their child, so it is important for them to be able to discuss their feelings and to feel supported, rather than judged. A&E departments can also take on a similar role. Paediatric liaison health visitors based in A&E departments can notify injuries to community health visitors who can undertake postaccident support visits to provide

---

Box 22.3

Age-specific advice at child health surveillance for families with children under 1 year

- Vehicle occupant injuries — encourage use of infant car restraints

- Burns and scalds — encourage smoke alarm use, do not drink hot drinks whilst holding child, check and reduce hot water temperature, use fireguards once child becomes mobile

- Choking — check toys for small removable parts

- Falls — avoid baby walkers, consider play pens instead, avoid placing babies on beds and tables, stair gates once child becomes mobile, do not place baby bouncers on high surfaces

- Suffocation — do not use pillow or duvet in cot, avoid dummies or toys on cords around neck

- Teach parents first aid

Box 22.4

Age-specific advice at child health surveillance for families with children aged 1–4 years

- Falls — stair gates, window locks, furniture corner protectors

- Burns — smoke alarms, fireguards, stair gates across kitchen doorways, coiled kettle flexes or cordless kettles, make an exit plan in case of fire

- Poisoning — cupboard locks, keeping cleaning products, chemicals and medicines out of reach, dispose of unwanted medicines, prescribe small quantities only, purchase cleaning products with child-resistant caps

- Cuts — store sharp objects out of reach, cupboard locks, use safety glass or film, make low-level glass visible by bright stickers, etc.

- Choking — check small toys for removable parts, avoid peanuts

- Drowning — do not leave child alone in bath, fence off, or cover, garden ponds and pools, teach children to swim

- Suffocation — keep plastic bags out of reach

- Road traffic injuries — child seats and restraints, fenced and gated garden, cycle helmets

- Teach parents first aid

---

support for the parent and child and to explore the prevention of future injuries.

Older children and their parents can be reached via schools and primary healthcare teams. School nurses have an important role to play in developing school injury prevention strategies, teaching pupils first aid, monitoring injuries occurring on the premises, and in working with other agencies, for example to develop safe routes to school and to increase cycle helmet use.

Working with others

It is clear from the evidence regarding effective injury prevention that we as health professionals need to develop our skills and confidence in widening our role. Engineering and enforcement have often achieved more than education, so we need to work with the agencies and professionals who can achieve change by these means. We need to ensure our representation on local injury prevention groups; we need to develop networks with relevant agencies and organisations and skills in lobbying and campaigning (Box 22.5).

Putting it all together — local and national strategies for unintentional injury prevention

A comprehensive injury prevention programme requires leadership, coordination and a high profile to ensure its place on the agenda of policy-makers and resources. The approach taken by many health and local authorities and other agencies has been to establish a multiagency and multidisciplinary injury prevention group. These groups have a wide representation including public health, paediatrics, accident and emergency medicine, primary care, health promotion, housing, environmental health, social services, the fire and rescue service, the police, highways, education, trading standards, the ambulance service and voluntary organisations. The role of these groups has been to develop and implement an injury prevention strategy. The key elements of such a strategy are outlined in Box 22.6.

'Saving Lives: Our Healthier Nation' (The Stationery Office 1999) emphasises that improvements in health and reductions in inequalities will only be achieved by re-focussing local services to increase the priority given to health, and by the establishment of local partnerships where people and organisations work together to improve health. Health authorities are charged with promoting action to improve health and reduce inequality through their Health Improvement Programmes (HIMP) that will be developed with local authorities and other relevant agencies and organisations. The programme will describe how national targets will be met locally, set out locally agreed targets, programmes of evidence-based action and provide measures for assessing progress. Primary care trusts are also expected to develop partnerships to ensure the delivery of shared goals for health

improvement, and must produce their own plans for implementing the HIMP and ensuring local targets are met. Setting a target for the reduction of unintentional injuries in 'Saving Lives: Our Healthier Nation' will ensure injury prevention is included in HIMPs and that progress towards achieving reduced injury rates is monitored, both nationally and locally.

REFERENCES AND FURTHER READING

Alwash R, McCarthy M 1988 Accidents in the home among children under 5: ethnic differences or social disadvantage? British Medical Journal 296:1450–1453

Avery J G, Jackson R H 1993 Children and their accidents. Edward Arnold, London

Beautrais A L, Fergusson D M, Shannon F T 1981 Accidental poisoning in the first three years of life. Australian Pediatric Journal 17:104–109

Bijur P E, Golding J, Haslam M 1988 Persistence of occurrence of injury: can injuries of pre-school children predict injuries of school-aged children? Pediatrics 82:707–711

Child Accident Prevention Trust 1989 Basic principles of child accident prevention: a guide to action. Child Accident Prevention Trust, London

Unintentional injuries

Child Accident Prevention Trust 1991 The health visitor's education and training resource. Child Accident Prevention Trust, London

Child Accident Prevention Trust 1992 The NHS and social costs of children's accidents: a pilot study. Child Accident Prevention Trust, London

Clamp M, Kendrick D 1998 A randomised controlled trial of general practitioner safety advice for families with children under 5 years. British Medical Journal 316:1576–1579

Coombes G 1991 You can't watch them 24 hours a day: parents' and children's perceptions, understanding and experiences of accidents and accident prevention. Child Accident Prevention Trust, London

Department of Health 1993 The health of the nation. Key area handbook: accidents. Department of Health, London

Department of Trade and Industry 1998 Home accident surveillance system: 20th annual report Department of Trade and Industry, London

Department of Transport 1996 Road accidents Great Britain: 1995. The casualty report. Government Statistical Service, London

DiGuiseppi C, Roberts I 1997 Injury mortality among children and teenagers in England and Wales, 1992. Injury Prevention 3:46–49

Elkan R, Kendrick D, Hewitt M et al 1999 The effectiveness of domicillary visiting: a systematic review of the literature and meta-analysis. Health Technology Assessment 4(13):

Eriksson M, Larsson G, Winbladh B, Zetterstrom R 1979 Accidental poisoning in pre-school children in the Stockholm area. Acta Paediatrica Scandmavica Supplement 275:96–101

Gofin R, Adler B 1997 A seven item scale for the assessment of disabilities after child and adolescent injuries. Injury Prevention 3:120–123

Heptinstall E 1996 Healing the hidden hurt: the emotional effects of children's accidents. Child Accident Prevention Trust, London

Kendrick D 1993 Accidental injury attendences as predictors of future admission. Journal of Public Health Medicine 15:171–174

Kendrick D 1994a Children's safety in the home: parents' possession and perceptions of the importance of safety equipment. Public Health 108:21–25

Kendrick D 1994b The role of the primary health care team in preventing accidents to children. British Journal of General Practice 44:372–375

Kendrick D, Marsh P, Williams E I 1995 General practitioners, child accident prevention and the Health of the Nation. Health Education Research 10:345–353

Lawson S D, Edwards P J 1991 The involvement of ethnic minorities in road accidents: data from three studies of young pedestrian casualties. Traffic Engineering and Control January: 12–19

Learmonth A 1979 Factors in child burn and scald accidents in Bradford 1969–1973. Journal of Epidemiology and Community Health 33:270–273

Marsh P, Kendrick D 2000 Near miss and minor injury information — can it be used to plan and evaluate injury prevention programmes? Accident Analysis 32:345–354

Marsh P, Kendrick D, Williams E I 1995 Health visitor's knowledge, attitudes and practices in childhood accident prevention. Journal of Public Health Medicine 17:193–199

Morgan P S A, Carter Y H 1996 Accident prevention in primary care: part 4: are the training needs of community nurses and health visitors being met? Royal Society for the Prevention of Accidents, Birmingham

Office for National Statistics 1996 Mortality statistics. Childhood, infant and perinatal. England and Wales. 1993 and 1994. Series DH3 no 27. Government Statistical Service, London

Office of Population Censuses and Surveys 1995 The health of our children. Decennial supplement. Series DS no 11. Government Statistical Service, London

Pless I B 1993 The scientific basis of childhood injury prevention. A review of the medical literature. Child Accident Prevention Trust, London

Roberts H, Smith S J, Bryce C 1995 Children at risk? Safety as a social value. Open University Press, Buckingham

Roberts I, Norton R 1995 Sensory deficit and the risk of pedestrian injury. Injury Prevention 1:12–14

Roberts I, Power C 1996 Does the decline in child injury mortality vary by social class? A comparison of class specific mortality in 1981 and 1991. British Medical Journal 313:784–786

Roberts I, Kramer M S, Suissa S 1996 Does home visiting prevent childhood injury? A systematic review of randomised controlled trials. British Medical Journal 312:29–33

Roberts I, Carlin J, Bennett C et al 1997 An international study of the exposure of children to traffic. Injury Prevention 3:89–93

Roberts I, Diguiseppi C, Ward H 1998 Childhood injuries: extent of the problem, epidemiological trends and costs. Injury Prevention 4 (suppl):S10–S16

Sibert J R 1975 Stress in families of children who have ingested poisons. British Medical Journal 3:87–89

Taylor B, Wadsworth J, Butler N R 1983 Teenage mothering, admission to hospital and accidents during the first 5 years. Archives of Disease in Childhood 58:6–11

The Stationery Office 1998 Independent inquiry into incqualities in health report. The Stationery Office, London

The Stationery Office 1999 Saving lives: our healthier nation. Cm 4386. The Stationery Office, London

Thompson R S, Rivara F P, Thompson D C 1989 A case control study of the effectiveness of bicycle safety helmets. New England Journal of Medicine 320:1361–1367

Towner E, Dowswell T, Simpson G, Jarvis S 1996 Health promotion in childhood and young adolescence for the prevention of unintentional injuries. Health Education Authority, London

Transport Research Laboratory 1992 Restraint use by car occupants. TRL, Crowthorne

Wadsworth J, Burnell I, Taylor B, Butler N 1983 Family type and accidents in pre-school children. Journal of Epidemiology and Community Health 37:100–104

World Health Organization 1957 Accidents in childhood — facts as a basis for prevention. Technical Services Report no 118. WHO, Geneva

World Health Organization 1982 The epidemiology of accident traumas and resulting disabilities. Report on a WHO symposium, Strasbourg 1981. EURO Reports and Studies 57. WHO, Copenhagen

23 | Health inequalities

The phrase 'inequalities in health' is used to describe the gradient in health that exists in society from the most privileged to the most disadvantaged. This may result from poverty, poor environment, lack of knowledge, neglect or unequal access to health care. Usually it is a combination of these factors. Current UK government health policy is very much directed at the reduction in health inequalities. Health inequalities have been highlighted in the Black Report (Black 1990) and more recently in the Acheson Report (Acheson 1998). The latter report has led to wide-ranging changes in UK Government policy, making reduction in health inequalities a priority. This is in stark contrast to the response to the earlier Black Report (Fig. 23.1).

Social class

Social class derived from the Registrar General's classification of occupation is in general use as the basis for comparison of health measures in different sections of the population. In child health it relates to the occupation of the parent, usually the father.

- social class I: professional, higher administrative
- social class II: administrative, managerial
- social class III: clerical and skilled manual (IIIn non-manual and IIIm manual)
- social class IV: semi-skilled
- social class V: unskilled.

It is, to some extent, an artificial classification of a continuum of social positions. Nevertheless it does allow helpful comparisons to be made. A weakness is that some children may be difficult to classify, for example children of single mothers who register a birth in their name only, or the unemployed. An extra category, 'Others', where included in analysis often shows poorer health than in social class V.

The Acheson Report: recommendations

Recommendations in the Acheson Report of Relevance to Child Health include:

- Increasing benefits to women of childbearing age, expectant mothers and young children.
- Additional resources for schools serving children from less well off groups.
- Development of health promoting schools, initially focused on disadvantaged communities.
- Measures to improve the nutrition provided at school.
- High-quality pre-school education and day care meeting, in particular, the needs of disadvantaged families.
- Policies that promote the social and emotional support to parents and children.
- Promoting sexual health in young people and reduce unwanted teenage pregnancies.
- Promoting the physical and psychological health needs of looked after children.

The term 'deprivation' is often used to describe the multiple dimensions of disadvantage experienced by children growing up in poor circumstances. According to the National Child Development Study (NCDS), of children born in 1958, 4% of families in the UK suffer 'deprivation' on the basis of low income, poor housing and single-parent or large families. This study (Wedge & Prosser 1973) sharply identifies the educational as well as the health consequences of deprivation. Deprivation

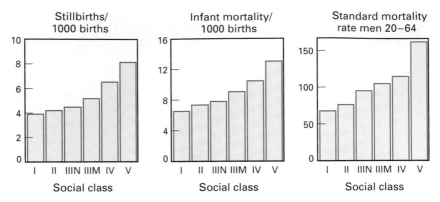

Fig. 23.1 Examples of 'inequalities in health': Black Report (Black 1980)

shows strong intergenerational continuities exhibited in areas such as poverty, employment, mental health, educational achievement and antisocial behaviours (Rutter & Madge 1976). Policy is now focused on how those cycles can be interrupted.

Poverty

Poverty is generally defined as less than 50% of the national average income. The Acheson Report, using this definition, shows the figure of 10% in 1961 rose to 20% in 1991, decreasing to 17% in 1995.

Deprivation

Deprivation is a relative lack of material and/or psychological support. In an attempt to direct resources according to need, measures of deprivation have been developed.

Jarman index

The Jarman index is derived from eight variables, each weighted according to how much GPs in a national study believed that it increased their workload (Table 23.1). Areas of low deprivation have a negative score, while high deprivation has a positive score. These are divided into four bands to describe increasing levels of deprivation: 20–30, 30–40, 40–50 and 50+.

The score is applied to electoral wards (average population in 1981 of approximately 5000) and the GP receives payment according to the level of the

Table 23.1

The eight variables (obtained from Census data) relating to the proportion of the population

Variable (population group)	% weighting
Old people living alone	6.62
Children aged under 5	4.64
Single-parent households	3.01
Unskilled people	3.74
Unemployed people	3.34
Overcrowded households	2.88
People who have moved house	2.68
Ethnic minority	2.50

score to reflect the workload implications (Jarman 1983). There has been criticism of this score: because of the size of the wards, there may be considerable pockets of deprivation within predominantly affluent areas and vice versa, and the scores are derived from census data which can become quickly out of date in a highly mobile population. Another criticism is that it is based on GP workloads and the list does not *necessarily* reflect the health *needs* of the population served.

Townesend index

The Townesend index containing only four indicators, is also commonly used; it is thought by some to be a better reflection of deprivation rather than GP workload. Negative scores reflect affluence, positive scores deprivation. The most deprived areas will have scores of 10 or 11. The four indicators used in the index are:

- % of those of economically active age who are unemployed.
- % of households that are overcrowded.
- % of households without a car.
- % of households not being buyers or owners.

Social index

The Social index was developed for use in the Child Health and Education Study and was designed to be more in tune with the home environment of the child than occupational class alone. It has been used to identify disadvantaged groups experiencing difficulties in health service use (Osborn & Morris 1979). By recognising these difficulties, resources can be targeted specifically at the most disadvantaged, for example, provision of a mobile immunisation service or an interpreter service. Indicators used in this index are:

- Father's social class.
- Highest known qualification of either parent.
- Type of neighbourhood.
- Tenure of accommodation.
- Persons per room ratio.
- Presence of a bathroom.
- Accommodation self-contained.
- Availability of a car or van.

Inverse care law

The availability of good medical care tends to vary inversely with the need for it in the population served. The 'Inverse Care law' holds that market forces lead to this situation where the higher income groups are more able to obtain and use services; they receive more specialist attention, occupy more of the beds in better equipped and staffed hospitals, receive more elective surgery, have better maternal care, and are more likely to get psychiatric help and psychotherapy than low-income groups — particularly the unskilled (Tudor

Hart 1971). Additionally the disadvantaged may feel uncomfortable in their relationship with health professionals, perceiving a difference in status that might make them reluctant to seek health care. We need to be aware of these potential barriers, and endeavour to create a welcoming, friendly and open atmosphere in our clinics. Previous negative experiences need to be uncovered and addressed. Fear of going to see the doctor can be very real in both parents and children, based upon previous contacts, fears of the unknown or the doctor being presented to children as a bogeyman or threat. For some, services are not accessed, because parents or young people do not know they are there or they do not know how to access them. Health care may not be a priority and other more pressing concerns, for example debt, might take precedence. Common problems with access might be the lack of a telephone to make an appointment, not knowing the number to call, lack of transport to get to an appointment, lack of child care for other children, not knowing where the clinic is, clashes with work or other appointments. Poor self-organisation and time keeping can prove fatal in accessing health care in an unforgiving world. For other parents lack of strong commitment merges into neglect of their children's healthcare needs, and child protection procedures may be required (Table 23.2). Conflicting beliefs in alternative medicine must be handled sensitively to avoid complete alienation from conventional health care.

The reasons for poorer health and lower uptake of services are complex. There is no single explanation and no simple solution. More resources may be required to achieve the same outcome. General practitioners whose practice population has a high Jarman score quality for extra deprivation payments. Programmes such as Surestart to provide opportunities for the pre-school child, Health Action Zones, Education Action Zones and the New Deal for Communities and Inner City Regeneration Programmes are all based upon policies with the intention of reducing inequalities through targeted intervention.

Many children who come within the framework of inequalities in health are also within the definition of 'Children in Need' under section 17 of the 1989 Children Act (Box 23.1). This covers a broad

Table 23.2
Impact of poverty on child health: the two main areas

Physical	Behavioural
Infant mortality	Educational attainment
Childhood deaths	Truancy
Childhood morbidity	Teenage conceptions
Height and weight	Conduct disorder
Iron deficiency	Child abuse and neglect
Protection from infection	Low self-esteem
Dental decay	Accidents
Admission to hospital	Low expectations
Homelessness and housing conditions	Lack of continuity in health care
Clothing	Separations and residential care
Conductive hearing loss	Unhealthy lifestyle
Enuresis	Juvenile crime

Box 23.1
Children Act 1989, section 17

A child is defined by the Act as being *in need* if:

a. he is unlikely to achieve or maintain, or to have the opportunity of achieving or maintaining, a reasonable standard of health or development without the provision for him of services by the local authority

b. his health or development is likely to be significantly impaired, or further impaired, without the provision

c. he is disabled

range of overlapping groups, from parents who requires assistance if they are to deliver an adequate level of child care to those whose children have disabilities. Social services departments are required to respond to referrals of 'Children in Need'. This is further discussed in Chapters 18 and 24.

Data on the effects of poverty on the 'outcomes' listed above is available with varying degrees of completeness and accuracy. The challenge of paediatrics in the future is in developing methods of recording the health status and determinants for children at disadvantage and developing effective interventions to promote positive outcomes. Community paediatricians are in a very good position to act as advocates for change.

FACTORS AFFECTING THE WELL-BEING OF CHILDREN

The factors we shall discuss are those that influence the outcome for individual children. Some are capable of being changed by personal practice, others require action by local authorities or government, but some such as genetic factors are not currently amenable to change. Graham (1988) lists the basic needs which if not met will impair health as: an adequate diet; adequate housing; adequate income; a stable, continuous source of affection and care, together with protection from physical, emotional and sexual abuse; cognitive stimulation and adequate education; safe environment; and access to preventive and curative health care (Fig. 23.2).

Genetics

Studies of families of both gifted children and those with learning difficulties show strong intergenerational continuities (Rutter & Madge 1976). In the Isle of Wight study, 37% of the families of children with learning difficulties had a family history of learning problems compared to 12% of the general population (Rutter et al 1970). Although it is difficult to dissect inherited factors from the care received from parents, there is a high correlation between the IQ of parents and children, even where they are reared away from their natural parents. We often talk about children reaching or failing to reach their 'full potential'. We describe the phenomenon of improvements in development when children's circumstances are improved. However, it is difficult if not impossible to predict the 'potential' of individuals and the degree of improvement to expect with improvements in care. The extent to which

these levels of development can improve depend upon the age at which adverse conditions are removed (Rutter 1980).

Environment

Housing

Housing conditions can have a profound effect upon children's health and development (Table 23.3). Peaks of ill health and mortality in the winter months, which are a prominent feature in the UK, are probably related to dampness (Platt et al 1989), and defects in heating and ventilation. It has been well known since the earliest days of public health, that overcrowding and poor sanitary conditions are related to the spread of infectious disease, particularly gastroenteritis and respiratory infections (Lowry 1991). Passive smoking will add to the risks of acquiring respiratory infections and secretory otitis media. Poor housing is also associated with an increase in childhood accidents. Children living in flats or in other circumstances where there is no safe, supervised play area, such as a private garden or a playground, are likely to be at risk through playing outside on roads and other dangerous areas. Poor housing can lead to maternal depression and adverse effects upon child development. Overcrowding can lead to conflict within the home and

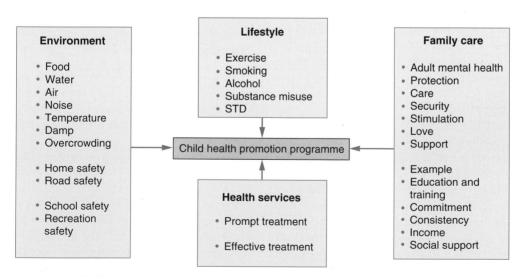

Fig. 23.2 Promoting health

Community paediatrics

Health inequalities

Table 23.3
Housing and children's health.

Housing Condition	Symptoms/child* (no.)
No damp	2.04
Damp	2.46
Mould	2.86

* Symptoms: aches and pains, diarrhoea, wheezing, vomiting, sore throat, irritability, tiredness, headaches, earache, fever, depression, tantrums, bedwetting, poor appetite, persistent cough, running nose
Source: Platt et al (1989)

children can suffer from lack of personal privacy, which is especially important for teenagers, and lack of space and proper conditions in which to do homework.

Homelessness

Homelessness may result in inadequate housing in bed and breakfast accommodation with very restricted facilities for play and for preparing meals. Frequent moves result in stress for families, insecurity for children and disrupt continuity of service provision in terms of changes in school, changes in medical practitioner and in social work support (Edwards 1991). Growing numbers of teenagers are sleeping on the streets of our towns. They are often the 'graduates' of disturbed family lives or inadequate local authority care.

Neighbourhood

Community paediatricians are well aware that health is not only powerfully affected by the quality of individual houses, but also by the nature of the neighbourhood as a whole. Within a neighbourhood there are often associated problems of lack of local amenities, public transport, adequate refuse collections and shops. Blocks of flats may have particular problems with security and vandalism (Coleman 1985). Deprived neighbourhoods are also associated with increased unemployment and increases in juvenile crime (Nottingham County Deprivation Survey) (Fig. 23.3). Profiles of neighbourhoods, case loads or practices can be used to target resources.

Income

Many indices of child health such as growth, mortality rates, respiratory infections, hospital admissions and educational attainments have been related to income. The problems of income and appropriate utilisation of income have been discussed by many. Those on a low income spend 30% of their money on food compared to 12% for the average family, and are more likely to provide a poor quality diet for their children with less fruit, fresh vegetables and fresh meat (Graham & Stacey 1984, Sheppard 1986).

Lack of disposable income leads to difficulties in budgeting. Skills in budgeting or getting value for money may not be sufficient to prevent families slipping into debt. For the families at the lowest income level, providing an adequate diet and remaining out of debt may be an impossibility. Debt or fear of debt puts large stresses on families. Poverty and the outward appearances of it may also have a detrimental effect on self-esteem and provide an obvious badge by which they can be identified by others. Health workers, therefore, should be aware of the limitations placed upon child care by low income and of the personal sensitivities related to poverty.

Family structure

In 1995 33.9% of live births were outside marriage; in 1984 it was 17.3%. Twenty per cent of children now live with a lone parent (18% mothers, 2% fathers); 55% of lone mothers have been previously married.

About one in five couples are now cohabiting. Of those who do marry, between one in two and one in three will divorce. For children born in the early 1980s, about one in five will have experienced parental divorce before their fourteenth birthday. These average figures hide the much higher rates that can be found in individual localities. An increasing number of children are growing up with either a lone parent or in a reconstituted family (i.e.

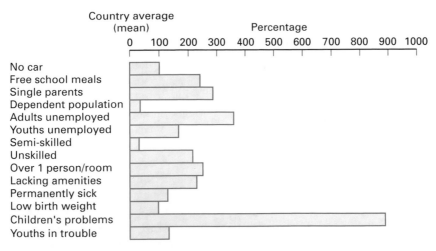

Fig. 23.3 Disadvantages of inner city areas: Nottingham Deprivation Study 1983

not living with both biological parents). What then is the effects of these differing family structures on children? Perinatal, neonatal and postneonatal mortality rates are higher for children born to lone parents. Educational attainments at age 7 are poorer in illegitimate children (Crellin et al 1971). In practice, the difficulties that the children have may arise from a number of factors associated with family structure; these may be economic due to low income, secondary to the stress or depression that an unsupported parent may experience or related to family tensions and arguments. The children show more evidence of depression, unhealthy lifestyles and are more likely to become a parent at an early age. Children from reconstituted families occupy an intermediate position between lone parent and intact dual-parent families (Rodgers & Pryor 1998). Professional help may need to be focused at all these three levels. Marital breakdown occurs more commonly in families where parents' childhoods were marked by divorce or separation. Skilled counselling is needed to explore family relationships.

Culture

In the UK, there are higher perinatal and infant mortality rates for some immigrant groups. Part of this may relate to lower socio-economic status and part to inherited disease, particularly where there is consanguinity. Health workers are often faced with

different childrearing practices and different family traditions (Henley 1979, Black 1990), which they need to understand before acceptable advice can be given. For example, understanding religious dietary restrictions or the contrasts between lifestyles or living conditions in their country of origin and the UK can form a basis for explaining some medical problems such as iron deficiency and appreciating the degree of adaptation required to a new environment. Interpreters and link workers recruited from the community to promote health care and explain customs are an essential part of the service to immigrant communities.

Stimulation

Children can only learn as a result of the stimulation that they receive. Lack of such early stimulation results in impaired language development and later educational difficulties. Bath (1981) found significant language delay in up to 50% of children attending social service day nurseries in Nottingham. Interventions may involve general advice to parents on the importance of language stimulation, the introduction of language programmes or help for underlying problems such as parental depression which may impair communication. Pollak (1979) found poor levels of development associated with inadequate stimulation from child minders in south London.

Nurture and affection

Bonding is a powerful, specific attachment between parents and child that enables care, protection, affection, sacrifice and empathy to take place. Its origins are in the parents' own childrearing experience. It is facilitated by early contact between mother and child and is inhibited by separations, malformations or unresponsiveness of the child or adverse circumstances such as an unwanted pregnancy. Children who do not receive affection and whose parents are consistently critical are likely to suffer low self-esteem and severe emotional problems. Facilitation and understanding of positive reactions between parents and children are important in the prevention and management of these behaviour problems (Fig. 23.4). Children in early life are often withdrawn (though often later having more outwardly difficult behaviour), fail to thrive and have characteristically cold extremities (deprivation hands and feet).

Diet

Non-organic growth delay is associated with developmental delay, as shown by Dowdney et al (1987) in a study of 4 year olds from an inner-city area. Children whose weight and height lay below the tenth centile were found to have a general cognitive index of 77.1 compared to 97.7 for controls. Two per cent of the caucasian inner city children fitted their definition of chronic non-organic growth retardation, and of these 35% had a cognitive index below 70 points. In these children an inadequate diet is the main cause of their failure to thrive. In Nottingham, Marder et al (1990) found 25% of inner city children to be iron deficient at 15–24 months with a rate of 39% in Asian children. In Birmingham, Grindulis et al (1986) found that two-fifths of their Asian toddlers were vitamin D deficient. Treatment of iron-deficient children in Birmingham led to improved weight gain and 42% of the children whose haemoglobin rose by 2g or more as a result of treatment achieved six or more new skills on the Denver scale compared to 13% in controls (Aukett et al 1986). There are conflicting claims for improvement in IQ by giving vitamin and mineral supplements to school children (Whitehead 1991).

Poor nutrition is clearly common in a relatively wealthy country such as the UK and is associated with poor development. Causes, however, may be complex and can relate to low income, inadequate knowledge about diet or, as described by Skuse (1985), a maladaptive behavioural interaction between caregiver and infant, sustained by high emotional tensions. Barker & Osmond (1986) have suggested that poor nutrition in childhood may have long-term consequences in the incidence of ischaemic heart disease in adult life.

In the Jamaican Study (Granthan-McGregor et al 1991), the effects upon development of both nutritional supplementation and stimulation were investigated in stunted children, age 9–24 months. The authors were able to demonstrate the relationship between these two factors. The developmental quotient improved for stimulated and supplemented children, but not in the controls. Children who received both supplementation and stimulation did better than children who received only a single intervention. Children who received both had a mean IQ 13.4 points greater than controls after 24 months, with improvements of 6.5 and 7.9 for single interventions.

The first two years of life are a critical time for brain growth. In view of the developmental deficits in children whose growth is poor, active early management is required for children who fail to thrive.

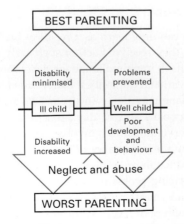

Fig. 23.4 It is difficult to overstate the effect of parenting on the well being of children

Access to services

Access to adequate child welfare services is not equal. Parents in disadvantaged areas face difficulties if they do not have a telephone to contact the doctor or personal transport to bring their child to clinic or surgery. Children from disadvantaged families are certainly much more likely to be admitted to hospital for preventable causes of ill health (Wynne & Hull 1977, Carter et al 1990, Conway et al 1990). The cause of this may be related to the ability to prevent or recognise ill health as well as to decision making with regard to medical consultation and access to health care.

Life events

Life events in a child's family may have profound effects upon the functioning of the family overall. Obvious examples are the death of a parent or the onset of disability in a parent. Unemployment, housing problems, family separations, convictions or being a victim of crime are also important. Life events can of course be positive as well as adverse — 'he hasn't looked back since . . .'. 'Medical records may with advantage have life event lists, which can usefully supplement problem lists and other summary sheets.

Temperament

Children of similar levels of intelligence given the same opportunities and the same quality of care do not always reach the same outcomes. An important factor is the individual child's temperament (Oberklaid 1991). Important characteristics of an individual child's temperament may be drive, adaptability to change, persistence, distractibility, regularity of behaviours such as sleeping and thresholds of responsiveness. The child's temperament needs to match or be compatible with the lifestyles and expectations of the rest of the family. For example a child who is quiet and thoughtful may be of concern in a family whose general characteristics are boisterous and outgoing. In other situations an 'average' child born into a quiet and thoughtful family may be viewed as hyperactive. Our assessment of individual children and their families must take temperament into account and must also recognise that our own individual temperaments may also influence our judgment at times.

EARLY INTERVENTION SCHEMES

This section outlines examples of community programmes that are designed to prevent the consequences of disadvantage or at least to minimise its effects. These aims are central to any 'mission statements' of community paediatric services. Research to demonstrate the effectiveness of these programmes is difficult in securing sufficient numbers of children and long enough follow-up to demonstrate outcomes.

Pre-school education

Osborn & Milbank (1987) in the Child Health and Education Study of a cohort of 13 000 children born in 1970, found better attainments in the children who had received pre-school education. Children who attended nursery schools and playgroups did best and children from disadvantaged families did best when they had attended nursery schools. Children who had attended day nurseries had the poorest attainments in reading and mathematics. This important study supports community health workers who advocate both the availability and the uptake of pre-school education. It also indicated the importance of pre-school education for disadvantaged groups and the need to improve educational provision in day nurseries.

The Radford Family Centre (Box 23.2)

Family centres are designed for parents and children to attend. They provide support for parents, but also education in child care and an important element of 'parenting of the parents'.

The Radford Family Centre was staffed by a multidisciplinary team which included a social worker, a nursery teacher, a playgroup leader and a health visitor. Additional help was obtained from adult literacy teachers, a cook (who also taught), a hairdresser and a paediatrician!

Some family centres work with families with severe multiple problems or those where there has been child abuse. For example of 22 parents attending the Radford Family Centre, 14 had literacy problems of which nine received special education, 13 had court appearances, 11 had been in care as children and seven had psychiatric problems. Work in the centre included individual reviews and counselling, a daily rota organised for tasks such as washing up and serving food, and group work and practical activities including health education, budgetting, literacy, child care, play, family life, bereavement and cooking. The focus of work was on decision-making, self-help and personal responsibility as well as the acquisition of knowledge and skills. Improvements in self-esteem and in self-care and appearance were important elements in the functioning of the centre. Results are variable: some

children 10 years later are in care, but other families are performing much better with no special professional involvement and with their children making normal physical, emotional and developmental progress.

Perry Pre-school Program

In the Perry Pre-school Program in the USA, children whose mothers had been engaged in an early intervention programme when their children were infants were found to have better educational attainments (Fig. 23.5,) better chances of employment on leaving school and less chance of having been in care or in trouble with the law (Schweindart & Weihart 1980). The crucial features were an early start and parental involvement. It involved weekly home visits and a daily pre-school programme extending over 2 years. The authors in this study were also able to demonstrate that their programmes were cost effective. They estimated that for each $1000 invested in the programme, $4130 would be returned to society because of the costs that would have been associated with juvenile crime, special education and unemployment. The authors conclude that the child-positive attitudes and increased parental aspirations were important factors in the success of the programme.

Long-term effects of nurse home visits (Olds et al 1998)

More recent is the 15-year follow-up of children of 116 mothers who received an intensive home visit-

---

> **Box 23.2**
> ## The aims of the Radford Family Centre
>
> To promote practical parenting skills
>
> To promote better home management
>
> To promote literacy
>
> To provide insight for parents into the needs of children, both in family life and in education
>
> To promote satisfaction for parents in parenting, and enjoyment of their children
>
> To reduce dependence on agencies for day-to-day care and acute problems
>
> From: Polnay 1985

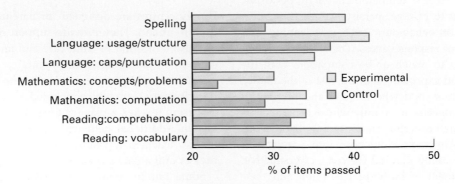

Fig. 23.5 Educational attainments: the Perry Preschool Program

ing programme during pregnancy and the first 2 years of life. Mothers received on average nine antenatal and 23 postnatal visits lasting around 1 hour 15 minutes. These visits focused on promoting positive health-related behaviours, competent child care and maternal personal development. During the 2-year programme, it was observed that mothers and children enrolled in the programme had a safer and more stimulating home environment and had fewer visits for injury or ingestion (Olds et al 1995). When followed-up at age 15 children who had been enrolled in the programme, in comparison with controls, had fewer episodes of running away, fewer arrests and convictions, fewer sexual partners, smoked less and consumed less alcohol. As in the Perry Program, the length, intensity and skill applied in the intervention may be important factors in achieving positive long-term outcomes.

Cope Street

In the Cope Street centre in Nottingham's inner city referrals were mainly teenage parents (Billingham 1989). The core staff were health based, consisting of a health visitor, a midwife and nursery nurses. The programmes at Cope Street centred around parents defining their own needs and groups and topics chosen by parents were set up. Increasing self-confidence was an important theme in the work of the centre. The centre staff recognise that parents may learn more from others in the same situation than from traditional teaching by health professionals. They also stress that people learn by doing, hence the practical activities in the centre. Parents were involved in the planning, organisation and evaluation of group sessions. The groups include teenage antenatal, teenage mothers, food, Open University using the Open University Courses for parents, craft, coping with kids and a literacy summer school.

The approach of Cope Street has been most successful. Examples of achievements have been all the members of the 'Open University' group going on to attend college; the 'teenage mothers' group giving talks in local secondary schools and featuring on a local radio programme; the 'food' group producing their own cookery book; groups

addressing meetings of health visitors and midwives; and the 'coping with kids' group continuing to meet in each other's houses after the group at the centre had finished.

Cope Street and other similar centres break away from the mould of conventional health service provision. They provide a much more intensive service than is available from routine programmes and a message and medium which is acceptable to their target group. Short-term follow-up has suggested that the programmes can not only impart knowledge and skills, but also overcome the consequences of the teenagers' own deprived childhoods, their own emotional needs and the difficulty of combining adolescence with parenthood.

Bristol Programme

The Child Development Programme has been developed by the Early Childhood Development Unit of the School of Applied Social Sciences at the University of Bristol. This is a structured programme carried out by specially trained health visitors. It is focused on first-time parents usually during the antenatal period and the first 8 months of life, but can be extended up to the age of 3 years. The parents receive more frequent home visits and the health visitor uses attractive cartoon-style materials that encourage parents to develop their own skills rather than be passive receptacles for advice. Important issues covered are early health, nutrition, language, socialisation, early education and parent's own health and self-esteem. The programme includes a system for monitoring of results.

The programme claims increased parental self-esteem, improved diet and immunisation rates, reduced hospitalisation of children and greater job satisfaction for health visitors.

Language schemes

Language delay is a common finding among children in disadvantaged families. For this reason language programmes have been developed to prevent language delay or to manage children from these groups who are already delayed. Bath (1981) developed the use of language programmes in day nurseries by nursery nurses. She used programmes developed along the lines of the Wolfson Developmental Language Programme (Cooper et al 1978). This follows a sequence through attention control, comprehension and symbolic understanding to expression. Assessment preceded enrolment on the programme and careful records were kept on each child. Results show rapid progress in the majority of children and maintenance of a normal rate of language development 1 year after their involvement in the programme ended.

The Burnley, Pendle and Rossendale Language programme was developed in 1983 by the speech therapy department of Burnley, Pendle and Rossendale Health Authority. It is designed for use with groups of children in day nurseries and comprises five daily topics covering 8 weeks. The programme is prepared on two levels to meet individual abilities. It is designed for children who are linguistically deprived, rather than those who have specific language problems. Examples of the topics covered are: name and use of common objects; listening and attention (sound sequences, rhythm, stories); classification (identifying like or related objects, e.g. cups, spoons, books on shelf, coats on hooks, bricks by colour); action day (demonstrate use of objects, identify objects by mime); positioning (understanding use of 'on', 'under', 'in', etc.); size and shape; and sequencing (e.g. putting objects in requested order). This programme is now used throughout the family centres in Nottingham.

The WILSTAAR programme (Ward Infant Language Screening Test Assessment Acceleration Remediation) is designed to help speech and language therapists to identify babies at risk of language delay and provide early intervention (Awcock & Habgood 1998). Of 122 language-delayed children who had received an intervention programme, only 5% continued to show delay at age 3 years, in comparison to 85% of controls (Ward 1999).

Portage

The Portage scheme was developed in Portage, Wisconsin as a home-based scheme to help the development of pre-school children with moderate learning difficulties (Cameron 1982). It is very widely used in the UK and other countries. A trained portage worker visits the family for about an hour a week. A developmental checklist covering social, language, cognitive, self-help and motor skills is then filled out by the parent and the portage worker. Targets are then chosen and broken down into stages with a series of activities that can be completed within the week. The portage materials include cards with suggestions for activities that will lead towards the target. The portage worker shows the parent that stage of the programme including important techniques such as reinforcement and will also observe the parent carrying it out. Progress records are kept by the parents so that skill levels before and after teaching are known. The system works well for children whose developmental delay is related to their deprived backgrounds as well as for those with intrinsic causes for their learning difficulties.

Correcting iron deficiency

Intervention programmes may also very successfully be targeted on important clinical problems. James et al (1989) set up a programme of education and screening to reduce iron deficiency in an inner city general practice. Dietary information was provided antenatally and in the first year of life. An information sheet on foods rich in iron, including those suitable for vegetarians, was given to all mothers. Haemoglobin was measured at the time of MMR immunisation in the second year of life. Iron deficiency in the practice dropped from 25% to 8% following the introduction of the education programme. This study, conducted from general practice, is an instance of the effectiveness of a community-based nutrition education programme.

YOUNG CARERS

Introduction

Young carers are children and young persons under 18 who provide or intend to provide care, assistance or support to another family member. They carry out significant or substantial caring tasks, often on a regular basis, and assume a level of responsibility which would usually be associated with an adult. The person receiving care is often a parent but can be a sibling, grandparent or other relative who is disabled, has some chronic illness, mental health problem or other condition connected with a need for care, support or supervision.

Where young carers and their families lack appropriate health- and social-care support, and adequate income, some children experience impaired health and psychosocial development. This includes physical injury, stress-related symptoms, poor educational attendance and performance, restricted peer networks, restricted friendships and opportunities, and difficulties in making the transition from childhood to adulthood. All these will have implications for the young carer's health and well being as well as for their security and stability in adulthood.

Most children, not just young carers, will care about and care for others and this caring needs to be encouraged and nurtured if children are to value caring both during childhood and later in adult life. Learning to care is part of a child's socialisation and is a prerequisite for healthy psychosocial development. But what of children who take on caring tasks and responsibilities which have a negative impact on their own health and development or on their own opportunities to engage fully in the parameters of childhood? It is this group of children who are specifically referred to as 'young carers' and who are eligible for help and support under existing children's and carers' legislation.

Not all children in families where there is illness or disability will become young carers. In many families another adult may provide care from within, or from outside, the family unit. The family may also receive support and services from the so-called 'mixed economy of welfare' — from health, social services, the voluntary and private sectors — working with families as part of the state's policies and provision for health and community care, or as part of the welfare infrastructure which exists to protect children and support families. Clearly, the involvement of health- and social-care professionals will be critical in determining the quality of life and autonomy of young carers and family members who are ill or disabled.

Definitions, numbers and tasks

The Department of Health definition refers to young carers as being children and young persons who are providing or are intending to provide a substantial amount of care on a regular basis. The definition is principally framed in terms of the quantity of care provided by children.

In the UK, almost three million children under the age of 16 (equivalent to 23% of all children) live in households with one family member hampered in daily activities by a chronic physical or mental health problem, illness or disability. It is impossible to estimate the proportion of these children who take on, or do not take on, caring responsibilities within the family. However, Office for National Statistics figures indicate that there are up to 51 000 children who can be classified as young carers, i.e. children who take on substantial or regular care. The figure will be significantly higher if the definition of a young carer is constructed more broadly, to include the significance or impact of caring as well as the quantity of care provided.

Characteristics and caring tasks

Since the early 1990s there have been many small-scale studies of the characteristics, experiences and needs of young carers. The findings of these studies have been remarkably uniform and have provided a picture of what young carers are, what they do, and the outcomes caring has for their lives. The findings of these small-scale studies have also been confirmed by the largest survey of young carers, 'Young Carers in the United Kingdom: a profile' (Dearden & Becker 1998). This study provides a profile of the characteristics, needs and experiences of 2303 young carers aged 18 or under, all of whom are supported by specialist young carers projects. The research also enables comparisons to be drawn between the position of young carers in 1998 and in 1995, when the results of a similar but smaller survey of 641 young carers was published (Dearden & Becker 1995). The average age of young carers supported by projects remains the same, at just 12 years. Over half are from lone-parent families and most are caring for ill or disabled mothers. In 1995, 10% of young carers were

Table 23.4
Percentage of young carers performing various caring roles: 1995 and 1998.

Tasks	1995	1998
Domestic tasks	65%	72%
General care, giving medication, lifting etc.	61%	57%
Emotional support	25%	43%
Intimate care (toiletting, bathing, etc.)	23%	21%
Child care to siblings	11%	7%
Other tasks (translating, dealing with professionals, money management, etc.)	10%	29%

Source: Dearden & Becker (1995, 1998)

Table 23.5
Proportion of young carers of school age experiencing educational difficulties or missing school: 1995 and 1998.

Age group (yr)	1995	1998
5–10	20%	17%
11–15	42%	35%
All: 5–15	33%	28%

Source: Dearden & Becker (1995, 1998)

caring for more than one person, this had risen to 12% by 1998.

The tasks performed by young carers range along a continuum from basic domestic duties to very intimate personal care (Table 23.4). Most young carers (like other children who are not carers) do some level of domestic tasks within the home. However, where young carers differ substantially from other children is in the extent and nature of the personal caring tasks that they perform and the adult-like responsibilities that they take on. Over half of the young carers in 1998 were involved in general care, which includes giving medication, lifting parents, etc. About 43% provided emotional support, particularly to parents with mental health problems. One in five provided intimate care including toileting and bathing, while almost a third took responsibility for translating (where English was not the first language), dealing with professionals, money management, etc. A small proportion, about 7%, also took on child-care responsibilities in addition to their caring roles for other family members.

Outcomes

Research has also illustrated the outcomes for children of caring and of being inadequately supported by professionals (Table 23.5). These outcomes include:

- Limited opportunities, horizons, aspirations.
- Limited opportunities for social and leisure activities.
- A lack of understanding from peers, restricted friendships.
- 'Stigma by association', particularly where parents have mental health problems or misuse alcohol or drugs, or have AIDS/HIV.
- Fear of what professionals might do.
- 'Silence' and secrets.
- Emotional difficulties.
- Health problems.
- Difficulties in making a successful transition from childhood to adulthood.
- Some young carers are consistently late, miss a great amount of school or have other educational difficulties.

Since 1995 there have been some small improvements in the overall position of young carers in the UK. For example, fewer are providing personal intimate care such as bathing, showering and toileting — the type of caring tasks found most unacceptable by both parents and their children — fewer young carers are missing school or experiencing educational difficulties. However, these improvements are slight. The incidence of intimate care has reduced by only 2% (from 23% of all young carers in 1995 to 21% in 1998), while the overall incidence of educational difficulties has fallen by just 5% (from 33% of all young carers in 1995 to 28% in 1998). This is in spite of a Department of Health national initiative during 1996–97 to raise awareness of young carers.

The needs of young carers

The research on young carers identifies consistently the needs of young carers. When asked, young carers say they need:

- Recognition and respect:
  — to be acknowledged, valued and listened to
  — to be respected as an individual with their own needs and entitlements.
- Information:
  — on care planning and management
  — on medical conditions
  — on practical chores
  — on benefits, money, welfare rights
  — on services and support available to the care receiver and themselves.
- Support and services:
  — to be given practical help now and then
  — to be given time off.
- Choice:
  — the choice to care as well as choice of services.
- Someone to talk to:
  — a friend
  — a confidante
  — an advocate.

Young carers' rights

The Children Act

The 1989 Children Act proposes that children are best cared for within their own families and that intervention should only occur when necessary to safeguard the child's welfare. The emphasis is on 'parental responsibility', the combination of rights, powers, duties and responsibilities which parents have. The Act also stresses the 'welfare principle' which makes the child's welfare paramount. This principle would be applied in any court proceedings. Furthermore, courts must listen to the wishes of the child subject to their age and understanding.

Section 17 of the Children Act states that local authorities have a duty to 'safeguard and promote the welfare of children within their area who are in need; and so far as is consistent with that duty, to promote the upbringing of such children by their families'. A child is defined as being in need if:

(a) she/he is unlikely to achieve or maintain or to have the opportunity of achieving or maintaining, a reasonable standard of health or development without the provision for her/him of services by a local authority;
(b) her/his health or development is likely to be significantly impaired, or further impaired, without the provision for her/him of such services; or
(c) she/he is disabled.

While the Act does not specify what constitutes a 'reasonable' standard of health or development, there is some debate as to whether young carers should be considered as children in need of services and as children who may not have an equal opportunity of achieving a reasonable standard of health in relation to non-caring children. As we have already seen, the research evidence shows that many young carers are vulnerable to a range of health-related and developmental difficulties.

Many local authorities use predetermined groups to establish the numbers of children in need in their areas. These predetermined groups include children with disabilities, children from homeless families, children in low-income families, children in lone-parent families and children of unemployed parents. Few define young carers as a predetermined group of children in need, although this may change in the future as more authorities become aware of the needs and rights of young carers. Being defined as a child in need means that social services are able to provide a range of services and interventions, including advice, guidance and counselling; activities; home help (including laundry services); assistance with travelling to use a service provided under the Act; and assistance to enable the child or his family to have a holiday. These, and small amounts of cash, can be provided to the family of a child in need, rather than specifically to the child, if it will benefit the child.

Young carers and the Carers Act

Young carers may be assessed as children in need under the Children Act if they meet their local authority criteria, but their needs as carers may be overlooked. While the NHS and Community Care Act offers carers the opportunity to request an assessment of their needs, the Act is intended specifically for adults; young carers were not considered when the Act was drawn up. As a consequence, young carers have been unable to access this legislation but have been referred instead to social services children's sections for assessment of their needs under the Children Act. The Carers Act 1995 has closed this loophole, since it applies to all carers, regardless of age. For the first time, the needs of young carers as carers can be assessed.

The Carers Act is concerned with carers of any age who are providing, or intend to provide, a substantial amount of care on a regular basis and entitles them to an assessment of their needs when the person for whom they care is being assessed or re-assessed for community care services. The result of a carer's assessment must be taken into account when decisions about services to the user are made. The 'Practice Guide' to the Act recognises that 'denial of proper educational and social opportunities may have harmful consequences on [young carers'] ability to achieve independent adult life'. Consequently, 'the provision of community care services should ensure that young carers are not expected to carry inappropriate levels of caring responsibilities' (Department of Health 1996 p 10, 11).

However, while the Act imposes a duty on local authorities to recognise and assess young carers' needs, it does not oblige departments to provide any services to them. The Carers and Disabled Children Act 2000 plugs this gap by providing all carers, including young carers aged 16 and over, with a right to services and in some cases to direct cash payments in lieu of social services.

The major benefits of the 1995 Carers Act, as it relates to young carers, are in the way it gives formal recognition to this group of children and provides for an assessment of their needs as carers. Moreover, the Act allows for a wider interpretation of the definition of a 'young carer'. While the Carers Act refers to carers as people who provide a 'substantial amount of care on a regular basis', the term

'substantial' is not defined. The 'Practice Guide' clarifies the definition of a young carer and acknowledges for the first time that young carers should not be defined solely by reference to the amount of time they spend caring. The guidelines state: 'there may be some young carers who do not provide substantial and regular care but their development is impaired as a result of their caring responsibilities' (Department of Health 1996 p 11).

The needs of young carers identified under this piece of legislation will be met under local authorities' duties under section 17 of the Children Act, i.e. they will be treated as children in need. This will also be the case for those young carers who do not provide a 'substantial' amount of care but who are considered, nevertheless, to be in need of services which will promote their health and development. Thus, young carers — those who provide a substantial amount of care or those who provide less care but whose health or development is nonetheless impaired as a result of their caring responsibilities — can be defined as children in need and can expect support and assistance via the Children Act, even in the absence of resources available to deliver services under the Carers Act.

The assessment of young carers

Although young carers have rights under the Children Act and Carers Act, very few have ever been assessed by social services. Of the 2303 young carers surveyed by Dearden & Becker (1998), only 249 had received any form of assessment of their needs under the Children Act or Carers Act. These figures are particularly low considering that all of these young carers are supported by specialist projects and therefore have someone to act on their behalf (should they require it) to request an assessment of their needs. They are also low considering that one in five young carers still perform intimate caring tasks and almost a third have educational difficulties. The process of assessment by social services of young carers was found to be variable, ranging from very poor to excellent. The majority of young carers interviewed were unaware that they had been assessed by social services even after the event and few had been actively involved in the process.

While the process of assessment is variable, the outcomes tend to be positive. Of those young people assessed, services were either introduced or increased following assessment and most children and families were satisfied with these outcomes. It is the availability of such external support services which has a key influence on what young carers have to do within the family, and why. While other factors such as age, gender, ethnicity, family structure and the nature of the illness or disability of care recipients all influence how and why some young people become carers (and what they do), it is the presence or lack of external support services, coupled with the adequacy or otherwise of a family's financial resources, that are the most important determinants of whether or not a child will become a carer in the first place and what tasks they will have to undertake.

Specialist young carers projects

The increasing awareness of young carers and their needs and rights is reflected on a practical level in the growing number of young carers projects now operating across the UK. In 1992 there were only two such projects in existence. By 1995 there were 37 projects and by 1998 there were 110 projects. All of these and their details are listed in the 'National Handbook of Young Carers Projects' (Aldridge & Becker 1998) on *www.ycrg.org.uk*.

The projects offer a range of services and are valued highly by young carers and their families alike, especially those families who resist professional assistance or are not entitled to it. Without the support of these projects a quarter of young carers and their families would have no outside support at all.

Research by the Department of Health has also suggested that the services offered by young carers projects are also equally valued by health and social care professionals for their 'specialist' response to the needs of young carers and their families, as a way of locating appropriate access to statutory services and of raising the profile of young carers.

Young carers projects offer a range of services based on the identified needs of the children themselves. Some projects are also adopting more of a family perspective when planning their services. Most provide information and avenues for accessing other forms of support as well as counselling, advocacy and befriending services. Befriending schemes can be informally arranged, providing young carers with a 'listening ear' when the need arises, or they can be formally organised, one-to-one friendships with volunteer befrienders.

Advocacy is a crucial part of the work of many projects as the majority of young carers are unaware of their rights. Project workers either work alongside young carers or advocate on their behalf to try and secure their rights under existing legislation, particularly the Children Act and Carers Act. In this way, project workers can also try to ensure that the needs and rights of other family members are met.

Providing leisure activities for young carers is a priority for most of the projects and is valued highly by the children themselves. Activities allow young carers some respite from caring and the opportunity for fun 'time-out' as well as the chance to meet and mix with other children in a similar situation. This also gives parents 'time off' from their children — an opportunity to have some privacy and time away from worrying about or having to deal with their children's needs.

Aside from service provision young carers' projects are also involved in awareness-raising strategies in order to ensure that the needs and rights of young carers are identified and met both within statutory and voluntary agencies. Projects are also keen to work in collaboration with, or advise other agencies in order to meet these needs and some aim to influence local policy and practice. Young carers projects are increasingly located within carers' centres or other carer support groups.

Tackling health inequalities for young carers

Young carers' experiences of caring, and the impact on their health, development and transition to adulthood, challenges common understanding of what childhood is about. Because young carers are involved in adult-like tasks which require maturity, responsibility and often a high degree of expertise, there is a question as to whether it is appropriate for children to be involved in such tasks at all, or whether there are appropriate ages at which children might be reasonably expected to take on these responsibilities. So, for example, at what age should children be allowed to toilet a parent or to carry them up and down stairs? Could we define an age for these and other tasks or responsibilities? Even if it was possible to determine an 'appropriate' age, would it be desirable to do so?

The key issue here is that for healthy psychosocial development children should *gradually* increase their responsibilities within, and outside, the home. Being responsible from an early age for caring and other tasks, especially those which would usually be associated with adult duties, can seriously compromise a child's health and development and can lead to a number of negative outcomes.

How can these negative outcomes be tackled or reduced for the benefit of young carers? There are a number of ways forward which need to be addressed by health- and social-care professionals, and others:

1. The definition of young carers needs to be broad and inclusive. It should not just be based on the amount of care provided by children but it should also relate to the significance of that care to individual families and to the impact of caring on children. Definitions are important. To be defined as a young carer can lead to a detailed assessment of need, which can provide access to services and support under children's or carers' legislation.

2. Awareness-raising and training on young carers' issues needs to be on-going within medicine, health and social care, and also for those in education and youth services. Professionals need to recognise and understand that their involvement and their interventions with families and children are those most likely to help young carers. They also need to ensure that young carers and their families are aware of, and understand, their rights to assessments under the various pieces of legislation. Currently few young carers are being assessed under any Act. Where children have been assessed and have received services or support this is usually beneficial.

3. Assessment processes will need to be viewed by families as a positive step. Disabled parents must feel that their needs and rights will be taken into account and promoted, and that their parenting abilities will not be questioned. Equally, young carers must feel that their abilities as carers are acknowledged and valued and that they are not patronised or ignored in decision-making processes.

4. While support of the whole family should be seen as a priority, rather than a focus on parents or children in isolation, young carers' projects do offer a highly focused way of recognising, valuing and responding to the specific needs of children who have care-giving responsibilities. However, there is scope for young carers' projects to take a more active role in supporting whole families. Moreover, young carers' projects should operate alongside and complement support services for ill and disabled people. The existence of such projects should not detract statutory organisations from their duties to arrange or provide services to ill or disabled people and to children in need as laid down by law.

5. Where health and social services are provided to assist ill or disabled parents and their young carers, this combination of provision is likely to reduce and in some cases remove the need for children to provide care on a regular basis. Moreover, if family support has been extensively and sensitively applied, a young carer's situation will rarely trigger child protection procedures.

6. Health, social services, education and other organisations, agencies and professionals need to consider the best way of working together, to deliver a seamless package of health- and social-care support. There is also a need for national standards for the quality and quantity of health- and social-care support to young carers and their families. There is currently no uniformity across regional boundaries in what families can expect in the way of help and support. Families should receive help that is based on their needs, rather than where they live.

7. Each family must be considered and treated as unique, with its own strengths, weaknesses and needs. Professionals must acknowledge, value and respect the reciprocal and interdependent nature of caring within families and support these relationships through a range of policies and services. Care must be taken to acknowledge and value the diverse cultural, religious and social expectations and experiences of families from minority ethnic communities whilst acknowledging the rights of children. The challenge for us all is to ensure that young carers have the opportunities for a healthy and happy childhood, and that their own health and welfare is not compromised by their caring roles and responsibilities.

LOOKED AFTER CHILDREN: THE PHYSICAL AND MENTAL HEALTH NEEDS OF CHILDREN LOOKED AFTER IN LOCAL AUTHORITY CARE

There are about 53000 children who are looked after in local authority care in the UK. About 11% of these young people are looked after in residential care, and about 65% are fostered (Davies 1998); about 13% of the looked-after population are believed to be black or dual heritage children (O'Hanlon & Ejioforj 1999). Although the majority of children come into the care system for short periods (i.e. no more than 6 weeks), those who are looked after for long periods often have multiple placements. For example, in one local authority over 15% of looked-after children had three or more different placements in one year (Cooper 2000).

Prior to coming into care, the majority of young people have experienced a range of traumatic and disrupted relationships. Some of these experiences are listed in Box 23.3. Subsequently, they have the added trauma of being removed from home and placed in a new setting with strangers. There are numerous physical and mental health implications of these highly damaging experiences, and these will be reviewed in more detail in the next section. There are, however, other social areas where young people in the care system are vulnerable and at a disadvantage, and these are shown in Box 23.4.

Box 23.3
Common experiences of young people prior to coming into local authority care

History of physical, sexual and/or emotional abuse

Parents with mental health and physical health problems

Family social deprivation (e.g. overcrowding, income support)

Disrupted family relationships (e.g. marital breakdown, domestic violence)

Increased likelihood of having a young mother

Decreased likelihood of having both parents at home

Box 23.4
Social risk factors associated with being in the care system

Increased risk of offending

Increased risk of school attendance problems and learning difficulties

Increased risk of homelessness when leaving care

Increased risk of unemployment

Being unprepared for independent living

National surveys have demonstrated that 41% of homeless young people have been in care (Derkevorkian 1997). Furthermore, the unemployment rate has been found to be 50–80% for 16–24 year olds who have been in residential care compared to 15% of a non-looked-after comparison group. Seventy five per cent of looked-after young people have been found to have no academic qualification in comparison to 6% of the comparison group (Evans 1996 cited in Polnay et al 1997), and over 45% of looked-after children have been found to be regular non-attenders at school (Coutts & Polnay 1997). Forty-two per cent of the prison population have a history of being in care.

It is clear, then, that those young people who are looked after in local authority care are an extremely vulnerable group. In the remainder of this section of the chapter, a more detailed review of the physical and mental health needs of this group will be made, followed by a summary of how their health needs have been met (or failed to be met) in the past, with a final section reviewing innovative models of health care that have been introduced in recent years.

Health needs

Physical health needs

Young people who are looked after are at an increased risk of poor health. Some of the main health difficulties are shown in Box 23.5.

There is evidence, for example, that over 85% of young people entering children's homes are smokers (with some smoking over 40 a day), and that only 17% of young people in care were completely immunised (Derkevorkian 1997). Further-

more, a very high proportion of young women become pregnant soon after leaving care. In one study this was as high as 33% (Derkevorkian 1997).

Some of the reasons for such poor health are that there has often not been one or more people intimately familiar with the young person's medical history or aware of their specific health needs as a parent would normally be. As a result medical histories have often been inadequate (de Cates et al 1995). Health assessments have also been undervalued by professionals in the past within the care system. Furthermore, young people themselves have often been reluctant to take part in medical examinations as trusting other adults to carry out intimate examinations can often be too threatening to this group of young people (Landon 1998).

Mental health needs

There is now consistent evidence in the literature to show that young people who are looked after in local authority care are at a significantly higher risk of experiencing psychological difficulties than the general population (McCann et al 1996, Lang & Goatly 1997, Dimigen et al 1999). For example, rates of significant psychological difficulty in the looked-after population range from 96% of adolescents in residential care and 57% in foster care, compared to 15% in the general population (McCann et al 1996). Research has also shown that these elevated levels are present when young people enter local authority care (Dimigen et al 1999). Some of the most prevalent psychological difficulties are shown in Box 23.6.

The co-morbidity of symptoms is common and in one study many young people who exhibited externalizing problems (e.g. aggression and conduct difficulties) also showed significant levels of depression (Lang & Goatly 1997). In the majority of these cases, however, only the externalizing symptoms had been identified by social services or health professionals, and the depression was missed. The authors described this as 'masked depression', and it illustrates the risk of missing internalizing symptoms in this group of young people. Interestingly, lower rates of self-harm and suicide risk have been observed in young people whilst in residential care, but there is a greater risk after leaving care. This

---

Box 23.5
Overview of the health problems of young people in community homes

Missed routine surveillance and immunisation

Lack of detection and follow-up of chronic medical conditions

Less access to health promotion and personal social education (PSE) due to poor school attendance

High prevalence of risk-taking behaviour

Higher rates of smoking

Increased risk of substance abuse (e.g. drugs, alcohol, solvents)

Higher prevalence of unwanted pregnancy and poor antenatal care

Risk of sexually transmitted infections

Poor diet

Tendency to be lighter and shorter than other children

Box 23.6
Common psychological difficulties of looked-after children

Depression

Anxiety

Attention and concentration difficulties

Conduct difficulties

Attachment and relationship problems

Anger and aggression

Low perceived control

Substance misuse

might suggest that the social availability and support in residential establishments by staff and young people is a protective factor.

In a recent study of social workers' views on the mental health needs of looked-after children, 80% of the children were thought to require treatment from a mental health worker (Phillips 1997). There was also a concern amongst many residential social workers about labelling young people with 'psychiatric' diagnoses, and the possible stigma associated with this. However, it was also recognized that carers needed to be prepared appropriately as to the level of need and vulnerability of the young person.

Traditional ways of meeting the health needs of looked after children

Use of existing services

The traditional way of meeting the *physical* health needs of looked-after children has been to use existing tier one health services. This has involved accessing GPs, health visitors, school nurses and community paediatricians within their general health service work. Whilst there have been examples of good practice using this model, it has not met the complex needs of looked-after young people. This is because carers have often not been aware of the health needs of the children they are looking after (Coutts & Polnay 1997, Dewhurst & Polnay

1997), and young people themselves are reluctant to use traditional health services which they feel are inaccessible. The statutory annual medical examination for all looked-after children has traditionally been the responsibility of the GP, but evidence suggests that only a small proportion of these are completed comprehensively (Landon 1998).

In a similar vein, the complicated *mental* health needs of looked-after children have traditionally been met using existing services. There is evidence, however, that field social workers and residential social workers have been less likely to refer to specialist mental health workers (e.g. clinical psychologist, child psychiatrists and members of CAMHS [Child and Adolescent Mental Health Services] teams) than other health professionals (Audit Commission 1999). In this research, more than 50% of referrals were from GPs and 15% from paediatricians, with less than 14% from social services and education combined. Furthermore, social workers reported feeling that a health service referral may not be an appropriate setting for vulnerable young people in the care system (Audit Commission 1999), and there is much anecdotal evidence of young people in the care system refusing to attend their mental health appointments.

Care staff concerns

Despite the low referral rate of many care staff from social services to the traditional health services, there is evidence of the high levels of concern that staff have for the emotional well being of the young people in their care. For example, research by Street (1998) indicates that residential social workers have been very concerned about the lack of specialist mental health resources for looked-after young people, and reported that the lack of continuity of care was a significant problem (i.e. seeing a different clinician in the community for each visit). Nearly three-quarters of the residential social workers interviewed also expressed concerns about the lack of specialist external resources available to them as professionals, and the difficulties in getting health professionals to attend planning or family meetings (Street 1998). Furthermore, there is evidence of young people in the care system being shifted around to different areas of health provision depending on resources (Malek 1993).

Recommendations for change

In response to the difficulty that existing health service provision has had in meeting the extensive health needs of looked-after young people, a number of Government guidelines and Department of Health reports and recommendations have been made in recent years. The House of Commons Health Select Committee produced a document in 1998 entitled 'Children Looked After by Local Authorities, which made a number of highly significant recommendations relating to health. These are listed in Box 23.7. The British Paediatric Association report *Health Needs of School Age Children* had already recommended in 1995 that the health needs of this group of vulnerable children should be met by a discrete and specialist service (British Paediatric Association 1995).

The Department of Health also launched a 3-year Quality Protects programme in 1998, in which all local authorities were expected to strengthen their management and quality assurance systems in their delivery of services to children (Department of Health 1998). One of the eight primary objectives is 'To ensure that children looked after gain maximum life chance benefits from educational opportunities, health care and social care'. Specific further health objectives include the take up of medical examinations required by statute, the take up of immunizations, and access to health information to a similar level as those young people from the same area who are not looked after. There are also expectations that there will be interagency working between specialist mental health services and local authorities.

Annual medical examinations are due to be replaced by a comprehensive health assessment leading to an action plan, with the implementation and outcomes of the plan being closely monitored. Comprehensive health assessment will include review of medical history, ascertainment and action on missed appointments, detecting unrecognised health, development and emotional needs and arranging specialist referral where needed. A high uptake will be expected compared to levels as low as 25% for the current service. A designated doctor and nurse will be appointed in each district with similar roles to the designated nurse and doctor in child protection (Department of Health 1999). Reducing placement moves, improvements in education attainment, better communication and joint working and addressing low expectations are key features of the strategy.

New developments in service delivery

Specialist looked-after health teams

Perhaps the most important new development in the provision of healthcare services to young people who are looked after is the setting up of specialist health teams. These teams have recently begun to be funded by joint social services and health funding following the priority given to these services by the Department of Health. Although many of these teams have only recently been formed, and therefore it is too soon to have any reliable or valid outcome data as to their effectiveness, there are a number of theoretical benefits to their formation. Firstly, they enable discrete amounts of time to be offered to these young people in the most appropriate setting. Secondly, they allow social services staff and foster carers to make relationships with a consistent set of people. Thirdly, they enable health staff to become specialists in a very challenging area. Finally, they set up the possibility for a creative form of intervention to be designed, evaluated and modified. In theory at least, these teams may stop the perceived separation of health care from social care.

Box 23.7
Some of the recommendations of the House of Commons Select Committee in relation to the health of looked-after children

---

Reform of the training of residential social workers to include increased heath awareness

Increased health promotion to young people

Increased funding for specialist health resources

Increased multidisciplinary working

A number of innovative ways of working with young people and staff have already developed out of this specialist provision. For example, creative ways of engaging young people in the health assessment process have been put into action. The Nottingham Community Health Team have been using lap-top computers to conduct their physical and mental health assessments and have seen a significant increase in the quantity and quality of health-related information as a result (Report of the Programme Team for Health Needs of Young People in Residential Care 1992–1997 in Nottingham 1997). The Nottingham team also have a specialist community paediatrician and two school nurses in post now, and they have developed an alternative to the looked-after medical examination which was so poorly attended in the past when it was conducted by GPs. Instead, they conduct a fitness assessment which can involve the use of sports centre facilities and is less 'medical' in its orientation. Both of these initiatives have enabled the young person to have an increased ownership of the assessment process. A final example of innovative approaches involves the joint working of the health team with the specialist education achievement team for looked-after children. In this way joint planning has occurred across three agencies (i.e. health, education and social services).

Consultation to staff and carers

One of the other implications for health staff of having discrete time to work within the looked-after system is the potential to work directly with care staff and foster carers. In the past the debate between social services departments and health workers has always concentrated on the appropriateness of taking direct referrals of young people. However, as we have seen in the previous sections, young people who are looked after are often hesitant to work individually with mental health specialists as well as doctors and nurses. Whilst there are undoubtedly some young people who need direct therapy and can access it emotionally whilst they are still in care, the majority find it extremely hard to engage on long-term therapeutic work. It is essential, therefore, to find an alternative way of meeting their needs. One particularly effective way is to provide regular consultation to staff and carers

to help those who have direct and regular contact with the young person to understand and help them. In the Nottingham Children Looked After Mental Health Team a group of 11 specialist mental health workers offer regular consultation to residential social workers, field social workers and foster carers across both the residential sector and the foster teams. Using a model adapted from working with teachers, the team help those carers share their problem in a safe environment, reflect on their own understanding of the issues, explore the emotional impact on themselves of being a carer for a particular child and share possible solutions (Newton 1995). Following consultation, a series of agreements are made about whether direct assessment and therapy might be appropriate, and whether other important members of the professional or family network might be involved in future consultations. In this way a much deeper and wide-ranging assessment of the needs of a young person can be gained, which can be revisited by the same team over time. This goes some way to avoiding the disjointed nature of the traditional process.

Health promotion and peer education

There have also been a number of initiatives aimed at directly influencing young people's health behaviour from within their community home. The aims of all these initiatives has been to encourage young people to take some responsibility for their own health and help them understand and use the health facilities in their area. Nottingham Community Health Trust has run a number of specialist health education groups with young people covering topics such as sexual health, drug awareness and hygiene and self-care (Coutts & Polnay 1997). They have been facilitated by a school nurse and have always had a co-worker present. Establishing ground rules has always been essential to maintain both a safe environment and confidentiality, and outcomes have been positive with young people engaging in the process and reporting that their health knowledge has improved.

Another initiative has been coordinated by the National Children's Bureau (NCB), and has been targeted at young people who are close to leaving care in the London boroughs of Islington, South-

Health inequalities

wark, Wandsworth and Westminster (Landon 1998). The groups were facilitated by project workers but the topics and format of the group were designed by the young people themselves. Common topics discussed in large groups included: (1) diet and nutrition, (2) hygiene and self-care and (3) first aid. The young people preferred to discuss sexual health and drug issues in small groups or in one-to-one adult pairs. As part of this project, some of the young people have themselves become peer educators and have been working with other young people in the care system. Another local initiative has been set up in community homes in Wandsworth and has involved stress management and relaxation groups (Landon 1998). The young people themselves have again set the agenda and have tested out aromatherapy, yoga, keep fit, as well as psychological relaxation techniques.

Training for carers and social workers

A number of innovative health training packages has been developed in recent years which have had the aim of increasing foster carers' and residential and field social workers' confidence in meeting some of the health needs of the young people in their care. A 6-day training course has been run for the past 6 years in Nottingham for residential social work staff and foster carers (Coutts & Polnay 1997). Over 140 staff and carers have now completed the training package and feedback has been positive. Staff have reported increased knowledge and confidence in dealing with health problems and knowing who and when to refer to for additional help. The course is coordinated by a school nurse and has eight other health professionals who facilitate individual sessions. Details of the course contents are provided in Box 23.8.

Similar packages of training have also been developed in Northamptonshire Health Authority (Derkevorkian 1997), and by the NCB with four local authorities: Bedfordshire, Croyden, Havering and Hertfordshire (Landon 1998). A comprehensive training manual for residential social workers and foster carers has now been produced by the NCB covering five main areas: (1) understanding and promoting health; (2) managing health within the care system; (3) child development, childhood ill-

---

Box 23.8
Health training programme for social work staff and carers of looked-after children

Growth and development

Child health surveillance

Common childhood illnesses

Sexual health

Substance use/misuse

Mental health

Diabetes

The health promoting community home

Note: Future developments on this course include integrating specialist education teaching within the curriculum and linking the contents to formal non-vocational qualifications, NVQs

---

nesses and health problems; (4) understanding mental health, and (5) promoting health lifestyles (Lewis 1999).

REFERENCES

Acheson D (Chairman) 1998 Independent inquiry into health inequalities. HMSO London

Aldridge J, Becker S 1993 Children who care: inside the world of young carers. Young Carers Research Group, Loughborough University, Loughborough

Aldridge J, Becker S 1998 The national handbook of young carers projects. Carers National Association, London

Audit Commission 1999 Children in mind: child and adolescent mental health services. Audit Commission, London

Aukett A, Parks Y A, Scott P H, Wharton B A 1986 Treatment with iron increases weight gain and psychomotor development. Archives of Disease in Childhood 61:849–857

Awcock C, Habgood N 1998 Early intervention project: evaluation of WILSTARR, Hanen and specialist playgroup. International Journal of Language and Communication Disorders 33(suppl):500–505

Barker D J P, Osmond C 1986 Infant mortality, childhood nutrition and ischaemic heart disease in England and Wales. Lancet ii:1077–1081

Bath D 1981 Developing the speech therapy service in day nurseries: a progress report. British Journal of Disorders in Communication 16:159–173

Billingham K 1989 45 Cope Street: working in partnership with parents. Health Visitor 62:156–157

Black D 1980 Inequalities in health: report of a research working group. DHSS, London

Black J 1990 Child health in a multicultural society. British Medical Journal Books, London

British Paediatric Association 1995 Health needs of school aged children (chairman, Polnay L). BPA, London

Cameron R J (ed) 1982 Working together: portage in the UK. National Foundation for Educational Research-Nelson, Windsor

Carter E P, Drew A G, Thomas M E, Mohan J F, Savage M O, Larcher V F 1990 Material deprivation and its association with childhood hospital admission in the East End of London. Maternal and Child Health 15:183–186

Coleman A 1985 Utopia on trial: vision and reality in planned housing. Hilary Shipman, London

Conway S P, Phillips R R, Panday S 1990 Admission to hospital with gastroenteritis. Archives of Disease in Childhood 65:579–584

Cooper A 2000 Looked after children. In: Richardson J, Joughin C (eds) The mental health needs of looked after children. The Royal Collage of Psychiatrists, London

Cooper J, Moodley M, Reynell J 1978 Helping language development. Edward Arnold, Sevenoaks

Coutts J, Polnay L 1997 Children in residential care: a healthier future. Primary Health Care 7(3):12–16

Crellin E, Pringle M L, West P 1971 Born illegitimate. Social and educational implications. National Foundation for Educational Research, Windsor

Davies C 1998 Developing interests in child care outcome measurement: a central Government perspective. Children and Society 12:155–160

de Cates C, Trend U, Buck S, Ng Y, Polnay L 1995 Services for children in Residential Care. In: Spencer N (ed) Progress in community child health. Churchill Livingston, Edinburgh, pp 153–169

Dearden C, Becker S 1995 Young carers: the facts. Reed Business Publishing, Sutton

Dearden C, Becker S 1998 Young carers in the United Kingdom: a profile. Carers National Association, London

Department of Health 1996 Carers (Recognition and Services) Act 1995: policy guidance and practice guide. Department of Health, London

Department of Health 1998 The Quality Protects Programme: transforming children's services. Department of Health, London

Department of Health 1999 Promoting health of looked after children. Department of Health, London

Derkevorkian G 1997 Teenagers leaving care: their health needs. Rapport 4(2):4–19

Dewhurst T, Polnay L 1997 Here's health. Community Care 19–25 June

Dimigen G, Del Priore C, Butler S, Evans S, Ferguson L, Swan M 1999 Psychiatric disorder among children at time of entering local authority care: questionnaire survey. British Medical Journal 319:675

Dowdney L, Skuse D, Hepstinstall E, Puckering C, Zur-Szpiro S 1987 Growth retardation and developmental delay amongst inner-city children. Journal of Child Psychiatry and Child Psychology 28:529–541

Edwards R 1991 Homeless families, highlight no 99. National Children's Bureau, London

Evans A 1996 We don't choose to be homeless: report of the national enquiry into preventing youth homelessness. CHAR, London

Graham H, Stacey M 1984 Socioeconomic factors related to child health. In: MacFarlane J A (ed) Progress in child health, vol 1. Churchill Livingstone, Edinburgh, pp 167–178

Graham P 1988 Social class, social disadvantage and child health. Children & Society 2:9–19

Grantham-McGregor S M, Powell C A, Walker S P, Himes J H 1991 Nutritional supplementation, and mental development of stunted children: the Jamaican study. Lancet 338:1–5

Grindulis H, Scott P H, Belton N R, Wharton B A 1986 Combined deficiency of iron and vitamin D in Asian toddlers. Archives of Disease in Childhood 61:843–848

Henley A 1979 Asian patients at home and at hospital. King's Fund, London

House of Commons Health Select Committee 1998 Children looked after by local authorities. The Stationary Office, London

James J, Lawson P, Male P, Oakhill A 1989 Preventing iron deficiency in pre-school children by implementing an educational and screening programme in an inner city practice. British Medical Journal 299:838–840

Jarman B 1983 Identification of under privileged areas. British Medical Journal 286:1705–1709

Landon J 1998 Children in care: responding to their health education needs. Healthlines Magazine 50:13–14

Lang J, Goatly J 1997 Assessing the mental health needs of children looked after in the care of the local authority. In: Report of the Programme Team for Health Needs of Young People in Residential Care 1992–1997 in Nottingham. Nottingham Community Health NHS Trust, pp 3–4

Lewis H 1999 Improving the health of children and young people in public care. National Children's Bureau, London

Lowry S 1991 Housing and health. British Medical Journal Books, London

McCann J, James A, Wilson S, Dunn G 1996 Prevalence of psychiatric disorders in young people in the care system. British Medical Journal 313:1529–1530

Malek M 1993 Passing the buck. The Children's Society, London

Marder E, Nicoll A, Polnay L, Shulman C E 1990 Discovering anaemia at child health clinics. Archives of Disease in Childhood 65:892–894

Newton C 1995 Circles of adults: reflecting and problem solving around emotional needs and behaviour. Educational Psychology in Practice 11(2):8–14

Oberklaid F 1991 The clinical assessment of temperament in infants and young children. Maternal and Child Health 16:14–17

O'Hanlon L, Ejioforj J 1999 Should we encourage

transracial adoption? The Guardian 23 October

Olds D, Henderson C R, Kitzman H, Cole R 1995 Effects of prenatal and infancy nurse home visitation on surveillance of child maltreatment. Paediatrics 95:365–372

Olds D, Henderson C R, Cole R, et al 1998 Longterm effects of nurse home visitation on children's criminal and antisocial behaviour: 15 year follow-up of a randomised controlled trial. JAMA 280(14):1238–1244

Osborn A S, Morris A C 1979 The rationale for a composite index of social class and its evolution. British Journal of Sociology 30(i):39–60

Osborn AP, Milbank JE 1987 The effect of early education: a report of the Child Health and Education Study. Oxford University Press, Oxford

Philips J 1997 Meeting the psychiatric needs of children in foster care: social workers' views. Psychiatric Bulletin 21:609–611

Platt S D, Martin C J, Hunt S M, Lewis S W 1989 Damp housing, mould growth and symptomatic health state. British Medical Journal 298:1673–1678

Pollak M 1979 Nine year olds. MTP Press, Lancaster

Polnay L 1985 A service for problem families. Archives of Disease in Childhood 60:887–890

Polnay L, Glaser A, Dewhurst T 1997 Children in residential care; what cost? Archives of Disease in Childhood 77:394–395

Report of the Programme Team for Health Needs of Young People in Residential Care 1992–1997 in Nottingham. 1997 Nottingham Community Health NHS Trust

Rodgers B, Pryor J 1998 Divorce and separation: the outcome for children. Joseph Rowntree Foundation, York

Rutter M 1980 The long-term effects of early experience. Developmental Medicine and Child Neurology 22:800–815

Rutter M, Madge N 1976 Cycles of disadvantage. Heinemann, London

Rutter M, Tizard J, Whitmore K 1970 Education, health and behaviour. Longman, Harlow

Schweindart L J, Weihart D P 1980 Young children grow up. The effects of the Perry pre-school programme on youth through age 15. Monographs of High Scope Educational Research Programme, no 7

Sheppard J 1986 Food facts. London Food Commission, London

Skuse D H 1985 Non-organic failure to thrive: a reappraisal. Archives of Disease in Childhood 60:173–178

Street C 1998 Residential treatment and care: the professional perspective. Young Minds Magazine 36:10–11

Tudor Hart 1971 The inverse care law. Lancet i:405–412

Ward S 1999 An investigation into the effectiveness of an early intervention method for delayed language development in young children. International Journal of Language and Communication Disorders 34:243–264

Wedge P, Prosser H 1973 Born to fail. Arrow Books, London

Whitehead M 1987 The health divide: inequalities in health in the 1980s. Health Education Authority, London

Whitehead R G 1991 BMJ 302:548

Wynne J, Hull D 1977 Why are children admitted to hospital. British Medical Journal 2:1140–1142

FURTHER READING

Barker D J P 1998 Mothers, babies and health in later life, 2nd edn. Churchill Livingstone, Edinburgh

Becker S, Aldridge J, Dearden C 1998 Young carers and their families. Blackwell Science, Oxford

Blaxter M 1981 The health of the children. A review of research on the place of health in cycles of disadvantage. SSRC/DHSS Studies in deprivation and disadvantage, vol. 3. Heinemann, London

British Medical Association 1999 Growing up in Britain: ensuring a healthy future for our children. BMJ Books, London

Browne K, Davies C, Stratton P (eds) 1988 Early prediction and prevention of child abuse. John Wiley, Chichester

Burnley, Pendle and Rossendale Health Authority 1984 Speech therapy language programme

Crittenden P 1988 Family and dyadic patterns of functioning in maltreating families. In: Brown K, Davies C, Stratton P (eds) Early prediction and prevention of child abuse. John Wiley, Chichester, pp 161–193

Department of Health 1996 Young carers: making a start. Department of Health, London

Department of Health 1996 Young carers: something to think about. Report of Four SSI Workshops, May–July 1995. Department of Health, London

Dowling S 1983 Health for a change. Child Poverty Action Group, London

Idjradinata P, Pollitt E 1993 Reversal of developmental delays in iron-deficient children treated with iron. Lancet 341:1–4

Lindstrom B, Spencer N (eds) 1995 Social paediatrics. Oxford University Press, Oxford

Marmot M, Wilkinson R G 1999 Social determinants of health. Oxford University Press, Oxford

Murphy J F, Jenkins J, Newcombe R G, Sibert J R 1981 Objective birth data and the prediction of child abuse. Archives of Disease in Childhood 56:295–297

Office for National Statistics 1996 Young carers and their families. The Stationery Office, London

Polnay L, Glaser A, Rao V 1996 Better health for children in resident care. Archives of Diseases in Childhood 75:263–265

Powers J 1998 Long-term effects of nurse home visitation on children's criminal and antisocial behavior: 15 year follow-up of a randomised controlled trail. JAMA 280:1238–1244

Spencer N 2000 Poverty and child health. 2nd edition. Radcliffe Medical Press, Oxford

Stevenson O 1999 Child welfare in the UK. Blackwell Science, Oxford

Syla K 1989 Does early intervention work? Archives of Disease in Childhood 64:1103–1104

Wedge P, Essen J 1982 Children in adversity. Pan Books, London

Wicks M 1989 Family trends, insecurities and social policy. Children and Society 3:67–80

Woodroffe C, Glickman M, Barker M, Power C 1993 Children, teenagers and health — the key data. Open University, Milton Keynes, Buckingham

24 | Avoiding harm: child protection

The position of children in society has varied at different times in history which has influenced thinking about their welfare. In terms of work and punishment, children have sometimes been treated very much as powerless small adults. Child prostitution and the use of children for sex has been documented as an accepted and normal practice at various points in written history. In the seventeenth century, religious and social changes in Europe, paralleling the rise of Protestantism, meant that children began to be seen as innocent, not sharing in original sin, and in need of special treatment, education and protection until adulthood. Incest was made a crime under church law and in the nineteenth century the Factory Acts and universal primary education were instituted. In 1875 the use of children as chimney sweeps was ended. In 1870 a major issue was baby farming. For a fee, unwanted or illegitimate babies were handed to an adopter who, instead of care, was free to provide a lingering death from neglect, starvation and laudanum. In 1878 Tardieu in Paris described post-mortem findings of sexual abuse of children (Tardieu 1878). Incest was dealt with in ecclesiastical courts until it became a criminal offence with the passing of the Punishment of Incest Act in the UK in 1908. Various pieces of legislation followed relating to age and permitted relationships but even amongst experts the sexual abuse of children was thought to be confined to rare acts committed by perverts.

Cruelty to children

As philosophies have changed, fashions in names have changed to reflect the users' new thinking. In 1875, Mary Ellen was brought before the US supreme court wrapped in a horse blanket to test her case under animal protection laws. The adoptive parents were convicted and imprisoned. The ensuing outrage led to the New York Society for the Prevention of Cruelty to Children being formed. The concept of 'cruelty to children' was developed. It embodied the idea of deliberate and sustained mental and physical assault by an evil person, or institution, and the view that the child must be rescued. Ideas quickly crossed the Atlantic and a number of UK Societies for the Prevention of Cruelty to Children (SPCCs) were founded. The London SPCC, formed in 1884, expanded and adopted the title National Society (PCC) in 1889. One of the NSPCC's greatest triumphs was the passage of the 1889 Prevention of Cruelty to Children Act. Known as 'the children's charter', it allowed for the legal removal of a child to the care of a fit person in proven cases of cruelty. It was the first time the law had intervened in the conduct of parents to children. The NSPCC remains an independent body with statutory legal duties today.

Battered child syndrome

This syndrome was described by Henry Kempe, a paediatrician from Denver Colorado, in 1962 (Kempe et al 1962). It brought new medical knowledge to support previous social proofs of abuse. The concept that severe injury and death could be inflicted within a family with no externally obvious criminality or deviance was shocking and slow to be accepted by many people.

Non-accidental injury

Non-accidental injury (NAI) became the medically correct term used by doctors in the UK who now found themselves on the front line of an army previously staffed by police and social workers. Government circulars used the term NAI throughout the 1970s, and in 1974 recommended that each local authority set up an interagency committee to agree on procedures and review practice. These were named, interestingly, without any reference to their main agenda, Area Review Committees, or ARCs. Widespread public recognition of the extent of child sexual abuse swept across the USA in 1977 and 1978 and thence to the UK. Here sexual abuse was the province of the police as long as they had evidence, usually through witnesses or police surgeon examination, that a crime had been committed. Action was focused primarily on convicting a criminal and the victim was helped only to that extent.

Child abuse

Sexual abuse and severe neglect only came to acquire mandatory social work action under revised procedures in the 1980s. NAI became an inadequate description and the term child abuse was preferred, as the whole spectrum of abuse, with overlapping categories, became clear. Staff training programmes mushroomed and new jobs such as 'nurse adviser — child abuse' were created in the health service to implement child abuse procedures and work with social services and police.

Child protection

The late 1980s saw an increased emphasis on prevention and early intervention in child abuse. Child abuse was what adults did to children and not a term that described medical, social or police work. Child protection was the new title adopted by the register, the procedures and the nurse advisor. The first set of Department of Health guidelines, 'Working together', issued following the Butler Schloss enquiry into child abuse in Cleveland in 1988, recommended that ARCs be reconstituted as ACPCs (Area Child Protection Committees).

Organised or multiple abuse

Over the years it has become recognised that abuse of children can happen in an organised way. More recently there have been a number of well-publicised cases of child abuse happening in institutions such as children's homes. Organised or multiple abuse is the term used currently in the 1999 edition of 'Working Together to Safeguard

Children', a document issued by the Department of Health, Home Office and the Department for Education and Employment as guidance on interagency working in child protection. Previous terminology has included terms such as 'satanic abuse' and 'ritual abuse' when the abuse is thought to have had ritual elements.

A GLOBAL VIEW OF THE ILL TREATMENT OF CHILDREN

A conference in Berne in 1985 agreed the following definition.

Child abuse is any intended or unintended act or omission which adversely affects a child's health, physical growth or psychosocial development, whether or not regarded by the child or adult as abusive.

In the UK as in all industrial countries there has been a huge rise in the numbers of documented cases of child abuse and neglect in the last 20 years (Bankowski & Carballo 1986). In developing countries there has been much less reported abuse, but children's problems have been seen as a symptom of the economic and social state of the country, with widespread malnutrition and up to 20% mortality in the first 5 years. However even in developing countries specific abuse patterns are seen, for example the practice of child marriage in Bangladesh, child pawning and the use of children as beggars, prostitutes and street hawkers. In Latin America, poverty, urban drift and the abandonment of children has led to vagrant gangs of street children ruled by a brutal subculture of violence. In the Far East a whole industry exists supplying the demands of a paedophile tourist trade (Anon 1987).

War is another great abuser of children through physical injury and death and through the psychological stress of the survivors. Today's war children become tomorrow's militiamen and freedom fighters at very tender ages. Military spending as a priority directly reduces the investment in maternal and child health and education (Woolhandler & Himmelstein 1985).

Some aspects of the impact of abuse and neglect on children have long been recognised, for example death and permanent effects of injuries. However some of the longer-term effects, especially of abuse combined with neglect, on the affected children's development and abilities to function as adults have taken longer to be recognised (HMSO 1995, Department of Health 1999).

Origins of UK opinions

In this century opinions about child abuse in the UK have been shaped by three major forces.

Social and political change

This has been brought about by the work of reformers in legislating for improved education, work, social and health conditions, for example Lord Shaftesbury, and Benjamin Waugh, first director of the NSPCC, EPOCH (End Physical Punishment of Children), the campaign to end physical punishment of children, is a modern example.

The women's movement

As women have gained power over their work and home lives they have been able to speak about their childhood experiences of abuse. This has enabled people to look at the lives of today's children in order to identify abuse early and attempt to intervene.

Child abuse enquiries

One after another, starting with Lord Monckton's enquiry into the death of Denis O'Neil in foster care in 1945, these have galvanised public outrage and driven the passage of new legislation. The Department of Health has published an excellent digest of 20 enquiries over the decade 1980–89 (DH 1991). Studies of fatal child abuse such as described in 'Beyond Blame' (Reder et al 1993) and in their follow-up book 'Lost Innocents' (Reder & Duncan 1999) and documents such as 'Messages from research' (DH 1995) have been influential in guiding policy and practice. Sadly some problems persist in spite of recommendation after recommendation but gradually others improve (Tables 24.1, 24.2).

DEFINITIONS

Although books are written to describe the range of abuse, brief definitions are necessary for the purposes of research and communication and the framing of legal and criminal procedures. The following definitions are used for the purpose of the registration of abused children and have recently been updated in '*Working together* to safeguard children' (Department of Health 1999).

Table 24.1
Numbers of children on child protection registers in England (at 31 March 2000).

Age group (yr)						
	Under 1	**1–4**	**5–9**	**10–15**	**16+**	**All ages**
Numbers[a]						
Total[b]	2800	9200	9100	8400	600	30 300
Boys	1500	4800	4700	4200	200	15 400
Girls	1300	4400	4400	4200	378	14 600
Rates/10 000 population						
Total[b]	48	38	28	22	5	27
Boys	49	38	28	22	4	27
Girls	46	37	27	22	6	27

[a] Figures may not add due to rounding
[b] The 'All ages, Total' figures include 207 unborn children
Source: Department of Health 2000

Table 24.2
Registrations to child protection registers in England during the year ending 31 March 2000, by category of abuse: showing the mixed categories incorporated with the main categories.

Category of abuse	Registrations	
	No.	%
Neglect[a]	12 900	44
Physical abuse[a]	9 500	32
Sexual abuse[a]	5 100	17
Emotional abuse	4 800	17

[a] Three main categories also feature in the mixed categories. The total of the percentages will exceed 100 because children in the 'mixed' categories are counted more than once
Source: Department of Health 2000

A child or young person

The Children Act 1989 includes anyone under the age of 18 years old unless they are married.

Significant harm

The Children Act 1989 introduced the concept of significant harm as the threshold that justifies compulsory intervention in family life in the best interests of the children. There are no absolute criteria on which to rely when judging what constitutes significant harm, but consideration needs to be given to the severity of the ill treatment, including the degree and extent of physical harm, the duration and frequency of abuse and neglect and the extent of premeditation, considered alongside the family's and child's supports and strengths. The harm may be significant following a serious single event, or may be a series of events which affect a child's health and development.

Under section 31(10) of the Children Act, the question of whether harm suffered is significant rests on comparison with the health and development that could be reasonably expected of a child of similar age.

The local authority has a duty to make enquiries, or cause enquiries to be made, where it has reasonable cause to suspect that a child is suffering or is likely to suffer significant harm (section 47, Children Act 1989).

Child in need

A child is taken to be in need (under section 17 of the Children Act 1989) if:

a) he is unlikely to achieve, or maintain, or to have the opportunity of achieving or maintaining, a reasonable standard of health or development without the provision for him of services by a local authority;
b) his health or development is likely to be significantly impaired, or further impaired, without the provision for him of such services; or
c) he is disabled.

There is a general duty of every local authority, in addition to the other duties under section 17 of the Children Act, to:

a) safeguard and promote the welfare of children within their area who are in need; and
b) so far as is consistent with that duty, to promote the upbringing of such children by their families.

Physical abuse

Physical abuse may involve hitting, shaking, throwing, poisoning, burning or scalding, drowning, suffocating, or otherwise causing physical harm to a child. Physical harm may also be caused when a parent or carer feigns the symptoms of, or deliberately causes ill health to a child whom they are looking after. This situation is commonly described using terms such as factitious illness by proxy or 'Munchausen syndrome by proxy'.

Emotional abuse

Emotional abuse is the persistent emotional ill treatment of a child such as to cause severe and persistent adverse effects on the child's emotional development. It may involve conveying to children that they are worthless or unloved, inadequate, or valued only insofar as they meet the needs of another person. It may feature age or developmentally inappropriate expectations being imposed on children. It may involve causing children frequently to feel frightened or in danger, or the exploitation or corruption of children. Some level of emotional abuse is involved in all types of ill treatment of a child, though it may occur alone.

Neglect

Neglect is the persistent failure to meet a child's basic physical and/or psychological needs, likely to result in the serious impairment of the child's health or development. It may involve a parent or carer failing to provide adequate food, shelter and clothing, failing to protect a child from physical harm or danger, or the failure to ensure access to appropriate medical care or treatment. It may also include neglect of, or unresponsiveness to, a child's basic emotional needs.

Sexual abuse

Sexual abuse involves forcing or enticing a child or young person to take part in sexual activities, whether or not the child is aware of what is happening. The activities may involve physical contact, including penetrative (e.g. rape or buggery) or non-penetrative acts. They may include non-contact activities, such as involving children in looking at, or in the production of, pornographic material or watching sexual activities, or encouraging children to behave in sexually inappropriate ways.

The following categories are not defined as part of the 1989 Children Act.

Ritualistic abuse

This may be defined as repetitive, bizarre, sexual, physical, and psychological abuse of children that includes supernatural and/or religious activities (Snow & Sorensen 1990). Three forms have been typified (Finkelhor et al 1988).

- True cult based, type 1, involves child abuse as an expression of an elaborate belief system.
- Pseudo, type 2, has the sexual abuse of children as the primary motivating factor.

- Psychopathological, type 3, includes abuse as part of an obsessive or delusional system of an individual or group.

Child sex rings

Organised networks of abusers may not use ritual. A study of 11 such rings (Wild & Wynne 1986) showed that most perpetrators used child ring leaders to recruit victims. Others became a 'family friend' or obtained a position of authority over children. Secrecy was encouraged and bribery, threats and peer pressure used to induce participation in sexual activities. Detection is difficult, and conviction of such a ring, particularly when extrafamilial, is often the subject of much media interest. Many early cases in the USA revolved around children's day-care nurseries.

Interfamilial rings, particularly with a ritual element, are even harder to detect and act upon. Several large sex abuse rings alleged in Nottingham, Rochdale and the Orkneys have had such bizarre details as to be beyond general public credibility and understanding. Matters are even worse when agencies cannot agree, and instead of going forward together sharing the difficulties, retreat to opposing professional moral high ground (Her Majesty's Inspectorate of Constabulary and Social Services 1991, La Fontaine 1994, Gallagher 2000).

THEORIES OF CAUSATION

Psychopathic

Early research focused on mentally disordered parents as a cause of the problem. Kempe reported only 10% of the parents of abused children as mentally ill, however other personality traits were noted in some abusing parents. These included a distorted perception of their own children, impulsive behaviour which could also be extremely aggressive, depression and preoccupation with self and lack of empathy with the child. Many were also either victims of, or witness to, abuse themselves. Another feature was transference from parent to child. The child was seen as hostile, manipulating or persecuting and as the cause of parental problems and a focus for anger. Other features were low self-

Avoiding harm: child protection

esteem, isolation and lack of social support and problems of alcohol and drug abuse (Kempe et al 1962).

Social and environmental

This approach looks at external factors causing stress which are clearly not accounted for in the psychopathic model. These are low wages, unemployment, marital breakdown, overcrowding and poor housing. Violence is seen as an adaptation to stress. Extreme violence must be seen against the general background culture. Is violence an expected part of child rearing, either in institutions or in the home? How much of what happens inside the home is open to public interference? (Table 24.3).

Special victim

By contrast, work in the 1970s looked at how much factors in the child might be responsible for making them vulnerable or an attractor of abuse. When abused children were compared with their unharmed siblings they were found to be more likely to have had an abnormal pregnancy, to have experienced neonatal separation and to have suffered illness in the first year of life. Disability has also been associated with increased finding of abuse.

Psychosocial

This combines simpler explanations in suggesting that certain stress factors and adverse background

Table 24.3
Abusing and neglecting families.

	Neglecting families	Neglecting and abusing families
Skills	Illiteracy common Depression common Unemployment common	Wider range of skills Unemployment or frequent job changes
Family structure	Young family Partner present 'Empty' relationship	Unstable, partner changes Violent relationships
Parents' childhood	Neglected	Maltreatment
Expectations	Low	Very high or nil 'Just want peace and quiet'
Network support	Poor	Poor relationships Isolated
Parental coping strategies	Withdrawal	Violent outbursts or withdrawal Punishment is an expression of frustration
Children	Passive in infancy Can be very active, when older Developmental delay	Out of control
Prognosis	?Poor Limited skills and 'vision' of change	Variable

After Crittenden 1988

influences may serve to predispose individuals to violence which will occur in the presence of precipitating factors such as a child misbehaving. Rather than seeing 'abusers' as distinct from 'non-abusers' it is more helpful to think of a continuum of behaviour and outcome.

Integrated model

Today it is broadly accepted that a combination of social, psychological, economic and environmental factors interact together to result in abuse and neglect (Fig. 24.1).

Model for sexual abuse

Finkelhor (1984) outlined four preconditions for sexual abuse to take place, and these are described below.

1. The perpetrator needs to be motivated to abuse

Motivation may derive from one or more of three distinct sources:

a. *Emotional congruence*, whereby relating sexually to the child satisfies some important emotional need. This may be due to arrested emotional development, or the need to feel powerful and controlling. It may be a re-enactment of childhood trauma or a narcissistic identification with self as a young child.

b. *Sexual arousal*, where the child becomes a potential source of sexual gratification. In an individual perpetrator this may be due to: childhood experiences that were traumatic or strongly conditioning; modelling of sexual interest in children by someone else; misattribution of arousal clues; biological abnormality. On a social and cultural level it may be due to: child pornography; erotic portrayal of children in advertising; the male tendency to sexualise all emotional needs.

c. *Blockage*, where alternative sources of sexual gratification are not available or are less satisfying. This may be true of an individual who: has an Oedipal conflict; has a castration anxiety; fears adult females; has had traumatic sexual experiences with an adult; suffers marital problems; has inadequate social skills. There may be blockage in societies with repressive norms about masturbation and extramarital sex.

2. Whatever the motive, the perpetrator needs to overcome inhibitions within himself

In the individual, inhibitions are lowered by alcohol, psychosis, senility, impulse disorders, and by failure of the incest inhibition mechanism in family dynamics. On a social or cultural level inhibitions are weakened by social toleration of sexual interest in children, weak criminal sanctions against offenders, ideology of patriarchal prerogatives for fathers and social toleration for deviation committed while intoxicated.

3. The perpetrator needs to overcome inhibitors beyond himself

In the individual these environmental protections are lowered when the mother is absent or ill, or the mother is not close to or protective of the child. They are also reduced if the mother is dominated or abused by the father or the family is socially isolated. Other risk factors are unusual opportunities to be alone with the child, i.e. babysitting, lack of supervision of the child and unusual sleeping or rooming conditions. At a social and cultural level, environmental protective factors are overcome by child pornography, male inability to identify with the needs of children, lack of social supports for mothers, barriers to women's equality, erosion of social networks and the ideology of family sanctity.

4. The perpetrator needs to overcome resistance by the child

Although the perpetrator is completely responsible for the abuse there is no doubt that children themselves play an important part in whether or not they are abused. This goes beyond the ability to shout 'no' to an abusive approach. Subtle aspects of behaviour, personality and a 'front of invulnerability' may cause an abuser to select an alternative victim.

On an individual level a child's resistance is lowered when the child is emotionally insecure

Avoiding harm: child protection

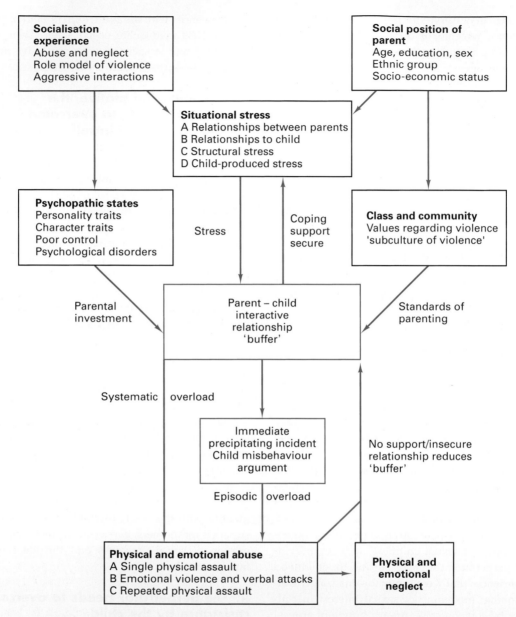

Fig. 24.1 An integrated model of child abuse and neglect. This integrated model assumes that violence in the family is influenced by situational and structural stress but that whether this stress results in violence depends upon a family buffer in the form of the strength of interpersonal relationships within the family. Insecure and anxious relationships will fail to buffer the family during stress and episodic overload may result in a physical or emotional attack. From Browne et al (1988)

or deprived or lacks knowledge about sexual abuse, where there is a situation of unusual trust between perpetrator and child, or there is bribery or coercion.

On a social and cultural level resistance is lowered by the social powerlessness of children and the unavailability of sex education for children.

This model is useful in that it is as applicable to family system models for father–daughter incest, as it is to abuse by the stranger paedophile, or abuse between children. It can also serve as a guide to work with abusive families and individuals, analysing the weak areas and serving as a guide to intervention.

This model assumes a male perpetrator. However about 5% of perpetrators are female. These divide into those who cooperate with an abusive male partner and those whose behaviour can be framed as above, but with differences. Women have much greater access to children, and because they are usually the protectors, precondition three does not apply. Society has an ambivalent attitude and is less likely to perceive that a woman who seduces a boy might harm him.

RECOGNITION OF ABUSE
Acceptance

Recognition first needs an acceptance by society that physical and sexual abuse occurs, and support for the work of professionals who make the diagnosis. Acceptance occurs in stages at different rates in different societies. All staff who work with children and families should be alert to signs that a family is under stress and in need of help in the care and parenting of their children.

General considerations

Abuse occurs to children of both sexes, at all ages and in all cultures, religions, social classes and both to children with and without disabilities.

Identification of child abuse may be difficult, with the paediatric assessment contributing to a full assessment led by social services and/or the police. The following possible indicators of abuse in the section below should be considered as part of the assessment.

Sources of stress within families may have a negative impact on a child's health and development. This is particularly so in families who are multiply disadvantaged by poverty and social exclusion. Domestic violence, parental mental illness and drug and alcohol misuse, may also have serious implications for children.

CLINICAL FEATURES OF PHYSICAL ABUSE

The interpretation of whether or not an injury has been caused by physical abuse is important in community paediatric practice.

Bruises

The following may be indicative of non-accidental bruising:

- Bruising or other injury to the face of a non-mobile child.
- Bruising to one or both eyes.
- Bruises or other injury in or around the mouth (including the labial frenulum).
- Fingertip marks (grasp marks) on the face, limbs or on the chest of a small child.
- Symmetrical bruising.
- Bruising to the ear.
- Outline bruising (e.g. belt marks, hand prints, shoe marks).
- Linear bruising (particularly on buttocks or back).
- Bruising on soft tissue without obvious explanation.
- Different ages of bruising.

Uncommon sites for accidental bruising include: mouth, cheeks, behind the ear, neck, abdomen, chest, under the arm, back, back of legs, buttocks, genital area, rectal area and soles of the feet.

Petechial haemorrhages are rashes of tiny discrete bruises which may be found on many body parts after pressure has been applied, particularly through clothes. After strangulation they may be found on the face and particularly the eyelids. Here there may also be symmetrical grip marks around the neck.

Ageing of bruises
This is not easy. The bruise is a collection of free blood cells undergoing degradation and resorption with a characteristic haem colour change sequence. Blood may track along tissue planes to show up

days later in a different site. For example a blow on the top of the head may show as colour changes under the eyes. The rate of resolution depends on the site and the amount to be resorbed. Ageing of bruises particularly from photographs is imprecise (Stephenson & Bialas 1996).

Easy bruising

Clotting disorders may not show until the child is several months old and should always be excluded in cases of unexplained bruising. Other children who are said to bruise easily may prove to be hyperactive or beyond the control of their parents. Still others seem to develop bruising that is unaccountably more severe than that of siblings following trivial trauma without any measurable abnormality of blood, skin, blood vessels or connective tissue. Here diagnosis is not usually a problem when site, distribution and explanation for the injury are evaluated.

Bruising in black children

At one time the myth that bruising would not be visible in Afro Caribbean or Asian children meant that diagnoses were missed. In fact with skins of varying depths of brown, bruises are quite clear to see in all but the faintest and oldest lesions. Injuries may also be raised, tender or accompanied by breaks in the skin. These children often react to inflammation with a deepening of skin pigmentation which can be quite marked, for example after chickenpox.

Fractures

These need to be looked for and their interpretation is definitely the realm of the experienced paediatric radiologist. Skull fractures are particularly difficult, and may cause diagnostic confusion, with differences of professional opinion. Complex, rather than simple, skull fractures are much more likely to be non-accidental. Skull fractures are rare after falls from a height of 2–5 feet (0.60–1.5 m). Kravitz (1969) found three skull fractures, all simple and linear, in 256 infants falling from this height.

Other fractures which are highly suggestive of non-accidental injury include metaphyseal fractures, rib fractures and spiral midshaft (diaphyseal) fractures.

Metaphyseal fractures

These occur particularly around knees, ankles and wrists, and are caused by gripping, pulling or twisting. There is usually no associated swelling or bruising, and they are difficult to date as there is often no callus.

Rib fractures

Rib fractures are seen posteriorly, in the mid axilla, or anteriorly. They are usually the result of severe compression, and may occur with a shaking injury. Occasionally a direct blow results in an anterior fracture, particularly in association with visceral injury.

Children who received cardiopulmonary resuscitation, prior to death, did not suffer rib fractures in two reviews of 50 and 91 infants, mean ages of 27 months and 2.4 months respectively (Feldman 1984, Spevak 1994).

Birth-related rib fractures are also extremely rare. Risk factors include birthweight more than 4000 g, shoulder dystocia and forceps delivery. A study of chest X-rays in 10 000 infants included 25 patients with rib fractures. Only one of these was due to birth trauma (shoulder dystocia) (Thomas 1997).

Long bone diaphyseal fractures

These are usually accidental, but are highly suggestive of NAI if the fracture is a spiral type. There is increased specificity for NAI if there is an inappropriate history, delay in presentation, evidence of healing or an additional injury.

Unusual fractures, for example of the hands, feet, pubic ramus, acromion or spine, may also suggest NAI.

Conditions that may lead to spontaneous fractures in infancy

The false accusation of abuse in these cases is extremely upsetting for families. A full family history, an examination of sclera and teeth, and review of X-rays should prevent error (Taitz 1991).

Profound prematurity

This is usually babies born weighing less than 1500 g. They are likely to show evidence of rickets and/or osteoporosis on X-ray. There will probably be a raised alkaline phosphatase.

Osteogenesis imperfecta
(Paterson & McAllison 1989)
Type 1 is the commonest form. The sclera are always blue, and in 90% of cases one parent will have blue sclerae and a history of multiple fractures. Some normal infants have blue sclerae, which become white at about 1 year of age.

Type 2 and 3 are very severe autosomal recessive conditions with either death or gross deformity in early infancy.

Type 4 is usually quite severe but with normal sclerae. There is controversy as to whether the condition may occur with a normal radiological appearance. Most cases have a family history of multiple fractures, odontogenesis imperfecta and deafness. It is very rare.

Patterson (1993) has suggested that a temporary collagen defect may cause fractures due to 'temporary brittle bone disease'. Thirty-nine infants had skeletal findings suggestive of NAI in association with anaemia, vomiting, neutropenia and apnoeic attacks. There was no biochemical abnormality, and this paper has had no scientific corroboration.

Copper deficiency
Fractures have been described only in preterm babies fed copper-deficient formula or given parenteral nutrition lacking in copper, or full-term infants over 5 months suffering from severe malabsorption and fed copper-deficient diets. It does not occur in normal healthy infants. All affected babies with fractures have had severe haematological abnormalities and radiological evidence of osteopenia.

Burns and scalds

These are common accidents where the precautions which protect children fail. There may be negligence on the part of the carer. More rarely they may be deliberately inflicted, perhaps as a form of punishment. They are found in 10% of physically abused children and 5% of sexually abused children. Of all children presenting at hospital with burns, between 1% and 16% receive inflicted injuries; however the differentiation from accidental aetiology is very difficult and abuse certainly goes underrecognised, particularly where the burns unit doctors are not paediatrically trained.

Scalds
Scalds have a shape which is related to dripping or splashing and are often altered to follow the contours of clothes. They most commonly occur when a toddler pulls a container of hot fluid from a high kitchen surface, causing irregular burns on the face, arms and upper trunk. Similar patterns can occur if, for example, a cupful of hot tea is thrown over a child. Scalds on the extensor surfaces are more likely to result from abuse. Symmetrical glove and stocking burns are also suspect. One characteristic pattern is the doughnut burn which results from forced immersion of the buttocks in a sink of hot water. Extensive burns occur but there is sparing of the centre of the buttocks which is cooled by contact with ceramic.

Dry contact burns
These burns cause a well-defined mark of uniform depth in the shape of the object that touched the skin.

Cigarette burns
Cigarette burns produce characteristic superficial elliptical and usually solitary marks when accidental. The marks of inflicted burns are deep circular ulcers and their coincidence with other injuries is quite significant. They are not common and the lesion the doctor is likely to be asked about will usually come from the long differential diagnosis including impetigo, old chickenpox, insect bites, eczema, psoriasis and excoriated spots.

Bites

There may be clear impressions of teeth on the skin, or oval- or crescent-shaped marks from a bite. Distinguishing between adult and child bites can be difficult, as an adult can produce a bite mark of small diameter. Rapid access to a forensic odontologist is invaluable in establishing the perpetrator.

Scars

Most children have scars, but an exceptionally large number of scars of differing ages or those of an unusual shape should raise the likelihood of physical abuse.

Other injuries

Deliberate poisoning occurs mainly in children below the age of two and a half years. The child may be presented as having ingested the drug accidentally, they may present with inexplicable symptoms of acute onset, or with recurrent unexplained illnesses as in fabricated disorder by proxy. Poisoning is a cause of sudden unexpected death.

Conditions which may be mistaken for child abuse

Striae in various parts of the body associated with obesity, adolescence or steroids may resemble stick marks. *Specific ethnic practices* such as hot cupping, coin rubbing and tribal tattooing need understanding in their correct context. *Mongolian blue spots* are patches of blue/black pigmentation classically found on the lumbar and sacral regions of Afrocaribbean children at birth. They continue to be mistaken for the marks of inflicted injury. What is less well known is that the markings can also be found in caucasian children of every skin tone, more commonly in Indian and Pakistani children, less commonly in Mediterranean children. The marks may be on other parts of the body, for example shoulders and hands.

FACTITIOUS DISORDER BY PROXY ABUSE

Factitious disorder by proxy abuse was previously referred to as Munchausen by proxy. It occurs when an adult deliberately fabricates the history of an illness, its symptoms, or induces signs of such an illness in a child in order to gain medical attention (usually hospital admission).

This is a form of child abuse as there is a likelihood of this behaviour causing significant harm to the child. This harm may be indirect as the consequence of multiple investigations and hospital admissions, or direct due to the inducing of physical signs in the child. It may lead to the death of the child.

Fabrications, verbally of histories or active induction of illness in a child, can involve: descriptions of apnoeic attacks, description of vomiting, diluting feeds, passing blood in stools or urine, failure to thrive, placing blood on a nappy, description or induction of fits, induced skin lesions, specimen contamination, poisoning. In addition, children may be referred to child mental health services with reports of disturbed behaviour. There is usually a significant discrepancy between parental reports and observed behaviour. Factitious pregnancy and miscarriages are associated with sudden unexpected death in infancy. Sometimes the perpetrator may have a history of factitious disorder (15–20%), or may make false allegations of child abuse. There may be frequent and often inappropriate consultations for the child or siblings.

Factitious disorder by proxy can best be regarded as a spectrum of abusive behaviour, with at its core a deviant group of dangerous abusers, merging out at its boundaries to a group of mothers who are having difficulty with parenting, and who inappropriately seek help or relief by expressing their problems through their child's physical health.

NON-ACCIDENTAL HEAD INJURY

Child abuse is the most common cause of serious head injury in children under 1 year of age. Accidental injury (other than serious trauma such as a car accident) rarely causes intracranial injury in infants. Non-accidental head injury (NAHI) should be suspected when there are other features of serious abuse (visceral/bony injuries) or if there is a history of shaking in a baby under 2 years of age. In addition NAHI may be identified on imaging during investigation of an undiagnosed intracranial problem, retinal haemorrhages, an enlarged head or in the unconscious or encephalopathic child.

The establishment of the aetiology of a subdural haemorrhage requires a full multidisciplinary social assessment, ophthalmic examination, a skeletal survey, a coagulation screen and imaging by MRI or CT scan, both on initial assessment and subsequently at 7–10 days depending on local radiology arrangements.

SUDDEN UNEXPECTED DEATH IN INFANCY

The incidence of 'cot death' has dropped dramatically from 1.8 in 1000 live births in 1989 to 0.68 in 1000 live births in 1994, due principally to the 'Back to sleep' and 'Reduce the risk' campaigns.

As the incidence has fallen, so more of these deaths must be regarded as suspicious. Features that should raise suspicion of an unnatural infant death include: previous unusual or unexplained events reported by parents (stopping breathing, looking blue, twitching), external signs at death (frank blood in the mouth, nose or on the face, unusual bruising or petechiae), fractures, or foreign bodies in the upper airways or stomach found at post-mortem, factitious disorder in parents, particularly factitious obstetric disorder, and a history of sudden unexplained death of another child of one or both parents.

NEGLECT

Children suffering from neglect may present to the doctor in many ways. The paediatrician's role is firstly to assess the child's growth, development and physical health and to identify and treat any medical conditions which may be affecting the child's welfare. The paediatric assessment contributes to the assessments of other professionals such as health visitor, social workers and teacher. Secondly the paediatrician may contribute to interventions to help the child and family and thirdly will be able to monitor and review the effect on growth and development. Furthermore the doctor must be able to recognise when interventions are not changing anything for the child and be able to act accordingly.

Frozen watchfulness

This is the apt description of a child who has become emotionally damaged from prolonged abuse. The face is expressionless and the child is motionless and afraid to speak. The eyes are wary that the next adult encounter may be painful. 'Radar gaze' describes the searching eyes of a neglected child hungry for any human contact.

'Pick me up and cuddle me someone' describes the behaviour of the neglected child who by toddler age has not developed close bonds with family adults and therefore shows no wariness for strangers.

Failure to thrive (see also Chapter 9)

Failure to thrive (FTT) implies both a failure to grow and a failure of emotional and developmental progress. There are many medical causes for this, but when due to parental neglect and abuse the term 'non-organic failure to thrive' (NOFTT) is used. The diagnosis of NOFTT is synonymous in many health visitors' minds with the presence of severe social deprivation.

There has been considerable debate as to whether emotional deprivation in the presence of adequate calories may cause abnormal growth in children under two. The current feeling is that the lack of calories is the cause. The problem is that this is often difficult to prove. Maternal dietary histories are notoriously unreliable and families quickly learn to provide the answers that health professionals wish to hear. The food may have been offered as stated but studies have shown that poor weight gain may be associated with a number of poor feeding practices: irregular and unpredictable mealtimes; very rapid spoon feeding; lack of age-appropriate supervision; lack of interpersonal contact during feeding; distraction such as watching television during feeding; inappropriate seating (Skuse & Wolke 1992).

Hospital inpatient investigation is often arranged to confirm the diagnosis by showing a continued poverty of growth and development in the face of adequate calorie intake. A positive diagnosis of NOFTT may also be made when there is a very rapid weight gain whilst in hospital. Similar catch-up of both weight (and height over the longer term) is also seen in children moved away from abuse and neglect into a substitute family environment, for example with relatives or foster parents.

Often FTT is applied loosely to growth measurements alone where use of the term 'failure to grow' is more accurate. This is understandable as height, weight and head circumference are easy and objective data to gather. In very young infants particularly, weights are the most sensitive indicator of well being and may change quite rapidly.

Certain growth changes should make people consider a risk of FTT: a child falling away from a previously maintained percentile; a child whose weight percentile drops well below his/her length percentile; any child below the third percentile. Older children may show fall off in linear growth, 'deprivation dwarfism'. Because the main growth is in the long bones, such children tend to maintain relatively infantile proportions of trunk to limbs. Wasting of muscles and frequent infections and reduced actively levels are further signs of protein-energy malnutrition. In extreme starvation the picture may be of frank marasmus. The weight loss and muscle wasting may be somewhat masked by ascites and peripheral oedema in the child whose diet is protein deficient though adequate in fluid, carbohydrate and fat, for example a diet of sweets, juice, bread, butter, chips and tea. Other features which make this similar to the kwashiorkor of developing countries are thin pale weak hair, iron-deficiency anaemia and general apathy.

Deprivation hands and feet

Cold purple and red swollen extremities are found in children subjected to severe neglect. The cause is not known though it may be a form of disuse atrophy. It improves when the children's needs are met again (Glover et al 1985).

Developmental delay

Although there are many recognised medical causes of delayed development, it must be remembered that slow progress and late attainment of milestones may be part of the picture of neglect. In some cases, the child's developmental needs are not being met, for example there are no appropriate toys available in spite of advice and opportunities given to parents. In other situations the child may have special needs and/or disabilities requiring extra input which the parents are unable to give even with extra support being provided to them.

Failure to attend or poor attendance at school may also come to the paediatrician's notice. There are many reasons for this but it may be part of a picture of neglect.

Failure/reluctance to take up health services

On its own this is not necessarily a sign of neglect. However when the appointments are for treatment and follow-up of potentially life-threatening conditions it is essential to take appropriate action, which could include applying the child protection procedures if necessary where there is risk of the child suffering significant harm. Assessment of possible neglect should include a careful chronology of health appointments offered and whether they were taken up or not. A medical opinion about the likely effects of failed appointments on the child's health and development forms part of the assessment.

Behavioural difficulties

Neglected children can present with a variety of behavioural problems to paediatricians or to other agencies. Such children have also usually suffered emotional harm. It is essential when working with such children and young people that paediatricians work closely with the other professionals involved (see also section on 'Emotional abuse' below).

EMOTIONAL ABUSE

Emotional abuse refers to a persistent pattern of parental behaviour unrelated to a child's needs, together with severe emotional or behavioural problems in the child. The *sustained repetitive inappropriate* response to a child's experience and expression of emotion provokes persistent negative emotions, such as fear, humiliation, distress, despair and inhibits appropriate emotional expression. It leads to serious impairment of social and emotional development.

Cognitive and educational impairment also occur particularly when *sustained repetitive inappropriate* behaviour (such as domestic violence, desertion, unpredictability, exploitation) damage intelligence, memory, perception, attention and imagination.

The recognition of emotional abuse can be difficult as it refers to a parent–child relationship, not an event or single interaction. All parents at times act or behave undesirably towards their children, but the concern in emotional abuse is the pervasiveness, persistence and inflexibility of relationship patterns (Glaser 1993). There is a problem of threshold, i.e. it is open to opinion when a particular behaviour, such as criticism, becomes abusive.

Impairments of development seen in emotionally abused children include:

- Emotional state — unhappiness, low self-esteem, fear, distress, anxiety.
- Insecure attachment.
- Behavioural change — attention-seeking, oppositional, responsibilities inappropriate for age.
- Peer relationships — withdrawn or isolated, aggressive.
- Developmental/educational attainment and opportunity — developmental or educational underachievement, non-attendance or persistent lateness.
- Physical state — non-organic pains and symptoms, physical neglect, poor growth.

Concern about emotional abuse often arise not just from observation of a child's impaired development, but also from both knowledge of harmful parental attributes or behaviours, and/or the witnessing of abusive patterns of interaction.

Alcohol and drug abuse, domestic violence and mental ill health are important risk factors, and featured singly or in combination in 61% of families registered for emotional abuse in four different local authorities (Department of Health 1996). The same study revealed common categories of ill treatment to the children: denigration or rejection in 31%, emotional neglect in 28%, inappropriate expectations in 23%, repeated separations in 11%, the use of a child for parental emotional needs in 6% and mis-socialisation in 1%.

A community paediatrician is well placed to recognise emotional abuse, particularly when gaining an understanding of a child's development or emotional/behavioural difficulties. Emotionally abusive interactions may be observed in a clinic when a child is seen for a general paediatric problem. After recognition comes the more difficult task of helping the family to understand the abusive nature of the interactions, and then to help them bring about change in the relationship with their children.

The dimensions shown in Box 24.1 provide a helpful framework for describing the nature and quality of parental harmful behaviour.

CLINICAL FEATURES OF SEXUAL ABUSE

The presentation of sexual abuse occurs in a number of ways, some clearly indicating a high probability of abuse, whilst others (a more common situation) raise this as a possibility. A clear disclosure of abuse is the most important single factor in making a diagnosis. Physical signs of sexual abuse are rare, and a substantial proportion of sexually abused children have no abnormal physical signs, the proportion depending on the type of abuse, and the time elapsed from the last abusive episode to the time of examination.

Normal anatomy must be familiar to any doctor attempting to interpret signs of possible abuse (Fig. 24.2). This chapter does not attempt to duplicate the excellent colour atlas illustrations now available (Chadwick et al 1989, Meadow 1997) nor more specialist texts (Royal College of Physicians 1997, Hobbs, Hanks and Wynne 1999).

External injuries/physical abuse

A proportion of children (10–20%) suffer both physical abuse and sexual abuse (Hobbs & Wynne 1990). Grip marks on the thighs and pelvis, and bruising or other signs of perianal, oral or genital trauma are particularly suspicious. Penile bruising and laceration may be due to sexual abuse but the distinction from accidental causes may be difficult. Oral injury should be specifically excluded.

Non-specific perianal appearances
Perianal erythema
This may result from the friction of unlubricated or intracrural intercourse but it is non-specific. Com-

Box 24.1
Dimensions of emotionally abusive or inappropriate relationships (Glaser 1993)

A. Persistent negative attitudes
Persistent negative attitudes towards the child may be expressed both verbally and non-verbally and may take various forms. These include:

1) Negative attributions and attitudes:
   Persistent denigration
   Persistent blame
   Ascribing inherent (possibly inherited) badness to the child with an expectation of the expression of this attribute by the child
   Belittling
   Mocking

2) Harsh discipline and over-control:
   Terrorising through threats of severe physical punishment
   Threats of abandonment, including placing the children 'in care'
   Isolating the child in confined or frightening situations
   Discipline by imitative retaliation

B. Promoting insecure attachment
Through conditional parenting:
Making the child's continued care by the parent contingent on the child's good behaviour
Making parental benevolence conditional on the child's gratitude

C. Inappropriate developmental expectations and considerations
Inappropriate imposition of responsibility on the child associated with blame for mishaps and perceived failures
Expectation of young children to accommodate to parents' needs
Frequent unexplained or unpredictable separations
Age-inappropriate exposure to experiences and failure to protect from inappropriate experiences
Failure to contain, or inappropriate expectation of self-control by the child
Overprotection — deprivation of opportunities to explore, individuate, learn (including collusion with school non-attendance) and form peer relationships
Deprivation of opportunities to gain emotional strength through modifying innate disabilities or combating (discomfort of) fears and anxieties
Failure to offer age-appropriate, honest and consistent explanations and cognitive explorations

D. Emotional unavailability

E. Failure to recognise child's individuality and psychological boundaries
Active involvement of the child in expression of delusional or overvalued ideation
Deployment of the child in pursuit of the carer's emotional needs
Projective identification
Failure to acknowledge the child's personality, worth and wishes
Failure to accommodate (age appropriately) to the child's personality and wishes
Attempts to modify coercively the child's personality

F. Cognitive distortions and inconsistencies
Presenting internally contradictory messages
Mystification
Inconsistent parental expectations
Unpredictable parental responses

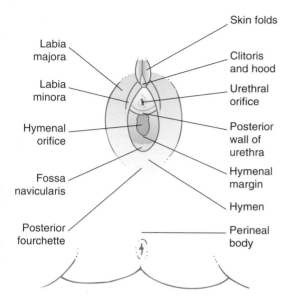

Fig. 24.2 Normal anatomy of the pre-pubertal vulva. Vestibule = area enclosed by labia minora

(Labels, clockwise from top): Skin folds; Clitoris and hood; Urethral orifice; Posterior wall of urethra; Hymenal margin; Hymen; Perineal body; Posterior fourchette; Fossa navicularis; Hymenal orifice; Labia minora; Labia majora

moner causes are infection with candida or thread-worms or streptococcus, poor hygiene and faecal soiling.

Vulvovaginitis

Vulvitis (soreness, itchiness, burning on micturition) or vaginitis (vaginal discharge, symptoms of vulvitis) or both is not uncommon in prepubertal girls. There are a number of causes, of which sexual abuse is one.

Causes of vulvitis

Poor hygiene, skin sensitivity (e.g. bubble baths), eczema, threadworms, excessive washing, infections (e.g. streptococcus), sexually transmitted disease, child sexual abuse.

Causes of vulvovaginitis

Non-specific, infection with group B streptococcus, *Staphylococcus aureus*, *Haemophilus influenzae*, *Gardnerella vaginosis*, sexually transmitted disease, rarely a foreign body.

Anal signs in abuse

There may be no physical changes seen in the anus even with a clear admission of abuse.

Examination is usually done in the left lateral position with hips and knees well flexed. To perform the buttock separation test, the buttocks are gently parted to show the anal area and observation is made for 30 seconds, during which time the external sphincter contracts briefly and is often subsequently seen to relax. A positive test i.e. one which shows reflex anal dilatation, involves a dynamic relaxation of the internal as well as the external sphincter so that the anus looks like a central hole with a clear view into the rectum.

Reflex anal dilatation (RAD)

This phenomenon is not clearly understood (Royal College of Physicians 1997). It has been linked with abuse (Hobbs & Wynne 1986) but interpretation of this sign should be done with caution. As an isolated sign, RAD does not have diagnostic significance. However, persistent well-marked RAD in an otherwise normal child should be followed up.

Anal laxity

Reduced anal tone producing a lax anus may be found in children with neurogenic bowel problems such as spina bifida. Anal dilatation has been described in association with myotonic dystrophy and may also be seen in children having a general anaesthetic and in seriously ill children, for example on a ventilator in intensive care. It has also been described as a post-mortem finding when the sphincters are relaxed. Without any other explanation, anal laxity is supportive but not diagnostic of abuse.

Anal fissures

Acute anal fissures are not unusual in young children who have not been abused (Royal College of Physicians 1997) and may be associated with constipation, diarrhoea, eczema, threadworms, nappy rash or lichen sclerosis. They are usually in the midline, either in the anterior or posterior position.

Anal lacerations

In the absence of a reasonable alternative explanation, a fresh laceration or a healed scar extending onto the perianal skin beyond the anal margin is the only specific indicator of anal abuse (Royal College of Physicians 1997).

Acute changes

Acute changes such as venous congestion, swelling, erythema, fissures and bruising are supportive but not diagnostic of abuse.

Chronic changes

Chronic changes such as reduced anal verge skin folds as a result of thickening of the skin of the anal verge, increased elasticity and reduction in the power of the anal sphincter, are supportive but not diagnostic of abuse (Royal College of Physicians 1997).

Vulval and vaginal signs in abuse

It is usual in the UK to examine the child in the supine, frog-leg position using separation and then gentle traction of the labia between the thumb and index finger. If the posterior hymen is not clearly seen, then the prone knee–chest position which allows relaxation of the pelvic floor muscles will usually enable this area of tissue to become more visible. Digital examination of the vagina is indicated only in exceptional circumstances, and mainly in postpubertal young people. A colposcope which provides a good light source, magnification and a convenient means of photography, may be helpful in the examination but is not essential.

Accidental injuries such as the classic straddle fall usually cause superficial and anterior damage. Typical findings would be a linear bruise or laceration across the labia and swelling and bruising in the clitoral area. With the specific and rare exceptions of falls onto a sharp object, damage to the hymen and other internal vaginal structures are not accidental. Though children may in experiment or in imitation of abuse insert objects into the vagina, they avoid hurting themselves. Masturbation in young girls is common but clitoral stimulation cannot be used to explain abnormalities of the hymen. Bruising, swelling, erythema, abrasions and tears of the external genitalia and introitus may result from attempted penetration. In addition there may be damage to the posterior fourchette, periurethral structures, hymen and vaginal mucosa. Healing can occur rapidly and there may be little to see in the way of abnormalities even when there is a clear history and admission of abuse.

Signs diagnostic of penetrating trauma are: hymenal tears and deficits and tearing or scarring of the posterior fourchette or vaginal wall. Also longstanding and gradually escalating abuse may produce a one-sided or generalised attenuation or absence of the hymenal tissue.

Findings which are supportive of abuse but are not in themselves diagnostic are: a notch or cleft in the posterior hymenal edge which may be associated with scarring, evidence of acute injury such as localised oedema and erythema or minor abrasions; a posterior fourchette scar. Labial fusion may follow labial inflammation both from infection and from trauma. Its presence often complicates interpretation.

Lichen sclerosus et atrophicus

This is a very rare condition. Its pearly, friable and sometimes excoriated and purpuric or bruised appearance can be mistaken for signs of sexual abuse.

SEXUALLY TRANSMITTED DISEASES

In children the presence of any sexually transmitted organism indicates that sexual abuse may have occurred. However, unlike in adults, other modes of transmission have to be considered. Some organisms have long and variable latent periods and can be transmitted vertically, so it is important to consider the age of the child and look for information about parental infection, especially if the child is less than 3 years of age (Royal College of Physicians 1997). Although not frequent, cases of non-sexual transmission have been reported (Neinstein et al 1984). The presence of a sexually transmitted disease (STD) cannot be used as an absolute indicator that abuse has taken place but it may be used as corroborative evidence and indicate a high probability of child sexual abuse (Royal College of Physicians 1997).

Genital warts

These are caused by human papillomavirus (HPV). In adults they are usually sexually transmitted and have an incubation period of several months. Transmission in children is more complex than in the adult. Vertical transmission in utero or at birth can occur, and due to the prolonged incubation period warts may not appear for 1–2 years. Transmission from a carer's hands and also autoinoculation from hands to genitals has been documented (Fleming et al 1987). It was hoped that advances in DNA typing might help in tracing the route of infection (types 1–4 are usually found in skin whilst 6, 11, 16, 18 are typically genital), but this remains a research tool.

The reported correlation with sexual abuse in children over 2 years old is too high to ignore but not high enough to be useful in its own right. Examination of the child's parents/carers and siblings for evidence of clinical or subclinical evidence HPV infection may provide useful information. There is an association with cervical intraepithelial neoplasia in some of the mothers. The diagnosis will depend on the presence of other indicators such as a known offender in the household or other physical or behavioural signs such as a second STD or a direct disclosure of abuse. The possible implications of the diagnosis should be discussed with the family prior to referral for surgical or dermatological treatment.

Neisseria gonorrhoea

Neisseria gonorrhoea is a fragile bacterium that requires intimate contact with mucus-secreting or epithelial cells for transmission. Perinatal vertical transmission into the conjunctiva of the newborn eye is a cause of neonatal ophthalmia. All other documented infection is by direct sexual inoculation into for example, urethra, cervix, anus or oropharynx. Non-sexual transmission remains a technical possibility but has never been demonstrated in vivo. The incubation period is 3–7 days and both adults and children (up to 45%) may be asymptomatic. In girls the commonest symptoms are vaginal discharge and vulvovaginitis. Gonorrhoea in children over 1 year of age is highly suggestive of sexual abuse. Appropriate treatment should be given in consultation with genitourinary medicine colleagues.

Chlamydia trachomatis

This is an obligate intracellular bacterium whose lifecycle is such that there may be prolonged subclinical infection. The infection can be transmitted vertically during birth and sexually. There is some evidence that rectovaginal infection may persist for several years after birth or after sexual contact. Current thinking is that if the organism is present over the age of 2 years it is likely to be due to abuse, particularly if the alleged abuser is also infected and asymptomatic infection of the mother has been excluded.

In adults infection with *Chlamydia* is commoner than gonorrhoea. In studies in the UK *Chlamydia* infection has been found in about 10% of adolescents attending at genitourinary clinics. Clinical presentation may be with discharge or cervical inflammation but many girls are asymptomatic. There is a high risk of subsequent pelvic inflammatory disease in girls with its resultant complications (e.g. future infertility). Screening for *Chlamydia* infection should therefore be seriously considered for all girls who have been sexually abused, particularly as testing can now be carried out using urine samples. Treatment should be given in consultation with specialists in genitourinary medicine.

Trichomonas vaginalis

This is a unicellular flagellate thriving only in the genitourinary tract of humans. If found in children older than 6 weeks, sexual contact is almost certain and evaluation for sexual abuse is indicated, together with screening for other STDs. The organism does not survive very long in the alkaline prepubertal vagina so that the finding of *T. vaginalis* is suggestive of recent abuse.

Genital herpes

Herpes simplex (HSV) types 1 and 2 can cause genital herpes. The virus is transmitted by close personal contact. Genital herpes infection in children and adolescents is uncommon. Primary infection is usually clinically obvious, causing vesicular and ulcerated genital lesions which are painful, with tender inguinal lymphadenopathy and systemic symptoms. The presence of genital herpes is likely to be due to sexual contact.

Bacterial vaginosis

This is one of the commonest causes of vaginal infection in adults. It is a polymicrobial infection with a mixture of vaginal anaerobes, *Gardnerella vaginalis* and other Gram-negative organisms. Bacterial vaginosis and the isolation of *G. vaginalis* is uncommon in healthy non-abused children. On its own, the probability of abuse is not high and it should not be considered more than weak support for a diagnosis of abuse (Royal College of Physicians 1997).

Syphilis

Fortunately syphilis is very rare in pre-pubertal children in the UK and if not congenital should be presumed to be the result of abuse.

HIV

HIV infection in children in the UK to date has been acquired congenitally or by infected blood products, and not from sexual activity. However transmission through sexual assault has been reported (Gutman et al 1991, Gellert et al 1993). Now that there is increasing evidence of benefit from the use of antiviral agents and the early treatment of complications, screening for HIV should be carefully considered for children at high risk, for example when the perpetrator has had multiple partners, is an intravenous drug user, or comes from an area where HIV is endemic, or when the young person is engaged in prostitution or drug abuse.

Screening for hepatitis B and possibly also for hepatitis C should be included.

Testing should not be done without appropriate discussion and consent given either by the young person or their parents or carers.

INTERAGENCY WORKING IN CHILD PROTECTION

Promoting the welfare of children and safeguarding them from harm, depends crucially on effective information-sharing, collaboration and understanding between agencies and professionals. Cooperation in this area of work is *mandatory*. The Department of Health (DH) has clear expectations of agencies (including health service organisations and their staff) in relation to safeguarding children and joint-working. These expectations are outlined in the following guidance: 'Working together to safeguard children' (Department of Health 1999), 'Child protection — medical responsibilities — guidance to doctors working with child protection agencies' (1996), 'Child protection — clarification of arrangements between the NHS and other agencies' (1995).

Area child protection committees

'Working together to safeguard children' (1999) provides a *national framework* within which agencies and professionals at local level, both individually and jointly, draw up and agree on their own, more detailed ways, of working together. Each local authority (with social services responsibility) has to ensure that there is an area child protection committee (ACPC) in their area. Membership is agreed locally but should consist of representatives of all the main agencies, as well as professionals responsible for helping to protect children from abuse and neglect. The health authority ensures that there is suitable health service involvement in, and commitment to, the work of the ACPC. The ACPC agrees how different services and professional groups should cooperate and has responsibility for developing, monitoring and reviewing child protection polices, and standards of practice. Subgroups or working groups may also be set up locally to carry out specific tasks on behalf of the ACPC, for example, to represent a defined geographical area within the ACPC's boundaries, to maintain or update procedures and protocols, to review child deaths and serious cases, or to identify interagency training needs and arrange/deliver training.

It is imperative that all health staff have easy access to, and are familiar with, their ACPC child protection procedures plus any organisational policies, protocols or guidelines. Whilst these are not an end in themselves, they do promote safe, effective practice and better outcomes for the child.

Roles and responsibilities

Local authorities (social services) have specific legal duties in respect of children under the Children Act 1989. Two very important areas of responsibility are firstly, under section 17, they have a general duty to safeguard and promote the welfare of children in their area who are in need by providing appropriate support and services. Secondly, under section 47, they have a duty to make enquiries if they have reason to suspect that a child in their area 'is suffering, or is likely to suffer significant harm', to enable them to decide whether they should take any action to safeguard or promote the child's welfare.

It is important to note that the Children Act 1989 also places other agencies *including health services* under a duty to cooperate in the interests of vulnerable children, by assisting the local authority in providing support and services to children in need (section 27) and by assisting local authorities with their enquiries, where it is suspected that a child is suffering, or is likely to suffer significant harm (section 47).

Children in need

Child protection practice has been re-focused in response to research commissioned by the Department of Health ('Child protection — messages from research' 1995). This suggested that too many children and families were being referred and managed within a child protection process, rather than being seen as children 'in need'. This often resulted in alienation of families, a lack of ongoing support and poor outcomes for the child. Agencies were criticised for using a 'sledge-hammer to crack a nut' by using heavy child protection 'investigation' processes inappropriately, which were often seen as the only means of unlocking much-needed resources for children and families. There is now

much more emphasis on conducting 'enquiries', rather than 'investigations' into individual circumstances and improving the quality of assessments. This is turn informs decision-making about the most appropriate course of action to take, resulting in the provision of 'needs-led' services. 'Working together to safeguard children' (Department of Health 1999) also refers to 'safeguarding' children, rather than 'child protection' which signifies that the needs of the child and family should been seen in a much broader context, giving consideration to the *overall* welfare needs of the child.

Work with children and families where there are concerns about a child's welfare is sensitive and difficult. Good practice requires effective joint-working, information-sharing, and sensitive working with parents and carers, in the best interest of the child. Competent professional judgements need to be based on a thorough assessment of the child's needs and consideration of the parent's capacity to respond to those needs (including their capacity to protect the child from harm) and the wider family circumstances.

In order to facilitate this process, the Department of Health has issued new guidance, 'The framework for the assessment of children in need and their families' (Department of Health 2000) which provides a tool for collecting and analysing information to support quality assessments and professional judgements. The 'Framework' looks at a broad spectrum of a child's developmental needs, family and environmental factors, and parenting capacity (Fig. 24.3). The Framework is to be used nationally within social services departments (and other agencies) for the assessment of *all* children in need, including those for whom there are concerns about significant harm. The Framework will be used to inform professional assessments from the first point of contact through the processes of 'initial' and more detailed 'core' assessments (where appropriate). By improving the quality of assessments, it is envisaged that referrals to social services will be more appropriate and that subsequent interventions, decision-making and service provision will lead to better outcomes for the child and family. The Framework will be very relevant to community paediatricians and a wide range of community and acute health service practitioners.

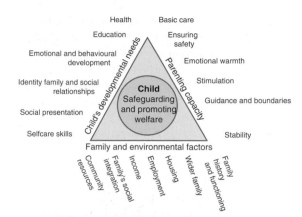

Fig. 24.3 The assessment framework. (Adapted from Department of Health 2000)

There are major training implications for all agencies to implement the 'Assessment Framework' during 2001/2002. Obviously, some situations will still need to be managed promptly within the ACPC child protection procedures and the Framework will not detract from this. For those children who are suffering, or at risk of suffering significant harm, joint working is essential to safeguard the children and, where necessary, to help bring to justice the perpetrators of crimes against children.

HEALTH PROFESSIONAL INVOLVEMENT IN CHILD PROTECTION

Because of the universal nature of health provision, health professionals are often the first to be aware that families are experiencing difficulties in looking after their children. In view of this, 'Working together to safeguard children' (Department of Health 1999) emphasises that the involvement of health professionals is important in all stages of work with children and families, for example:

- Recognising children in need of support and/or safeguarding, and parents who may need extra help in bringing up their children.
- Contributing to enquiries about a child and family.
- Assessing the needs of children and the capacity of parents to meet their children's needs.

- Planning and providing support to vulnerable children and families.
- Participating in child protection conferences.
- Planning support for children at risk of significant harm.
- Providing therapeutic help to abused children and parents under stress (e.g. mental illness).
- Playing a part, through the child protection plan, in safeguarding children from significant harm.
- Contributing to case reviews.

Individual children, especially some of the most vulnerable children and those at greatest risk of social exclusion, will need coordinated help from health, education, social services, and quite possibly the voluntary sector and other agencies, including youth justice services.

Referrals

If anyone has concerns about a child's welfare and/or believes that a child may be suffering from, or at risk of suffering from harm, then these concerns must always be referred to the social services department without delay, in accordance with local ACPC Child Protection Procedures. For professionals making a referral, internal arrangements may apply about who makes the decision to refer and how this is done, but it is important that this is undertaken *promptly*. At the end of any discussion about a child and family, the referrer and social services should be clear about who will be taking what action and when, or that no further action is necessary and why. Telephone referrals should always be confirmed in writing and a contemporaneous record made of the nature of the concerns and any discussions or actions undertaken by the individual practitioner.

Individual accountability for making referrals

Where there is uncertainty about an individual case, or perhaps a conflict of opinion between professionals about whether or not the concerns meet the criteria for referral under the procedures, specialist advice and support should be obtained from the named or designated professionals for child protection. There are named professionals in each health trust and designated professionals for each health authority. Having said this, if following these discussions the individual practitioner remains concerned about the welfare and safety of the child, they must *act independently* and refer their concerns to social services, in the best interests of the child.

Talking to parents/carers

Whilst professionals are encouraged to discuss any concerns they may have with the family and, where possible, seek their agreement to making a referral, this should only be done where such discussion and agreement-seeking will not place a child (or member of staff) at increased risk of harm, or jeopardise a possible criminal enquiry. Failure to gain parental agreement to a referral where a child may be at risk of harm should not prevent the professional from contacting social services about their concerns at the earliest opportunity.

The child protection register

Enquiries should be made to the child protection register where there are concerns about a child but this should not replace the need to make a formal referral to social services. The register contains information about children in the area who are at continuing risk of significant harm, and for whom there are active child protection plans in place. If the child is registered, the enquirer will be given information about the category of registration and the name and contact details of the key worker. All register enquiries are logged, which enables concerns shared by other sources/agencies to be linked together. If a second enquiry is received about a child who is not registered, the custodian of the register will refer this to social services as a child who may be 'in need'.

Social services response to referrals

Social services will gather information from other sources, including checking existing records, or speaking to other professionals (this may include the police where a criminal offence has been com-

mitted), and then within 24 hours decide on what further action to take.

Referrals may lead to no further action (the referrer will be notified of this), or to the provision of support and help (by social services or other agencies), or to a fuller initial assessment of the needs and circumstances of the child, which may, in turn, be followed by section 47 enquiries.

Immediate protection

At any point in the process, if there is a risk to the life of a child, or a likelihood of serious immediate harm either to the subject child, siblings, or other children who may be in contact with the alleged perpetrator, emergency action will be taken by an agency with statutory child protection powers (e.g. social services, the police or the NSPCC). *Note*: a child may need immediate protection where a parent does not follow medical advice or refuses urgent medical treatment for a child. This may also apply where children are removed from hospital care, placing them at grave personal risk. In these circumstances, medical staff will need to make a professional judgement about the implications for the child and decide if an urgent referral to social services is required. The police may also need to be contacted where an *immediate response* is required, either to prevent a child being removed from a hospital/clinical setting (police protection), or to trace a child who has been removed and there is an urgent need for medical treatment.

Initial assessment

Referrals to social services will usually lead to an *initial assessment*. This will apply to all children in need, whether or not there are child protection concerns, and should be completed within 7 working days. The Department of Health document, 'Framework for the assessment of children in need and their families' will be used to assess whether the child being referred is a child 'in need' (under section 17 of the Children Act) or whether the child is 'in need of protection' (section 47 of the Children Act). The assessment will involve social services speaking to the child and family, and analysing information from historical records and others involved in working with the family.

Note: Even if the initial reason for a referral was a concern about abuse or neglect, and this is not subsequently substantiated, a family may still benefit from support and practical help to promote a child's health and development. In fact, where the initial assessment indicates that a child may be 'in need', the 'Framework for assessment' enables a *core assessment* to be undertaken to look at the child's overall health and development, and the parent's capacity to respond to their child's needs. This assists in deciding which services are most likely to result in good outcomes for the child and family.

Suspected actual or likely significant harm

In some cases it may be obvious at the point of referral, that a child is in need of protection, in which case enquiries will proceed immediately under section 47 of the Children Act. However, this may only become apparent during the assessment process. Where a child is suspected to be suffering from, or is at risk of suffering from significant harm, social services will undertake a core assessment by way of section 47 enquiries to decide whether intervention is needed to safeguard a child and promote their welfare and, if so, how this can best be achieved. The 'Framework for assessment' is equally relevant here, as it provides a structure for collecting and analysing information about the child and family.

Strategy discussion

Whenever it is suspected that a child is suffering, or likely to suffer significant harm, a strategy discussion should take place between social services, the police and other agencies as appropriate (e.g. education and health). This may take place at a meeting or over the telephone. *Where a medical examination is required, a senior doctor from the providing service should be included.* The discussion enables information to be shared and decisions made regarding whether section 47 enquiries should begin (or con-

tinue, if already started), and how enquiries should be conducted. *Note*: The Children Act 1989 places a statutory duty on health and other agencies to help social services with these enquiries.

Consideration is given to the need for medical examinations/assessments, the need for any emergency action, which interviews may be required and which agencies should be involved. Where it is necessary for social services and the police to conduct joint enquiries (in serious cases of abuse particularly sexual abuse, neglect, abandonment or complex circumstances) police input will be provided by officers from specialised units.

Outcome of section 47 enquiries

There are three likely outcomes;

Concerns not substantiated

No further action may be required, although the need for further help or support should be considered. Sometimes an interagency meeting will be necessary to formulate a plan for the provision of services and on-going monitoring.

Concerns substantiated but the child is not at continuing risk

Agencies may agree that the child's safety and welfare can be ensured *without* the need for a child protection conference or child protection plan. This may arise if the perpetrator leaves the household, or if it is thought that harm was caused through an isolated incident and that such an event is unlikely to be repeated, with the provision of support and services. In these circumstances an interagency meeting should be convened to consider what action is required to complete the core assessment (under section 17 child 'in need') and formulate a plan for the provision of support and services. This will need to be reviewed to ensure it is effective.

Note: Professionals and agencies involved with the child and family, particularly those having taken part in the enquiries, *can and should* request that social services convene an initial child protection conference where it is felt that a child may not be adequately safeguarded.

Concerns are substantiated and the child is at risk of continuing harm

In such cases, an initial child protection conference should be convened.

THE INITIAL CHILD PROTECTION CONFERENCE

Purpose

The criteria for convening an initial child protection conference (ICPC) are that a judgement has been made that a child may continue to suffer, or be at risk of suffering *significant harm*. The aim of the ICPC is to enable those professionals most involved with the child and family, and the family themselves, to assess all relevant information, and plan how to safeguard the child and promote their welfare.

Timing

The ICPC should take place within 15 days of the strategy discussion.

Attendance

Professionals who have a significant contribution to make, arising from professional expertise, knowledge of the child or family, or both, should attend *and* provide a written report. Whenever possible and appropriate, the contents of the report should be shared verbally with the parents/carers and, where age appropriate, the child, prior to the conference. In *exceptional circumstances*, professionals may have confidential information which they feel cannot be shared at the conference, particularly if family members are present. It is imperative that this information is discussed with the chairperson, prior to the conference. Decisions can then be made regarding the relevance of the information and how this may be shared, strictly on a 'need to know' basis. The significance of information held by individuals in contact with the family can only be assessed when drawn together by social services during their enquiries, or on-going discussions and assessments. Participants in conferences are often surprised, when information is shared by others, at

how the 'overall picture of concerns begins to emerge' and should never underestimate the value of their own contribution to the assessment and decision-making process.

Involving child and family members

Parents and the child (subject to age and understanding) should be given the opportunity to attend and advised that they may wish to be accompanied by their advocate, friend or supporter. Where the child does not wish to attend, or their attendance is inappropriate, the social worker should ascertain the child's wishes and feelings, and make these known to the ICPC. The child may prefer their views to be shared by means of a letter, or taped message. Obviously, the involvement of family members needs to be planned carefully and assistance should be given to enable them to participate fully. Whilst it may not always be possible to involve all family members at all times in the conference, decisions about exclusion rests with the chairperson, acting within the ACPC procedures.

Action and decisions for the conference

If the conference decides that a child is at *continuing risk* of significant harm, the child's name will be entered on the child protection register. This decision, made by the chair, is based on the views of *all* the agencies represented. Differences of opinion will be recorded in the minutes. The chair also determines under which category of abuse the child's name should be registered (i.e. physical, emotional, sexual or neglect). Registration alone cannot protect a child. Safeguarding a child at *continuing risk of harm* requires interagency help and intervention, provided through a formal child protection plan. This plan will be developed as far as possible within the initial conference.

The conference will make recommendations about how agencies, professionals and the family should work together in the future, to protect the child from harm. All those involved should understand their role in safeguarding the child and know exactly what is expected of them. The conference is charged with specific tasks such as: appointing a key worker, a social worker and identifying members of the 'core group' (i.e. those professionals and family members who will have on-going responsibility for developing and implementing the child protection plan). Time-scales will be set for future meetings of the core group, production of the child protection plan and for the first child protection review conference. Consideration will also be given to what further core or specialist assessments of the child and family may be required. In addition a contingency plan will be outlined in case circumstances change quickly.

Minutes

All initial and review conferences should have a dedicated person to take notes and produce minutes. A copy should be sent as soon as possible to all those who attended, or were invited to attend, including family members (censorship may be required where family members have had to be excluded from certain aspects of the conference). Conference minutes are confidential and should not be passed to third parties without the permission of the chair or key worker.

Core groups

The first meeting of the core group should take place within 10 days of the ICPC. The purpose is to 'flesh out' the details of the child protection plan and decide what steps need to be taken by whom to complete the core assessment on time. All members are jointly responsible for the formulation and implementation of the child protection plan, refining the plan and monitoring progress against the agreed objectives. Thereafter, core group meetings should take place sufficiently regularly to allow monitoring and any necessary changes in the protection plan to take place. A written record of these meetings should be circulated to all members.

Assessment

Within 42 working days of beginning the initial assessment, social services should have completed a core assessment in respect of every child whose name is on the child protection register. Where a child is not registered, but meets the criteria for a core assessment as a 'child in need', then, provided the parents agree, this assessment should take place within the same time-scale. For children for whom there is a child protection plan, the core assessment should be carried out in accordance with the recommendations of the ICPC, as developed by the core group, and should be consistent with guidance in the 'Framework for the assessment of children in need and their families'. This assessment should include an analysis of the child's developmental needs and the capacity of the parents to respond to the child's needs and protect them from harm. Specialist assessments may need to be commissioned (e.g. from child and adolescent mental health services) which may not be able to be completed within the time-scale of 42 days. In this event, it is still important to pull together the rest of the findings at this point in time. Decisions about how to intervene, including what services to offer, should rest on what is likely to bring about good outcomes for the child. Intervention may include action to make the child safe, action to promote a child's health and development, action to help a parent/carer to protect a child or promote their welfare, therapy for an abused child, and support or therapy for a perpetrator of abuse.

The child protection review conference

The first review conference should be held within 3 months of the ICPC. Further reviews should take place at intervals of not more than 6 months, for as long as the child's name remains on the child protection register. *Note:* Where the primary presenting concern about a child has changed since initial registration, a child protection review conference should be convened to change the registration category.

Attendance should be similar to that of the ICPC, in that those most closely involved with the child and family (including members of the core group) should be invited.

The purpose of the conference is to review the *safety, health and development* of the child, against the outcomes identified in the child protection plan.

The review will determine if the child is being adequately safeguarded, whether there is a need for the protection plan to continue, or whether the plan needs amending. Research indicates that professional attendance at meetings diminishes after the initial conference. This is extremely worrying given the decision-making powers of the review conference and the potential implications for the child if a decision is made not to continue with a protection plan.

A child's name may be removed from the register if they are *no longer at continuing risk of harm* requiring an interagency protection plan. This may be as a result of the effectiveness of the protection plan, a significant change in the circumstances of the child or family, or as a direct result of a reassessment indicating that a child protection plan is no longer necessary. Under these circumstances, only a child protection review conference can decide that registration is no longer necessary. A child's name may also be removed from the register if he moves permanently out of the area (and the receiving authority have held their own child protection conference), or if the child has died, has reached the age of 18 years, or has permanently left the UK. De-registration should not automatically result in the withdrawal of family support. Ongoing provision of appropriate services should be discussed with the child and family.

Children looked after by the local authority

Where children 'looked after' are also subject to a child protection review conference, the systems must be integrated and carefully monitored in a way that promotes a child-centred approach. Timing is important, so that important information from the review conference can also be considered by the 'looked after' review meeting and therefore contribute to the overall planning process.

Pre-birth child protection conferences

Where section 47 enquiries suggest that an unborn child may be at future risk of significant harm, an ICPC may need to be convened prior to the child's birth. The involvement of midwifery services is vital in such cases.

THE PAEDIATRICIAN'S ROLE IN SAFEGUARDING CHILDREN

Diagnosis

The paediatrician's role in diagnosing child abuse requires an awareness of the possible signs and symptoms and a careful consideration of the history and examination findings in the context of the child's general, physical and emotional condition including his social history and circumstances. It follows that it is not appropriate for a doctor to perform a limited examination in restricted conditions without access to clinical and social information. In those situations where it is not possible to make a definite medical diagnosis of abuse the doctor may need to remind other professionals involved with the child that there could still be child protection concerns which need attention. For example, when a young child is presented with yet another set of bruises which are not typical of non-accidental injury and the child also lives in a chaotic home, the doctor should draw attention to the possibility of lack of adequate supervision in the home. One of the problems identified in several child death enquiries has been of inappropriate weight being given to doctors, both to their opinions which may be based on little evidence, but also to the value of intermittent medical examination as a method of monitoring child care.

In some cases it will be the doctor who is the first person to identify the abuse and makes the referral to the statutory agencies, according to local child protection procedures.

Assessment

When a child or young person who has suffered abuse is already known to the paediatric services, the doctor and other health professionals involved with the child will usually be asked to contribute to the child protection enquiries. When there are concerns about the health and/or development of such a child, a request to a paediatrician for a medical assessment will be made. An assessment may include advice about the possible medical effects of the abuse, diagnosis of previously unidentified conditions, advice about medical management, and recommendations for ongoing health care. The medical assessment will form part of the wider assessment as described in 'Working together' and the 'Framework for assessment'.

Contribution to case conferences

As mentioned above, the paediatrician may contribute his findings and assessment of injuries in a child seen once, or in the assessment of a child who is well known to him. It is essential for a written report to be prepared for case conferences even if the doctor is attending. In some instances the paediatrician may be the only doctor at the case conference and may be asked to interpret other medical information presented to the conference. Whilst the medical contribution is important, it should not be given greater or lesser weight than any of the other assessments. The lack of medical findings supportive of abuse does not necessarily mean that abuse has not occurred. If there is medical evidence for abuse this must be taken seriously, particularly if other assessments have not yet been carried out.

Specifically, a paediatrician may be asked to:

- contribute to risk assessment
- contribute to decision-making
- contribute to the child protection plan/core group.

See also the section on 'Interagency working in child protection' above.

Treatment and prevention

The paediatrician may have a role in these, depending on the circumstances.

Legal

In child protection cases that enter the court arena (criminal or care proceedings), the examining paediatrician or the paediatrician whose patient the child is may be asked to give evidence as a witness of fact.

Research

There is still much to be learnt about the many facets of child protection work and much research remains to be done, in medicine as well as in allied fields such as social science, if we are to improve the protection of children.

Interventions

It may be helpful to consider these in a similar way to disease prevention, i.e. as primary, secondary and tertiary types.

Primary interventions

These are aimed at whole populations, for example 'Don't shake the baby' campaign run by some ACPC, parenting programmes run in school for young people, 'Domestic violence' awareness campaigns, initiatives on aspects of parenting such as 'Positively no smacking'.

Secondary interventions

These are aimed at individuals or groups considered to be at risk, for example 'Positive parenting' groups run at many social services family centres for parents and carers who are identified as having difficulty managing their children's behaviour, Homestart which is a voluntary organisation that directly helps families who are struggling with parenting, helplines for parents such as Parentline.

Tertiary interventions

These are aimed at reducing further harm and preventing recurrences of the undesired event, for example ACPC procedures, treatment and support facilities within the statutory and voluntary sectors for victims and perpetrators of child abuse, helplines such as Childline.

Voluntary and self-help groups

These provide essential resources which cannot and perhaps should not be provided by the statutory agencies who provide the legal and professional general framework for child protection. A local directory of voluntary groups is as useful to a community paediatrician as a stethoscope.

PRACTICE ISSUES

Domestic violence and its effects on children

Domestic violence refers to physical, sexual or emotional abuse inflicted on a spouse or partner (or ex-partner) by the other. In most cases the abuser is male, and the victim female, although this is not always the case. The link between domestic violence and child abuse is well known. In at least half the cases of domestic violence the children are also suffering abuse, with this occurring in a number of ways: domestic violence can pose a threat to an unborn child, because assaults in pregnancy often involve punches and kicks to the abdomen, older children may get caught up in, or be put in the way of violence and be physically hurt. Children who live with parental or family violence may also be seriously psychologically and emotionally harmed, particularly when they witness the violence or are pressurised into concealing the assaults. The negative impact of domestic violence is also exacerbated by drink or drug misuse.

All health staff must be alert to the common problem of domestic violence, and know how to respond (Making an impact, BMJ).

A paediatrician should consider asking specifically about domestic violence in children who exhibit a wide range of behavioural and social adjustment problems. For example, children may have traumatic symptoms (anxiety, a sense of helplessness, sleep disturbance), they may be very passive, isolated from their peers with poor social skills, or conversely impulsive or aggressive. Poor concentration, distractibility and overactivity are also common, particularly in boys.

Confidentiality and child protection

Professionals can only work together to safeguard children if there is an exchange of relevant information between them. Health staff do however have a legal and ethical duty to maintain confidentiality to their patients, and should not disclose information without consent unless disclosure can be justified in the public interest, or is required by court order or statute. Disclosure of information to prevent, detect or prosecute in a serious crime is also justifiable, and this includes the abuse of children. 'Confidentiality: protecting and providing information' (GMC guidance 2000) is clear that if a doctor believes giving information to an appropriate responsible person or statutory agency is in the child's best interests, this is justifiable without the child's or their parents' consent.

Disability and child abuse

Any child whose progress to autonomy is delayed or who has to rely upon caretakers becomes more vulnerable to all forms of abuse. Recent studies indicate that the risk of abuse is about three times higher for children with disabilities. Congenital abnormality such as cleft lip increases the risk of assault. In sexual abuse the issue is power and dependency, and the extent of the problem has been hampered by a mistaken belief that the disability might somehow make abuse less attractive to abusers (McCormack 1991).

Children with neuromuscular conditions such as cerebral palsy may have extreme difficulties with feeding. Faced with such a child who is failing to grow there is a question of what is good enough parenting when huge demands are placed on the family. Early identification of stresses and appropriate support to these children and their families is increasingly recognised as helpful.

Problems of mobility may prevent escape. Problems of communication may prevent disclosure. Problems of intellect or the fact that the child is subjected to intimate personal care, for example because of chronic constipation, may mean that the child is not aware that abuse is even taking place.

The care of someone with disabilities may alter the usual social boundaries and thus make it easier for inhibitors of abusive behaviour to be removed or ignored. The response of the caring/protecting agencies may be altered, for example the parents of a severely disabled child may be viewed as 'saints' and this may hinder recognition, or a child with moderate learning difficulties is likely to have the validity of his testimony questioned and disallowed in court. How society views people with disability also has an effect, for example if a disabled person is considered to be 'not a person' then he could have things done to them that wouldn't be done to an able-bodied person.

There are also difficulties around the chronically sick or terminally ill child. It may be very hard for parents to apply normal discipline and so difficult and challenging behaviour may result. The situation may be further complicated by the effects of the illness or the treatment, producing bruises or other signs similar to the appearances of abuse.

Cultural and racial issues and child abuse

A general principle is that minority communities must be expected to obey the laws of the country in which they live. However the protection of the child needs to be placed inside the protection of the whole family's standing in the community. Here agencies can create more problems than they solve. For example, to shield the family from stigma the transfer of a child within the extended family may be preferable to a placement in a (usually white) foster home. The practice of co-opting religious or community leaders as intermediaries in child abuse cases should be avoided because of the issues of confidentiality and vested community interests.

On a case level many western *indicators* of possible abuse need to be given different weight. For example the role of an older female child as *little mother* is frequently normal in families with traditionally distinct gender roles. The white model of the incest family where skewed children's roles extend to a sexual role with the father cannot be applied.

The figure of the *collusive mother* needs to be reinterpreted. An Asian mother may be disadvantaged when it comes to disclosure. She may be isolated and have poor English. She may have no experience or confidence in dealing with the welfare bureaucracy. The child who is known to be violated may have no marriage prospects and this stigma may cross several generations.

Poverty also plays a large part. The perpetrator may be the sole bread-winner for a large extended family both in the UK and abroad. It is not so much

that the abuse is condoned, just that the whole family is trapped in it.

It is hard to make generalisations, because ethnic minority communities across the UK are quite diverse. The employing of link workers and social workers is in principle good but may cause conflicts if they are drawn from the communities they serve. It is important to recruit and train more foster carers from the various communities and in some areas family group homes staffed by social workers from those communities have been established and are particularly useful for those women who need a refuge from domestic violence (Moghal et al 1995).

Female genital mutilation

This is practised by a number of ethnic minority communities. It is an offence in this country to carry out such surgery.

Record-keeping and communication

Over the years many child death enquiries have highlighted a recurrent theme of poor documentation and communication within agencies as well as between agencies (HMSO 1991, Notts. ACPC Part 8 reviews). Sometimes much communication has taken place but it has not been effective in protecting children for a variety of reasons, such as not understanding each other's jargon, or misunderstanding roles or not having clear and agreed plans of action. Sometimes there has been the added problem of multiple sets of notes in each health district, none of which has complete information. Sometimes child protection information is wrongly regarded as too sensitive to be kept with the main record with the result that important information is missing when it would most serve the child. Some of these difficulties can be addressed locally but others require a change in national policy and culture. For example, some record-keeping difficulties can be tackled within local clinical governance systems through staff training. However the issue of the multiplicity of health records requires guidance and resources from central government to develop health records for individuals that can be used by all health disciplines. Better understanding of each other's roles in child protection can be promoted by interagency and multiprofessional training. However these require commitment of time and other resources and a culture shift amongst workers which is not always easy to obtain. Nevertheless the current national guidance is for increased 'joined-up' working between all the different governmental departments so this may help improve working together.

The writing of reports is an essential part of communication between everyone involved in child protection work. Doctors and other health professionals should try to use plain clear English and remember to explain in lay people's language the medical terminology necessarily used in our reports.

Supervision and support

The DH and professional organisations have consistently emphasised the need for professional supervision for staff involved in children in need/child protection work. The nature of the work is stressful and distressing, often requiring individuals to make difficult and sometimes risky professional judgements. The more complex situations become, the more risk there is of practitioners losing objectivity and being drawn into family circumstances, often resulting in a lack of focus on the needs of the child. Effective supervision is important in promoting safe standards of practice, ensuring that work is evidence based and in accordance with agreed policies, and procedures. Reflective practice also enables individuals to evaluate the work carried out and think about the effectiveness of their decision-making and actions, in relation to assessments of risk and need. It promotes professional development, allowing any gaps in knowledge and skills requiring training input to be identified.

REFERENCES

Anon 1987 Ill-treatment of children. Leading article. Lancet i: 367–368
Bankowksi Z, Carballo M (eds) 1986 Battered children — child abuse. WHO and Council for International Organizations of Medical Science, Berne
Browne K, Davies C, Stratton P (eds) 1989 Early prediction and prevention of child abuse. John Wiley, Chichester
Chadwick D L, Berkowitz C D, Kerns D, McCann J, Reinhart M A, Strickland S 1989 Colour atlas of child sexual abuse. Year Book Medical Publishers, Chicago
Crittenden P 1988 Family and dyadic patterns of functioning in maltreating families. In: Browne K, Davies C, Stratton P (eds) Early prediction and prevention of child abuse. John Wiley, Chichester
Department of Health 1991 Child abuse, a study of inquiry reports 1980–1989. HMSO, London
Department of Health 1995 Child Protection — Clarification of Arrangements Between The NHS and other Agencies. HMSO, London
Department of Health 1995 Messages from research. HMSO, London
Department of Health 1996 Child Protection — Medical Responsibilities — Guidance to Doctors working with Child Protection Agencies. HMSO, London
Department of Health 1999 Working together to safeguard children, a guide to inter-agency working to safeguard and promote the welfare of children. The Stationery Office, London
Department of Health 2000 Children and young people on child protection registers. HMSO, London
Department of Health 2000 Framework for the Assessment of Children in Need and their Families. HMSO, London
Feldman K W, Brewer D F 1984 Child abuse, cardio-pulmonary resuscitation and rib fractures. Pediatrics 73:339–342
Finkelhor D 1984 Child sexual abuse, new theory and research. Free Press, New York
Finkelhor D, Williams L, Burns N 1988 Nursery crimes, sexual abuse in day care. Sage, Newbury Park, CA
Fleming K, Venning V, Evans M 1987 DNA typing of genital warts and diagnosis of sexual abuse in children. Lancet ii: 454
Gallagher B 2000 Ritual, and child sexual abuse, but not ritual child sexual abuse. Child Abuse Review 9:321–327
Gellert G, Durfee M, Berkowitz C, Higgins K, Tubiolo V 1993 Situational and sociodemographical characteristics of children infected with human immunodeficiency virus from pediatric sexual abuse. Pediatrics 91:39–44
General Medical Council 2000 'Confidentiality: Protecting and Providing Information'
Glaser D 1993 Emotional abuse. In: Hobbs C J, Wynne J M (guest eds) Clinical paediatrics, vol 1, No 1. Ballière Tindall, London, edn pp 251–269
Glover S, Nicoll A, Pullan C 1985 Deprivation hands and feet. Archives of Disease in Childhood 60:976–977
Gutman L T, S T Claire K K, Weedy C, et al 1991 Human immunodeficiency virus transmission by child sexual abuse. American Journal of Diseases of Children 145:137–141
Her Majesty's Inspectorate of Constabulary and Social Services Inspectorate 1991 Report on Joint Police and Social Services Investigation of Child Sexual Abuse in Nottinghamshire. Home Office and Department of Health, London

Avoiding harm: child protection

Hester M, Pearson C, Harwin N 2000 Making an impact: children and domestic violence. Jessica Kingsley, London

Hobbs C J, Hanks H G I, Wynne J 1999 Child Abuse and Neglect: a clinician's handbook, 2nd edn. Churchill Livingstone, London

Hobbs C J, Wynne J M 1986 Buggery in childhood — a common syndrome of abuse. Lancet ii: 792–796

Hobbs C J, Wynne J M 1990 The sexually abused battered child. Archives of Disease in Childhood 65:423–427

Kempe C H, Silverman F N, Steel B F, Droegmueller W, Silver H K 1962 The battered child syndrome. Journal of the American Medical Association 18:17–24

Kravitz H, Drissen G, Gomberg R, Korach A 1969 Accidental falls from elevated surfaces in infants from birth to one year of age. Pediatrics suppl 44:869–876

La Fontaine J 1994 The extent and nature of organised and ritual sexual abuse: research findings. HMSO, London

McCormack B 1991 Sexual abuse and learning disabilities. British Medical Journal 303:143–144

Meadow R (ed) 1997 ABC of child abuse, 3rd edn. BMJ Publishing Group, London

Moghal N E, Nota I K, Hobbs C 1995 A study of sexual abuse in an Asian community. Archives of Disease in Childhood 72:346–347

Neinstein L S, Goldenring J, Carpenter S 1984 Nonsexual transmission of sexually transmitted diseases: an infrequent occurrence. Pediatrics 74:67–75

Paterson C R, Burns J, McAllion S J 1993 Osteogenesis imperfecta: the distinction from child abuse and the recognition of a variant form. A J Med Genetics 45:187–192

Paterson C R, McAllison S J 1989 Osteogenesis imperfecta in the differential diagnosis of child abuse. British Medical Journal 299:451

Royal College of Physicians 1997 Physical signs of sexual abuse in children, 2nd edn. Report of a working party. RCP, London

Reder P, Duncan S, Gray M 1993 Beyond blame: child abuse tragedies revisited. Routledge, London

Reder P, Duncan S 1999 Lost innocents: a follow-up study of fatal child abuse. Routledge, London

Skuse D, Wolke D 1992 The nature and management of feeding problems and eating disorders in young people. Monographs in clinical paediatrics. Harwood Academic Publications, New York

Snow D, Sorenson T 1990 Ritualistic child abuse in a neighbourhood setting. Journal of Interpersonal Violence 5(4)274–287

Spevak M R, Kleinman P K, Belanger P L, Primack C, Richmond J M 1994 Cardio-pulmonary resuscitation, and rib fractures in infants. JAMA 272:617–618

Stephenson T J, Bialas Y 1996 Estimation of the age of bruising. Archives of Disease in Childhood 74: 53–55

Taitz L 1991 Child abuse: some myths and shibboleths. Hospital Update May: 400

Tardieu A 1878 Etude medico-legale sur les attentats au moeurs. Balliere et fils, Paris

Thomas P 1977 Rib fractures in infancy. Annales de Radiologie 20:115–122

Wild N J, Wynne J M 1986 Child sex rings. British Medical Journal 293:183–185

Woolhandler S, Himmelstein D U 1985 Militarism and mortality. Lancet i: 1375–1378

Further reading

Cook A, James J, Leach P 1991 Positively no smacking. Health Visitors Association, London

HMSO 1974 Report of committee of enquiry into care and supervision provided in relation to Maria Colwell. HMSO, London

HMSO 1988 Report of the inquiry into child abuse in Cleveland. HMSO, London

Hobbs C J, Wynne J M 1993 Child abuse. In: Clinical paediatrics. International practice and research, Vol 1, no. 1. Ballière Tindall, London

Hobbs C J, Hanks H G I, Wynne J 1999 Child abuse and neglect: a clinician's handbook, 2nd edn. Churchill Livingstone, London

Jenny C, Kuhns M L D, Arakawa F 1987 Hymens in newborn female infants. Pediatrics 80:399–400

Mtezuka M 1989 Towards a better understanding of child sexual abuse among Asian communities. Practice Autumn: 248–260

NCH 1991 The National Children's Home factfile, children in danger. NCH, London

Newson J, Newson E 1989 The extent of physical punishment in the UK. Approach Ltd, London

Porter R (ed) 1984 Child sexual abuse within the family. CIBA Foundation. Tavistock Publications, London

Shemmings D 1991 Family participation in child protection conferences. Report of a pilot project in Lewisham Social Services Department. University of East Anglia, Norwich

25 | Young adults

Adolescence may be defined as the process of growing up. The age span is variable as young people mature at different ages and speeds. *The World Health Organization puts the ages between 11 and 21.*

As well as the profound physical and emotional maturational changes that occur, adolescence is also a time of seeking independence, of risk-taking to 'imitate' adult behaviour and of establishing a personal identity. Family structure and the level of its support, peer group and educational environment influence adolescent behaviour. Most young people traverse adolescence without problems. If difficulties do arise, then those of early adolescence are primarily associated with physical and developmental changes, and those in late adolescence with identity change.

In order to establish personal identity young people may search for their cultural roots at this time, or for their biological parents if adopted. The question of sexual orientation may arise with the ensuing struggle to recognise and 'come out'. Many young people begin to question the fundamental values of parents and other adults, and develop a critical awareness of the world around and its social injustices. Disabled or chronically ill young people may become increasingly aware of how their condition impacts on their lives, which may lead to feelings of aggression, depression or even suicide. Those from ethnic minority groups may become aware of unequal opportunities, and the impact of racism. Social changes on leaving school may range from further education, to financial independence or to unemployment. Homelessness and poverty may contribute to depression and low self-esteem.

The struggle to become independent is often too threatening to accomplish alone, so many adolescents choose to go through the process in the same way as their peer group with all its pressures.

PUBERTY

Puberty is defined as the stage in life when gonadal maturation occurs. It involves the acquisition of secondary sexual characteristics and an associated growth spurt, and ends with the achievement of fertility.

There is a wide variation in the age of onset and duration. The trigger factor, which initiates this maturation, remains unknown. The hypothalamus is responsible for the synthesis and release of gonadotrophin releasing hormone which in turn stimulates the synthesis and release of follicle stimulating hormone (FSH) and luteinising hormone (LH) from the pituitary. The secreted FSH and LH stimulate the production of gonadal testosterone and oestrogen.

Girls

The first signs of puberty in over 85% of white girls are the oestrogenic changes of breast development. Breast budding usually begins around 10.5–11 years and may be initially unilateral. Adrenal androgens produce growth of pubic and axillary hair, sweat gland activity and facial acne. Pubic hair development usually occurs about 6 months after the onset of breast development, but may be the first sign in Afro-Caribbean races. Both growth hormone and sex steroids appear to contribute to the growth spurt which occurs early in girls, and is almost complete by the time menstruation begins. From the Tanner series, the mean age of menarche is 13.4

Table 25.1
Breast development

Stage	Mean age (years)
1. Pre-adolescent: no development	
2. Breast and papilla elevated as a small mound; areola diameter increased	11.5
3. Breast and areola enlarged; no contour separation	12.5
4. Areola and papilla form secondary mound	13.5
5. Mature stage: nipple projects, areola part of general breast contour	

years; the range is 9–16 years (Marshall & Tanner 1969). The interval from breast development to menarche is 2.3 years with a range of 0.5–5.75 years. Menarche appears to be associated with a critical body weight. One theory suggests a minimum fatness level of about 17% body weight is necessary for the onset of the menstrual cycle, and a minimum fatness level of about 22% is necessary to maintain regular ovulatory cycles (Frisch 1996). Gymnasts, ballet dancers and long-distance runners with reduced weight often have significant delays in development and menarche, especially if their training began in the pre-pubertal years. Irregular and heavy menses are common in the first year following menarche and require no treatment. Adolescent girls who are not sexually active are less likely to be worried about mildly irregular or late menses. Primary dysmenorrhoea is relatively common and may cause absence from school.

Breast development occurs in five stages, which are described in Table 25.1.

Boys

The first sign of puberty in boys is testicular enlargement above the pre-pubertal size of $2.0\,cm^3$. Increasing testosterone secretion produces growth of pubic, axillary and facial hair, enlargement of the penis, deepening of the voice, ability to ejaculate and acne. The growth spurt is associated with an increase in body size and muscle bulk, and reaches its peak 2 years later in boys than it does in girls. Gynaecomastia occurs in 65% of normal boys. It is usually transient, frequently unilateral, and is thought to be due to increased end-organ sensitivity to normal oestrogen concentrations.

Genitalia development in boys is described in five stages in Table 25.2.

Pubic hair — girls and boys

The five stages of pubic hair growth in boys and girls are described in Table 25.3.

Delayed puberty

Delayed puberty is defined as the onset of puberty later than 14 years in a girl, and 14.5 years in a boy. Three per cent of children have some delay. In 50% of boys and 15% of girls it will be constitutional in origin. Of the rest, 30% will have pituitary problems, 10% of boys and 14% of girls will have gonadal failure and in the remaining 10–15% the delay is associated with chronic and severe disease such as cystic fibrosis, coeliac disease or renal failure. Another possible cause is anorexia nervosa (Merritt 1996).

Precocious puberty

Precocious puberty is defined as the onset of sexual maturation before 9 years in a boy and 8 years in a girl (Neinstein 1991a). It is more common in girls than in boys. In girls, the aetiology is usually idiopathic, whereas in boys it is commonly associated with an intracranial tumour (Neinstein 1991b). The precocious development may cause considerable embarrassment to the child and may lead to unrealistic expectations of the child in that emotional and intellectual maturity are not similarly advanced.

Premature thelarche

Premature thelarche or isolated breast development occurs in girls under the age of 3 years. The growth rate is normal. Reassurance only is required.

**Table 25.2
Genitalia development in boys**

Stage	Mean age (years)
1. Pre-pubertal, testes <2 cm^3	
2. Scrotal enlargement, skin reddens, texture alters, testes >2 cm^3	12
3. Lengthening of penis, further growth of testes and scrotum	13
4. Scrotum enlarges further, and darkens; penis broadens, glans develops	14
5. Adult male genitalia: testes average 15 cm^3	

**Table 25.3
Pubic hair — girls and boys**

Stage	Mean age Boys	Girls
1. No pubic hair		
2. Sparse growth of slightly pigmented hair along labia or at base of penis	12.5 years	11.5 years
3. Darker curled hair, increasing in amount	13.5 years	12 years
4. Coarse, curly hair, small adult configuration	14.5 years	13 years
5. Adult configuration, complete triangle plus spread to medial surface of thighs		

HEALTH NEEDS

Young people's health needs are diverse and are affected by their gender, culture, ethnic group and sexual orientation. In planning services for their needs we must take account of their physical, mental and sexual health within the context of social issues and legal rights. *Confidentiality is a key issue identified by young people whatever their needs.*

Physical health problems of adolescence

The physical health problems specific to adolescence fall into three main groups: disorders of puberty, diseases of adolescence (e.g. acne, bone tumours, anorexia nervosa) and problems of chronic disease during puberty associated with changing needs and poor compliance (e.g. asthma, diabetes, cystic fibrosis, renal failure). The incidence of illness in this age group is lower than that at any other time in life. Nevertheless there has been an increase in self-reported illness in the last decade (Department of Health 1994). The General Household Survey suggests adolescents visit their GP three to four times a year, mainly for respiratory tract disease, but also for skin disorders, allergies, injuries and contraception (Churchill et al 1997).

Adolescents are concerned about a wide range of health and environmental issues, feel responsible

---

Box 25.1
Health and behaviour of 11–16 year olds.

- 15% drank moderate amounts of alcohol
- 22% had been bullied in present school term
- 22% of girls and 16% of boys currently smoking
- 30% of year 11s had tried cannabis
- 33% of boys and 16% of girls did sport every day
- 75% watched television for more than 2 hours per day
- 84% said using a condom would protect against sexually transmitted infection
- 93% considered themselves healthy

Box 25.2
Factors affecting nutritional status in adolescence

- Growth spurt
- Increased physical activity
- Changes in eating habits (e.g. irregular meals, high sugar snacks)
- Inadequate vegetarian/vegan diet
- Sports
- Menstruation
- Pregnancy
- Drug abuse

---

for their own health and acknowledge that good health is mainly due to sensible living. Even though the majority consider themselves to be healthy, evidence suggests that they are at increasing risk from the harmful effects of smoking, alcohol consumption, using drugs and unsafe sex (Coleman 1997). Many of the accidents that occur in this age group are the result of risk-taking behaviour, for example excess alcohol consumption and driving, dangerous sports or not wearing protective clothing (Box 25.1).

Nutrition

This is discussed further in Chapter 7. There are increased nutritional requirements in adolescence for iron (for muscle mass and blood volume in males and for menstrual loss in females), calcium (for skeletal growth) and zinc (for adequate sexual maturation). Dietary status is an important part of health evaluation in adolescence (Neinstein 1991c). (Box 25.2).

Mortality rates

Death rates in young people are highest in the 15–19-year age group. The major causes are shown in Table 25.4.

Table 25.4
The major causes of death in young people: 15–19 years

Cause of death	%
Heart disease	20
Injury, poisoning and transport accidents	54
Neoplasm	10
Nervous system	7
Other causes	9
Mortality Statistics 1997	

Hospital admissions

In early adolescence admission rates are divided fairly evenly between general paediatrics, general surgery, ENT and trauma and orthopaedics. By around 16 years less than 1% are admitted for general paediatrics. Twenty-four per cent of girls are admitted for gynaecological reasons, mainly termination of pregnancy (Henderson et al 1993). Forty per cent of young men are admitted for trauma and head injuries. Self-poisoning is common in older teenage girls (Kerfoot 1996).

SOCIAL AND MENTAL HEALTH ISSUES

Social and mental health issues are intricately entwined. The Mental Health Foundation (1999) estimates that 20% of children and adolescents are experiencing significant psychological problems. Social issues, such as homelessness and poverty, are relevant. There are individual and family factors. Three risk factors predict emotional problems for 8%, but four risk factors predict problems for 20%. Adolescents who have been sexually abused become more aware of the significance of their trauma after puberty. Self-harm and drug use became more prevalent, and either may be considered coping strategies (Herman 1998). Other traumas include bullying, changing family structure and bereavements. The Trent Lifestyle Survey reported that 8% of young people in 1994 did not feel good about any of the following: their health, the future, how they looked, what happened at home, schoolwork or friendships. Nine per cent stated there was no one to talk over problems with (Roberts et al 1995).

The risk factors that affect young people's mental health are outlined in Box 25.3.

Mental health issues may be expressed as:

- Drug use.
- Self-harm and suicide.
- Depression.
- Truancy and offending behaviour.

Box 25.3
Risk factors that affect young people's mental health

- Experience of abuse and other traumas, bullying and rascism (often not expressed)
- Family breakdown, hostile parenting, psychiatric illness, alcoholism, bereavement
- Poverty, homelessness, disaster, discrimination
- Physical and learning disability, illness, academic failure, low self-esteem

---

Alcohol

Under-age drinking and problems associated with it are increasing in the UK. Surveys show that children drink alcohol earlier, and by their teens, drinking is a regular part of their lives. Between 92% and 98% of 15 years olds have tried alcohol (Miller & Plant 1996, Gabhain & Francois 2000). Up to 9% of 11-year-old girls and up to 12% of 11-year-old boys have tried alcohol (Gabhain & Francois 2000). Goddard (1997) reports that more than 50% of 15 year olds drank alcohol the previous week. Girls drank on average 7 units and boys 9.7 units. Home is the major source of the alcohol, but 5.5% of year 10s buy it from a supermarket and 23% buy it from an off-license (Balding 1996). McKeganey (1996) reports more than 50% of 14 year olds saying they have been drunk. This fits in with the World Health Organization study (Gabhain & Francois 2000) that reports between 53% and 72% of 15-year-old boys in the UK have been drunk at least twice, and 10% of 11-year-old boys. The way alcohol is used at home influences the development of drinking behaviour as young people mature. Young inexperienced drinkers have a lower tolerance to alcohol and even small amounts of alcohol significantly lower their judgement and control. One would expect drinking to be associated with unwanted sex, unprotected sex and violence.

The Confiscation of Alcohol (Young Persons) Act 1997 permits police to remove alcohol if the person is considered to be under 18 years and in a public place (Swade 1997).

Smoking

The health hazards of smoking are well recognized. The younger children are when they begin smoking, the more likely they are to die from it as adults. Children starting to smoke at the age of 15 years are three times more likely to die from smoking than adults starting in their mid twenties (Doll & Peto 1981).

The prevalence of smoking in children aged 11–15 years has increased from 8% in 1988 to 13% in 1996. This is higher in girls, having increased from 9% to 15% (Thomas et al 1998). Eighty-two per cent of adult smokers began when they were teenagers. Is smoking a paediatric disease?

Children are more likely to smoke if parents and siblings do. Friends may influence them. It helps them feel independent and more attractive. They do not consider that the risks of smoking apply to them (Sutton 1998). There is an association with poverty, use of alcohol and drugs and educational under-achievement (McKee 1999).

Seventy per cent of children buy cigarettes from shops; 33% use vending machines. Ninety-six per cent of school children report seeing cigarette advertising in the last 6 months. Children smoke brands that are heavily advertised. Fifty per cent consider they have seen advertising on the television in the last 6 months — there has been none for 33 years (Jarvis 1997).

The UK government aims to reduce smoking in 11–15 year olds from 13% to 11% by 2005, and to 9% by 2010. The policy is aimed at reducing access to cigarettes and making smoking less desirable in this age group (Smoking Kills — A White Paper on Tobacco 1998). It is a worthy aim, but innovative methods on changing young people's attitudes need evaluation.

Illegal drug use

Britain has the highest use of illicit drugs in the European Union (European Drugs Monitoring Centre 1998). McKee (1999) links this to educational underachievement, poverty and family life with parents working the longest hours in Europe. The Police Research Group reported in August 1998 that heroin was flooding the market and being sold for £10 in areas where it had not appeared before. The majority of users are in socially deprived areas, but increasing numbers have an affluent background (Evans 1998).

Many drugs are illegal (Misuse of Drugs Act 1971), and there are penalties for being in possession or for intending to supply them.

Classification of illegal drugs

The classification of illegal drugs is shown in Box 25.4. There are heavier penalties for Class A drugs than Class C drugs. The police may be willing to caution for simple possession of cannabis if the

---

> **Box 25.4**
> ## Misuse of Drugs Act 1971 classification of illegal drugs
>
> *Class A*: LSD; ecstasy; cocaine; heroin and other strong opiates; magic mushroom if dried or processed; any Class B drug prepared for injection.
>
> *Class B*: Cannabis (resin and herbal); amphetamines; barbiturates; codeine and other weaker opiates
>
> *Class C*: Tranquillisers and sleeping pills such as diazepam, chlordiazepoxide, temazepam, and anabolic steroids.

---

offence is admitted. This still means a criminal record. Users may not realise ecstasy is in the same class as heroin with the same penalties as a Class A drug. The maximum sentence is life imprisonment for supply of a Class A drug. This includes buying for or giving to friends.

Recreational drug use

Recreational use of illegal drugs like cannabis, ecstasy, LSD, is prevalent amongst young people. Surveys report between 35% and 45% use in 15–16 year olds (Roker 1995, Miller & Plant 1996, Parker et al 1998). Most use cannabis. Some drugs are more associated with the dance scene. These include ecstasy, LSD, magic mushrooms and nitrites. The Trent Lifestyle Survey suggests many young people use them to be like their friends (Roberts et al 1995). Experimentation and curiosity motivate others. For some, the effects will help block out difficult feelings or provide an escape from painful life experiences. These young people may then move on to using drugs with more risks, for example smoking or injecting opiates.

Solvent abuse

Solvents are volatile compounds that may be inhaled, causing intoxication. They include toluene-based adhesives, aerosols, fuel gases and solvents. An extensive range of household products is used. Solvent abusers are mainly boys between the ages of 11 and 17. Between 4% and 8% of secondary school children try it. The profile is lower than it was in the 1980s, perhaps because other drugs are more readily available. Most will only experiment a few times, but others may carry on sniffing regularly for some time, usually with friends.

There are still more deaths associated with solvents than with ecstasy. The majority of deaths are associated with fuel gas or aerosol abuse. Over 75% of the deaths are sudden. This may be from the direct toxic effect on the heart due to increased sensitivity to adrenaline (epinephrine). Others die from suffocation by plastic bags, choking from vomit or acute laryngospasm, or through injury or accident while intoxicated. More than half the deaths occur at home or in the house of a friend.

It is not illegal to possess or to sniff substances, but it is an offence for retailers to supply such products knowingly to a person under the age of 18 (1989 Intoxicating Substances Supply Act). In July 1999 the UK government also banned the sale of lighter fuel to under 18 year olds.

Serious drug use

Opiates, crack cocaine and injecting drugs cause serious health consequences. Tolerance and dependence develop quickly. Injecting drug users risk hepatitis B and C infection, human immunodeficiency virus (HIV) infection, thrombophlebitis, heart disease and lung disorders. Doctors in England are required to notify treatment demands of drug misusers to their local drug misuse database. This is not limited to opiates and cocaine (Tregoning 1998). Heroin use in teenagers has increased, with over one-third of new users being under 16 years of age (childRIGHT 1998).

Clinical conditions arising from drug use

Five clinical conditions arising from the use of drugs are:

1. Acute intoxication — may lead to injuries.
2. Harmful use — a pattern of use that results in physical or mental harm, e.g. hepatitis.
3. Dependence syndrome — the need for the drug dominates the user's life.
4. Withdrawal — may cause convulsions with some drugs and needs medical treatment.

5. Psychotic disorder — any drug may produce hallucinations, delusions or behaviour characteristic of psychosis. This may include flashbacks, personality change and cognitive deterioration. (From Gerada & Ashworth 1998.)

Drugs in common use and their effects

Table 25.5 outlines the drugs most frequently encountered. The information is summarised from drugs information agencies such as Lifeline and The Institute for the Study of Drugs and Dependency (ISDD). Tranquillisers are also used for recreational purposes. They are depressants and Class C drugs. Anabolic steroids are illegal to supply, but not to possess or use. They are supplied as tablets or liquid for injection. They are classed as stimulants but are usually taken for their body-building effects.

Not all drugs affect people in the same way. It depends on the individual, how they are taken, the mood, etc. Cannabis usually makes people feel relaxed and giggly. It can also produce paranoia. Very few drugs when bought are pure. Mixing drugs may be dangerous, particularly barbiturates and alcohol. There are deaths with first-time use, mainly ecstasy and solvents. If people experience drug-induced 'highs', then a 'low' usually follows. This is likely to be accumulative. There is some evidence that ecstasy depletes serotonin in the brain. It is uncertain whether it is neurotoxic and whether regular use may lead to major depression (Green & Goodwin 1996, Merrill 1996, Gouzoulis-Mayfrank et al 2000, Kelly 2000).

Mortality

The main source for drug deaths was from the Home Office. Statistics were discontinued in 1997. There is no regular publication of statistics on drug-related mortality in the UK. Information about deaths comes from a variety of sources which combine to present a patchy and incomplete picture. Data is now held by The Office of National Statistics and the General Register Offices (GRO) for Scotland and Northern Ireland.

Individual researchers and/or agencies also collect data. ISDD has been informally tracking ecstasy deaths since 1989. St George's Hospital

Young adults

Table 25.5
Commonly used drugs

	Also known as	Legal status	How used	How long it lasts	Effects	Long-term problems	Comments	Mortality — all ages 1985–1994	Urine test +ve for drug for
Amphetamine	Speed, whizz, dexies, billy, sulphate, uppers	Stimulant Class A	Swallowed, licked from finger, sniffed or injected	Up to 3–4 h	Exhilaration, increased energy, confidence, panic, paranoia	Tolerance, dependence, high BP, injecting dangerous	May not be pure, people react differently	97	2–4 days
Barbiturates	Barbs, sleepers, downers	Depressant Class B	Swallowed, sometimes with alcohol, cannabis or amphetamines	3–6 h	Relaxation, sleepy, slurred speech, clumsy	Loss of memory, fatigue, depression	Easy to misjudge dose, could be lethal with alcohol	See heroin	1–2 days
Cannabis	Grass, dope, blow, spliff, ganja, hash, weed, skunk	Depressant Hallucinogenic Class B	Smoked with tobacco in a joint or on its own in a pipe, eaten or used in cooking	Several hours	Relaxed, giggly, anxious, sick or paranoid, skunk is stronger	Lethargy, short-term memory loss, possible paranoia, tobacco risks	People react differently		2–7 days casual use 30 days heavy use
Cocaine	Coke, snow, charlie, freebase	Stimulant Class A	White powder, sniffed, licked, injected	After 15 min lasts 30 min	Euphoria, less fatigue, increased heart rate	Paranoia, anxiety, depression, lethargy, mucosal damage	Large doses may cause convulsions and death	67	12 h to 3 days

Drug	Street names	Class	Form	Duration	Effects	Negative effects	Risks	Deaths	Detection
Crack cocaine	Rocks, crack	Stimulant Class A	White lumps as chalk or crystal, smoked or inhaled	Immediate effect Lasts 10–20 min	As cocaine, but more intense	Rapid tolerance, distressing come-down symptoms	As cocaine		As cocaine
Ecstasy	E, MDMA, ADAM, XTC	Hallucinogenic Class A	Pill or capsule, swallowed	Peaks 2 h Lasts up to 8 h	Mental calm, heightened perceptions	Unable to sleep, heat-stroke, depression	Death from hyperthermia, dehydration	Approx. 60 from 1989 to 2000	2–4 days
Heroin	Smack, skag, junk, Henry	Depressant Class A	White or brown powder, sold as wraps injected, sniffed or smoked	Lasts 5–7 h	Feeling of warmth, reduced physical, emotional pain	Nausea, vomiting, sedation, unconscious, death	Withdrawal symptoms last 7–10 days, increasing tolerance	2395 for all opiates	1–2 days
LSD	Acid, trips	Hallucinogenic Class A	Liquid or on blotting paper, swallowed, sniffed or injected	Lasts 8–12 h Peaks 2–3 h	Vivid colours, etc. mood change, delusions, anxiety, dizziness	Increased heart rate, BP, bad trips and flashbacks, paranoia long-term disorientation			2–4 days
Magic mushrooms	Liberty cap	Hallucinogenic Class A (if dried or processed)	Cooked or dried and infused as tea	Lasts up to 9–12 h Starts 30 min	Similar to above	Can have bad trips and be very frightened	Some mushrooms are poisonous		2–3 days
Nitrites	Poppers, rush, liquid gold	Not illegal	Yellow liquid in bottle or capsule sniffed	Immediate Lasts 5 min	Relaxes muscle sexual enhancement	Headache, vomiting	Dangerous with heart condition		

BP = blood pressure

Young adults

Medical School produces an annual survey of solvent deaths.

Deaths associated with drug use in teenagers aged 15–19 years have increased consistently by 8% each year from 1985 (Roberts et al 1997). There were 436 deaths from 1985 to 1995, with twice as many boys as girls. The highest death rate is from opiates. Psychostimulants like ecstasy were responsible for 1 death from 1985 to 1989 and 16 deaths from 1991 to 1995. Misuse of solvents led to 152 deaths in 1990. This reduced to 73 in 1997. Deaths from glue and aerosols were reduced following an intense educational campaign, but deaths from butane gas remained static (Taylor et al 2000).

Drug-related deaths from amphetamine, cocaine, ecstasy and opiates given in Table 25.1 are best estimates from available statistics, and are total deaths for all ages from 1985 to 1994, except for ecstasy which is from 1989 to 2000.

Services for drug users

A government task force was set up in 1994, to report on services for drug users. It reported in 1996 and issued 80 recommendations that have been passed on to local authorities. Information is available from ISDD.

Drugs education

Between 1986 and 1993, the Department of Education supported local initiatives to develop drugs education and appoint drug education coordinators. After this funding ended, most local education authorities appointed health coordinators to provide health education and in-service training on the misuse of drugs, tobacco, solvents and the transmission of HIV. Peer group education initiatives were also developed. From 1995, central government funding was provided to train teachers and support new projects. In 1996 funding became available to train youth workers. Aspects of drugs education are included in the national curriculum. Funds are available for training, and resources are becoming available (Teachers' Advisory Council on Alcohol and Drug Education, (TACADE), www.tacade.com).

As well as providing information, education should aim to promote a climate of respect and understanding, the development of self-esteem, decision-making skills and the ability to cope with adverse situations when they arise. Some drug-prevention strategies are aimed at primary prevention. 'Project Charlie' is aimed at children in primary education (McGurk & Hurry 1995). Early evaluation suggests that it is showing a positive effect. Other projects aim to give young people accurate information about what they are using and the effects, in a way that is acceptable. The Lifeline — Manchester's publications include leaflets with cartoon characters such as 'Peanut Pete' (Fig. 25.1) and 'Skunk-Weed Tom', with serious messages that avoid patronising young people. Young people are saying they want to talk about drugs, but will not listen to teachers (Young 1997). Evaluations of different approaches suggest peer-led methods may be most effective (Black et al 1998). Most reports indicate drug use is increasing, but Plant & Miller (2000) report a recent decrease in the use of all drugs except heroin.

Homelessness and poverty

Homelessness refers to young people living on the streets, in shelters or hostels, or on friends' or relatives' floors. Estimates of numbers vary enormously. It is agreed that the numbers have increased over the last 12 years, and that the reasons for homelessness have changed. At Centrepoint, 41% are aged 16 and 17 years, with no automatic rights to benefits (Havell 1999). Young black and mixed race people make up 43%. One in four of the young people have been in local authority care (Anderson et al 1993). As many as 86% of young homeless people have been forced to leave home by violence, abuse, family breakdown or being thrown out (Nassor & Simms 1996).

Local authorities only house small numbers of vulnerable young people. Being homeless has devastating consequences. Up to 80% of homeless young people are unemployed, 70% report poor health and they are twice as likely to suffer from mental health problems (The Mental Health Foundation 1996). There are high rates of alcohol and drug misuse (Fleman 1995). There are strong links with offending behaviour (Association of Chief Officers of Probation 1993). These crimes are

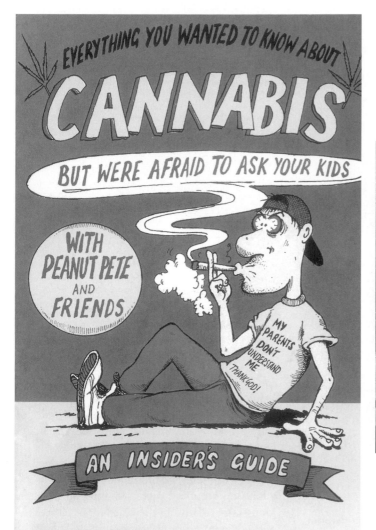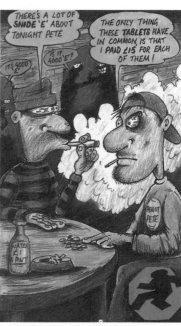

Fig. 25.1 'Peanut Pete' (Reproduced with permission from Lifeline — Manchester)

usually for self-preservation or related to alcohol and drugs.

Young homeless women are vulnerable to sexual exploitation. Many have been sexually abused as children (Hendessi 1992). The lack of appropriate housing puts them at risk and some will be coerced or forced into prostitution (The Guardian 1998, Nottinghamshire Country Council Social Services 1998).

Truancy and offending behaviour (Fig. 25.2)

Truancy is often associated with crime, and so the effects extend beyond school. Schools have obliga-tions under the Education Act to monitor atten-dance and investigate unauthorised absences. The Department for Education and Employment issues guidelines. There is no agreed level where inter-vention is automatically triggered. Boys are over-represented in the statistics. Public concern about youth crime has increased in this decade, and parents have been made responsible in law for the offences of their teenage children (Coleman 1997). They may be ordered to pay fines or compensation for their children's offences. There is no signifi-cant increase in the level of crime committed by teenagers from 1985 to 1995, but the number of 14–17 year olds in prison has doubled from 1993 to 1998 (Russell 1999). Male teenagers commit the

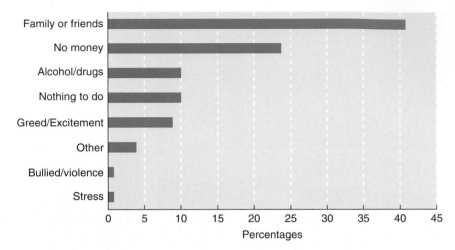

Fig. 25.2 Reasons given by young offenders for their behaviour. From Coleman (1999); statistics from Audit Commission (1996)

majority of crimes of theft and burglary. At the same time, they are most at risk of becoming victims of violent crime outside domestic violence (Criminal Statistics, England and Wales 1999).

Coleman (1997) discussed the Audit Commission publication 'Misspent Youth'. One-quarter of the sample said lack of money was a reason for offending — we return to poverty as a significant contribution.

The Social Exclusion Unit

The UK government recognises the overlapping issues that affect vulnerable groups in this country, including young people, and has formed this Unit to report and make recommendations. All relevant government departments are involved. New guidance to housing authorities recommends better liaison with social services regarding vulnerable young people, which automatically includes those leaving care. The Department of Health has also announced more support to young people leaving care. There will be new opportunities for 16–18 year olds in education, employment and training. Policies for reducing truancy have been presented, which includes providing alternative education outside school for children who see the current curriculum as irrelevant (Social Exclusion Unit 1998).

SEXUAL HEALTH ISSUES

Surveys among adolescents have shown that there is a trend towards more sexual activity, and from an earlier age, than in the past. Although 90% of sexually active teenagers appear to have some experience of using contraception, first intercourse and casual relationships are particularly likely to be unprotected. Contraceptives are often not used because sexual intercourse is viewed as an unpremeditated and infrequent act. Alcohol is often an important factor in unplanned teenage pregnancy. Many 14–15-year-old adolescents do not seek contraceptive advice until they have been sexually active for 6 months or more because of the fear of parents finding out and doubts about the confidentiality of any advice they seek (Johnson et al 1994).

Early teenage sexual activity is best helped by:

- Confidential counselling.
- Access to advice.
- Encouraging personal worth.
- Developing skills in personal relationships.
- Developing decision-making skills.

Sexually transmitted infections

Associated with sexual activity are the whole range of sexually transmitted infections (STIs), including

Table 25.6
Conception rates England and Wales.

Year	Total	Conception rates/1000	
		→Maternities	→Abortions
13–15 year olds			
1972	9.3	5.5	3.8
1982	7.8	3.4	4.4
1990	10.1	5.0	5.1
1994	8.3	3.9	4.4
1996	9.4	4.6	4.8
15–19 year olds			
1970	82.4	71.4	10.9
1980	58.7	40.5	18.2
1990	69.0	44.4	24.6
1994	58.6	38.0	20.6
1996	63.0	40.0	23.0

From Office for National Statistics, Teenage conception rates, England and Wales

HIV, and their potential effect on future fertility. *Chlamydia* is now the commonest bacterial STI in the UK in women of childbearing age (Public Health Laboratory Service 1999). Screening has now been adopted in some teenage health clinics (e.g. in Nottingham City Primary Care Trust), in addition to genitourinary medicine (GUM) clinics. The risk of sexual dysfunction in the future is increased if the initial sexual experience is unhappy, for example in cases of sexual abuse (Wyatt & Powell 1988, Herman 1998).

Teenage pregnancies

The UK has the highest teenage pregnancy rate in Western Europe, twice that of Germany and six times that of the Netherlands. The reasons cited for the lower rates in the Netherlands are earlier sex education, greater contraceptive accessibility, greater openness between mothers and daughters and society in general regarding sexual issues, and a different peer group attitude that regards unplanned teenage pregnancy as not acceptable (European Union of Schools and Universities for Health and Medicine Conference 1997, personal communication).

Although there is a reduction overall in the pregnancy rates compared with the 1970s, the downward trend in the 1980s was halted by fears surrounding confidentiality (the Gillick case — see under 'Legal issues Concerning Services for adolescents') and in the 1990s by the 'contraceptive pill scare' (Spitzer et al 1996) (Table 25.6).

The Social Exclusion Unit's report on teenage pregnancy (June 1999) contends that there are three main factors contributing to the higher rates in the UK:

1. Teenagers have lower expectations due to increasing social deprivation and lack of employment prospects.
2. Teenagers are less informed about contraception, sexually transmitted infections, relationships and parenthood.
3. There are mixed messages from the media and peer group pressure that sexual activity is the norm, but there is reluctance by parents and society to acknowledge and discuss sexual matters.

The UK government's plan is to halve the rate of conceptions in under 18 year olds by the year 2010, and to reduce the risk of long-term social exclusion

Box 25.5
The categories of young people most at risk from pregnancy

- Those who have started to be sexually active in their early teens. They may not have developed the skills to talk about sex with a partner, negotiate a contraceptive method and use it effectively

- Those who lack self-esteem and have a poor self-image. They may seek to become pregnant for reassurance of their femininity and fertility

- Those from unhappy or unstable backgrounds. A baby is seen as someone who will give the love denied them by others and the pregnancy may be a means of establishing independence

- Those in care; the complexity of their problems makes them a particularly vulnerable group

- Young women not in education, training or employment

for teenage parents and their children. They aim to achieve this by:

- A coordinated national campaign.
- Greater prevention through issuing new guidance on sex education in schools and the provision of contraception for under 16 year olds, with better advice for parents and targetting of particular groups — boys and young men, those in and leaving care, young offenders and ethnic minority groups.
- Providing better support for teenage parents through appropriate services, education, training and child care.

The categories of young people most at risk from pregnancy are listed in Box 25.5.

Consequences of teenage pregnancy

There appear to be two distinct groups of pregnant schoolgirls, those who become pregnant inadvertently, and those who try to become pregnant, and who want to continue their pregnancies and keep their babies. Teenage mothers are more likely to come from large families (more than four children), broken homes and be low achievers educationally. Their mothers are more likely to have been preg-

nant as teenagers. Siblings of teenage mothers are also affected: loss of bedroom, noise, added family financial strains and emotional upheavals, and the time devoted to sharing baby care, all impinge on their study time, with lowering of achievements and expectations (Seamark 1997).

Termination of pregnancy is likely to have a considerable emotional effect on the pregnant girl, and adverse effects are more likely where the girl has a poor relationship with her parents. Those undergoing termination of pregnancy, under the age of 16 years particularly, need very careful counselling and support, to help them understand fully the benefits of future contraception.

Teenage maternal morbidity

In early teenage pregnancies some investigators have reported an increased risk of obstetric complications such as pre-eclampsia, prematurity, pelvic insufficiency and prolonged labour (Irvine 1997). Contributing factors are late booking for antenatal care, poor nutrition and poor attendance at antenatal clinic and mothercraft classes. There appears to be an increased risk of postnatal depression, and even suicide, in this group, particularly in those who have little support from family and friends (Wilson 1995). Perinatal mortality rates in England and Wales for babies born to teenage mothers tends to be higher (Dattani 1999). Also children born to teenage mothers are more at risk from a number of factors, as detailed in Box 25.6 (Social Exclusion Unit 1999).

LEGAL ISSUES CONCERNING SERVICES FOR ADOLESCENTS

The Children's Legal Centre in association with the University of Essex publishes 'childRIGHT', a journal of law and policy affecting children and young people in England and Wales. The Centre also provides a telephone advice line.

Confidentiality and people under 16 years of age

The British Medical Association, the Health Education Authority, the Brook Advisory Centres, the Family Planning Association and the Royal College of General Practitioners issued guidance for this collectively in 1993. In summary: 'The duty of confidentiality owed to a young person under 16 is as great as that owed to any other person. Any competent young person, regardless of age, can independently seek medical advice and give valid consent to medical treatment.' Confidentiality for under 16 year olds should be maintained wherever possible, unless there are child protection issues where the young person is deemed to be at risk of harm. The reasons for breaking their confidentiality should always be discussed with the young person.

Consent to treatment

Following the Gillick case in 1985 (*Gillick* vs. *West Norfolk and Wisbech Area Health Authority*), young people under the age of 16 can give consent to treatment, medical (including contraception), surgical and dental, provided they are deemed to be competent to understand fully what is proposed. This consent can only be overridden by the court. Refusal to consent to treatment can be overridden by someone with parental responsibility and by the court (Family Planning Association 1996).

The law in relation to sexual intercourse

The duty to report unlawful sexual intercourse was removed in 1967. At the age of 16 a girl can consent to heterosexual intercourse. She does not commit a crime if she is younger. Once over 16 she may be charged with assault if the boy is under 16. A boy aged 10 and over can be convicted of a criminal offence against a girl. It is an absolute offence for a man to have sexual intercourse with a girl under 13. There is no defence even if she consents. If the girl is between the ages of 13 and 16, he may defend himself on the grounds of: (a) he thought he was validly married to her (marriage in legal jurisdiction of another country); (b) he had reasonable grounds to think she was over 16; (c) he is under 24 years with no previous offence. When both parties are young there is usually no prosecution if there is no evidence of exploitation (Sexual Offences Act 1956, sections 5 and 6, Criminal Law Act 1967, section 2 and schedule 2). At 16 years of age a man can consent to a homosexual act with another man (also over 16) in private (Sexual Offences Act 1956, section 12, amended November 2000).

Age-based legislation

Confusion is caused by the variation in legal rights of the adolescent at different ages. In England and Wales they can apply at any age for access to personal information held on a computerised system, and for access to medical information about them (under the Access to Health Records Act 1990). At 16 years they are allowed to have access to their school records, leave school, marry with parental consent, legally have sex and ride a motorcycle. They must wait until 17 to drive a car and donate blood, 18 to drive a lorry, marry without parental consent, own property (land or house), vote and legally buy alcohol (Hamilton 2000).

SERVICES FOR ADOLESCENTS
Background

In 1976 the Court Report stated 'adolescents have needs and problems sufficiently distinguishable from those on the one hand of children, and on the other of adults, to warrant consideration as a distinct group for health care provision'.

In 1985 the British Paediatric Association's (BPA) Working Party on the needs of adolescents said

---

Box 25.7
Vulnerable adolescents

- Those with chronic illness
- Those who are physically disabled
- Those who are learning disabled
- Those with visual or hearing impairment
- Those with language development problems
- Those whose parents suffer chronic physical or mental illness
- Victims of physical, emotional or sexual abuse
- Those who are sexually exploited
- Those who are homeless, unemployed or experiencing poverty
- Pregnant adolescents and young teenage parents
- Those who are bereaved, from disrupted homes or who are unwanted
- Minority groups

Box 25.8
Teenage health clinics: Services that should be provided

- Easily accessible service with opportunity for drop-in consultations
- Friendly staff who are approachable and sympathetic
- Confidentiality
- Immediate help and advice on all health matters
- Counselling for emotional and personal problems
- Contraceptive advice including emergency contraception
- Provision of free condoms
- Instant pregnancy testing
- Pregnancy counselling and abortion referral
- Advice about sexually transmitted infections

'physical illness was not the predominant problem, but there was a need for self-referral clinics to provide advice on: a) growth and development, b) sexual problems, c) emotional difficulties including drug abuse' (British Paediatric Association 1985). Services for adolescents need to be multidisciplinary, friendly, discrete, attractive and easily accessible, recognising that adolescents have the right to confidentiality, to be respected and valued, set their own agendas, define their own needs and make decisions and choices for themselves. Services also need to be sensitive to the particular needs of vulnerable groups (Box 25.7).

In the last 15 years a variety of self-referral clinics for adolescents have been developed within local community centres, family planning services and general practices, particularly providing contraceptive and general health advice, or advice on drugs.

Teenage health clinics

These clinics need to provide the services listed in Box 25.8.

Health services for adolescents in hospital remain poor. Although data on bed usage by young people 12–19 years suggest that each district health authority should provide an adolescent ward of around 15 beds, still only about 10% of health authorities recognise their specific health needs in hospital (Viner 1999).

School health services for adolescents

The foundations for involving children in their own health are laid down during health appraisal at primary school. This continues during the adolescent years, the emphasis being on explanation of health indices, self-awareness and accepting responsibility for one's own health. Secondary school pupils should be able to self-refer to the school nurse or doctor to discuss any health, personal or social problems that may be worrying them (Polnay 1995).

Sex education

The importance of sex education has been increasingly recognised. As well as providing biological information, it should promote sexual health covering personal relationships, values and attitudes.

Since the introduction of the 1993 Education Act, sex education has become a compulsory component of the curriculum in all UK state secondary schools (Sex Education In Schools, Department For Education 5/94 circular). Recognising that teaching should be complementary and supportive to the prime parental role, parents have the right to withdraw their children from sex education lessons except that required by the National Science Curriculum. School governors are required to formulate and maintain their school sex education policy and they must have a written statement of this available to parents.

Mode of sex education

A flexible curriculum is necessary, and should be an ongoing part of personal and social education, and not dealt with as a separate subject on one occasion. Teachers need appropriate training and advice.

Impact of sex education programmes

School-based sex education can be effective in reducing teenage pregnancy, especially when linked to access to contraceptive services (Effective Health Care 1997). In 19 studies by the World Health Organization, none showed that they led to earlier or increased sexual activity. Two studies showed delayed onset of first intercourse (Mellanby et al 1995) and increased use of condoms at first intercourse (Johnson et al 1994).

Sex education programmes are more effective when there is:

- A narrow focus on reducing specific risky behaviours.
- Greater than 14 hours instruction plus small group work.
- A variety of interactive teaching methods to personalise information.
- An opportunity to practise communication and negotiation skills.

Information

Adolescents need to be provided with adequate information directed at boys as well as girls. It needs to be easily understood whatever their intellectual ability. Young people should be helped to understand the implications of sexual activity without moralising or censuring, but with obvious concern for their future happiness. Although behaviour is much more strongly influenced by family attitudes and experience than by formal teaching, a great many parents prefer someone else to teach their children about sex. Most young people learn from their friends or books. Publicity of services should also be aimed at professionals and the public in general.

Disability

Adolescent goals of independence, good self-image, vocation and sexual identity are achieved with more difficulty by those physically disabled. Chronic conditions present challenges to school and career development.

Transition to adult services

For young people with chronic disorders, transition to adults services needs to be effective and with appropriate information passed on (Kurtz & Hopkins 1996). If difficulties arise these may be around:

- Coping with change (girls more than boys).
- Relinquishing of control by parents and paediatricians.
- The differing emphasis placed by paediatricians (school progress, family relationships) and adult physicians (avoiding long-term complications).
- The timing of transition may be variable, for example a set age or dependent on physical and emotional maturity.
  There are various models of transition
- Continuation of paediatric service.
- Direct transfer to adult clinics.
- Young adult clinics.
- Joint clinics.

In conclusion

- Young people's health needs are diverse and affected by gender, culture, ethnicity and sexual orientation.

Young adults

- Services for adolescents must take account of their physical, mental and sexual health needs within the context of social issues and legal rights.
- Confidentiality is crucial, and should be maintained unless there are child protection issues.
- Reducing teenage pregnancy is a priority.

REFERENCES AND FURTHER READING

Anderson I, Kemp P, Quilgars D 1993 Single homeless people. Department of the Environment, London

Association of Chief Officers of Probation 1993 Youth crime: problem solved. Study quoted in National Association for the Care and Rehabilitation of Offenders (NACRO) Occasional Paper. Report available from NACRO, London

Audit Commission 1996 Misspent Youth: young people and crime. Audit Commission Publications, Abingdon, Oxon. Online. Available: *www.audit-commission.gov.uk/ac2/NR first.htm*

Balding J 1996 Young people in 1995. Schools Health Education Unit, University of Exeter

Black DR, Tobler NS, Sciacca JP 1998 Peer helping/involvement: an efficacious way to meet the challenge of reducing alcohol, tobacco, and other drug use among youth? Journal of School Health 68:87–93

British Paediatric Association 1985 Working party on the needs of adolescents. Royal College of Paediatrics and Child Health, London. Online. Available: *www.rcpch.ac.uk*

Brook C 1993 The practice of medicine in adolescence. Edward Arnold, London

childRIGHT: See Appendix 1

Churchill R D, Allen J, Denman S et al 1997 Factors influencing the use of general practice based health services by teenagers: a descriptive study in the East Midlands. Final Report for the NHSE R&D Mother & Child Health Programme. Division of General Practice, University of Nottingham

Coleman J 1997 Key data on adolescence. Trust for the Study of Adolescence, Brighton

Coleman J 1999 Key data on adolescence. Trust for the Study of Adolescence, Brighton

Court D 1976 Fit for the future Report of the Committee on Child Health Services. The Stationery Office, London. Online. Available: *www.statistics.gov.uk*

Criminal Statistics, England and Wales 1995 The Stationery Office, London. Online. Available: *www.statistics.gov.uk*

Dattani N 1999 Mortality in children aged under 4. Health statistics quarterly 02, Office for National Statistics, London. Online. Available: *www.statistics.gov.uk*

Department of Health 1994 On the state of the public health 1993. HMSO, London

Doll R, Peto R 1981 The causes of cancer: quantitative estimates of avoidable risks of cancer in the United States today. Journal of National Cancer Institute 66:1191–1308

Drugscope: see Appendix 1

Effective Health Care 1997 Bulletin on the effectiveness of health service interventions for decision makers. NHSS Centre for Reviews and Dissemination, University of York

European Drugs Monitoring Centre 1998 Annual report on the state of the drugs problem in the European Union. European Monitoring Centre on Drugs and Drug Addiction, Lisbon. Online. Available: *www.emcdda.org*

Evans K 1998 Tackling heroin amongst young people: an holistic approach. childRIGHT 150:10–11

Family Planning Association 1996 Family Planning Association factsheet 5E: the legal position regarding contraceptive advice and provision to young people. Family Planning Association, London

Fleman K 1995 Smoke and whispers. Turning Point Hungerford Project. Turning Point, London

Frisch R E 1996 The right weight: body fat, menarche and ovulation. Ballière's Clinical Obstetrics and Gynaecology 4:419

Gabhain S N, Francois Y 2000 Substance use. In: Currie C, Hurrelmann K, Settertobulte W, Smith R, Todd J (eds) Health behaviour in school-aged children: a WHO cross-national study (HBSC) international report. World Health Organization, Copenhagen, ch 9. Online. Available: *www.who.dk/document/e67880.pdf*

General Household Survey, Office for National Statistics, London. Online. Available: *www.statistics.gov.uk*

Gerada C, Ashworth M 1997 ABC of mental health: addiction and dependence 1: illicit drugs. British Medical Journal 315:297–300

Goddard E 1997 Young teenagers and alcohol in 1996, vol 1: England. Office for National Statistics, London. Online. Available: *www.statistics.gov.uk*

Gouzoulis-Mayfrank E, Daumann J, Tuchtenhagen F et al 2000 Impaired cognitive performance in drug free users of recreational (MDMA). Journal of Neurology, Neurosurgery and Psychiatry 68:719–725

Green R R, Goodwin G M 1996 Ecstasy and neurodegeneration, [editorial]. British Medical Journal 312:1493–1494

The Guardian 1998 29 December, p 1

Hamilton C 2000 At what age can I? The Children's Legal Centre, University of Essex. Online. Available: *www2.essex.ac.uk/clc*

Havell C 1998 Homelessness: a continual problem for young people in the UK. childRIGHT 148:12–14

Henderson J, Goldacre M, Yentes D 1993 Use of hospital inpatient care in adolescence. Archives of Disease in Childhood 69:559–563

Hendessi M Investing in Young People Programme 1992 Four in Ten. Report on young women who become homeless as a result of sexual abuse. CHAR — the housing campaign for single people, London

Herman J L 1998 Trauma and recovery, 2nd edn. Rivers Oram Press, London Institute for the Study of Drug Dependence, London (now Drugscope): See Appendix 1

Irvine H 1997 Pregnancy and motherhood: the implications for primary health care: unresolved issues. Journal of Royal College of General Practitioners 47:323–326

Jarvis L 1997 Smoking among secondary school children

in 1996. Office for National Statistics, London. Online. Available: *www.statistics.gov.uk*

Johnson A, Wadsworth J, Wellings K, Field J, Bradsay S 1994 Sexual attitudes and lifestyles. British survey. Blackwell Scientific, London

Kelly PAT 2000 Does recreational ecstasy cause long-term cognitive problems? Western Journal of Medicine 1173:129–130. Online. Available: *www.ewjm.com*

Kerfoot M 1996 Suicide and deliberate self-harm in children and adolescents. Children and Society 10:236–241

Kurtz Z, Hopkins A 1996 Services for young people with chronic disorders in their transition from childhood to adult life. Royal College of Physicians, London

Macfarlane A, McPherson A, Ahmed L 1987 Teenagers and their health. Archives of Disease in Childhood 62:1125–1129

McGurk H, Hurry J 1995 Project Charlie: an evaluation of a life skills drug education programme for primary schools. The Home Office, London. Online. Available: *www.homeoffice.gov.uk/dpas/charliec.htm*

McKee M 1999 Sex and drugs and rock and roll [editorial]. British Medical Journal 318:1300–1301

McKeganey N, Forsyth A, Barnard M, Hay G 1996 Designer drinks and drunkenness amongst a sample of Scottish school children. British Medical Journal 313:401

Marshall W A, Tanner J H 1969 Variations in pattern of pubertal changes in girls. Archives of Disease in Childhood 44:291

Mellanby A R, Phelps F A, Crichton N J, Tripp J H 1995 School sex education: an experimental programme with educational and medical benefit. British Medical Journal 311:414–417

The Mental Health Foundation 1996 Off to a bad start. The Mental Health Foundation, London. Online. Available: *www.mentalhealth.org.uk*

The Mental Health Foundation 1999 The big picture. The Mental Health Foundation, London. Online. Available: *www.mentalhealth.org.uk*

Merrill J 1996 Letter: ecstasy and neurodegeneration. British Medical Journal 313:423

Merritt D 1996 Paediatrics and adolescent gynaecology. In: Putorny S (ed) Current Topics in obstetrics and gynaecology. Chapman & Hall. New York, ch 5

Miller P, Plant M 1996 Drinking, smoking and illicit drug use among 15 and 16 year olds in the United Kingdom. British Medical Journal 313:394–397

Mortality Statistics 1997 The Stationery Office, London. Online. Available: *www.statistics.gov.uk*

Nassor I A A, Simms A 1996 The new picture of homelessness in Britain. Youth affairs briefing. Centrepoint, London. Online. Available: *www.centrepoint.org.uk*

Neinstein L S 1991a Adolescent health care. Urban and Schwaarzenberg, Baltimore, ch 8, p 156

Neinstein L S 1991b Adolescent health care. Urban and Schwaarzenberg, Baltimore, ch 8, p 157

Neinstein I S 1991c Adolescent health care. Urban and Schwaarzenberg, Baltimore ch 6, pp 110–114

Nottinghamshire County Council Social Services 1998 Sexual exploitation of children. Resource and Strategy Pack

Office for National Statistics: see Appendix 1

Parker H, Aldridge J, Measham F 1998 Illegal leisure: the normalisation of adolescent recreational drug use. Routledge, London

Plant M, Miller P 2000 Letter: drug use has declined among teenagers in United Kingdom. British Medical Journal 320:1536

Police Research Group 1998 New Heroin outbreaks amongst young people in England and Wales. The Home Office, London. Online. Available: *www.homeoffice.gov.uk/prgpubs.htm*

Polnay L 1995 Report of a joint working party on health needs of school age children. British Paediatric Association, now Royal College of Paediatrics and Child Health, London. Online. Available: *www.rcpch.ac.uk*

Public Health Laboratory Service 1999 Data from PHLS Communicable Disease Centre. The Stationery Office, London. Online. Available: *www.statistics.gov.uk*

Report of the Royal College of Obstetrics and Gynaecology (RCOG) Working Party on Unplanned Pregnancy 1991. RCOG, London. Online. Available: *www.rcog.org.uk*

Roberts H, Dengler R, Magowan R 1995 Trent Health Lifestyle Survey of Young People: report to Trent Regional Health Authority 1994. Department of Public Health Medicine and Epidemiology, University Hospital and Medical School, University of Nottingham

Roberts I, Barker M, Li L 1997 Analysis in trends in deaths from accidental drugs poisoning in teenagers, 1985–1995. British Medical Journal 315:289

Roker D 1995 Young people and drugs in Surrey. The Trust for the Study of Adolescence, Brighton

Russell F 1999 Juvenile Crime and Youth Justice. childRIGHT 155:7

Seamark CT 1997 Pregnancy in teenagers. Like mother, like daughter: a general practice study of maternal influences. Journal of Royal College of General Practitioners 47:175–176

Smoking kills — a white paper on tobacco 1998 The Stationery Office, London. On line. Available: *www.doh.gov.uk/public/wgpaper.htm*

Social Exclusion Unit 1998 Bringing Britain together, a national strategy for neighbourhood renewal. The Stationery Office, London. Online. Available: *www.cabinet-office.gov.uk/seu/1998/bbt/nrhome.htm*

Social Exclusion Unit 1999 Teenage pregnancy. The Stationery Office, London. Online. Available: *www.cabinet-office.gov.uk/seu/1999/teenpar.pdf*

Spitzer W, Lewis M, Heinemann L, Thorogood M, Macrae K 1996 Third generation oral contraceptive and risks of venous thromboembolic disorders: an international case-control study. British Medical Journal 312:83

Sutton S 1998 How ordinary people in Great Britain perceive the health risks of smoking. Journal of Epidemiology and Community Health 52:338–339

Swade R 1997 The confiscation of alcohol (Young Persons) Act 1997. childRIGHT 137:2

Taylor J C, Field-Smith M E, Norman C C, Bland J M, Ramsey J D, Anderson H R 2000 Trends in deaths associated with abuse of volatile substances 1971–1998. Department of Public Health Sciences and

Young adults

the Toxicology Unit, Department of Cardiological Sciences, St George's Hospital Medical School, London. Online. Available: *www.sgmhss.ac.uk/depts/phs/vsamenu.htm*

Thomas M, Walker A, Wilmot A, Bennett N 1998 Living in Britain: results from the 1996 General Household Survey. Office for National Statistics, The Stationery Office, London. Online. Available: *www.statistics.gov.uk*

Tregoning D 1998 Letter — Home Office addicts index no longer exists. British Medical Journal 316:151

The Trust for the Study of Adolescence: see Appendix 1

Turtle J, Jones A, Hickman M 1997 Young People and health: health behaviour in school-aged children. Health Education, Authority, London

Viner R 1999 Youth matters. Royal College of Paediatrics and Child Health Newsletter June: 3. Online. Available: *www.rcpch.ac.uk*

Wilson J 1995 Maternal policy. Professional care of mother and child. 5:139–142

Wyatt G A, Powell G J 1988 Lasting effects of child sexual abuse. Sage, London

World Health Organization 1997 young people and health: health behaviour in school-aged children. A WHO Cross National Study. WHO, Copenhagern

Young L 1997 Young people and drugs: knowledge, experience and values. childRIGHT 138:5–6

26 | General paediatrics in the community setting

This chapter is designed to discuss some of the common problems that community paediatricians face in clinics in the community. It is *not* designed to replace standard textbooks of paediatrics but to complement them. As models for paediatric practice change the types of problems we see are potentially changing, with general paediatric problems becoming more common in the local clinics. The chapter has been divided into system-based areas and focused on the common problems.

RESPIRATORY PROBLEMS IN CHILDHOOD

Asthma

Asthma is the commonest chronic disease in childhood. Epidemiologists agree that the prevalence and severity of asthma globally is on the increase. In the UK the prevalence of asthma has increased from around 4% in the 1960s to 14% in the late 1990s. Although this increase may reflect a more readiness to diagnose and give a label of asthma, there has been a true rise in wheezing illness in children. Corresponding with an increase in the prevalence there has been an increase in the severity, with a higher level of hospital admission and mortality.

What is asthma?

The definition of asthma has recently incorporated the principal role played by inflammation in the pathogenesis of asthma and is currently defined by the presence of the following:

- Airway inflammation.
- Airway obstruction that is reversible either with medications or spontaneously.

- Increased airway responsiveness to stimuli that would not effect non-asthmatics (airway hyper-responsiveness).

This inflammatory process causes recurrent episodes of wheezing, breathlessness, coughing and tightness of chest.

Pathophysiology

Although asthma is a well-recognised clinical syndrome, its pathogenesis is not well understood. Inflammation is an early event in asthma, and inflammatory cells are always present in tissue biopsies obtained from newly diagnosed asthmatic patients. Eosinophils and lymphocytes infiltrate into the airway wall. Lymphocytes bearing the Th2 subtype produce various cytokines, some of which further aid the allergic response. Mast cells sensitised with immunoglobulin E (IgE) against specific antigen are abundantly present. Smooth muscle in the airways undergoes histological changes leading to reduction in the airway lumen eventually leading to its remodelling. Mast cells and eosinophils are also responsible for the production of not only histamine but also leukotrienes and platelet-activating factor. These molecules have the various properties including airway muscle constriction and stimulation of the airways nervous system. The hypersecretory state produced by these chemicals worsens airways' obstruction.

Epidemiology, genetics, mortality, race, risk factors

A number of factors are associated with increased risk of developing asthma.

- **Genetics.** There is genetic predisposition to developing asthma and atopy, the risk of a child developing asthma being two to three times greater if one or both the parents had asthma. Monozygotic twins are more likely to have concordance for asthma than dizygotic twins. Current studies show that a locus on chromosome 5 and 11 may be responsible for susceptibility for atopy. However the prevalence of atopy is 33%, being two to three times the prevalence of asthma, indicating that additional factors predispose to the development of asthma.

- **Race.** There have major differences noted in the prevalence of asthma across various racial and ethnic groups. In the UK asthma is commoner in children of Afro-Caribbean or Asian origins that in the white Caucasian population. Similarly in the USA asthma is up to 2.5 times more common in Afro-American children than white Caucasian children. Studies from the UK and New Zealand demonstrate no racial differences in the prevalence of asthma in children from similar socio-economic and environmental backgrounds.

- **Socio-economic.** Poor and socially disadvantaged children are more severely affected than affluent children, this being more obvious in urban settings.

- **Boys are more commonly affected than girls**, being up to two times as common in the under 10 years old, although after puberty the incidence begins to equalise. It also appears to be more severe in males, possibly explained by greater prevalence of atopy in young boys and reduced relative airway size in boys compared to girls.

- Energy-efficient building has led to **increased indoor air pollution** especially house dust mite (requiring high relative humidity for optimal growth) and animal allergens (cat and dog allergens). In deprived neighbourhoods cockroach allergen and fungal spores may play a major part in the development of asthma.

- **Air pollution.** There is increased nitrogen dioxide and sulphur dioxide in the environment, although there is no clear association between air pollution and asthma.

- It is not known whether **viral respiratory infections** in infancy induce asthma or whether severe viral respiratory infections occur in infants with underlying predisposing factors, e.g. small lungs. There is however some epidemiological evidence that frequent respiratory infection during infancy may protect against the later development of asthma.

- **Prenatal exposure to cigarette smoking** is associated with reduced pulmonary function in the infant, increasing the risk for wheezing and subsequent development for asthma later in life.

- **Prematurity and infants with chronic lung disease.** Children of young mothers have a higher risk of developing asthma.

Both parents and physicians are becoming increasingly aware of asthma and diagnosis is made earlier than in the past (Box 26.1).

Natural history of asthma

Most parents wish to know whether their child will grow out of his asthma or whether it continue into adulthood. Recent work by Martinez and his col-

---

Box 26.1
Triggers of asthma: in children a variety of factors either precipitate or worsen asthma

- Commonest precipitating factor — intercurrent upper respiratory tract infection

- Exercise

- Pollen sensitivity; associated with other allergic symptoms such as allergic rhinitis, conjunctivitis or eczema

- Indoor allergens — house dust mite, animal hair or secretions, moulds and cockroaches in very deprived housing estates

- Environmental tobacco smoke

- Foods, e.g. citrus fruits and ice cream amongst Asians

- Sulphites or the colouring tartrazine

- Gastro-oesophageal reflux may be a trigger for nocturnal symptoms

- Menstrual periods or pregnancy in adolescent girls

- Emotion

leagues from Tucson, Arizona has helped us to understand wheezing in the early years of life. It appears that wheezing in infancy is not a homogeneous condition. A substantial group of infants will have transient wheezing associated with low lung functions; maternal smoking seems to play a major part in this. However by the age of 6 years 60% of children with wheezing in the first 3 years of life will have no wheezing. A further subgroup will have persistence of symptoms into adolescence, this being determined by frequency of symptoms early in life, infantile eczema and a maternal history of asthma. Elevated levels of IgE and maternal smoking seem to be significant factors in predisposing to asthma persisting into adolescence and adulthood. Severe untreated asthma appears to result in lower lung function than those with less severe symptoms.

Diagnosis and management

In children coughing and wheezing are the most common symptoms:

- **Cough.** A dry usually unproductive cough is the commonest symptom in children. Occasionally sputum may be present. Wheezing may or may not be present and hence may lead to inappropriate treatments such as cough suppressants or antibiotics being prescribed. Symptoms are usually worse at night or first thing in the morning and may indicate more severe asthma.
- **Wheezing.** Expiratory wheeze may be present, although in severe obstruction it may be biphasic. A silent chest in an asthmatic child indicates a severe medical emergency.
- **Tightness of chest**, or pain on breathing associated with breathlessness, may be presenting symptoms in older children.

Box 26.2 gives differential diagnoses when investigating a possible case of asthma.

Physical examination

Although physical examination is usually normal in most asthmatics certain abnormal findings would suggest asthma:

- Other signs of atopy:
  - ☐ eczema

> Box 26.2
> ## Asthma: differential diagnoses
>
> - Bronchiolitis
> - Cystic fibrosis
> - Immune disorders
> - Ciliary dyskinesia
> - Bronchiolitis obliterans
> - Interstitial lung disease
> - Bronchopulmonary dysplasia
> - Anatomical anomalies of upper airways, e.g. tracheomalacia
> - Vascular rings
> - Congestive heart failure
> - Vocal cord dysfunction

  - ☐ rhinitis/nasal crease due to itching
  - ☐ dry skin.
- Chest deformity:
  - ☐ Harrison's sulcus
  - ☐ increase in antero-posterior diameter of the chest.

Investigations

- **Chest X-ray.** A chest X-ray is essential only as an **initial** investigation. Congenital malformations may be identified or rarely a malignancy observed. Features of asthma may be identified although in most patients the investigation is normal.
- **Sweat chloride test.** In infants failing to thrive or in those with diarrhoea and respiratory symptoms a sweat test should be carried out to establish a diagnosis of cystic fibrosis.
- **Barium swallow.** A barium swallow may be helpful in diagnosing vascular rings or tracheo-oesophageal fistula. This is especially useful in the under 1 year old. Oesophageal pH monitoring may be useful in diagnosing gastro-oesophageal reflux.
- **Skin testing.** Skin testing may be helpful only when used in selective patients.

Principles of treatment

The goals of asthma treatment:

- To bring relief to symptoms of asthma with minimal medications and to bring *normality* to daily life, including participation in sporting activity both at home and school.
- Minimise nocturnal symptoms and maximise school attendance.
- Minimise acute exacerbation's and prevent hospitalisation.
- Active participation of parents and the child in his management at home and tailoring treatment for the individual child.
- Optimise growth by minimising side effects of drugs.
- Improvement in lung function.
- Asthma and anti-smoking education for the child and family.

Pharmacological management

(Table 26.1)

The stepwise approach in therapy is adopted based upon asthma severity. The dosage and frequency of drugs administered is increased as necessary to achieve optimal control. Once this has been achieved, attempts should be made to reduce the dosage at 1- to 2-month intervals as tolerated. The lowest dosages of medications are maintained to optimise control and minimise side effects. Acute exacerbations of asthma require a more aggressive management at any time, including the administration of oral steroids.

Impact on child and family

The impact of asthma on both the patient and his family's lives can, depending upon severity, be at the least disruptive and at the worst devastating. In a recent asthma survey more than 25% of respondents felt that asthma totally dominated their lives, with some of the problems stated as:

- Sleep disturbance due to coughing.
- Bad tempers and loss of concentration at school.
- Failure in academic or sporting field (29% had to give up sport altogether).
- Loss of time from work or, more importantly, the loss of a job for parents.

- Repeated visits to GP, hospital, hospital casualty or clinics.
- Parental anxiety with loss of social life and difficulty in planning holidays.
- Restriction on owning a pet.
- Visiting relatives or friends with a pet can be out of the question.

Developing specialised clinics can enhance communication between patients and health professionals. Nurse-run asthma clinics have been shown to be successful because:

- Nurses are more readily approachable and accessible.
- Nurses are less judgmental yet still in a position of trust.
- Regular follow-up by specialist asthma nurses both in hospital and general practice have reduced crisis management of asthma by management through education and training.
- Specialist asthma nurses empower patients and parents to manage the situation themselves.

Patient education

The efficacy of inhaled medications especially metered dose inhalers can be compromised if the patient uses the device inaccurately. For optimal asthma care, time must be spent with the patient in order to develop appropriate treatment and to tailor it to the patient's needs. The choice of the correct device initially will in the long run deliver better treatment, resulting in less morbidity and fewer consultations. Choosing an inhaler is a complex decision depending on:

- age of the child
- drug to be delivered
- patient preference.

There are basically two types of inhaler:

- **Metered dose inhalers** (MDIs) can deliver a variety of inhaled medications, including beta-agonists, anticholinergics, corticosteroids and cromolyn. The MDI device in conjunction with a holding chamber (spacer) is the method of choice for infants regardless of drug and for all ages

Table 26.1
Pharmacological management of asthma

Drug	Mechanisms	Indications	Side effects observed
Anti-inflammatory agents			

1. Inhaled steroids
  a. Beclomethasone
  b. Budesonide
  c. Fluticasone
	Controls inflammation
	Reverses down-
	regulation of beta-
	agonists
		Long-term control of
		symptoms
			Adrenal suppression with high
			dose
			Growth suppression
			Osteoporosis
			Cataracts and glaucoma in
			the elderly

2. Sodium cromoglicate	Stabilises mast cells Blocks early and late reaction to allergen Inhibits acute response to exercise, cold air		A long trial may be necessary to determine efficac
Inhaled bronchodilators	Smooth muscle relaxant		Tachycardia, tremors, headaches
Short acting 1. Salbutamol 2. Terbutaline		Acute relief of symptoms For exercise- induced symptoms	
Long acting 1. Salmeterol 2. Formoterol (eformoterol)		Long-term prevention of symptoms Prevent exercise- induced bronchospasm	
Anticholinergics Ipratropium bromide	Reduces vagal tone Inhibits cholinergic receptors	Acute relief of bronchospasm	Dry mouth and blurred vision
Leukotriene antagonists Montelukast Zafirlukast	Antagonises leukotriene receptors	Prevention of mild symptoms Exercise-induced symptoms	Headaches, reversible hepatitis

(Modified from National Asthma Education and Prevention Program — NIH publication 1997 *http://www.ginasthma.com*)

when inhaling steroid therapy, ensuring a better deposition in the lungs and better airway response. Spacers also minimise topical side effects such as oral candidiasis and vocal changes by decreasing the oral deposition of medicine from 80% to 8%. Children under the age of 2 usually require a soft silicone face mask to be used with a large volume spacer. In general, larger sized spacers appear more effective than smaller ones, but proper technique and frequent cleaning of the spacer to minimise static electricity may be more important for obtaining optimal drug delivery.

- **Powder devices** (Rotahalers, Easibreathe, Turbohalers) are breath-actuated dry powder medications. Newer devices eliminate the need to coordinate inhalation and hand actuation in one study, patient timing errors were reduced by the breath-activated inhaler in inexperienced volunteers from 32% to 6.5% and in experienced patients from 21.5% to 5%.

Teaching patients the correct inhaler technique is important for better control and minimisation of side effects. The trained asthma nurse has a major role in ensuring this. In addition to using the correct technique, patients should be taught to rinse their mouths after using an inhaled steroid and to spit the water out rather than swallow it to minimise oral deposition.

Other respiratory disorders

Upper airway

The community paediatrician needs to be aware of other difficulties, particularly those of the upper airway and those of an atopic nature. The upper airway can be the cause of a number of problems including hearing loss, poor sleep and eating difficulties. The behavioural management of these can be found in various texts but without addressing the underlying pathology this will be difficult to undertake.

Up to 25% of 5 year olds snore but only a small proportion of these will have sleep apnoea of a clinically significant degree. Many however will have disturbed sleep. The lymphoid tissue increases in size in the late preschool years and this is the most common time for problems to be identified. Generalised problems are often identified, for example 'glue ear', large tonsils and adenoids and a 'blocked nose'. A good history and diary can be very helpful in assessing the problem. The clinical assessment for sleep apnoea/tonsillar size can be unreliable and if there is doubt then more objective tests should be carried out.

For many older children treatment with a nasal steroidal spray can offer relief particularly in those with an atopic element. In some, particularly those with recurrent illness, courses of antibiotics on a long-term basis (i.e. once daily) may help. In some children (those with more severe problems and concurrent problems, e.g. conductive deafness affecting speech), adenotonsillectomy and grommet insertion may prove beneficial. The natural history is that the size of adenoids and tonsils reduce with time. Therefore in those with minor difficulties who do not have concurrent problems an expectant approach is appropriate.

GASTROINTESTINAL AND NUTRITIONAL PROBLEMS

Coeliac disease

This gluten-sensitive enteropathy is more common in children of European origin. The average incidence in Europe is about 1 in 1000 live births.

Coeliac disease arises as a result of immunologically mediated structural damage to the mucosa of the small intestine leading to malabsorption. The cereals responsible for producing the mucosal reaction are wheat, barley, rye and oats. The specific antigen is gliadin. There is a strong genetic association, with HLA types DR3 and DR5 being significantly more common in patients with coeliac disease.

The symptoms of the condition vary. Few children nowadays present with classic signs, i.e. diarrhoea, abdominal distension and gross malabsorption. More commonly children present with chronic diarrhoea, mild failure to thrive, irritability, recurrent abdominal pain, short stature and iron deficiency. Children presenting at less than 2 years tend to have more marked gastrointestinal symptoms, whereas older children present with milder more insidious symptoms such as anaemia, short stature and recurrent mouth ulcers.

A child may show extra-intestinal manifestations such as dermatitis herpetiformis, insulin-dependent diabetes, autoimmune thyroid disease, Down's syndrome, arthritis, infertility or rarely epilepsy thought to be due to intracerebral calcification.

Definitive diagnosis is made by small intestinal biopsy but the diagnosis may be strongly suspected if positive IgA antigliadin and IgA antiendomysial antibodies are found in blood. The classical histological changes are subtotal villous atrophy.

The only treatment for coeliac disease is a life-long gluten-free diet to minimise the recognised increased risk of intestinal lymphoma. A strict gluten-free diet may protect against the increased risk of malignancy. The advice of a dietician is therefore essential in the management of such children.

Cows' milk protein intolerance

The true prevalence of cows' milk protein intolerance (CMPI) is unknown. Most affected infants have multiple symptoms which develop in the first 3 months of life (Box 26.3). The condition is often familial.

CMPI is an immune-mediated reaction between the food protein antigen and the intestinal mucosa. Most immunological investigations are unhelpful, including skin prick tests and RAST for circulating IgE. The most reliable diagnostic tool is the elimination — rechallenge test, whereby an improvement is seen in symptoms when cows' milk is completely eliminated from the diet followed by recurrence of the symptoms when cows' milk is reintroduced. Failure of the symptoms to remit when cows' milk is excluded from the diet may occur because the diagnosis is incorrect or because cows' milk exclusion is incomplete.

Box 26.3
Symptoms of cows' milk intolerance

- Vomiting
- Diarrhoea leading to anal excoriation
- Blood in stool leading to iron deficiency anaemia
- Poor weight gain
- Crying, irritability
- Less commonly wheeze, cough, eczema

Soya milk or a protein hydrosylate (e.g. Pregestimil) should be substituted and the advice of a dietician may be necessary. Infants who are fed proprietary infant soya formulas do not need calcium supplements, although it is recommended that older children on a soya milk diet should receive such supplements. Note there is considerable cross-reactivity between cows', goats', sheep and soya milks.

The majority of children with cows' milk protein intolerance outgrow the condition by the end of the first year of life, but it may persist.

Lactose intolerance

Lactose intolerance is caused by a deficiency of the enzyme lactase in the intestinal mucosa. This most often occurs after an episode of gastroenteritis, when the intestinal mucosa is temporarily damaged (the so-called postgastroenteritis syndrome). The main clinical feature is diarrhoea after ingestion of milk. Diagnosis is made by finding reducing substances in the stool. As with cows' milk protein intolerance the diagnosis is confirmed by eliminating lactose from the diet followed some weeks later by a rechallenge.

Toddler diarrhoea

This is the most common cause of chronic diarrhoea in preschool aged children in developed countries. Typical symptoms are frequent foul-smelling, watery stool which contains undigested food particles. There are usually few or no other symptoms (e.g. poor weight gain), although abdominal pain may rarely be a feature.

The diarrhoea is thought to be due to a reduced colonic transit time resulting in less water being absorbed from the colon causing the stools to be more watery than expected. Additionally toddler diarrhoea is more common in young children who consume large quantities of fruit juice particularly apple juice as part of a 'healthy eating' diet at the expense of a reduced fat intake.

A complete examination should reveal an otherwise healthy, thriving child. If the diagnosis is clear then no further investigations are required and an explanation and reassurance can be given. Advice

General paediatrics in the community setting

should be centred around dietary modification so that the amount of juice is reduced and fat intake increased to 35–40% of total intake.

Recurrent abdominal pain

The overall incidence is about 10% of older children and adolescents. The definition (after Apley 1959) is of at least three episodes of pain severe enough to interfere with daily activity, occurring over a 3-month period in a child at least 3 years of age. Organic disorders are found in a very few (<5%) children. A careful history is essential. The pain is usually described as central, cramping or dull ache and may be associated with pallor, anorexia, headache or vomiting. Despite this clinical examination is almost always normal. The cause remains obscure and the majority of children with recurrent abdominal pain do not have any psychological difficulties.

Family history may reveal other family members with similar symptoms. Some children with recurrent abdominal pain go on to suffer with irritable bowel syndrome as adults but this is not universal.

There is some overlap between this condition and recurrent headaches and leg pains in children.

Childhood constipation and soiling

Constipation: a standard definition does not exist because of the wide variation in the normality of frequency of stool passage.

Encopresis or soiling: repeated involuntary or voluntary passage of stool into clothing or other places not intended for that purpose, for at least 1 month's duration, in a child of 4 years or greater.

Ninety-five per cent of newborns pass meconium in the first 24 hours after birth. In early infancy the average baby has his bowels open three to six times a day, although it may be as little as once a week in breast-fed babies. The normal range of frequency of bowel motions for children 1–4 years is from three times a day to three times a week. Infrequent bowel motions alone do not indicate constipation (Fig. 26.1). The gender ratio is approx 3:1, males to females.

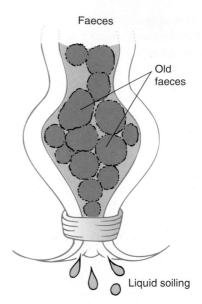

Fig. 26.1 Chronically constipated child. Firm stools become impacted in the rectum which becomes dilated. This dilated rectum loses its sensation as the nerve fibres are stretched, and soiling occurs, often unknowingly, as the liquid stool leaks around the large solid mass

Pathophysiology

History is fundamental to further management (Box 26.4). The urge to defaecate helps to distinguish chronic constipation from Hirschsprung's disease. In Hirschsprung's there is no urge as the faecal mass is above the anorectum. A distended rectum also causes bladder compression causing enuresis (Box 26.5). Other factors such as school toilet facilities should be considered, especially for children whose soiling started around the time of school entry.

Encopresis occurs in 2.8% of 4 year olds and 1.5% of 8 year olds.

Family stresses, for example death, separation, birth of a sibling, may interfere with normal toilet training. Children may be frightened by the thought of drowning or falling down the toilet. Children may not wish to use an unfamiliar toilet (e.g. at school) and thus hold on.

Encopresis may adversely affect the child's self-esteem. This is referred to in the chapter on emotional and behavioural problems (see Chapter 28).

Box 26.4
Constipation: important points in history taking

- Family history in as many as 55%
- When meconium was first passed
- Lack of fibre in diet and/or inadequate fluid intake, fever
- Associated loss of appetite, urinary tract infections (UTI), enuresis — up to 20% of girls with recurrent UTIs have underlying chronic constipation
- Timing of soiling — most frequently in the afternoon, during exercise or walking home from school
- Stool frequency, consistency and size
- Presence of blood streaking
- Anxieties around sitting on the toilet
- Difficulties around the time of toilet training

Box 26.5
Physical examination in constipation

- Abdomen for distension, palpation for faecal masses
- Inspection of perianal area for fissures, excoriation
- Lower spine for pigmented or hairy patches
- Digital examination for anal tone and faecal masses may be necessary

Differential diagnosis

- Hirschsprung's disease — 90% of affected babies are male, presenting in the neonatal period with delayed passage of meconium. Rectal examination reveals an empty rectum compared with constipation when the rectum is usually full.
- Anal stenosis.
- Cerebral palsy — reduced motility, poor diet.

- Spinal cord lesions, e.g. spina bifida occulta.
- Metabolic, e.g. hypothyroidism, hypercalcaemia.

Management

It is useful to explain the mechanism of the constipation to the child and his parents and to reassure the child that he is not to blame. The parents should be encouraged to alter the child's diet as necessary to a high fibre diet and to increase the fluid intake with water or juice.

Laxative medication should be commenced (e.g. lactulose and senna twice daily), although in some cases an enema or oral medication (e.g. picosulphate) may be required to empty the rectum before laxatives are started. In addition a behavioural approach should be followed, i.e. a star chart for the child to monitor his own progress. Regular review every few weeks is essential to keep up morale and to assess the need for a change in the dose of medication.

Gastro-oesophageal reflux (GOR)

This is the passive regurgitation of stomach contents into the oesophagus and is due to poorly developed lower oesophageal sphincter tone in infants and young children. It presents with effortless vomiting, discomfort during or soon after feeding and occasionally screaming. In normal individuals gastric contents (acid) are present in the lower oesophagus 1–5% of a 24-hour period but in children with GOR this is greatly increased.

There are various complications with GOR. In severe cases infants may fail to gain weight due to large vomits. The presence of regular acid in the oesophagus can lead to oesophagitis and blood-stained vomiting. Children with cerebral palsy are particularly prone to GOR and there is a risk of aspiration because of a poor gag reflex.

Diagnosis is usually made on the history but where doubt exists or trial of treatment has failed oesophageal pH monitoring can define the extent of the problem.

For a child who is well and growing satisfactorily the only treatment necessary may be reassurance and the addition of a feed thickener (e.g. Carobel) to feeds. In more severe cases an alginate compound such as Infant Gaviscon is used. The presence of oesophagitis often warrants the use of H_2 antagonists or omeprazole.

Typically children outgrow GOR within the first year of life as they naturally assume a more upright position and take an increasingly solid diet.

Iron deficiency anaemia

Anaemia in childhood is defined as a haemoglobin less than 11 g/dl. The commonest cause of anaemia in childhood is iron deficiency. The prevalence varies with age and is most common in the infant and toddler age group, with estimates of up to 40% of toddlers in inner city areas and 3–10% of school-aged children.

Iron deficiency anaemia (IDA) develops as a result of diminishing neonatal iron stores and an increasing red cell mass. A high index of suspicion is required as young children are often asymptomatic and have no physical signs although IDA may be associated with poor growth, poor appetite, lethargy, pallor, pica, recurrent infections, behavioural problems and developmental delay. A detailed dietary history should be taken.

Particular factors are associated with an increased risk:

- prematurity
- delayed weaning beyond 6 months of age
- early introduction of cows' milk
- excessive intake of cows' milk in the second year of life
- children from ethnic minorities.

At diagnosis the haemoglobin is less than 11 g/dl with low a MCV and MCH. The ferritin level is low, which helps distinguish IDA from thalassaemia in which a normal or raised ferritin level is seen. However it should be remembered that ferritin levels may be raised acutely after a recent infection which may give a false impression of normality despite IDA. Features of the management of IDA are detailed in Box 26.6.

Peanut allergy

The true incidence of peanut allergy is not known but it is estimated to be at least 1 in 200 of the population and is thought to be becoming more

---

> **Box 26.6**
> ### Management of iron deficiency anaemia
>
> **Dietary modification** — e.g. reducing amount of cows' milk consumed. In infants under 1 year a fortified formula or follow-on milk may be used. Iron absorption is increased in the presence of vitamin C and is inhibited by foods containing tannin, e.g. tea, coffee and bran. Iron-rich diets are those which contain good quantities of meat, fish and dark leafed vegetables
>
> **Iron supplements** — Sytron solution 1 ml/kg/day (equivalent to 5 mg/kg/day) for a period of 3 months after which Hb should be rechecked. Failure to respond to treatment suggests poor compliance but also requires review of the child, re-examination and consideration for further investigation. It is important to warn parents of the risks of accidental ingestion of iron

---

common. The typical symptoms are: urticaria, contact urticaria, angioedema, vomiting, diarrhoea, abdominal pain, wheezing or anaphylactic shock.

Diagnosis is usually made on the history alone. Skin prick or RAST tests may be positive in the absence of any clinical symptoms, especially in atopic children, therefore these tests should be interpreted with caution.

All children with a suspected severe reaction to peanuts should be referred to a paediatrician or allergy clinic. For children with mild allergic reactions non-sedating antihistamines may be used.

In severe cases the child will be given an adrenaline (epinephrine) containing EpiPen to be used in the event of any future reaction, and thus both parents and school teachers require instructions on its administration. Parents should be encouraged to liaise closely with their child's school. The education of school staff is most easily facilitated by the school doctor or nurse. An individualised protocol for the management of a particular child is very useful and should be readily available for all staff members to access. Parent and patient education is the cornerstone of prevention. Awareness should be raised of the presence of peanut in many manufactured foods such as vegetable burgers and cake icing.

It is uncommon for children to outgrow peanut allergy. It is also common for there to be a strong family history: 'Pregnant or breastfeeding mothers with a family history of peanut allergy may want to avoid eating peanuts' — is a recommendation made by the UK Chief Medical Officer 1998.

ENDOCRINOLOGY

Hypothyroidism

Hypothyroidism presents as two distinct entities in childhood: congenital and acquired.

Congenital

This affects approximately 1 in 3500 live births. The majority of cases are due to dysgenesis of the thyroid gland, i.e. absence or hypoplasia of the gland or an ectopically placed gland. The remainder are due to abnormalities of thyroid hormone synthesis (dyshormonogenesis) or to a transient drop in thyroid hormone levels as a result of transplacental passage of maternal antibody or anti-thyroid medication.

Population screening of all newborns in the first week of life, for raised TSH levels in heelprick blood specimens, was introduced in the late 1970s and the prognosis for intellectual development is very good if treatment is commenced as soon as possible before 3 weeks of age.

Treatment with L-thyroxine should be commenced by a paediatrician or paediatric endocrinologist with regular monitoring of serum T4 and TSH levels over the first few months.

Children with early treated congenital hypothyroidism now achieve IQ scores within the normal range, although more recent studies have suggested that there still may be up to a 10 point deficit in IQ between affected children and normal controls. There is also some evidence to suggest that children treated with high doses of L-thyroxine have a slightly increased incidence of attentional problems and mild hearing impairment (Grant 1997).

Acquired

This is most commonly seen in older children and adolescents, more often in females. Autoimmune thyroiditis accounts for a large proportion of cases and may be diagnosed by detecting raised titres of antimicrosomal, antithyroglobulin and antiperoxidase antibodies in serum. A family history of thyroid disease is obtained in up to 30% of cases. Autoimmune thyroiditis is particularly associated with Down's and Turner's syndromes.

The child may present with poor growth and delayed bone age, dry scaly skin, cold intolerance, muscle weakness and lethargy. Hypothyroidism may also occur after thyroid surgery or irradiation of the thyroid gland for tumours of the head and neck or during work up for a bone marrow transplant.

Acquired hypothyroidism should also be treated with L-thyroxine and parents should be advised about potential behavioural problems including a temporary deterioration in school performance when treatment is first introduced.

Hyperthyroidism

The most common cause of hyperthyroidism in childhood is Graves' disease which is an autoimmune condition associated with the presence of long-acting thyroid stimulating antibody (LATS) and thyroid stimulating immunoglobulin (TSI). There is a peak in the adolescent years with a female preponderance of $5:1$.

Hyperthyroidism usually presents insidiously with increased appetite without weight gain, emotional disturbance, irritability and excitability, motor hyperactivity, tremor, and deteriorating school performance may be noted. The affected child is likely to be tall with an advanced bone age but not sexually more mature.

Diagnosis is confirmed by a raised T4 and T3 and a low TSH.

Treatment is initially with medical therapy (e.g. carbimazole). Subtotal thyroidectomy may be necessary in resistant cases.

Diabetes

Diabetes in childhood is almost always insulin dependent and is due to autoimmune destruction of pancreatic beta cells. The prevalence in childhood is approximately 1 in 500 under 16 years. There is a peak in incidence in early to mid puberty

General paediatrics in the community setting

and a seasonal variation with a peak in winter and spring suggesting an additional possible viral link. Males and females are equally affected.

Diabetes often presents insidiously with poor appetite, malaise, polyuria, polydipsia and weight loss.

Over recent years there has been a shift from hospital to community management of children with diabetes and the paediatric diabetic liaison nurse plays a key role particularly with regard to education and motivation.

It is known that tight diabetic control during childhood significantly reduces the frequency of long-term complications, for example retinopathy, neuropathy and renal disease. There is also some evidence to suggest that type 2 diabetes is becoming more common in children as the incidence of childhood obesity increases. This raises serious public health concerns. The most important treatment for these children is weight reduction.

HEART DISEASE IN CHILDHOOD

Congenital heart disease

Congenital heart disease is the commonest congenital malformation — 8 per 1000 live births — but most babies are asymptomatic at birth (Box 26.7).

If a baby is noted to have a murmur at the newborn examination then further investigation including echocardiography should be performed (Box 26.8). In one study up to 50% of babies with a murmur on neonatal examination had an underlying structural cardiac abnormality, the remainder having normal physiological variants, for example patent ductus arteriosus or left pulmonary artery branch stenosis (Hall 1996, Ainsworth et al 1999).

According to UK recommendations in 'Health for all Children' (*www.health-for-all-children.co.uk*) a further screening examination should be carried out at 6–8 weeks of age. Babies found to have a murmur at this age should also be referred for investigation if this has already not been performed. It is important to remember that absence of a murmur does not exclude significant heart disease.

It is essential that all babies and children with congenital heart disease receive a full course of immunisations.

Box 26.7
Common cardiac conditions in childhood

- Ventricular septal defect
- Coarctation of aorta
- Patent ductus arteriosus
- Pulmonary stenosis
- Tetralogy of Fallot
- Atrial septal defect
- Aortic stenosis
- Atrioventricular septal defect
- Hypertrophic obstructive cardiomyopathy

Box 26.8
Distinguishing factors between innocent and pathological heart murmurs in childhood

Innocent
- Asymptomatic
- Normal pulses
- No thrill
- Mid-systolic
- Usually soft, musical
- Variable with position
- Normal heart sounds

Pathological
- Cardiac symptoms
- Normal, collapsing, delayed pulses
- May be a thrill
- Pan or diastolic
- May be loud
- Consistent
- May be abnormal heart sounds

From: Jordan 1994

Ventricular septal defect

This is the commonest congenital heart lesion in childhood. Diagnosis is made by finding a harsh, loud pansystolic murmur over the lower left sternal edge which may be accompanied by a systolic thrill. The child is usually asymptomatic. Referral to a paediatrician or paediatric cardiologist is necessary if the diagnosis is uncertain. A small ventricular septal defect (VSD) will close spontaneously. Antibiotic prophylaxis for invasive procedures is necessary.

Cardiac lesions in Down's syndrome

The incidence of congenital heart disease in children with Down's syndrome is 40–50% with the commonest lesions being atrioventricular septal defect (AVSD), secundum atrial septal defect (ASD), patent ductus arteriosus (PDA) and ventricular septal defect (VSD).

It is recommended that every baby with Down's syndrome has cardiac ultrasound performed in the first few days of life to exclude a major cardiac defect which may be asymptomatic. There is also known to be a higher incidence of mitral valve prolapse and aortic regurgitation in adults with Down's syndrome who may also be asymptomatic, which puts them at risk of infective endocarditis particularly as the incidence of periodontal disease is also increased.

Information for parents in written or video form can be obtained from the Down's Heart Group.

For details of other cardiac conditions in childhood the reader should refer to a general paediatric or paediatric cardiology text.

Hypertension in childhood

Hypertension defined as systolic and diastolic blood pressures (BP) above the 95th centile when plotted on a BP for height or BP for age chart may be picked up at a routine screening session, for example school health appraisal, new patient check at the GP's surgery or during examination for a related problem, for example headaches. It affects 1–3% of the childhood population. It is important to ensure that the correct sized cuff is available, i.e.

one covering at least two-thirds of the upper arm with the bladder completely encircling the arm (a cuff which is too small produces an artificially high BP). In children with severe and persistent hypertension 80–90% will have an underlying renal condition, the most common being renal scarring as a result of reflux nephropathy, although signs of primary cardiovascular disease, particularly coarctation of the aorta, should be sought.

Minimal investigations, which can be carried out in the clinic, should include urinalysis for blood and protein and urine culture.

Treatment advice for severe hypertension should be sought from a paediatric nephrologist. For milder degrees of hypertension the consultation should be an opportunity for advice on lifestyle, i.e. diet, salt intake and exercise.

COMMON RENAL PROBLEMS

Enuresis

Enuresis may be primary or secondary, nocturnal, diurnal or just daytime and management differs accordingly (Box 26.9).

Diagnosis can usually be made by taking a detailed history and a thorough examination (Box 26.10).

It is useful to obtain an idea of the impact that the wetting has on the child and his family by asking what each one's response is to the wetting.

Most children with enuresis require only a minimum of investigations, namely urinalysis looking for blood, protein and glucose and urine culture (Box 26.11). Urinary tract imaging is not necessary in most cases.

Box 26.9
Incidence of enuresis in children

- 15% of 5 year olds
- 5% of 10 year olds
- 1–2% of 15 year olds
- Spontaneous resolution rate is 15% per year

Box 26.10
Diagnosis of enuresis, through history taking and examination

History
- Onset
- Duration
- Pattern — day or night
- Urinary stream (in boys)
- Family history
- Constipation
- Possible stress factors

Examination
- Growth
- Blood pressure
- Abdominal examination
- Genitalia
- Lumbrosacral spine
- Perianal sensation
- Lower limb neurology

Box 26.11
Other conditions which may cause wetting

- Detrusor instability
- Urinary tract infection
- Neurogenic bladder
- Posterior urethral valves
- Ectopic ureter
- Diabetes mellitus
- Chronic renal failure

Nocturnal enuresis treatment

Generally it is felt that children under the age of 5 do not require specific treatment as the likelihood of spontaneous resolution is still quite high. Between 5 and 7 years a star chart or other reward system is appropriate. After the age of 7 a number of treatment options are available. The range of treatments and their relative merits should be explained to the child and his parents, allowing them to become involved in the child's management plan.

Following the exclusion of physical causes, details of management are to be found in Chapter 28 on emotional and behavioural problems.

Daytime wetting

This is most commonly due to detrusor muscle instability. This muscle in the bladder wall contracts intermittently during the filling/storage phase when it should normally be relaxed, resulting in leakage of urine and urge incontinence. Clinically it presents as minor degrees of wetness that are often worse in the afternoon and are commoner in girls. Treatment involves regular bladder emptying (e.g. every 2 hours) as well as star charts or other reward system. Medical treatment with oxybutinin which stabilises the detrusor muscle may be required.

Neuropathic bladder

This condition is commonly seen in children with spina bifida and causes severe continuous wetting as well as soiling. Occasionally a neuropathic bladder is found in children who may have a lumbosacral dimple or naevus, abnormal lower limb neurology and a palpable bladder. The majority of affected children are managed in specialist clinics and benefit from the support of specialist nursing. Many are taught intermittent catheterisation which promotes continence as well as relieving the functional obstruction.

Urinary tract infections

Approximately 1% of boys and 3% of girls experience a urinary tract infection (UTI) in the first decade. The younger the child is at the first infection the higher the risk of long-term complications, namely renal scarring and hypertension as a result of vesicoureteric reflux (VUR). Reflux nephropathy as a result of VUR is responsible for 25% of end-stage renal failure in childhood, thus it is essential that UTIs are diagnosed and treated as soon as suspected.

Escherichia coli is responsible for over 80% of childhood UTIs. Breast feeding and circumcision have been shown to reduce the incidence of UTIs in young children.

Investigate all children by renal ultrasound (US) after their first UTI to look at the anatomy of the renal tract and to check for renal scarring. The results of the scan and the age of the child determine whether further investigations are necessary. In children under 1 year a micturating cysto-ureterogram (MCUG) is also routinely performed to look for VUR and may also be indicated in children over 1 year with recurrent infections. For a child with an abnormal US, DMSA and DTPA isotope scans give differential renal function between the two kidneys and demonstrate scarring and urinary tract obstruction.

Advice for preventing UTIs:

- Treat and avoid constipation.
- Ensure good hygiene especially in girls and avoid irritating soaps and bubble baths.
- Ensure correct wiping technique, i.e. from front to back to avoid introduction of pathogens from the bowel.
- Encourage regular bladder emptying, i.e. every 2–3 hours.
- Encourage the child to drink regular clear fluids.
- Recommend the child wears cotton underwear which is not too tight to allow ventilation.
- It is worth remembering that 20–30% of siblings of children with VUR are also affected.

COMMON SURGICAL PROBLEMS
Undescended testes

The incidence is approximately 6% of males born at term but up to 20% of preterm births. A significant proportion will descend spontaneously in the first 3 months so that the incidence at 3 months of age is 1–2%. Testes noted to be not well down in the scrotum at or after the 6–8-week check should be referred directly to a paediatric surgeon. The nearer the pubic tubercle the less likely the testis is to descend fully. There is still some controversy as to

whether retractile testes are abnormal. Surgical intervention is only necessary if the testis never resides in the scrotum. Undescended testes confer a greater risk of fertility problems, testicular tumours, trauma and torsion and may be a cosmetic problem.

Hypospadias

Hypospadias describes an ectopic urethral opening in boys. The incidence is 1 in 300 male births. Referral to a paediatric surgeon should be made as soon as the defect is detected. The optimum age for operation is 6–18 months of age.

Inguinal hernia

This is most commonly seen in infancy in boys. The hernia is due to a persistently patent processus vaginalis. There may be a history of intermittent abdominal pain or screaming or just a lump noted in the groin. On examination unilateral or bilateral swelling is seen which is reducible in the supine position unless incarcerated. In view of the high incidence of strangulation, especially in the younger age group, immediate referral for herniotomy is required.

Umbilical hernia

Umbilical hernias are commonly noted in the newborn period especially in infants of Afro-Caribbean origin — most resolve spontaneously in the first year of life. On examination there is a thick-edged circular ring and the hernia may be reduced easily on pressure. Umbilical hernias may also be seen in older children with Down's syndrome, hypothyroidism and mucopolysaccharidoses.

Hydrocoele

Hydrocoeles are most commonly seen during infancy. Scrotal swelling occurs due to a very narrow persistent processus vaginalis. At this age most hydrocoeles will resolve spontaneously and surgery is not required. The recent appearance of a hydrocoele in an older child with no history of trauma requires urgent referral to exclude a tumour or leukaemic infiltration.

ABNORMAL HEAD SIZE AND SHAPE

Microcephaly

Head circumference is an important measurement throughout the first year of life. It should be measured using a Lassoo tape measure and plotted on the 1994 centile charts.

Microcephaly is defined as a head circumference 2 or more standard deviations below the mean. If an abnormal head size is found it is essential to measure both parents' head circumferences if possible (Box 26.12).

Box 26.12
Causes of microcephaly

Prenatal
- Genetic
  - autosomal dominant (generally less severely learning impaired)
  - autosomal recessive (generally more severely learning impaired)
- Chromosomal
  - particularly trisomy 13 and 18 — may be associated with holoprosencephaly and midline defects and other migrational defects
- Intrauterine infections, e.g. TORCH
- Fetal alcohol syndrome
- Placental insufficiency, e.g. due to maternal smoking, chronic systemic disease
- Undiagnosed or untreated mother with phenylketonuria

Perinatal
- Hypoxic ischaemic insult (head size normal at birth)
- CNS infections

Postnatal
- CNS infections
- Severe chronic disease causing malnutrition

Macrocephaly

The definition of macrocephaly is a head circumference greater than 2 standard deviations above the mean. Causes are:

- familial
- hydrocephalus — particularly if head circumference crossing centiles upwards
- subdural effusions (possible non accidental injury)
- megalencephaly (large brain size)
- skeletal or cranial dysplasia, e.g. achondroplasia.

Craniosynostosis

Craniosynostosis is defined as premature fusion of one or more cranial sutures resulting in deformation of the skull and face. Ridging of the affected suture may be noted. It is a rare condition in childhood but confusion may arise in distinguishing it from benign postural deformations as most commonly seen with plagiocephaly.

Plagiocephaly

This term describes a skull that is skew or oblique in shape. It is due either to an external deforming force (e.g. intrauterine position), or as has been noted increasingly since the Back To Sleep campaign due to babies sleeping in the supine position. Less commonly it is caused by unilateral coronal or lambdoid synostosis (Fig. 26.2).

If necessary the two conditions may be distinguished on skull X-rays where synostosis is diagnosed by absence of the involved suture and perisutural sclerosis. The majority of non-synostotic deformities are non-progressive and improve with time.

FITS, FAINTS, FUNNY TURNS

A number of episodic neurological problems present in childhood, many of which are benign, but it is important to recognise those that have underlying pathology (Box 26.13).

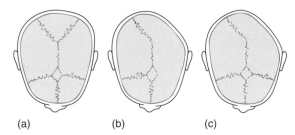

Fig. 26.2 Plagiocephaly (flattened forehead) due to (a) deformation, (b) unilateral coronal stenosis and (c) unilateral lamboid stenosis

> **Box 26.13**
> **Differential diagnosis of fits, faints and funny turns**
>
> - Neurological, e.g. tics
> - Myoclonic jerks
> - Migraine
> - Cardiac
> - Behavioural, e.g. pseudoseizures
> - Parasomnias

> **Box 26.14**
> **Key questions in the history of epilepsy**
>
> - Does the child experience an aura before the seizure?
> - What is the child doing when the seizure begins?
> - What are the child's movements like during the fit?
> - How long does the fit last?
> - How does the fit terminate?
> - What is the child's behaviour like afterwards?
> - How often do the fits occur?

Epilepsy

Epilepsy affects 1 in 200 of the population. Diagnosis is made largely on the history and investigations are confirmatory. Epilepsy may be primary or secondary (i.e. syndromic (e.g. Lennox–Gastaut syndrome), infantile spasms)

Box 26.14 provides a list of key questions to be asked when history-taking in a possible case of epilepsy. For further details of epilepsy classification and management refer to a paediatric or paediatric neurology text.

Epileptic children in school

Learning difficulties are common in children with epilepsy and should be looked for. Seidenberg showed that 30% of epileptic children with normal or low normal abilities had significant difficulties with reading, spelling and arithmetic (Seidenberg

1989). In addition, antiepileptic medication may affect a child's performance in school, for example phenytoin can affect learning, ethosuxamide can affect reaction times, benzodiazepines may affect memory and the majority of medications can cause drowsiness and behavioural changes. The epilepsy itself can lead to behavioural or psychiatric disturbance in 20–30% of children depending on seizure control, type of epilepsy, use of drugs and family response.

It is important to give clear advice to the child's parents and school about which activities the child may or may not participate in. The following guidelines may be used:

- Swimming is encouraged with one-to-one supervision.
- Cycling should be supervised as appropriate to the child's age. Busy roads are best avoided and cycle helmets should always be worn — non-affected siblings too.
- Watching TV. A child with photosensitive epilepsy should sit at least 6 feet (1.8 m) from the TV in a well-lit room.
- Computer games may induce seizures if the child is tired.
- Socialising. Both sleep deprivation and excessive alcohol ingestion reduce the seizure threshold.

- Bathing is associated with a slightly increased risk of death, especially if the child is left unsupervised. Showering is a safer alternative.

Syncope

Syncope or fainting is a common symptom in school-aged children experienced by approximately 15% children by late adolescence.

Causes of syncope can broadly be divided into three groups:

- Neurovascular, e.g. vasovagal, postural hypotension.
- Cardiac, e.g. hypertrophic cardiomyopathy, aortic stenosis, arrhythmias secondary to Wolff–Parkinson–White syndrome, prolonged QT syndrome, reflex anoxic seizure, Marfan's syndrome.
- Other, e.g. epilepsy, hyperventilation, cyanotic breath-holding attack.

The majority of cases are due to vasovagal response or postural hypotension. Vasovagal attacks are usually preceded by a stimulus, for example fear, pain, hunger, high room temperature. Recovery is rapid after the attack. A strong family history is often obtained. If the syncope is exercise induced it is much more suggestive of a cardiac abnormality (Box 26.15).

Box 26.15
Key points to consider in the history of syncope

- What was the precipitating event?
- Was there any prodrome or warning?
- Was the child standing still or exercising?
- Is there any family history of similar events?
- Did the child turn blue?
- Did the child recover immediately or were they drowsy and confused afterwards?
- Were there any other associated symptoms, e.g. weakness, tingling

---

HEADACHES IN CHILDHOOD
Migraine

Migraine affects 5% of school-age children. In 90% of cases there is a positive family history of migraine. The headaches may take the form of classic migraine with an aura but more commonly no aura is reported. Migraines tend to be exacerbated by various dietary factors such as cheese or chocolate, as well as anxiety and sometimes exercise. The headache is described as throbbing and may be accompanied by nausea, vomiting and blurred vision. In childhood the headache is not always unilateral.

The diagnosis is usually evident after taking a careful history. Physical examination should include examination of blood pressure and optic fundi. It is useful for the child or parent to keep a headache diary noting time of day, antecedents to the headache, duration of headache and relieving factors. For infrequently occurring headaches simple analgesia with paracetamol or codeine which may be combined with an antiemetic (e.g. Migraleve) is usually sufficient. Many children find benefit from lying in a dark room. For frequently occurring headaches, i.e. more than once a week, prophylaxis with pizotifen or propranolol is appropriate. The former drug may cause weight gain.

In up to 40% of children and young people their migraine may extend into adulthood.

Tension headaches

Tension headaches are also very common in children and are defined as being bilateral and tightening in quality, lasting typically from 30 minutes to 7 days and occurring on average 15 days a month (International Headache Society, Olesen 1988). They are not associated with nausea or vomiting and photophobia is uncommon.

As the name suggests these headaches are usually triggered by stressful events in the child's life, although the child may be unaware of these stresses. Common factors may be school problems, for example bullying or worrying about falling behind in class due to learning difficulties. Pressures may come from within the home, for example parental conflict or excessively high expectations put upon the child to perform well. These avenues should be explored sensitively.

Physical examination should include examination of the optic fundi and blood pressure measurement. Once again a headache diary is useful to try and elucidate an underlying cause. Simple analgesia may be given, although often this does not have an impact on the headache. If possible the precipitating factors should be avoided but generally this is not possible and the child will need to be taught coping mechanisms such as relaxation techniques. The assistance of a clinical psychologist may be helpful. It is important to remember that depression may be a cause of persistent headaches in older children.

COMMON ORTHOPAEDIC PROBLEMS

A number of orthopaedic problems present to the community paediatrician (Box 26.16). It is important to be able to recognise those that require orthopaedic review, however a number of common conditions present in the first years of life that are of concern to parents and require reassurance only.

Developmental dysplasia of the hip or congential dislocation of the hip

It is important to be aware that not all cases are picked up at birth as some cases develop in the

---

Box 26.16
Orthopaedic problems presenting to the community paediatrician

Common conditions

- Intoeing
- Genu valgus/varus

Requiring orthopaedic review
- Spinal abnormalities

- Hip abnormalities

---

first year. The community paediatrician should be aware of the child presenting with hip problems in the first year of life. The incidence is reported as 1–2 per 1000 live births (Hutson et al 1999). The condition is best diagnosed by examination in the neonatal period and supplemented by hip ultrasound examination. Hip X-rays are not useful until after the age of around 8 months when the femoral ossification centre develops. The examination is best performed using the traditional Ortolani and Barlow tests of hip instability (See Jones Clinical Paediatric Surgery). All cases where concern exists should be maintained in a stable gentle abduction and referred for orthopaedic management. If diagnosed early then most will resolve, however if this is missed it can have devastating consequences for the hip development.

DERMATOLOGY

The paediatrician is often consulted about skin conditions. These have not been included in this chapter. The reader is referred to the appropriate reference books for up-to-date treatment and management. Management of these conditions in the community must include addressing medical, genetic, environmental and psychosocial aspects of care and the impact on education and future career.

OTITIS MEDIA WITH EFFUSION OR GLUE EAR (see Chapters 20, 34)

Recent research has demonstrated that otitis media with effusion (OME) is even more prevalent in young children than previously thought. Between 15 and 20% of children will have OME in at least one ear for more than half of their first year, while the cumulative proportion of children developing one or more episodes of OME between 2 and 24 months of age is in excess of 91% (Paradise et al 1997). Between 2 and 6 years approximately 10–20% of children will have OME at any one time, with a sharp drop in prevalence after 6 years of age (Centre for Reviews and Dissemination 1992).

Concern about the possible contribution of OME to academic, social and behavioural difficulties has highlighted this problem in childhood. The primary mechanism is thought to be the conductive hearing loss.

OME usually presents with inflammation and persistent fluid (effusion) in the middle ear cavity without pain, fever or malaise. Fluid may persist for some months and many children will have a fluctuating hearing loss throughout this period. Hearing loss averages 20–25 dB (range 0–60 dB) over several frequencies while the effusion is present. Although the hearing loss tends to fluctuate and is mild in most children, some children have a persistent moderate hearing loss for the duration of the effusion.

The main factors associated with OME are socioeconomic index and amount of exposure to other children, for example at day care centres. Although breast feeding is widely believed to protect against OME and smoking to predispose to OME, recent research suggests that these effects are weak and may operate in the first year of life only (Paradise et al 1997).

In some disorders such as Down's syndrome, cleft palate and other syndromes involving upper airway changes, OME is present in almost all of these children and increased vigilance is required and appropriate management instituted.

Diagnosis

The gold standard for diagnosis is myringotomy. However, in practice this occurs only with insertion of tympanostomy tubes (grommets).

Other diagnostic tools include tympanometry, audiometry and pneumatic otoscopy. **Tympanometry** can be used easily in the primary care setting. A Type B (flat) tympanogram has a sensitivity of 78–90% and a specificity of 63–94% in determining the presence of fluid in the middle ear. If Type B and C (shifted to the left) tympanograms are combined, sensitivity increases to close to 100% but specificity falls to approximately 75%. A Type A tympanogram has high specificity in ruling out OME (Fig 26.3). However, tympanometry does not measure hearing, so cannot be used to tell which children with OME have significant hearing loss. **Pneumatic otoscopy** (approximately 90% sensitivity and 75% specificity) is cheap, easy

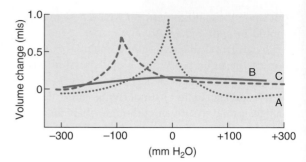

Fig. 26.3 Tympanometry

and quick to perform, and is used widely in the USA. However, it relies on individual judgement about the appearance and movement of the eardrum, so requires specific training, validation and regular re-validation.

Audiometry quantifies the hearing loss associated with OME. It requires skill, time, quiet conditions and cooperation on the part of the child and is therefore most useful in the child older than 4. Since the vast majority of hearing loss in early childhood is conductive, it can be used in screening 'sweep' audiograms in school and preschool children. The accuracy is dependent on the background level of ambient noise.

Refer to Chapter 34 for more discussion on screening and diagnosis. Despite common belief, parental perception is not a reliable predictor of conductive hearing loss or of change in hearing status (Rosenfeld et al 1998, Stewart et al 1999).

Treatment/management

Strategies for treatment/management may be directed either at resolution of middle ear effusion and/or hearing impairment, or at remediation of presumed adverse effects of OME (Box 26.17). In practice this is often dictated by degree, severity and chronicity of hearing loss. The few good studies investigating the long-term outcomes of OME suggest that OME contributes far less to adverse outcomes than previously thought. Therefore, many now elect to adopt a 'wait and see' approach

> **Box 26.17**
> **Treatment of otitis media with effusion**
>
> - Antibiotics
> - Autoinflation
> - Tympanostomy tubes
> - Steroids
> - Short-term hearing aids
> - Watchful waiting
>
> From: Centre for Reviews and Dissemination 1992

to the asymptomatic child (Peters et al 1997, Paradise et al 1999).

Children with mild hearing loss probably require no treatment, with ongoing review of the hearing loss. The optimum frequency for this is not known, but many would review approximately every 3 months until either the effusion clears or the hearing worsens to the extent that more active treatment may be justified. Antibiotics lead to only a small increase in clearance rates in the short term (<30 days) and their use is increasingly questioned because of the rise in resistant infections (Jensen & Lous 1998). Alerting the teacher to the child's hearing loss may enable implementation of classroom strategies, such as sitting close to the front of the class, getting their attention before giving instructions, etc.

The child with more severe hearing loss may require a more aggressive approach. This may include tympanostomy tubes (grommets) which dramatically improve hearing in the short term (mainly in the first 6 months after placement) but not thereafter. However, it is not at all clear from recent randomised controlled trials that tympanostomy tubes improve developmental outcomes. Many now suggest that significant hearing loss (e.g. >25–30 dB) should be documented over a 3–6-month period before deciding on this course.

Several other strategies are also available. Short-term hearing aids (from which parents report appreciable improvement in hearing) may benefit some children while giving the effusion time to

resolve spontaneously. Recent studies of auto-inflation using nasal balloons suggest overall improvement in children older than 4 years, despite considerable heterogeneity in the studies (Reidpath et al 1999). The use of steroids remains controversial. They appear to have some benefit in a small number of randomised controlled trials, but concern about their harm:benefit ratio limits their use, particularly in younger children. The 1994 US Guideline 'Managing otitis media with effusion in young children' (Anonymous 1994) recommended against their use for OME in children under 4 years (Anonymous 1994)

REFERENCES AND FURTHER READING

Ainsworth S, Wyllie J, Wren C 1999 Archives of Disease in Childhood 80:F43
Anonymous 1994 Managing otitis media with effusion in young children. The Otitis Media Guideline Panel Pediatrics. American Academy of Pediatrics 94:766–773
Apley J 1959 The child with abdominal pains. Blackwell Scientific Publications, Oxford
Ball T M, Castro-Rodriguez J A, Griffith K A, Holberg C J, Martinez F D, Wright A L 2000 Siblings, day-care attendance, and the risk of asthma and wheezing during childhood. New England Journal of Medicine 343:538–543
Centre for Reviews and Dissemination 1992 The treatment of persistent glue ear in children. Effective Health Care Bulletin Vol 4
Grant D 1997 Management of Hypothyroidism. Current Paediatrics 7(2)92–97
Hall DMB (ed) 1996 Health for all children, 3rd edn. Oxford University Press, Oxford
Holberg C J, Wright A L, Martinez F D, Morgan W J, Taussig L M 1993 Child day care, smoking by caregivers, and lower respiratory tract illness in the first 3 years of life. Pediatrics 91:885–892
Holt P G 2000 Key factors in the development of asthma: atopy. American Journal of Respiratory and Critical Care Medicine 161:S172–S175
The International Study of Asthma and Allergies in Childhood (ISAAC) Steering Committee 1998 Worldwide variation in prevalence of symptoms of asthma, allergic rhinoconjunctivitis, and atopic eczema: ISAAC. Lancet 351:1225–1232
Jensen P M, Lous J 1998 Antibiotic treatment of acute otitis media. Criteria and performance in Danish general practice. Scandinavian Journal of Primary Health Care 16:18–23
Jordan S C 1994 Innocent murmurs — when to ask a cardiologist. Current Paediatrics 4:59–61
Martinez F D 1999 Maturation of immune responses at the beginning of asthma. Journal of Allergy and Clinical Immunology 103:355–361

Maw R, Wilks J, Harvey I, Goldring J 1999 Early surgery compared with watchful waiting for glue ear and effect on language development in preschool children: a randomised trial. Lancet 353:960–963

NIH 1997 Global initiative for asthma. Online. Available: *http://www.ginasthma.com* 1997

Olesen J 1988 Cephalgia 8 (suppl 7):1–96

Paradise J L, Rockette H E, Colborn D K et al 1997 Otitis media in 2253 Pittsburgh-area infants: prevalence and risk factors during the first two years of life. Pediatrics 99:318–333

Paradise J L, Feldman H M, Colborn D K, et al 1999 Parental stress and parent-rated child behavior in relation to otitis media in the first three years of life. Pediatrics 104:1264–1273

Paradise J L, Feldman H M, Campbell T F et al 2000 Early vs late tube placement for persistent middle-ear effusion in the first 3 years of life: effects on language, speech, sound production, and cognition at age 3 years. Pediatric Research 47(Suppl 2):1157–1273

Peters S A, Grievink E H, van Bon W H, van den Bercken J H, Schilder A G 1997 The contribution of risk factors to the effect of early otitis media with effusion on later language, reading, and spelling. Developmental Medicine and Child Neurology. 39:31–39

Platts-Mills T A, Woodfolk J A 1997 Rise in asthma cases. Science 278:1001

Rach G H, Zielhuis G A, van Baarle P W, van den B P 1991 The effect of treatment with ventilating tubes on language development in preschool children with otitis media with effusion. Clinical Otolaryngology 16:128–132

Reidpath D D, Glasziou P P, Del Mar C 1999 Systematic review of autoinflation for treatment of glue ear in children. British Medical Journal 318:1177

Rosenfeld R M, Goldsmith A J, Madell J R 1998 How accurate is parent rating of hearing for children with otitis media? Archives of Otolaryngology: Head and Neck Surgery 124:989–992

Rosenfeld R M, Bhaya M H, Bower C M et al 2000 Impact of tympanostomy tubes on child quality of life. Archives of Otolaryngology: Head and Neck Surgery 126:585–592

Seidenberg M 1989 Neuropsychological, psychosocial and intervention aspects. In: Herman B, Seidenberg M (eds) Childhood epilepsies. John Wiley, Chichester, 105–118

Stewart M G, Ohlms L A, Friedman E M et al 1999 Is parental perception an accurate predictor of childhood hearing loss? A prospective study. Otolaryngology: Head and Neck Surgery 120:340–344

Taussig L M 1995 Conclusion. In: Early childhood asthma: what are the questions? American Journal of Respiratory and Critical Care Medicine 151(suppl 2):S32–S33

von Mutius E 2000 The environmental predictors of allergic disease. Journal of Allergy and Clinical Immunology 105:9–19

Wickens K, Crane J, Pearce N, Beasley R 1999 The magnitude of the effect of smaller family sizes on the increase in the prevalence of asthma and hay fever in the United Kingdom and New Zealand. Journal of Allergy and Clinical Immunology 104:554–558

BASIC RECOMMENDED TEXTBOOKS

Behrman R E, Kleigman R M, Jenson H B 1999 Nelsons textbook of pediatrics, 16th edn. WB Saunders, Philadelphia

Campbell A G M, McIntosh N (eds) 1998 Forfar and Arneil's textbook of paediatrics, 5th edn. Churchill Livingstone, Edinburgh.

Hall D M B 1996 Health for all children, 3rd edn. Oxford University Press, Oxford (Updates and 2001 recommendations are to be found at www.health-for-all-children.co.uk)

Hutson J M, Woodward A A, Beasley S W (eds) 1999 Jones' paediatric surgery diagnosis and management, 5th edn. Blackwell Science, Victoria, Australia

Milner A D, Hull D 1998 Hospital paediatrics, 3rd edn. Churchill Livingstone, Edinburgh

Rudolph A M (ed) 1996 Rudolph's pediatrics, 20th edn. Appleton & Lange, Stamford, CT

ADVANCED READING

Apley A G 1993 Apley's system of orthopaedics and fractures, 7th edn. Butterworth-Heinemann, Oxford

Brett E M (ed) 1997 Paediatric neurology, 3rd edn. Churchill Livingstone, London

David T J 1993 Food and food additive intolerance in children. Blackwell Science, Oxford

Fenichel G M 1997 Clinical pediatric neurology: a signs and symptoms approach. WB Saunders, Philadelphia

Harper J, Oranje A, Prose N 2000 Textbook of pediatric dermatology, Vols 1, 2. Blackwell Science, Oxford

Jordan S C, Scott O 1989 Heart disease in paediatrics, 3rd edn. Butterworths, London

Maw R, Wilks J, Harvey I, Goldring J 1999 Early surgery compared with watchful waiting for glue ear and effect on language development in preschool children: a randomised trial. Lancet 353:960–963

Rovers M M, Straatman H, Ingels K, van der Wilt G J, van den Broek P, Zielhuis G A 2000 The effect of ventilation tubes on language development in infants with otitis media with effusion: a randomized trial. Pediatrics 106(3):E42

Stephenson B P, King M D 1989 Handbook of neurological investigations in children. Wright, London

27 | Psychiatric disorder and emotional development

Child psychiatric disorders are one of the most frequent reasons for child consultations to paediatricians and GPs. Between 20% and 30% of all child health consultations involve a psychiatric disorder. A sound understanding of the causes and treatment of these common problems is therefore important for anyone dealing with children. This relatively high rate of psychiatric disturbance in children may seen surprising but similar rates are also to be found in adults who consult health practitioners and there is no reason to believe that children are somehow immune from mental disorder. Children who have a psychiatric disorder are often seen as difficult rather than disturbed. However the distinction between 'normal' and pathological behaviour is important because reassurance is appropriate in the first case and dangerous in the latter.

Behaviour, mood and cognition are the three main aspects of mental functioning and a disturbance in one is usually associated with an abnormality in the others. A psychiatric disorder may be diagnosed if the change in behaviour, emotions or thought processes is so prolonged or so severe that it interferes with everyday life and becomes a handicap for the child or those who care for the child (Box 27.1). The definition of a psychiatric disorder must also take into account the child's stage of development and the sociocultural context in which the behaviour occurs. For example, lying on the floor, kicking and screaming in a temper for 2 minutes several times a day would not be unusual in a 2 year old, but would be considered abnormal in most 10 year olds — unless the child was developmentally delayed or if everyone else around the child behaved in the same way.

Occasionally, a child's mental state may be so bizarre or extreme that a behaviour or thought only has to occur once to be regarded as abnormal. For example, deliberate self-injury or hallucinations are not part of normal experience and one event is enough to indicate mental dysfunction. Using the above definition of psychiatric disorder, the overall prevalence rate is 10% for child psychiatric disorder in the general population, which is much the same as in adults. This rate is influenced by a number of factors which are outlined in Table 27.1.

Assessment and aetiology

The assessment of child psychiatric disorders is a complex process in which the observations of others play a major part. Thus it is important to gain information about the child from as many sources as possible. Even so, a child's disturbance is often situation specific and there may be reports of difficult behaviour in one setting only. Psychiatric disorders that are only manifest in one situation do not necessarily mean that the cause of the problem must also be there: a child may be difficult at home due to academic failure at school. For example, a child who has been abused within the family may present major problems at school but not at home. However, if a behavioural problem only occurs in one setting, it generally means that the child is not too disturbed because there is still enough emotional strength to control their behaviour when necessary.

The temptation to identify a single cause for any psychiatric disorder should be resisted. The aetiology is likely to be due to multiple factors, each interacting with the others in such a way that the whole is greater than the sum of the separate factors. The different contributing factors act together as part of a pathogenic process. Thus a child with mild physical handicap may induce

Psychiatric disorder and emotional development

overprotectiveness in the mother, resulting in immature, demanding behaviour at home. This is turn leads to a relative withdrawal of the father that only serves to make the mother/child interaction more powerful.

Box 27.1
Definition of psychiatric disorder

- A change in the child's usual behaviour, emotion or thoughts
- Persistent — for at least 2 weeks
- Severe enough to interfere with the child's everyday life
- A handicap to the child and/or the carers
- Taking account of the child's stage of development
- Taking account of the sociocultural context

The assessment process will take account of a number of different factors, each interacting with the others in such a way as to generate the problem. It is helpful to start by considering the contribution that the child makes to the development of the disorder and then to go on to review the role of the family and finally the influence of school and the outside world.

THE CHILD

Labelling the child as the problem is often regarded as unacceptable and unfair because he is given responsibility for the problems that more correctly *may* belong to the parents or to the family as a whole. But 'labelling' is often more of an issue for professionals than it is for parents, and to identify the child rather than the parent as the problem will usually lead to a more positive and caring attitude on the parent's part.

Table 27.1
Summary of the main aetiological factors that increase the risk of child psychiatric disorder

Child factors	Family factors	Outside factors
Boys: more likely to develop behaviour problems when younger	Marital difficulties: separation and divorce	Bullying
Girls: more likely to develop emotional problems when older	Death of parent or close relative, or even loss of a favourite pet	School ethos/organisation
Physical illness/poor discipline: especially epilepsy	Sociocultural factors inconsistent, hostile or weak	
Difficult temperament	Abuse: physical, emotional, sexual and/or neglect	Peer group pressure
Developmental delay	Hostile rejection	Social policy
Communication problems, e.g. deafness/language disorder	Poverty: poor housing, unemployment, poor facilities	
Poor self-image, low self-esteem	Large family size — four or more children	
Mental handicap	Mother — psychiatric illness; father — criminal activity	

Temperament

Obvious differences in temperament between one child and another exist from birth, if not before. At this early stage, temperament is defined in relatively simple descriptive terms, but there is a strong tendency for these characteristics to persist. Some children have a stable temperament from the start. They are relatively easy to bring up and are mostly predictable in their reactions. Others seem to be difficult from the start and require extra care and attention. The 'difficult child syndrome' consists of strong negative emotions, unpredictable behaviour and difficulty adapting to new situations (Box 27.2).

Children who persistently show strong signs of adverse temperament from birth onwards are likely to prove especially difficult to bring up. However there is a tendency to improve spontaneously, and by 5 years old at least half of the children will no longer show the full syndrome. Those who have persistent problems will require 'super parenting'. This means more loving care, closer supervision, more consistency and routine in daily life and firm clear limit setting for their behaviour (Box 27.3).

Gender and age

There are clear gender effects that influence the prevalence of psychiatric disorders and these differences give some clues about the aetiology of psychiatric disorders. Gender seems to have a limited effect on the rate of disorder in toddlers, but by school age there is a noticeable increase in the frequency of all types of psychiatric disorders in boys where they outnumber girls by almost 2 to 1. Any

---

Box 27.2
The difficult child syndrome

- Intense emotions — *unhappy*, mainly negative reactions
- Slow to adapt to change — *unsettled* by any change in routine
- Variable physiological responses — *unpredictable* feeding, sleeping, etc.

Box 27.3
The requirements for parenting difficult children

- More structure and routine in everyday life
- More limit setting and clear boundaries for behaviour
- More intensive training of appropriate behaviour
- More love and affection

---

developmental disorder, such as enuresis, language disorder and clumsiness, is associated with an even higher ratio of males to females. In adolescence the ratio gradually reverses with increasing age to the normal adult ratio where females outnumber males in the prevalence of most types of psychiatric disorder.

The gender effects are influenced by the diagnostic category as well as by age. All forms of behaviour problem are more common in boys throughout childhood. Emotional disorders however occur with equal frequency in younger boys and girls and then become more prevalent in girls during adolescence. It seems that the most likely explanation for the age/gender differences is that younger boys are developmentally more immature and constitutionally more vulnerable than girls. This is most probably due to the reduced chromosomal material in the Y chromosome that allows unbalanced genetic influences to take effect. In adolescence, however, the sex hormone changes probably play a dominant role, making females emotionally more vulnerable and boys more likely to react aggressively. Knowledge of these age and gender influences may not affect the way in which emotional and behavioural disorders are managed, but many parents find it helpful to have their child's problems put in a framework that makes them more understandable.

Intelligence

A child's ability to solve problems and to use abstract concepts are important aspects of general

---

Box 27.4
The chief factors that increase the risk of psychiatric disorder in children with severe learning difficulties

- Isolation from 'normal' society
- Poor adaptability to new situations
- Limited problem-solving ability
- Organic brain dysfunction
- Low self-esteem
- Poor communication skills
- Low expectations of parents and others

---

intellectual ability that influence the development of psychiatric disorder. There is an inverse relationship between intellectual ability and psychiatric disorder that holds true right through the full range of intelligence. Psychiatric disorder is five times more frequent in children with an IQ less than 50. At this severely limited level of ability, the normal gender differences are not seen. There are many possible reasons for the increased prevalence of psychiatric disorder in mentally handicapped individuals, but abnormal brain function is probably the most important (Box 27.4).

Physical state

Young children who are tired, hungry, too hot or too cold are more likely to show signs of emotional stress or difficult behaviour. For example, tempers occur more frequently in the evening and before meals. Of course, this does not constitute a psychiatric disorder unless it is a persistent and handicapping problem. Nevertheless, it can be helpful to know that there are high-risk times for problem behaviour so that preventative action can be taken.

Physically ill children are also more likely to develop emotional and behavioural problems, but the effect is not as much as one might expect. This may be due to an emotionally strengthening and maturing effect of illness. In this case the child may actually gain skills and competence as a result of

having to cope with being ill. Even children with life-threatening conditions such as leukaemia and other malignant disease cope remarkably well. What does seem to have an adverse effect is the number and intrusiveness of any investigations. Repeated invasive tests that the child is unable to influence in any way are most likely to result in psychiatric disorder. But even then the majority of children manage without having significant problems.

In addition to the child's reaction to the illness, the parent's own feelings will have an effect on the child. Overprotectiveness and overindulgence are common responses to illness in a loved one. It is likely that conditions affecting a vital organ such as the lungs, the brain or the heart produce the strongest protective reactions in parents.

Emotional state

It may seem self-evident that a child's emotional state can alter the threshold for behavioural and emotional problems. However, it is frequently overlooked and in any case the relationship is often a complex one. For example, a jealous child may become defiant and attention seeking. This may lead to a negative, punitive parental response which in turn could eventually result in the child's depressive withdrawal or apparently unprovoked aggressive behaviour, all due to an original jealous emotional state.

The concept of emotional arousal is useful in explaining how stress can have a cumulative effect. A child starting at a new school can be expected to have an increased level of arousal. This will be raised even further if the child has previously experienced problems at school or if there are other current stress factors. Eventually, when the level of emotional arousal has reached a high level, a relatively small amount of additional stress, such as being mildly reprimanded, may trigger a major emotional outburst. Unless it is understood that the outburst has occurred in the context of high emotional arousal due to the accumulation of multiple stress factors, it will be difficult to work out why it happened and what can be done to prevent another episode (Box 27.5).

Children with immature emotions are more likely to present with emotional and behavioural

---

> **Box 27.5**
> ## Factors that cause emotional immaturity
>
> - Developmental delay
> - Exposure to a severe emotional stress
> - Repeated experience of emotional stress
> - Inconsistent parenting
> - Lack of affection or frank rejection
> - Lack of training in stress management

> **Box 27.6**
> ## Ways of coping with emotional stress
>
> - Talking with others about the stress
> - Conflict resolution (or avoidance if resolution impossible)
> - Graduated exposure to stress
> - Cognitive coping techniques
> - Relaxation

disorders. Emotional immaturity can occur as a result of a number of different factors. Emotional maturity can be promoted by graduated and carefully supervised exposure to stressful situations that are within the competence of the child to cope with. At the same time the child is taught a variety of strategies that can be used to help manage the stress (Box 27.6), but the details of these approaches are beyond the scope of this chapter.

Self-esteem

The sense of having a separate identity develops slowly during childhood. A clear sense of being a separate person has usually developed by $2\frac{1}{2}$ years of age, but it is not until around 7–8 years that most children develop self-concept and have an understanding of what kind of person they are. Before this age a child might describe themselves as bad after doing something wrong, but the feeling of being bad will not continue for long. By 7–8 years old it is possible for a child to feel permanently bad and to have a low self-esteem as a result.

Children who have experienced repeated failure, rejection or other negative experiences will eventually develop a low self-esteem and poor self-image. This makes children vulnerable to behavioural disorders. Children with low self-esteem often behave badly deliberately in order to have it confirmed that they really are bad. This results in a paradoxical feeling of pleasure.

Low self-esteem is therefore a powerful motivating factor for bad behaviour and emotional distress, as well as a strong force that actually maintains the problems. It is also an important reason why the usual methods for treating behavioural disorders are often ineffective in children with a poor self-image. Looked at the other way around, high self-esteem is a protective factor against emotional and behavioural problems and good self-image increases children's resilience to stress.

Communication problems

Anything that interferes with clear communication can easily lead to frustration and the development of difficult behaviour. All forms of speech and language disorder may cause problems, as can deafness. Unclear or inconsistent communications from parents and other adults have just the same effect and result in frustration and bad temper.

PSYCHIATRIC DISORDER AND THE FAMILY

Families come in all shapes and sizes, but there are distinct advantages of the traditional family with two natural or 'birth' parents. However a dysfunctional two-parent family may cause considerably more problems for children than a stable and caring alternative family arrangement such as the single parent. All families, however they are constituted, have a number of basic tasks to carry out, such as providing loving care and protection from danger, promoting learning and responding to the child's changing developmental needs (Box 27.7).

> **Box 27.7**
> ## The basic tasks for the family
>
> - Giving continuity of care throughout childhood
> - Providing food and protection from danger
> - Training children to be socially competent
> - Helping children adapt to life crises
> - Meeting the changing needs of children during development
> - Ensuring children have positive self-esteem
> - Encouraging children to reach their full potential
> - Promoting the child's physical and emotional health

Family breakdown

The institution of 'The Family' has undergone dramatic changes in recent years. Rates of divorce and separation are reaching epidemic proportions, with one in five children in the UK experiencing the break up of their family at some stage during their childhood. In the USA, up to 40% of children can expect to be separated from a parent before they reach adulthood. A high rate of psychiatric disturbance is associated with parental separation and divorce and in the year following parental separation, the rate of psychiatric disorder is as high as 80%. Nevertheless, it is clear that many of the problems were already present several years earlier, reflecting the dysfunction of the family prior to the eventual breakdown. Emotional and behavioural problems are particularly frequent in children who have been exposed to persistent quarrelling and ill feeling between parents and where children have been used as pawns in the marital conflict. The effect of family breakdown is generally greater in boys than in girls, but in older teenagers, it is the girls who are more likely to show overt emotional distress. The increased vulnerability of boys to the effects of family breakdown is seen most noticeably in an increase of aggressive and antisocial reactions on the one hand, or withdrawal and anxious behaviour on the other. Both reactions are often associated with academic underachievement in boys, but not in girls.

Overt parental conflict constitutes the most damaging aspect of the fraught relationships that are associated with family breakdown. Covert tension between parents seem to have much less of an adverse effect on children. There is evidence that some of the detrimental impact of marital breakdown on children is delayed as a 'sleeper' effect that only emerges many years later on in life. This is probably more likely to occur in women and to affect the parent–child relationship in the next generation. Most children who have experienced the separation of their parents continue to feel a deep sense of loss, even into adult life, and children who come from a broken home have a higher than expected frequency of marital failure themselves in adult life. Unfortunately, fathers often start to disengage from the family well before the divorce, and within a few years of the divorce more than 50% of children have little or no contact with their father.

Forming attachments

The process of forming a bond of attachment and affection between parent and child develops for the parents from the moment that pregnancy is confirmed and reaches a peak in the first few days after birth. However, the child's attachment to the parent only becomes noticeable at around 6 months old when separation anxiety is seen for the first time. The child–parent bond then continues to strengthen over the next few years and should be securely established by the time the child starts at school.

Immediately after birth some 10% of mothers have no feeling of affection for their baby, but within a fortnight this has reduced to less than 1%. A very small number of mothers fail to form an attachment to their child, with serious implications for the future development of childhood psychiatric disorder.

Attachment problems are more likely to occur if there has been reduced parent–child contact in the first few weeks after birth or if the mother has experienced a failure of attachment to her own parents. In spite of problems in the mother–child relationship, it is possible for fathers to compensate for the adverse effects of this on the child. It is also important for parents to know that it is not necessary to have affectionate and loving feelings for their child all the time and that it is possible to do a reasonable job of parenting without these positive feelings.

Bereaved children show a very similar range of emotional and behavioural disturbance to children who have experienced loss of a parent by separation or divorce. Nevertheless, the rate of psychiatric disorder following death is significantly less than that following divorce. In fact young children may show surprisingly little reaction to the death of their parent provided that they receive continuity of good quality care. It is not until 7–8 years of age that children develop the concepts of time and an understanding of the uniqueness of the individual necessary to comprehend death.

Boys appear to be more vulnerable to the death of a parent, particularly to the death of a father. The long-term consequences for children who have experienced the death of a parent have been hotly debated. There is some evidence that there is an increased risk for developing depression in adult life, but it is unclear whether this is directly due to the loss or the result of the many changes in family function and fortune that follow the bereavement.

Family size and structure

Children who come from families with four or more children have an increased risk for conduct disorder and other antisocial behaviour. There is also an increased risk of reading difficulties and decreased verbal ability in children from large families. The effect of sibship position is less than one might imagine. Eldest and only children may be academically more successful and youngest and only children are slightly more likely to experience separation anxiety. The age gap between siblings also has little effect, although there is some evidence that academic achievement and social adjustment is better if the age gap between siblings is

more than 4 years. A very close gap between the first born and the next child can be associated with a higher rate of anxiety and moodiness in boys.

Single-parent families

Approximately 1.5 million children in Great Britain are being brought up in a one-parent family. Of these families about 20% are headed by a lone parent who has never been married, 10% of one-parent families arise through the death of a parent and another 10% of lone parents are fathers. Although many children live for a while in a one-parent family, more than 50% of lone parents have either re-married or are co-habiting within 3 years of the family breakdown.

Most one-parent families live in deprived inner-city areas and 60% of them are dependent on local authority housing, compared with 20% for two-parent families. More than 50% of one-parent families are living in poverty. Therefore financial and social adversity have a major influence on children brought up in one-parent families (Box 27.8).

Box 27.8
Some of the adversities faced by children brought up in single-parent families

- Financial hardship
- Social adversity
- Difficulty in maintaining continuity of care
- Overinvolved relationships more likely to develop
- Less likely to have back-up for parent who is sick or tired
- Less opportunity for parent to have time for him/herself
- Full responsibility for the family is borne by one person
- Lack of modelling of normal male/female relationships

In spite of all the difficulties that single parents face, many are highly successful in the child care that they provide — against all the odds. But children brought up in single-parent families will continue to be at risk unless there are major social changes to provide more adequate support, and ways can be found for children to maintain satisfactory contact with their absent parents. The trend of dysfunctional parenting and broken relationships is likely to continue until training and help with relationships for children is given a higher priority by society.

Parental illness

There is a strong link between parental mental illness and psychiatric disturbance in their children. This is mostly due to adverse social factors and disturbed family relationships that are so frequently associated with illness. The degree of involvement of the child in the parental illness is the key factor in determining how disturbed a child may be. Thus, a child whose parent has schizophrenia may be less disturbed than one whose parent is suffering from obsessional neurosis or personality disorder involving the child in the parent's psychopathology. It seems likely that parents with psychotic disorders are readily understood to be ill and children are therefore able to distance themselves from the illness.

Maternal depression has been shown to have a particularly adverse effect on children. There is some evidence that emotional and behaviour problems persist in children even after the mother has recovered from the depression. This suggests that the disturbed parent–child interactions that occur during the period of depression set up a chain of disturbances that then become self-perpetuating. Although the depression probably has a direct effect on parenting ability, there is evidence that the often associated social and marital difficulties also play a significant part. The move towards care in the community for parents who are either physically or psychiatrically ill has led to a much greater exposure of children to the social adversity and emotional stress of illness. A child's temperament seems to be a key factor in determining the nature of their response to a sick parent. Children with intense emotional responses, generally negative mood and poor adaptability, have been found to react badly to stressful situations at home.

Social adversity

Social factors alone are rather weak determinants of childhood psychiatric disorder. They generally seem to act by making children more vulnerable to health and educational problems. The concept of a cycle of disadvantage is the most helpful way of understanding the way social adversity operates. For example, families who live in rented accommodation are frequently found to have a higher rate of delinquency in their children. The important factor here is unlikely to be the rented accommodation itself, but rather the process that leads to families using rented accommodation. The children of teenage mothers are another example. Many are brought up in adverse socio-economic circumstances, but the most important factor that determines the outcome for these deprived children is the amount of personal and educational support that the mothers receive, rather than the level of social adversity.

There is good evidence that unfavourable social influences tend to occur together and affect children from an early age — even in utero. In spite of this, many children from socially deprived backgrounds can be successful, provided they receive consistent affection and predictable child care. There is little doubt that ethnic origin and family culture make a significant contribution to children's everyday life. It is less clear what role these influences play in the aetiology of child psychiatric disorder, but there is some evidence to suggest that as children grow older, sociocultural factors become more significant. It might be expected that children from mixed race marriages would have a higher rate of psychiatric disorder, but there is little evidence to support this view once socio-economic factors are controlled for.

The birth of a child

The arrival of the first-born child leads to a radical realignment of relationships. The single 'diadic' relationship between the couple increases to three 'diadic' relationships and for the first time a 'triadic' relationship. It is the three-person relationship that provides the fertile ground where jealously can develop. A well-established bond between the parents is therefore necessary in order to maintain the family unit through this period of change and potential crisis. The birth of a second child leads to a further dramatic increase in the number of possible relationships within the family. The first-born typically becomes more naughty and confrontational and has to initiate more of the interactions with the mother. It is in this context that a previously satisfactory relationship between a mother and child can become strained, sowing the seeds for a longstanding behavioural problem. Once again, the key factors in determining whether or not the child will develop a psychiatric disorder are the child's temperament, the mother's state of health and the stability and security of the parents' relationship with each other.

Adopted and foster families

Children who are fostered have a higher rate of psychiatric disorder, but in the majority of cases this disturbance was present before the fostering took place. The breakdown of a fostering placement is associated with a particularly high rate of emotional and behavioural disturbance. Adopted children have a slightly increased rate of psychiatric disorder that becomes more noticeable during adolescence when young people are trying to come to terms with their origins in order to look to their future. There is also evidence from twin studies showing that genetic influences can have a powerful effect on behaviour which may only partially be compensated for by the environment within an adopted family.

Concerns have recently been raised about 'out of country' and 'mixed race' adoptions and anxiety is voiced about the adoption of children by homosexual adults. It seems reasonable to conclude that in each of these situations, an additional adversity is present. However, none of these conditions precludes the possibility that a child will receive a high standard of care. What evidence there is suggests that children brought up in these unusual families do not have a particularly high rate of emotional or behavioural problems.

CHILDREN'S EMOTIONAL DEVELOPMENT WITHIN THE FAMILY

Crying is one of the main methods that babies use for communication and most babies soon discover that crying quickly brings them full adult attention. Even so, it is difficult to be sure exactly what a newborn baby is feeling and later on it is still hard to know what young children are feeling. Describing and communicating feelings is a complex task for children — and for most adults! The strong feelings that parents experience when they hear their baby cry is helpful because it is a signal that the child wants attention. Thus the ability to manipulate parents develops early on in life. In fact, manipulating people by using emotional pressure is a very primitive way of getting what you want and even very young children soon learn how to do it. It is important to recognise it for what it is and to help children to develop more acceptable ways of making their needs known.

There are both positive (enjoyable) and negative (unpleasant) emotions. Each positive emotion has its mirror image — a negative aspect of the same emotion. So, for example, it is possible to cry with happiness. Love can easily turn to hate and it is not unusual to experience remarkably strong feelings of anger towards those who we also love the most. There are, of course, other more complicated emotions such as jealousy and grief. These are complex emotions and are made up of several different feelings. Thus jealousy includes both anxiety and anger; grief is a mixture of sadness, anger and anxiety (Fig. 27.1).

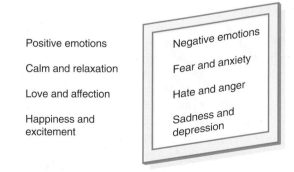

Positive emotions	Negative emotions
Calm and relaxation	Fear and anxiety
Love and affection	Hate and anger
Happiness and excitement	Sadness and depression

Fig. 27.1 Pleasant and unpleasant emotions and their mirror images

Psychiatric disorder and emotional development

Positive emotions

The first 'smile' may be seen soon after birth, but this is not the real thing since it often occurs when the child is completely relaxed or even asleep. By 2 weeks old it may be possible to elicit a smile by any form of gentle stimulation, although the smile often occurs as much as 8 seconds after the event. At about 6 weeks babies are smiling in direct response to sounds (especially the mother's voice) and to smiling faces. Even eyes on their own can produce smiling and the reaction time gradually becomes less as time goes by. By 8 weeks the child's smiling becomes an essential part of developing social relationships.

Laughter is usually seen for the first time around 4 months of age as a reaction to strong stimulation by touch, sound or movement. By 9 months laughter becomes more responsive to social situations such as hiding games or behaving in a very different way from usual. However, at this stage the same behaviour may easily result in either laughter or in tears. Older children gradually develop a sense of humour and by 6–9 years most children have found their own unique brand of humour. At this stage children go through a stage of loving jokes that almost no one else finds funny.

Fear and anxiety

Even very young babies show fear, but it is in a very uncomplicated form and is seen in the startle response to a loud noise or any sudden and unexpected change. It has the characteristics of a reflex response rather than an emotional reaction to a perceived threat and it is not until about 6–8 months old that babies show the first clear evidence that they are experiencing a definite and specific emotion. At about 6 months old the first signs of anxiety appear in the form of anxiety towards strangers and fear of separation. Anxiety is therefore the first emotion to develop in a specific way, so that it is absolutely clear what the child is feeling even though the emotion may be unreasonable because there is no actual threat to safety (Table 27.2).

Anxiety is associated with a high level of physiological arousal and a wide range of psychophysiological reactions. Young children complain a lot

Table 27.2
The relationship between age and the physical symptoms of anxiety and emotional distress

Age (yr)	Symptom
2–6	Generalised aches and pains
5–8	Limb pains
6–12	Abdominal pains
7 onwards	Headache

Table 27.3
The change of anxieties and fears with age

Birth onwards	Loud noise
6 months to 3 yr	Strangers
9 months onwards	Heights
2–4 yr	Animals
4–6 yr	Darkness, storms, imaginary monsters
6–12 yr	Mysterious happenings
12–18 yr	Social embarrassment, academic failure, death and war

about the physical symptoms of anxiety. Then as they grow older, their complaints become more specific and easier to relate to their worries. Table 27.3 gives an idea about how children's symptoms of anxiety change with age. At first, children's worries are to do with real dangers and specific objects, but later on in adolescence the anxiety becomes more to do with the imagination and ideas.

Anger

The first sign of obvious anger that is clearly directed against a specific person develops between 18 months and 2 years of age. Before that time children scream and yell in what seems an angry way, but it is more likely to be aimed at the general situation rather than aimed at a specific person. To be angry in a way that targets another person, it is necessary to be aware of oneself as separate from other people and from the rest of the outside world. This stage is not reached until between 2 and 3 years of age when children start to use 'I' when talking about themselves.

At first, anger is shown in a physical way by pushing, hitting, kicking and rolling on the floor, but by the time children are 4–6 years old, the anger is expressed more often in words. At the same time the outbursts of anger become shorter and are replaced with sulking instead. As children grow older they continue to react to frustration with anger and sulking which last much the same total length of time as a toddler's tempers. At all ages, anger is always associated with feelings of anxiety and the psycho-physiological reactions of anger are similar to those of anxiety.

Sadness and depression

Although children can become sad and miserable in a reasonably clear way at an early age, this is not the same as being depressed. Depression is different from sadness because it has two additional and essential components that are not necessarily part of feeling miserable.

1. Feeling of worthlessness (self-concept required).
2. Feeling of hopelessness (concept of time necessary).

Children who feel depressed come to believe that they are useless failures and that there is little hope that things will get better in the future. In order to feel a failure and to have a sense of worthlessness, it is necessary to have a concept of what sort of person you are (self-concept). This develops at about 7–8 years of age. A sense of hopelessness requires a concept of time which also develops around the age of 7–8 years.

This means that it would be very unusual for a child less than 8 years old to become 'depressed' in the strict sense of the word. Younger children can certainly be sad and tearful, but that is not the same as the specific emotion of depression which has a very different significance. Depression is always accompanied by the psychophysiology of anxiety. It is also associated with the behaviour of anger such as irritability, disturbed relationships and withdrawal of affection.

Grief

Grief is the normal emotional reaction to loss. The most obvious form of grief is seen in the bereavement reaction to the death of a close friend or relative, but the same reactions also occur in children after the loss of a pet or if a friend moves away to another area. Surprisingly strong grief reactions may also be felt when an older brother or sister leaves home. Before 7–8 years old, children have little real understanding of death and what it means. However, they quickly pick up how other people are feeling and react to that. Nevertheless, reactions to loss are clearly apparent in children over the age of about 6 months and the level of acute distress that is caused by loss and separation increases to a peak at around 3–4 years (Box 27.9).

As children grow older these three phases of emotional reactions to separation — protest, withdrawal, despair — develop into the bereavement reaction which also has three stages.

Box 27.9
The three phases for the response to separation

In younger children:

1. Protest — crying, screaming and actively searching for the absent parent
2. Withdrawal — becoming detached and quiet, showing few emotions
3. Despair — resignation, misery and listlessness

In older children:

1. Shock and disbelief (lasts up to 2 weeks)
2. Overwhelming emotions (lasts up to 6 weeks)
3. Readjustment (lasts up to 1 year)

Psychiatric disorder and emotional development

Grief is not the same thing as depression because self-esteem is normally preserved and there are no feelings of worthlessness, but in other respects the symptoms and signs are much the same. Grief contains large amounts of anger, sadness and anxiety. Bereaved children show grief in different ways depending on their stage of development. Before 7–8 years of age children may show very little response to a personal loss, provided that their basic needs for care and affection are being met. Young children tend to take their cue from adults and to a large extent they mirror the emotions and behaviour of those around them. Older children can experience the full range of grief and in adolescence the experience of loss can result in the most acute feelings of any age.

Slow emotional development

Some children seem to take much longer to develop mature emotions. Delay in emotional development is characterised by selfishness, rapid mood swings and poor impulse control. Of course any child will react with immature emotions when under stress, but children with slow emotional development will behave in this way all the time, even in the absence of stress. Immature emotions are associated with general developmental delay, but they may also occur where children have been exposed to emotional abuse or to repeated severe emotional stress over a long period, although this may also result in emotional maturation in some cases (Box 27.10).

Ways of promoting emotional maturity

Fortunately, the emotions of most children develop naturally along the normal lines without parents having to think much about it. However, no child will be able to mature properly without a feeling of emotional security which requires the type of care outlined in Box 27.11.

If a child is emotionally immature, it is important not to take any of these requirements for granted. None of them is easy to achieve and immature children need them even more than mature children do and it would be pointless to attempt to promote emotional development if one or more of these needs is unmet. Assuming that everything has been done to provide for a child's emotional security, then the following approaches given in Box 27.12 may assist emotional maturation.

Box 27.11
Emotional security requires

- A loving and affectionate atmosphere
- Predictability of care and relationships
- Consistent discipline and limit setting
- Age-appropriate expectations

Box 27.10
The major causes of emotional immaturity

- Generally slow development
- Temperamental characteristic
- Lack of training in emotional control
- Lack of emotional security

Box 27.12
Ways of promoting emotional maturation

- Setting a clear standard and model for emotional expression
- Planning a graduated increase in responsibility
- Avoiding any response to emotionally immature behaviour
- Praising any mature expression of emotions
- Training emotional control

FURTHER READING

Barker P 1986 Basic child psychiatry, 5th edn. Blackwell Scientific, Oxford

Bentovim A, Elton A, Hildebrand J, Tranter M, Vizard E (eds) 1988 Child sexual abuse within the family. Wright, Bristol

Garralda M E, Bailey D 1986 Psychological deviance in children attending general practice. Psychological Medicine 16:423–429

Goodyer I M, Kolvin I, Gatzanis S 1987 The impact of recent undesirable life events on psychiatric disorders in childhood and adolescence. British Journal of Psychiatry 151:179–184

Graham P 1987 Child psychiatry: a developmental approach. Oxford University Press, Oxford

Herbert M 1987 Conduct disorders of childhood and adolescence, 2nd end. John Wiley, Chichester

Hersov L, Berg I 1980 Out of school: modern perspectives in truancy and school refusal. Wiley, Chichester

Hill P 1989 Adolescent psychiatry. Churchill Livingstone, Edinburgh

Nicol A R (ed) 1985 Longitudinal studies in child psychiatry: practical lessons from research experience. Wiley, Chichester

Richman N, Landsdown R 1988 Problems of preschool children. John Wiley, Chichester

Rutter M 1983 Development neuropsychiatry. Guilford Press, New York

Rutter M 1985 Family and school influences on cognitive development. Journal of Child Psychology and Psychiatry 26:683–704

Rutter M 1989 Isle of Wight revisited: 25 years of epidemiological research in child psychiatry. Journal of the American Academy of Adolescent Psychiatry 28:633–653

Rutter M, Hersov L 1985 Child psychiatry: modern approaches. Blackwell Scientific, Oxford

Rutter M, Tizard J, Whitmore K 1970 Education, health and behavior. Krieber, New York

Rutter M, Hersov L 1985 Depression in young people: developmental and clinical perspectives. Guilford Press, New York

Taylor E A 1986 The overactive child. JB Lippincott, Philadelphia

Tonge B, Burrows G, Werry J 1990 Handbook of studies on child psychiatry. Elsevier, Oxford

28 | Emotional and behavioural problems

The range of emotional and behavioural problems presented by children is endless, therefore only the general issues and the most significant points will be discussed here. Each problem, however simple it may seem, occurs as the end result of complex interaction of numerous aetiological factors. An assessment of any particular behaviour or emotion must take into account these factors and also consider what other influences are at work in maintaining the disorder. It is often the case that a self-perpetuating cycle develops with a strong tendency to continue. The concept of a vicious circle is useful when discussing behavioural problems with parents and it may be helpful to actually draw up a list of the various contributing factors. Some of these will be difficult, if not impossible to influence. It is therefore important to focus therapeutic efforts on those parts of the cycle that are most likely to change in response to interventions. It may be helpful to use several different therapeutic approaches at the same time; for example supporting the parents whilst working directly with the child and at the same time attending to any problems that have occurred at school.

Some 7% of 3-year-old children have moderate or severe behaviour problems, as defined by their parents. At 5 years of age approximately 10% of children are reported to be often disobedient and 'quick to fly off the handle'. By 7 years old some 20% of children showed some form of antisocial behaviour such as destructiveness or disobedience, with or without hyperactivity. This steady increase of problems may be due to parent's changing perception of what is unacceptable at different ages and the fact that larger children make more of an impact, rather than to a true increase in bad behaviour. Generally, behavioural problems have been found to be more than twice as common at home than at school and boys are noted to show more difficult behaviour than girls.

Serious disturbance

The majority of difficult behaviour does not necessarily indicate a serious disturbance. For example, on the one hand children who steal may be doing this simply because they can get away with it, on the other hand it may be the outward manifestation of profound disturbance. Even something as serious as fire-setting could be seen as normal experimentation by an inquisitive child. Nevertheless this explanation can only be used once and further attempts at fire-setting would suggest pathology in family function. Although most emotional and behavioural symptoms are non-specific and may or may not indicate an underlying disorder, there are a few symptoms that are almost invariably indicative of significant abnormality. These are:

- Deliberate destructive behaviour that is repeated and apparently without purpose.
- Running off from home.
- Marked deterioration in function with no obvious cause.
- Repeated aggressive behaviour in all settings after the age of 5 years.
- Deliberate self-harm.
- Repeated fire-setting.

Generally, what determines the significance of any particular symptom is the severity, the duration and the associated symptoms. It is the pattern of symptoms that is the best indicator of risk for the child. For example, crying as a single symptom may have

Table 28.1
Childhood behaviours indicative of serious disturbance

Symptom	Disturbance
Deliberately destructive	Hostile relationships, low self-esteem
Deliberate messing	Lack of self-worth, inadequate care
Wandering off	Poor supervision
Running off	Lack of affection and/or intolerable distress
Deliberate self-harm	Low self-esteem or intolerable distress
Age-inappropriate sexual behaviour	Sexual abuse

little significance, but if it is associated with loss of interest, poor appetite, loss of sleep and morbid thoughts, it may well indicate a depressive disorder (Table 28.1).

GOOD HABIT TRAINING

Basic training in the habits of everyday life is an important developmental task that parents seem to find increasingly difficult because of the extensive demands on their time and energy. Most children go through a developmental sequence for establishing routines in the different areas of everyday life as shown in Table 28.2.

There is no doubt that some children have more difficulty getting into a daily routine than others, especially those with a difficult temperament. Nevertheless, it should eventually be possible to achieve a regular habit with even the most trying child, provided that the parents insist on keeping to a routine and a time-schedule. Once the routine is established, things can then be relaxed a little to allow family life to be more flexible and adaptable. The relevance of training a child in the routines of everyday life may seem obvious, but it is surprising how many parents find this difficult, and how many clinicians underestimate its importance. Failure to achieve an acceptable routine in everyday life will result in daily hassle and distress for the family.

Table 28.2
The development sequence of everyday habits

Habit	Time
Regular feeding	4–12 weeks
Good sleep routine	4–12 months
Dressing and undressing	1–2y
Toileting	2–4y
Eating	3–5y
Self-care	4–6y

Pervasive habit-training disorder

Some children present with a wide range of problems relating to the routines of everyday life. There will be problems getting the child to sleep at night, arguments over dressing, unsettled meal times and sometimes associated toileting problems. In such instances it is best to start by tackling the problem that comes earliest in the developmental sequence, before attempting to improve some of the others. The management of pervasive habit-training disorder involves agreeing a strict routine with the parents. It helps to write this down so that the parents can be reminded to keep to the strict time sequence, if necessary using timers or alarm clocks to keep everybody to schedule. Close supervision will be needed to ensure that the agreed routine is maintained.

Young children enjoy and benefit from routine and regularity in their life. It helps them to feel secure and makes argument and discussion over daily routines much less likely to occur. The benefits of establishing these routines at an early stage are all too obvious and parents need to understand that it is best to get in first and establish a routine which suits the family, rather than to follow the routine set by each child.

Unwanted habits

Unwanted habits are very common in young children and have no special significance in terms of underlying psychopathology. The repetition is familiar and therefore usually comforting. The fact that habits become more marked under stress does not mean that they are caused by stress — which exaggerates almost every behaviour. In addition to stress, habits are also worse by excitement and boredom.

Nail-biting and thumb-sucking

Large-scale surveys of children show that habits such as nail-biting and thumb-sucking occur quite frequently. Approximately 30% of 5-year-old children bite their nails, suck their thumbs or both and about the same number have eating or sleeping habit problems. These habit disorders are rather more likely to occur in girls than in boys. In addition, roughly one in four children experience twitches and tics at some time in their development.

Most of these habits are strongly age dependent. Finger-and thumb-sucking under the age of 3 years is quite normal, but there is evidence that after the age of four it may cause problems due to malocclusion (Box 28.1).

Nail-biting and thumb-sucking are particularly difficult habits to influence. Both require a cooperative effort between the parent and the child. Reassurance may not be sufficient in itself, since many parents find it difficult to ignore these behaviours. A recent approach to this problem involves identi-

---

> **Box 28.1**
> **The adverse effects of finger- and thumb-sucking**
>
> - Malformation of the mouth and face
> - Difficulty in responding to questions
> - Interference with spontaneous speech
> - Restricted use of play material
> - Negative interactions with parents
> - Perceived by others as being immature

---

fying the times and circumstances when the child is most likely to thumb-suck. Then the child is taught to make a clenched fist with the thumb inside the fist and to hold it in that position for a count of 20. The child has to repeat this whenever the circumstances arise where thumb-sucking may occur. If the child is actually found thumb-sucking at any time, then the fist-clenching exercise is repeated at least once. A similar approach can be used for other simple habits where first a behaviour is identified that makes the habit impossible to perform, then the child's cooperation is gained to perform that behaviour and, most important of all, the approach is kept playful and good humoured.

Masturbation

Although masturbation in young children provokes a range of strong feelings in parents and other adults, it is really just like any other habit. It occurs more frequently when children are bored, emotionally upset or excited. The principles of disrupting the habit are also the same. Hands need to be kept occupied and any satisfaction from the behaviour should be kept to the minimum by withdrawing attention or by dressing in clothes that make access more difficult.

TICS

Tics are simple, repeated and unwanted movements that, unlike habits, have no purpose and can only be controlled by will-power over a period of minutes (Box 28.2). However, like habits they are

---

Box 28.2
Features associated with tics

- Overactive behaviour
- Family history of tics (about 15%)
- Other habits
- Speech disorder
- Obsessional behaviour
- Emotional problems (more common in males)

---

strongly influenced by altered levels of arousal and are made worse by emotional stress, boredom and excitement. Tics are not present during sleep. The usual onset of childhood tics is between 2 and 15 years, with one peak around the age of 7 years old and another in early adolescence. Only a very small number continue into adulthood.

It seems likely that all tics are based on the neurophysiology of the startle response. The most common tic is eye-blinking and the next is the facial tic and then a head-twitch, and so on in the same progression as would occur when a person is startled. The most extreme from of tic known as Gilles de la Tourette's syndrome involves multiple and complex tics often including vocal expletives. There is evidence that neurotransmitter imbalance is an important factor in the production of tics and that environmental and psychological factors are also important in maintaining the movements. The end result is that neuronal inhibitory feedback is insufficient to stop spontaneous but simple movements.

A simple explanation of the nature of tics may reassure some parents, but many will want some more specific instructions. The primary goal is to deal with any stress and achieve optimal arousal levels. Any comments or actions that draw attention to the tic must be stopped, both at home and at school, since they will have a major influence in maintaining the symptom. Other approaches such as deliberately practising the tic or keeping a detailed diary of tic frequency may sometimes be helpful.

Treatment with drugs such as haloperidol to alter neurotransmitter release can be effective in controlling severe tics. Unfortunately, they all have potentially serious side effects and should only be used by clinicians with specialist experience, and only then if a tic is causing a severe handicap to the child's development.

EATING PROBLEMS

The close relationship between food and feelings is the underlying reason why children's eating habits are the cause of considerable concern for parents. Most of the worry about children's eating is unnecessary, because the majority of childhood eating problems resolve spontaneously. But at the same time most of the eating problems of adult life can be traced back to childhood. Significant feeding problems occur in 10–15% of very young children and are likely to be associated with having a young mother and being an only child with a low birthweight. By the time that the children start at school about one in four children are described as being faddy and are more likely to come from smaller and better off families. Children with feeding problems are more likely to have stomach aches, vomiting, and headaches, but there is no way of telling if this is due to a common factor such as food allergy. There is no difference between boys and girls in the overall rate of eating difficulties.

Obesity

Childhood obesity appears to be increasing in frequency in western countries. Some 10–15% of pre-school children are overweight. The follow-up of these fat children shows that there is a strong tendency for the obesity to continue. The onset of obesity after the age of 4 years seems to have a much worse prognosis than an onset in infancy. Weight control is notoriously difficult in childhood obesity and requires major changes in parental attitudes and dietary behaviour patterns. Parents need to understand that whatever they think may have caused the obesity, weight gain can only be reduced by eating less than the child actually needs. Parents must take full responsibility for their child's weight, since it is the parents who have bought, prepared and served the food that the child has grown fat on.

It should be made clear to parents that if a child is slimming, hunger is a positive sign that should be rewarded with praise and cuddles rather than more calories. Since children are still growing, weight stability is usually the goal rather than weight reduction and the nutritional quality of any special diet needs to be carefully monitored.

Food fads

Various factors such as parental attitude to food, family dietary and eating habits have been implicated in children's abnormal eating patterns. More severe eating problems are likely to be associated with problems in the parent–child relationship and by emotional stress affecting the child or parent. Most fussy children seem to do extremely well in other respects. Physical growth, haematology and biochemistry are usually well within the normal. It is essential to find ways of banishing emotions from mealtimes and to take a long-term view, gradually introducing new foods over a period of years. At the same time it is important for parents to avoid becoming a slave to the child's fads by allowing the fussy child to control family meals with demands for separate food. Some children seem to develop a 'phobia' of particular foods. Forcing a child to eat the feared food may make things worse, but avoiding it will only maintain the problem.

It is not unusual for toddlers to use food refusal as one way of asserting their independence or to find out how far they can push their parents. This type of negativism is best dealt with by a 'take it or leave it approach'. The hunger drive can be used to good effect and it is quite acceptable for children to miss two or three meals, provided that their weight is satisfactory and fluid intake (without calorific value) is kept within the normal range.

Anorexia

More extreme forms of food refusal can occur in a range of conditions, most of which are fuelled by emotional distress (Box 28.3). Symptoms that are similar to anorexia nervosa can occur in prepubertal children, in which case they are almost invariably the result of obvious stress factors at home or at school. Occasionally the food refusal may be part

> **Box 28.3**
> ## Characteristic features of anorexia nervosa
>
> - Loss of more than 20% of expected body weight in relation to height
> - Preoccupation with food and body weight
> - Concern about being too fat in spite of being underweight
> - Persistent refusal to maintain an appropriate weight
> - A tendency to set high standards and to be obsessional
> - A feeling of being out of control and difficulty in communicating feelings

of a more general despairing state where the child seems to give up completely sometimes described as 'pervasive refusal'. This condition often occurs after a flu-like illness in children who tend to set themselves high standards. It can best be understood as a failure to convalesce and usually responds well to carefully graduated rehabilitation with the parents playing a critical supporting role.

Mild or undeveloped forms of anorexia nervosa are quite common and are best dealt with before lack of food intake leads to the many secondary symptoms of starvation, such as lowered mood and amenorrhoea. Recent treatment approaches for anorexia have been aimed at encouraging the older child to take responsibility for their weight and eating, using 'eating and feeling' diaries. Young people with anorexia nervosa seem to find communication at an emotional level especially difficult. They are therefore encouraged to examine their feelings in relation to eating and it may help them to carefully record the details of what they have eaten and how they felt about it. At the same time a reasonable target weight range should be agreed and progress closely supervised. Younger children may benefit from their parents taking more active control of their eating and being prepared to be quite tough and determined that their child will eat appropriate amounts of food.

Food and behaviour

Undernutrition in the weeks just before and after birth can have an adverse effect on brain function which may be lasting and result in poor school performance and an increased rate of behaviour problems. The brain uses about two-thirds of the sugar available in the body. It has been claimed that sugar causes difficult and aggressive behaviour in school children and that it interferes with learning. There is some evidence that sugar might increase movement in children, but there is no convincing evidence that sugar affects other aspects of behaviour. Caffeine in coffee and tea does have a general alerting effect, but is unlikely to change children's behaviour.

Food allergies are quite common in young children during the first few years of life, but become less frequent as they grow older so that by the age of 5 years most of the problems have resolved. The chief symptoms are diarrhoea, abdominal pain and skin rashes. There are theoretical reasons why salicylates, occurring naturally in food, might have an effect on behaviour through their influence on the production of prostaglandins in the brain. Removing salicylates as well as artificial colourings and preservatives from the food of hyperactive children has been claimed to result in an improvement within a few days in at least 50% of cases. Unfortunately, in most cases this is likely to be due to the 'halo' effect of a special diet. Properly controlled research suggests that only a very small number of children are affected by food additives and an even smaller number improve on an exclusion diet (some estimates suggest 25 per 100 000 children). If parents are keen to try an exclusion diet to improve their child's behaviour it is as well to be supportive, rather than undermining of their efforts. Better behaviour often results, although in most cases this is more likely to be due to the child's experience of more consistent and firm management than to the removal of allergens or toxic substances.

CHILDHOOD SLEEP PROBLEMS

It is reported that one in three infants and children up to 5 years old have disturbed sleep and, of these, about 30% could be regarded as having a serious problem. Fortunately, children sleep better as they grow older and, by 8 years old, the frequency of sleep problems is down to one in 10. The newborn infant spends most of the day and night asleep, but has a short sleep cycle of about 20 minutes. By 3 months old children spend more time awake during the day than during the night, but there are still four to five periods of nocturnal wakefulness. Around the age of 6 months, most children spend up to 15 hours asleep during the night and a clear day/night sleep pattern is normally established. Therefore, it is better to wait until at least 6 months of age before taking any firm action to deal with a child's disturbed sleep pattern, although a regular bedtime and sleep routine can be helpful before this age.

Why worry

There is evidence that sleep deprivation adversely affects children and, indeed, their parents. Lack of sleep leads to poor concentration and irritability after 24 hours of wakefulness, followed by anxiety and feelings of depression after 48 hours. These symptoms are shared by both children and adults. But paradoxically, as children become more tired, they tend to speed up, becoming restless and apparently energetic, whereas most adults slow down and run out of energy. Parents also need time for themselves, time to communicate and to enjoy being together. A sleepless child can make this very difficult.

Since parents cannot force sleep on their child, they should concentrate on making sure that they are providing the right conditions for sleep: that the child is lying in bed with the light turned off and, if possible, the bedroom door closed. Resting in bed at night is almost as restorative as sleep itself. Sleep is therefore not the absolute goal for parents to aim for, rather they should aim to get their child to bed in good time and ensure that the child stays there.

The management

Children are quick to realise that by playing up at bed time, they can control their parents and obtain extra attention and cuddles. It often seems that children are better at training their parents into a night-time routine than the other way round. Hypnotic drugs are contraindicated because they have side effects and are ineffective in the long run. Complying with the child's wishes may seem an easy way out, but this too has side effects and is no long-term solution.

Establishing a good sleep habit

At 6 months, most children have settled into a reasonably stable sleep/waking cycle, but by 2 years this has often broken down, especially if a regular sleep routine has not been firmly established. Sleep, just like eating, toiletting and dressing, is a daily habit that requires regular training over a long period before it becomes properly established. How parents organise a good sleep habit is a good indicator as to how they will cope with other developmental tasks where the child's unreasonable demands have to be denied. It is important to focus on sorting out sleep problems before dealing with any other behavioural and management problems.

There is more to night time than merely sleeping — rest is also important, whether the child is asleep or not. Less obviously, night time is when children begin to learn to feel confident on their own. This is one of the very few times when children are completely alone for any length of time and, therefore, able to develop self-reliance. Children have to grow up relatively quickly in order to cope with our present-day society. It is therefore helpful to achieve a reasonable level of self-confidence and independence before starting at school. Sleeping in the parents' bed may seem like an easy solution to night-time problems, but it is difficult to mature while still dependent in this way. In addition, sleeping together exposes the child to a highly intimate experience of the parent's emotions. Children gain a sense of security from parents who are confident and predictable in their child care. Confusion about what is expected at night is likely to lead to feelings of insecurity and unsettled behaviour during the day. One of the main reasons why children do not settle quickly at night is because insufficient effort is put into getting the bed-time routine well established (Box 28.4).

This routine needs some explanation. It is important that the bed time is not fixed too late. The

---

> **Box 28.4**
> **The recommended approach for establishing a good sleep routine**
>
> 1. Take time to go through the routine carefully with parents
> 2. It may help to write it all down
> 3. Agree a bed time that can be kept to rigidly
> 4. Start the routine 1 hour before bed time
> 5. Gradually wind things down
> 6. Always do the same things in the same order
> 7. Once in bed, spend no more than 5 minutes with the child
> 8. Always say exactly the same words when saying goodnight
> 9. Turn the light out and shut the bedroom door

---

longer a parent stays in the bedroom the more the child is likely to complain when the parent leaves and also to wake during the night. A few quiet words together is all that is needed before saying the usual goodnight phrase and leaving the room. The same 'sleep phrase' can also be used at other times during the night if, for example, a child is woken by a nightmare. If the light is left on it gives the wrong message to the child: *that darkness is dangerous*. If the door is left open wide enough for the child to walk through, the message is: *come out anytime you like*.

Ensuring a successful outcome

Most parents can manage to get their children to bed. Any difficulty with this would suggest a disciplinary problem. The child has to be taught to stay in bed — or at least, in the bedroom. Of course, if the child is still in a cot, there is no problem. When children graduate to a bed it is best to aim for a 'psychological lock' on the bedroom door so that the child knows not to come out of the bedroom after having been put to bed, except to go to the toilet or in an emergency.

The quickest way of achieving a 'psychological lock' on the bedroom door is to catch the child at

Emotional and behavioural problems

the earliest possible moment after getting out of bed. Then to return the child immediately, with a tone of voice and facial expression and a manner that is so impressive that the child remains in bed. The child's reaction to this will let the parents know if the performance was good enough, or if they will have to practice a bit more. Parents who are unable to control their children enough to keep them in bed at night are also likely to have similar problems in other more dangerous situations. Children should be considered to be at risk until parents have achieved this first stage of discipline. If the child stays in bed, but calls out, cries or screams, it is important, *provided the child is safe and well*, that the parents do not respond in any way. This 'in at the deep end' approach is effective in a few days if parents can keep to it.

Parents often say they have done it all before and it has not worked, but on checking carefully it is usual to find that they have not really carried it through. Either the child has been allowed out of the bedroom or the parents have eventually responded to the crying which shows the child that it is worth carrying on crying because someone will respond in the end (Table 28.3).

This rather tough approach can only be justified if it is clear that the child is not ill or in discomfort, but is just crying to get his own way. It is best to carry it out any time between the age of 6 months old and starting at school. The difficulty of keeping to this sleep programme should not be underestimated, and parents will often need intensive support on a daily basis to help them persevere. It is always best to see both parents together before they tackle sleep problems. Any slight disagreement is likely to be magnified using this tough and demanding approach.

An alternative approach

Some parents lack the confidence and motivation to carry out the demanding approach described above. There is an alternative approach where the parent spends progressively less time in the child's bedroom each night, following a carefully worked out schedule. This can be effective, but many children soon grasp what is happening, and return to their previous ways.

There will always be a few who are against causing a child any distress at all, fearing that it must inevitably lead to long-term psychological

---

Table 28.3
Reasons for failing to establish a good sleep routine and possible solutions

The problem	Possible solutions
The child creeps out without parents knowing	Fit an alarm to the door or a movement detector
The child might suffer some harm	The bedroom must be totally safe
The room must be entered to check that the child is all right	Look through the keyhole or use a mirror or a baby alarm
The neighbours complain about the crying	Warn them first. They will normally be supportive
One parent gives in	Both parents must agree. The tougher parent should look after the one that gives in
The crying is too distressing	Try a personal stereo or ear plugs
The child will not stay in bed, but stays in the room	Dress in a warm all-in-one suit
The child vomits with screaming	Clear it up with the minimum of fuss, avoiding any eye contact

harm. There is no evidence to support this view which makes the unrealistic assumption that distress can somehow be avoided in life. In fact, children cannot have all their wishes met, so denying their unreasonable demands in the context of a loving family can have a positive and protective effect on children. Success in establishing a good night-time routine leads to increased confidence and happiness all round, making all the hard work well worth the effort.

ENURESIS AND ENCOPRESIS

Many of the issues related to enuresis and encopresis are similar. The one major difference being that soiling provokes much stronger negative reactions than wetting. Enuresis is much more common than encopresis and will therefore be dealt with in more detail. The 1946 British National Survey found that most parents started to sit their children on the pot well before the end of the first year and there is no evidence that early training has any adverse influence on the achievement of continence in any way. It may well be that delayed toilet training makes it more difficult for some children to gain continence.

Most of the usual explanations that parents use to help them understand enuresis have been shown to be mistaken. Deep sleep has not been found to play any part. Sleep electroencephalograms (EEGs) have shown that enuresis can occur at any stage of sleep, although wetting is more frequent in the stage just before waking and occurs less frequently during rapid eye movement (REM) sleep. The notion that incontinent children have a smaller bladder capacity than normal has a certain logic to it, but the issue is far from straightforward. The average urine volume voided is about 80 ml at 2 years of age, increasing to around 225 ml between 7 and 8 years old. The ability of the bladder wall (detrusor) muscles to relax as they become stretched keeps the pressure at around 15 cmH$_2$O water until micturition occurs when the pressure increases to about 50 cmH$_2$O. In young children the detrusor muscle contracts at relatively low volumes leading to a rise in pressure and an urge to micturate which has to be inhibited by contraction of the external urethral sphincter.

Urine volume per voiding has been found to be significantly less in enuretic children. However, under light anaesthesia bladder capacity is the same for continent and enuretic children at 40 cmH$_2$O pressure. The total output per 24 h is also the same. These findings suggest that it is the immaturity of bladder function that leads to small amounts of urine being voided, rather than small structural capacity.

The observation that wetting is frequently worse when a child is emotionally distressed has led to the commonly held view that it must be the emotion that actually causes the enuresis. However, enuresis presents in much the same way as other conditions, such as asthma, nail biting or toothache — they all get worse if a child is distressed for any reason. There are very few aspects of development that improve with emotional distress and regression under the influence of threatening or stressful influences is part of normal functioning.

Children who have experienced stressful life events do have an increased rate of incontinence, but there is also an increase in a whole range of maladaptive behaviour. What does seem to be important is the timing of the stress. For example, children admitted to hospital between the ages of 2 and 5 years are more likely to continue wetting than children who have not been admitted.

The relationship between stressful life events, emotional states and enuresis is highly complex. If enuresis is primarily a symptom of emotional disorder, one might expect more girls than boys to be affected or at least for the sex ratio to be equal, since the frequency of adverse life events is much the same for boys and girls. Enuresis in school-age children is at least twice as common in boys than in girls, although if girls do wet they tend to be more emotionally disturbed than boys.

Enuresis

Enuresis is a specific developmental delay and this implies that one or more aspects of maturation are significantly delayed by 20% or more in relation to the rest of the child's general development. The commonly recognised specific delays in development involve speech and language, reading and arithmetic, fine and gross motor skills, bowel and bladder development. It is likely that hyperactivity and some forms of impulsiveness also occur as specific delays in development (Box 28.5).

There is a 68 per cent concordance rate for enuresis in monozygotic twins compared with 36 per cent concordance for dizygotic twins. The steady improvement of enuresis with age is well documented as is the superiority of treatments involving training over other therapies. These findings all support the view that enuresis is primarily a specific developmental disorder as defined above (Fig. 28.1).

The implications of enuresis

The developmental model of enuresis is essentially an interactive one that takes account of a range of different factors and at the same time is capable of integrating a wide range of different theories. The outlook for a specific developmental delay is good in the sense that it improves with time, but ineffective training or stressful experiences will delay the attainment of skill competence. According to this model the delayed skill will remain vulnerable and is likely to be the first skill to be lost as a result of regression under stress.

Secondary enuresis may not at first appear to fit the model, since it characteristically follows a stressful event after a period of continence. However, the concept of children being either continent or incontinent is unhelpful because conti-

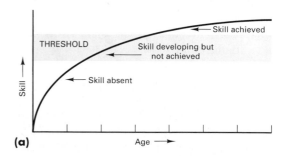

(a)

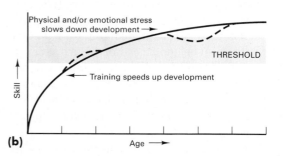

(b)

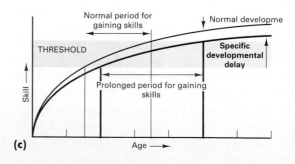

(c)

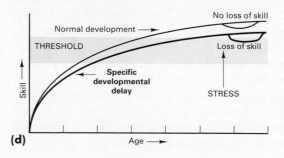

(d)

Box 28.5
Specific developmental delays share the same characteristics

- A higher incidence in boys

- A tendency to be more serious in girls

- Normal progression through maturational stages

- Evidence of heritability

- Good response to specific training and little response to other treatments

- Early regression under stress

- A tendency to be associated with other specific delays

- Increased vulnerability to psychosocial stress

- Associated with secondary emotional distress, frustration and low self-esteem

- Normal development in most other areas

- A strong tendency to improve spontaneously

Emotional and behavioural problems

nence is only gradually achieved and is always dependent on the relationship between bladder maturity and emotional or physical stress factors that can have an adverse effect on bladder control. This is why the main features of primary and secondary enuresis are the same, the treatment is the same and the outcome is much the same as well.

Day wetting is more common in girls and they in turn are also more likely to have bacteruria. Diurnal wetting is also linked to a higher rate of psychiatric disturbance, but none of these findings is contrary to enuresis being primarily a specific developmental delay.

Deliberate urination that causes wetting of the bed or elsewhere is very different from accidental incontinence and should be seen as a provocative antisocial act. Clinical impression suggests that children who indulge in this unusual behaviour are disturbed and are using it to signal their distress about their care within the family.

The feeling of failure and the development of a low self-esteem resulting from the many negative experiences associated with enuresis is likely to become apparent around the age of 6–9 years of age, when children start to have a more clearly developed concept of self-image. It is also difficult for children to feel grown up and mature while they are still wetting the bed. Treatment should, therefore, not be postponed in the hope that the child will grow out of it.

Toilet training

Less than 1 in 10 children with enuresis have some physical cause for the wetting, most commonly a urinary infection. This needs to be excluded before any continence training programme is put into effect. Toilet training in one form or another is the most effective way of managing enuresis. However, it is important that toilet training is undertaken at the appropriate age. Some parents start potting their children around the age of 9 months, an age at which most children can sit unsupported. Another accepted sign of readiness for toilet training is the ability to indicate a wish to pass urine and showing signs of distress when wet. There is some evidence that if training is delayed beyond 2 years the likelihood of persisting incontinence is significantly increased.

The first step in the treatment of day- or night-time wetting is to record the frequency of accidents, while at the same time giving high praise for being dry. Simple explanation of the significance of wetting and its developmental nature should also be given. If this fails to produce improvement after 2 weeks, daytime wetting is then best dealt with by visits to the toilet at intervals that are frequent enough to ensure that the child remains dry and then gradually increase the gap between the visits. The use of individually designed reward charts with stars or smiley faces indicating success is generally helpful, but takes a lot of organisation to do properly. In order to maintain motivation, it is best to limit the use of charts to 4–6 weeks, followed by a rest period before starting again.

Increasing a child's involvement in the clearing-up process after accidents is also helpful. Cleanliness training helps to increase children's awareness of the inconvenience of wetting. When wetting occurs, the child has to remove the wet clothes or sheets and put them to soak or in the laundry. They are then replaced with dry items. The more the

Fig. 28.1 An explanatory developmental model of enuresis. Any explanatory model of enuresis has to be able to integrate all the research findings and provide a satisfactory explanation for the complex relationship between enuresis and psychosocial stress too
(a) The typical relationship between the rate of skill acquisition and age, with a high rate of development early on eventually reaching a plateau. The normal course of development is not smooth, rather it is characterised by advances and regressions under the dual influences of training and stress
(b) Specific training speeds up the rate of development of skill competence and stress of any kind (physical and emotional) may slow down development or lead to regression and loss of skills
(c) The developmental curve of a typical example of specific developmental delay
(d) In a child with a specific developmental delay, a prolonged period is spent passing through the threshold and the plateau is established nearer the threshold than normal. In the event of a stressful experience, the specifically delayed skill is likely to be lost before other abilities

child takes responsibility for this 'cleaning up' process the better. Parents must understand that this is a training technique and not a punishment. They will also need to supervise the cleaning up and provide assistance at an age-appropriate level. This training approach helps children to become more aware of the wetting and less inclined to pretend that it does not exist. It also makes any success more noticeable for the child.

Moisture-sensitive electric buzzers that sound the alarm on micturition are available in many different forms, although they all make use of urine to complete an electric circuit. These gadgets can be used for day- or night-time wetting and if used according to the instructions, should result in an 80% improvement rate. However, social and motivational factors are crucially important in determining the outcome of these training interventions.

The so called dry-bed technique seeks to maximise motivation and raise social rewards for dryness. On the first night the child is woken up every hour, given a drink and guided to the toilet. If urine is passed in the toilet the child is praised and appropriately rewarded. The dry-bed training programme also includes a buzzer apparatus that is used to identify a wetting incident. If wet, the child has to do the '20 times routine'. This involves going to the toilet 20 times, counting up to 20 on each occasion. For the first week the child has to perform the 20 times routine every night before going to sleep even if the bed was dry the night before. But after that, it is only performed after wetting. There are several variations of this approach, but they all have in common an emphasis on overlearning, i.e. repeating something more times than might seem necessary. This rather extreme approach is remarkably successful if carried out properly, but is best reserved for the highly motivated families.

Lifting or waking children at night to go to the toilet may be quite successful, but it fails to train the child and the improvement is purely symptomatic. Bladder training techniques are occasionally helpful, but are not worth spending too much time and effort on. Bladder training includes voluntarily prolonging the intervals between voiding, or stopping and starting the flow during micturition.

Medication

Desmopression (desamino-D-arginine vasopressin), a vasopressin analogue, is currently more favoured than imipramine as the drug of choice for symptomatic treatment of enuresis. Desmopressin has been found to be effective for short-term symptom suppression. It is administered as a single intranasal dose of 20–40 µg or 200–400 µg by mouth before bed time. This recommended dose is independent of age and body weight and can be expected to produce improvement in 80% of children, half of whom will stop wetting altogether. The efficacy of desmopressin seems to be related to its ability to concentrate urine and thus decrease the output of urine during the night. Desmopressin is relatively free of side effects, in comparison with other drugs such as tricyclics which are no longer considered appropriate in the routine treatment of enuresis. Excessive drinking with desmopressin can lead to hyponatraemia.

Encopresis

The term encopresis implies that formed faeces are deposited in abnormal places. This distinguishes it from overflow related to constipation and accidental soiling due to diarrhoea. It is best conceived of as a specific delay in the development of bowel control, having all the characteristic features already outlined. A simple explanation of these issues is usually very reassuring for parents. The management of encopresis is relatively straightforward unless there are secondary emotional or physical factors that may perpetuate the symptom.

The programme outlined in Box 28.6 may seem rather basic, but it is usually very effective if it is applied to the letter. It is the strong emotions generated by the soiling that undermine treatment by making parents feel angry and children feel unlikable failures. Successful treatment normally reverses these negative processes, but where symptoms continue in spite of treatment interventions, the underlying, disturbed emotions will need attention.

HYPERACTIVITY AND ATTENTION DEFICIT DISORDER

Attention deficit and hyperactivity disorder (ADHD) is a condition that causes considerable

Box 28.6
Main steps in the treatment of encopresis

1. Train the child to sit on the toilet for up to 5 minutes at regular times. The use of charts and timers may be helpful

2. Plan for the child to sit on the toilet frequently enough to avoid soiling. Four or more times a day may be necessary

3. First reward regular sitting and when this is well established, reward passing a stool in the toilet

4. Use diet, laxatives or enemas to keep the lower bowel as empty as possible. Soiling will be less likely to occur

5. The child should take some responsibility for clearing up the mess with help and supervision as appropriate

6. If dirty pants are hidden, the parent should take control of all pants and only provide clean ones for old ones returned

Box 28.7
Main characteristics of ADHD

- Short attention span
- Distractibility
- Poor impulse control
- Marked overactivity

confusion amongst parents and professionals. It is characterised by marked overactivity and restlessness, impulsivity and poor concentration with distractibility (Box 28.7). Each of the three symptom groups is developmentally normal in younger children aged 2–6 years. This makes assessment difficult because there are no generally accepted measures of hyperactivity and the diagnosis is therefore a subjective one. Parents are often quick to diagnose hyperactivity if they find their child difficult to manage. Nevertheless, about 2% of children are noticeably restless and inattentive, many

of whom go on to have learning problems at school and pervasive behaviour problems as a result of their symptoms.

It seems likely that the condition will eventually be seen as the final common pathway of a number of different causes, including genetic, developmental, neurochemical and adverse psychosocial factors. The effect of diet on overactive behaviour remains less than certain. What is more certain is that at least 30% of hyperactive children seem to do particularly badly on a range of measures when followed up into adult life. It seems likely that a cycle of adverse relationships, low self-esteem and negative experiences is set up at an early age leading to progressively more antisocial behaviour. One way of conceptualising ADHD is as a developmental disorder of self-control. Like all developmental difficulties it becomes more obvious with age (until the skill has been achieved), it is more common in males and responds best to training. Self-control progresses through the following developmental sequence:

1. Activity control — normally achieved by 5–6 years.
2. Attention control — normally achieved by 7–8 years.
3. Impulse control — normally achieved by 9–10 years.

Although the potential to develop ADHD may be present from earliest childhood, it cannot be diagnosed for certain before the age of 6–7 years. This is similar to specific reading difficulty (or dyslexia) where there may be early indicators such as a positive family history, male gender and delay in language development, but it is not possible to make a diagnosis until a significant delay has been demonstrated. Many young children with early symptoms of ADHD will not go on to develop the disorder. They will either grow out of it normally, or be helped with training in self-control. One of the reasons why ADHD has become such a problem in recent years may be due to important changes in society where free expression and energetic activity are valued more than self-control and conforming to social norms. These changes are often reflected in both home and school.

The diagnosis of ADHD is much more difficult

than it might seem. Simply ticking off a checklist of symptoms as in Conner's Rating Scale may help in screening for the condition but is no help in diagnosis. Because the signs and symptoms of ADHD are on a continuum from normal through to very severe and disabling, it is always going to be difficult to decide where to draw the line for abnormality. The key issues in the decision-making process are:

1. Is there evidence of severe problems with overactivity, attention and impulse control to the extent that they significantly interfere with the child's everyday life?
2. Are the symptoms abnormal — taking into account the child's stage of development?
3. Is there confirmation from objective observers other than the parents?
4. Are the symptoms disabling and pervasive — present at school and home and adversely affecting learning and/or relationships?
5. Are there alternative explanations such as emotional distress, learning difficulty, overtiredness or poor parental management?

The treatment of ADHD should be focused on encouraging self-control and the training of appropriate behaviour. No one method has been shown to be better than another and it is best to create individually tailored programmes that address the most obvious problems at school and at home. Hyperactive children benefit from routine and regularity in everyday life, with firm boundaries set for their behaviour. A system of positive discipline is also helpful in preventing the inevitable negative responses engendered by their socially disruptive behaviour. This involves the simple principle of getting the child to put right whatever he has done wrong. It also has the advantage of teaching children what they should be doing. For example: the mess has to be cleaned up; what is broken has to be mended; someone has been upset or offended and apology should be given followed by doing something to make the person feel better and so on.

Concentration exercises can also help: the child is asked to concentrate on a task for a few seconds, timed by the clock, and the time is gradually increased over several weeks, always ensuring that each concentration session gives an experience of success. Simple games such as snap or snakes and ladders can be used and reading involves all the skills that need to be trained in ADHD. To begin with very high levels of control and supervision may be required, but this can gradually be reduced as the child is more able to keep self-control. Stimulants derived from amphetamine have a paradoxical calming effect in children and have been shown to be effective in the symptomatic treatment of ADHD in up to 80% of cases when used appropriately in conjunction with training and family support. It is all too easy to resort to drugs as an easy means of control for high-spirited, energetic children or emotionally distressed, restless and distracted children. The use of such drugs should be restricted to clinicians with special experience in this field. Each child with suspected ADHD requires a full and detailed assessment together with a carefully monitored treatment programme that includes support for the family and school and a training approach for the child as a basic minimum. Methylphenidate is the drug of choice, starting at a dose of 5 mg twice daily and then adjusting the dose 5 mg every 2 days up to a maximum of 20 mg three times daily or 1 mg/kg/dose. Methylphenidate is short acting and has an effect that lasts for 5–6 hours, often followed by a short rebound of symptoms. The timing of the doses is quite critical and the following factors need to be taken into account:

- The maximum benefit will occur between 1 and 2 hours after a dose.
- The maximum benefit should be used to improve concentration and learning.
- There is often a withdrawal effect at about 4 and 5 hours after the dose, lasting about 1 hour. This should not coincide with a high-risk time for disruptive behaviour.
- It may be better to give a smaller dose more frequently i.e. three to four times a day.
- The last dose of the day should not be given too late in order to avoid sleep problems.

Monitoring for side effects is important, even though methylphenidate is remarkably well tolerated by most children. Decreased appetite, poor

Emotional and behavioural problems

sleep, anxiety, crying and irritability are all quite common, as are aches and pains. Generally these symptoms are quite mild and can be expected to reduce further after a week or so. Alternatively the dose can be reduced. Less than 1% of children on stimulant medication develop tics but the reason for this is complex. It seems likely that a pre-existing tendency for tics is exacerbated. Reduced growth and weight loss appear to be reversible in the few case where they occur. However, there are concerns about what the long-term effect of stimulants might be on brain function generally and possibly on the cardiovascular system. For this reason it is important to monitor height, weight, blood pressure and pulse. A further 'side effect' to be aware of is the tendency for the carers of a child with ADHD on stimulants to use the medication to control natural exuberance and spontaneous behaviour with a dose that is greater than necessary or by prolonging treatment. Stimulants should only be prescribed where the child's learning and development is clearly impaired by the ADHD and where other treatments have failed. As soon as a child is put on medication plans should be made for how and when it will be stopped and a programme for continuing self-control training and family support must be maintained.

In the majority of cases ADHD occurs in association with other problems, the most common of which are specific developmental delays and various forms of family dysfunction. The complexity of the interactions between social, neurodevelopmental and personal factors is why it is best for the condition to be diagnosed, assessed and treated by specialist clinicians backed by an expert multi-professional team.

AUTISM

This is possibly one of the most difficult of diagnostic areas for many clinicians. The autistic spectrum describes a wide clinical spectrum of disorders. In general they include a triad of manifestations that have life long effects. The triad consists of impairments in: social interaction, communication and behaviour (poor imagination and narrow repetitive play and behaviour).

Clinical picture

The original descriptions of Kanner (Kanner 1943) and Asperger (Asperger 1991) are largely useful in a historical context.

Autism may manifest in infancy as abnormal attachment. However in most the diagnosis is made around 18–30 months of age when abnormalities in speech and play development are noted. Manifestations can be broadly categorised into abnormalities of behaviour, communication, play, social interaction and cognition.

Behaviour

Children demonstrate deficits in reapricocity both verbal and non-verbal, sociability and have a narrow range of interests. They can show affection but often on their terms and often without the expected happiness associated. These children may be extraordinarily shy, fearful or anxious. The older child or adolescent may become more withdrawn or depressed. Sensorimotor patterns of behaviour include handflapping, spinning, running in circles and other unusual motor stereotypic behaviour. These children often show abnormal sensory awareness either heightened or decreased particularly with auditory stimuli.

Communication

Children with autistic disorders have a wide range of language and communication difficulties including a lack of drive to communicate as well as a variety of language disorders. These may include in extreme cases verbal auditory agnosia, mixed receptive expressive disorders through to milder forms of language difficulty with literal, repetitive and poorly articulated speech.

Play

Autistic children have difficulty with pretend play and often have fairly stereotypic play consisting of repetition and lining small toys up, flicking light switches or other stimulatory behaviour.

Cognition

In general a large proportion (approximately 75%) of autistic children have deficits in cognitive skills.

Neuropsychological testing reveals an uneven profile with most having better skills in nonverbal areas. This pattern may be reversed in Asperger's syndrome. Some children can develop surprisingly good skills in musical, mathematical or visuo-spatial areas despite severe deficits in other areas.

Prevalence

Autism is thought to be present in the general population at between 0.3–1.7 per 1000 depending on the definitions used and whether milder definitions of autistic spectrum are included. Many feel that the incidence is increasing but there is a lack of evidence currently to support this.

Causes

Autism is diagnosed with behavioral criteria and as such is not specifically related to any one disorder and may well be the result of abnormal brain function after any one of a number of problems.

There is a wide range of conditions that can be associated with autism. Parents will most often recognise differences in their child from birth but a number will also recognise a change in their child usually between the first and second years. In many of these cases where a child has been apparently developing normally small changes that existed prior to the set back may be noted on specific and detailed questioning.

There are many defined biological causes and these include intrauterine rubella, tuberous sclerosis, as well as genetic causes such as fragile X, Cornelia de Lange's, Angelman's, Rett's and Down's syndromes. Postnatal conditions such as herpes simplex encephalitis and infantile spasms can also be associated. In general structural lesions are rare. EEGs are helpful when frankly epileptiform and are seen when the child has had a period of more normal development initially.

Immunological theories around immunisation and diet as a cause are controversial.

Diagnosis

The most important factor in making a diagnosis is a detailed developmental history from birth. A

Box 28.8
ICD-10 classification into subgroups

F84   Pervasive developmental disorders

F84-0 Childhood autism

F84-1 Atypical autism

F84-2 Rett's syndrome

F84-3 Other childhood disintegrative disorder

F84-4 Overactive disorder associated with mental retardation and stereotyped movements

F84-5 Asperger's syndrome

F84-8 Other pervasive developmental disorder

F84-9 Pervasive developmental disorder, unspecified

---

number of semi-structured interviews exist and these with the ICD-10 (World Health Organization 1992) or DSM IV (American Psychiatric Association 1992) research criteria can be useful to look at the subgroups and substantially increases the diagnostic reliability. Many of these however do require training to be used appropriately (Box 28.8).

Differential diagnoses include general learning disability, specific learning disability, semantic pragmatic disorder (where the child has good speech but finds it difficult to engage in reciprical conversation), attention deficit and hyperactivity disorder and Tourette's syndrome.

Investigations are often not helpful unless there are other findings especially neurological. These may include chromosomal studies and fragile X. Imaging is not generally helpful. EEGs may be indicated if there is clinical suspicion or where the child has regressed or has fluctuating abilities. In particular sleep EEGs can be helpful (Rapin 1997, Wing 1997). However the usefulness of treatment if uncertain in the group found to have paroxysmal abnormalities on EEG.

Management-interventions

Management of the child with autism or autistic spectrum disorder requires a multidisciplinary approach. There is no curative process for autism but behaviours can be modified through educational and behavioural approaches. Many children will cope in mainstream schools with appropriate resources however some will need a specialist and structured approach as in special school situations. Professionals involved may include educational psychologists, specialist teachers, clinical psychologists, preschool support (in developing play preschool), speech and language therapists and medical teams. The medical role after diagnosis and investigation may involve continuing support in the educational process, treatment if required of other difficulties e.g. Seizure disorders, sleeping issues, hyperactivity some of which may require medicational support. There are a number of controversial treatments in the community and these vary from intensive educational and behavioural programmes (e.g. Lovass method) (Matson et al 1996), dietary management with gluten and casein free diets (personal communication Shattock PE 2000) as well as various medications e.g. Secretin (Sandler et al 1999), Vitamin B6 and Magnesium (Pfeiffer 1995). The multifactorial nature of the likely aetiology of autism is reflected in the varying response of these treatments.

DIFFICULT AND DISOBEDIENT BEHAVIOUR

It is obviously important to focus on prevention as the primary aim of any therapeutic work with childhood behaviour problems. Ultimately it is good parenting that provides the most help for children in the long run. The risk of developing antisocial behaviour is greatly reduced if the child is provided with high-quality care (Box 28.9).

Difficult behaviour occurs frequently in children and is often due to the parents' misunderstanding of their behaviour or their mishandling of the child. It is all too easy to reassure parents that there is really nothing wrong with their child, or to offer the opinion that 'the child will soon grow out of it'. Unfortunately there is good evidence that many behaviour problems have a strong tendency to continue. Indeed, aggressive behaviour is a very stable characteristic and is almost as unchanging as IQ.

> **Box 28.9**
> **Parental qualities that reduce the risk of behaviour problems**
>
> - Routine and regularity in everyday life
> - Clear limit setting
> - Unconditional love and affection
> - A high level of supervision
> - Consistent care and protection
> - Age-appropriate discipline and rewards
> - High levels of supervision

Coping with problems

It is not difficult to see that many children's problems are actually caused or at least maintained by their parents. Sometimes parents actually provide examples of the unwanted behaviour and model it for their children. For example, argumentative children have frequently gained experience and been tutored in this style of interaction by their argumentative parents. Similarly, children who are aggressive have frequently experienced at first hand their parent's own aggression. It is important to identify this mechanism where it occurs and to be prepared to point it out to parents in a supportive and factual way. This is a delicate task because any approach that is seen to be critical of parent's actions is unlikely to produce positive results. The task of parenting is difficult enough as it is and impossible to get right all the time. The consequent feeling of guilt that parents experience much of the time is the main driving force for the majority of inappropriate and potentially harmful responses that occur between parent and child. Great effort, therefore, needs to be devoted to helping parents feel less guilty, while at the same time encouraging and supporting parents in the use of more effective methods of child care.

Antisocial behaviour in children is closely associated with aggressive behaviour in their parents. This leads to a predictable sequence of events called 'the coercive system' as follows:

Emotional and behavioural problems

1. Badly behaved children make it difficult for their parents to use the more subtle forms of management of deviant behaviour and to encourage good behaviour.
2. The naughty child frequently produces an aggressive response from the parent, which then serves as a model or example for the child to follow. Alternatively the parent may give in 'for a quiet life', in which case the child will learn that it pays to be bad.
3. The level of disturbance and aggression in the family rises and anarchy follows, leading to a further breakdown of caring and positive, helping behaviours in family interactions.
4. As a result, the parents tend to become fed up and irritable. They lose their confidence and self-esteem and their children also become frustrated and fed up.
5. Family members disengage from each other, the parents become disunited and the control of anti-social behaviour breaks down, resulting in still further problems and so the cycle continues.

Helping with discipline

Standards of parental discipline vary a great deal from one family to another. What seems to be the crucial issue is for each family to agree and set standards of acceptable behaviour. It is inconsistent discipline that causes far more problems for children than discipline that is consistently too lax or too strict. The word discipline comes from the Latin *disciplina* meaning teaching or training which gives an indication of how behaviour problems are best dealt with.

One of the most typical ineffectual parent–child interactions that occur in everyday family life is where parents ask their child to do something. When nothing happens they ask again and again and yet again. On each occasion the demand becomes more hostile until eventually the parent is driven to screaming pitch. At this point the child wonders what all the fuss is about. After all, it was only a relatively minor thing that was being asked in the first place. Unfortunately this type of interaction actually trains children to take little or no notice of their parents until they become furious.

Nagging is tiring and can lead to fraught and hostile relationships within the family. It is therefore best to have a rule that in general instructions are only given once. If it is unimportant, there is no need to repeat it again. If, however, it is important then a warning should be given about the consequences of not doing what has been asked. Most parents are very successful in using this training approach to protect their child from potentially dangerous situations such as playing with fire, running into the street and sticking fingers into electric sockets. Clearly until parents are able to gain this level of control, their children are at risk of accidental death.

Parents who have been able to gain compliance from children in order to protect them from danger can then use the same training approach for other areas that they feel are important. If parents feel uncertain or uncomfortable about being quite firm with and controlling their children, it may help to point out what they have already achieved in keeping their child safe. If their ultimate aim is for their child to gain self-control then this can only be achieved by the parents giving this control in the first instance. Children are not born with self-control and it does not develop spontaneously without it being provided externally first.

Most discipline used by parents is 'negative' in that it is aimed at stopping the bad behaviour. It usually involves depriving the child of something or saying 'NO'. This has its place in the management of younger children, but from school age onwards it is better to use 'positive' discipline. This involves getting the child to put right whatever has been done wrong following the principle of making the punishment fit the crime. For example:

- What is broken should be mended.
- The mess should be cleaned up.
- Any wrong doing should be apologised for.
- Anyone who is upset should have something done for them to make them feel better, e.g. making a cup of tea, drawing a picture, buying some flowers, cleaning the car.
- Anything stolen should be returned with an apology.

- Late return home should be followed by an earlier deadline by the same amount.
- Rude children should be expected to be extra polite.

ATTENTION-SEEKING BEHAVIOUR

Disruptive behaviour is often labelled attention seeking as a way of identifying the aetiology. Unfortunately this explanation is not a particularly helpful one because any behaviour could be called attention seeking. Even total conformity or doing nothing at all could be described in this way. An additional problem is that identifying behaviour as attention seeking does not provide any helpful insight as to what might be done about it. Giving the behaviour more attention is likely to make it worse. Alternatively, removing attention and ignoring the behaviour is also likely to lead to an exacerbation of the behaviour until the child does eventually get noticed. It is often best to assume that the attention seeker does actually need extra attention, in which case it is important to get in first and provide this in an appropriate caring way, rather than waiting for the child to demand it. One effective way of doing this is by giving 'quality time' where the child is given undivided and undisturbed attention for a period of 5–10 minutes on a regular basis.

SCHOOL-BASED PROBLEMS

Boys are more likely to be excluded from school than girls, with aggressive behaviour being the most common reason for suspension from school. Once excluded, few will return to normal schooling. Boys are also more at risk for specific reading problems which are associated with a higher rate of behaviour problems when compared with children who have no difficulty with reading. There is a highly complex relationship between the bad behaviour and the reading problem, with both having some causative factors in common.

The school itself may have characteristics that encourage or at least allow the development of antisocial behaviour. Even if school intake factors are controlled for, there remain consistent differences

---

> **Box 28.10**
> ### School factors which are associated with a high rate of antisocial behaviour
>
> - Unclear system of discipline
> - Children not known by name
> - Homework not marked
> - High turnover of teachers
> - Work not displayed in public areas
> - Bullying tolerated

> **Box 28.11**
> ### Factors associated with a poor outcome for antisocial behaviour
>
> - High frequency and wide range of antisocial acts, especially aggressive, argumentative and disruptive behaviour
> - Truancy and lying
> - Fire setting or running off
> - Mixing with other antisocial children
> - Growing up in extreme poverty
> - Misuse of drugs
> - Early onset of problems
> - Family members with antisocial behaviour or alcohol problems

---

between schools in the rate of children's antisocial behaviour. The most likely explanation for these differences is that they have been caused by factors within the school itself. These include the factors listed in Box 28.10 that increase the likelihood of antisocial behaviour:

From 5 years onwards, antisocial behaviour has an increasingly strong tendency to continue as a very stable characteristic (Box 28.11). About 50% of the children with bad behaviour continue to cause problems over long periods.

Assessment of school-based problems

When considering problems that arise within a school setting, it is important to distinguish the five main areas (school, home, self, peer relationships, social and cultural influences) where problems can arise. It is all too easy for schools to believe that any problems at school must be due to difficulties at home but children spend a considerable amount of their daily life at school (approximately 1500 hours in all). It would therefore be surprising if factors within school did not play a considerable part in the aetiology of childhood emotional and behavioural problems (Box 28.12).

Teasing and bullying

The majority of all bullying takes place in school or near the school. There are marked differences in the rate of bullying between schools, this is probably because some schools have an antibullying, anti-aggression ethos that makes bullying totally unacceptable. Overall about 10% of children report being bullied at least once a week, and approximately 7% of children are identified as bullies. Bullying is more common in primary than secondary school and becomes more subtle and verbal as children grow older. Girls use less physical means of bullying such as exclusion and spreading rumours, but are almost as aggressive as boys. Roughly 20%

of the victims are also bullies and this group of children tends to be particularly disturbed. The typical bully, on the other hand, tends to have high self-esteem, has less empathy and is generally aggressive and dismissive of authority. At least 75% of bullying goes undetected by parents or teachers, and it should be considered as a possible cause for any child whose symptoms of distress do not seem to have a sufficient explanation.

Bullying occurs where there is an unequal power relationship and where any form of aggression is deliberately used to humiliate someone and cause distress. This definition distinguishes it from fighting and aggression between two equals. Bullying should never be tolerated and should always be directly confronted and dealt with immediately. It is unacceptable to maintain that it is just part of normal life. A whole-school policy on bullying that includes a commitment from children, parents and teachers to identify and stop bullying has been shown to be the most effective approach. In addition, the bully should make reparation to the victim. Close supervision of bullies and victims is also helpful.

Non-attendance at school

The causes of school non-attendance are multiple and complex. Leaving aside those children who are kept at home by their parents, there are three main reasons for not attending school. It is most important to immediately exclude a genuine and acceptable reason for avoiding school such as being bullied by peers or teachers or being unable to cope with the work. The other two causes are the neurotic disorders of school refusal due to separation anxiety (worse on leaving the parent) or school phobia (worse on arrival at school) and the conduct disorder of truancy. Children with school refusal or separation anxiety — or both — tend to be model pupils at school and come from stable homes, whereas truants are disruptive at school and come from unsettled homes where there is often a history of antisocial behaviour (Table 28.4).

Management

Because the reasons why children do not attend school are multitudinous, it is important that the problem is not tackled in a piecemeal way. Close

---

> **Box 28.12**
> ## School-based sources of disturbed behaviour
>
> - The child's own problems, e.g. separation anxiety
> - Difficulties with peers, e.g. bullying
> - Problems with academic work, e.g. too easy, too difficult
> - Problems with teachers, e.g. poor discipline
> - Problems outside of school, e.g. family breakdown
> - Any combination of the above

Table 28.4
Main differences between school refusal and truancy

School refusal	Truancy
Well behaved at school	Antisocial behaviour in and out of school
No academic problems	Poor academic achievement
Associated neurotic behaviour	Associated antisocial behaviour
More frequent at primary school	More frequent towards the end of secondary schooling
More often youngest or only child	More often in children from large families
Stable home background	Unsettled family background
Child remains at home — overinvolved relationships	Child's whereabouts unknown — poor supervision
Prognosis generally good	Poor prognosis

collaboration is required between parents, teachers and other professionals, and after a detailed assessment of the problem, a comprehensive treatment package should be drawn up involving all the relevant people. In most cases of school refusal, except where there are genuine reasons for fear of school, the child should be returned as quickly as possible in a firm and determined way. At the same time that the child is returned to school, the underlying causes need to be dealt with, but it is often true to say that 'the treatment of school refusal is to return to school'. This is because once back at school most children usually settle into the routine quite quickly, almost as if nothing had ever happened. The advantage of returning a child to school rapidly is that if it does not work, the underlying causes can be expected to become clear for all to see. Should the rapid approach not work, the alternative is for a gradual return. This must be steadily progressive because it is easy to get stuck in an awkward halfway stage.

Truancy also requires a total treatment package involving all the relevant professionals. The most effective approach here is to construct a programme of education that is appropriate for the needs of the child, while at the same time monitoring and supervising the young person throughout the school day. Any learning problems must also be addressed.

EMOTIONAL DISORDERS

Anxiety states of one kind or another are the most common emotional disorders. The normal stages of anxiety development are described in Chapter 27. Each of these stages can develop into a pathological state and become a disorder if the symptoms are severe, prolonged, handicapping and developmentally inappropriate.

Simple anxiety states

Extreme shyness and separation problems become more significant as children grow older and at school age they can be a serious handicap to a child. In addition some children have a very high level of general anxiety that relates to a wide range of situations. These children usually have a 'sensitive' or 'highly strung' temperament that makes them highly reactive to stress of any kind, including exciting and happy events. The management of generalised anxiety has some important elements which are described below:

1. *Facing the anxiety*. This involves helping the child to learn how to manage the anxiety-provoking situation by facing up to it rather than by avoidance. There are two main approaches:
   a. The 'in at the shallow end' approach. The

child is gradually exposed to the feared situation, step by step. Anxiety must always be kept to a manageable level. Perseverance over a long period is essential and the process may fail if any of the steps are too large. If that happens it is then necessary to go back a stage and start again from there.

b. The 'in at the deep end' approach. The child is exposed directly to the feared situation and remains with it until the anxiety has reduced to a tolerable level. This approach carries a higher risk if it is not carried through to completion. In addition, everyone concerned must agree that this is a reasonable way to deal with the problem. The advantage of this potentially distressing approach is that it can be rapidly effective, especially in younger children. However, the supervising adults must feel confident in what they are doing.

2. *Anxiety is catching.* It helps to be aware of the powerfully infectious nature of anxiety. This is seen in the way parents cling to their child who has separation anxiety or where a parent keeps the bedroom light on because the child is afraid of the dark. Such anxious responses only confirm that there is indeed something to be frightened about. Professionals may also 'catch' anxiety from children or parents, or even from each other.

3. *Linking behaviour and thinking.* There is a strong connection between thinking and behaviour. For example, a child who has been helped to think through all the positive things about attending school for the first time is likely to cope better than a child who has heard about all the things that might go wrong. A child who has been taught to behave in a confident way at school is less likely to be picked on by other children. Most children respond well to role-play exercises where they practice coping with the feared situation.

4. *Thought control.* Anxiety is primarily due to the anticipation of feared situations before anything has happened. Thoughts are therefore an important trigger for anxiety. In fact, children are surprisingly good at controlling their thoughts, but they will need encouragement and practice to do this. This cognitive approach requires creative solutions that are tailormade for the child. For example, the child with a fear of spiders could be encouraged to name spiders after a close relative in order to change the perception of spiders to something friendly.

5. *Relaxation.* There are many types of relaxation, any of which may help a child cope with anxiety. Again, it is best to use a method of relaxation that makes sense to the child and is enjoyable. The relaxation technique can then be used to counter anxiety as it arises in the real world, or in the imagination.

6. *Keeping a sense of humour.* It is difficult to laugh and be anxious at the same time. Laughing and joking is a common strategy used to combat anxiety and all anxious children can be helped if the adults around them avoid becoming too serious with them. For example, the child who is anxious about monsters is not helped by the parent who looks under the bed and checks the wardrobe in order to demonstrate that they are monster free.

Phobias

A phobia is an overwhelming irrational fear of an object or a situation which is then avoided as far as possible. Simple phobias of animals and insects are very common and occur in more than 5% of children. It is the avoidance behaviour that tends to maintain the phobia because the child never has a chance to find out that there is nothing to fear. Most phobias can be traced back to an occasion when there was a genuine reason to be frightened or where the child has witnessed another person reacting in a fearful way. Phobic children may therefore have parents with similar fears. Phobias are best tackled along the same lines that have been outlined above for dealing with anxiety.

Obsessional compulsive disorders

There is a particularly strong association between phobias and obsessions, so it is possible to describe one in terms of the other. For example, a dirt phobia can be seen as an obsession with cleanliness or obsessional thoughts about harming someone can be viewed as a phobia of death. There is some evidence that obsessional compulsive disorder (OCD) is associated with other problems of repetition and impulse control such as ties and other habits, suggesting a neurophysiological basis for the condition. There is also evidence for an inherited genetic contribution to both OCD and phobias. Although drugs that inhibit 5-hydroxytryptamine (5-HT) re-uptake have been claimed to be effective, behavioural approaches are usually more effective in children. The aim is to find some way of disrupting or time limiting the obsessional thoughts or behaviour, sometimes called 'response prevention'. Thus, the child who insists on compulsively checking is prevented from doing this more than once or the child who repeatedly asks the same question is given one answer only.

Post-traumatic stress disorder

It is now clear that children experience post-traumatic stress disorder (PTSD) following exceptionally severe stress outside the normal range of experience in the much the same way as adults. Sexual abuse and near-death ordeals are typical of such events. The three characteristic features are vivid memories and avoidance reactions to the event, together with symptoms of hyperarousal (Table 28.5). The symptoms may not be present immediately after the stressful event, but develop within a few days. They would normally be expected to gradually reduce after 6 weeks, but can persist for many months and be complicated by other psychiatric disorder.

It is helpful to understand PTSD as the equivalent to an emotional wound. It may seem awful at the time but it can be expected to heal eventually. There will always be an emotional scar, but if the healing process is satisfactory the scar need not seriously interfere with function. The emotional wound must be cared for, but not covered up or it could become infected. Thus, exposing the wound to the fresh air is helpful, i.e. talking about the stressful event. However, scratching around in the wound is not, i.e. forced and unwanted counselling. Like a physical wound, the emotional wound may take a couple of weeks to heal over, but it is not until around 6 weeks that it is possible to function reasonably normally. The wound may continue to be painful when 'touched' and this gradually gets less with time, but the emotional scar always remains — although it may not interfere with function.

ANGER AND AGGRESSION

Much of our everyday understanding of anger stems from the work of the psychoanalysts. Freud, Jung, Klein and others highlighted the importance of anger as a normal, and sometimes unconscious, motivating force. Unfortunately these ideas underestimate the importance of learning and life experiences in shaping behaviour. A better understanding of children's moods and tempers has come from surveys and research, mostly using parental questionnaires, though some also use reports from teachers and/or direct observation of the children.

Tempers occur more often at bedtime, at the end of the morning and the end of the afternoon, that is, when children are hungry or tired. After the age of 2 years tempers gradually become shorter and less violent, but whining and sulking increase.

Table 28.5
Symptoms of post-traumatic stress disorder

Re-experiencing	Avoidance	Hyperarousal
Nightmares	Denial of event	Insomnia
Flashbacks	Social withdrawal	Irritability
Preoccupation with the event	Avoidance of memory triggers	Vigilant and over-reactive
Panic attacks	Regression	Easily started

Emotional and behavioural problems

Table 28.6
Associated features of temper tantrums

Child characteristics	Family and social factors
Speech and language problems	Young or elderly mothers
Wetting and soiling	Single or step parent present
Feeding and sleeping problems	Poor social conditions
Hyperactive and difficult	4 or more children in family
Miserable and tearful	Mothers smoke heavily
Frequent aches and pains	Poverty and unemployment
Frequent minor illnesses	Inner city areas

Overall, the main cause for tempers is attempts to get the children to conform to accepted standards of social behaviour and relationships. Tempers are generally more frequent in children aged from 2 to 5 years with a peak around 2–3 years old.

Tempers and difficult behaviour are more common in boys than in girls and after the age of 5 years problem behaviour tends to persist. In fact, about 70% of the children who have significant behaviour problems at 3 years of age still have them a year later. Children with temper tantrums and their families have been shown to have a wide range of associated characteristics.

Table 28.6 lists statistically significant associations, but they must be interpreted with some care. For example, the link between tempers and mothers who smoke heavily may be a direct one: the inhaled cigarette smoke may have an effect on the child or it may be the effect of a difficult child causing the mother to smoke more. Alternatively the link might be an indirect one, such as poor living conditions, which could cause stress reactions in the child leading to tempers and, in the mother, leading to heavy smoking.

About 10% of 5-year-old boys have temper tantrums at least once a week, but the same frequency of tempers is only reported in 2% of 15 year olds (Table 28.7). However, irritability and other forms of angry behaviour tend to continue. It would seem that although tempers usually

Table 28.7
Three main approaches to the management of childhood tempers

The approach	The methods
Prevention	Avoid high-risk situations (e.g. tired or hungry) Plan in advance Divert if possible
Training children to express anger in a more acceptable way	Teaching by example Rewarding self-control Training anger management
Ignoring the behaviour	Remove any audience Time out Leave until calm

decrease with age, there is no evidence that children's experience of anger diminishes over time — it just changes in the way it manifests itself. Thus while anger becomes less obvious, depression becomes more apparent.

CHILDHOOD DEPRESSION AND DELIBERATE SELF-HARM

Epidemiological studies of depression have noted a gradual increase in the incidence of depression in children starting from about 8 years of age, with a rapid increase of frequency during adolescence. The emergence of depressive disorder in the middle childhood years coincides with the development of clear concepts of 'self-image', 'time' and 'death' around the age of 7–9 years. Thus, younger children may experience misery and distress, but the essential ingredients of depressive disorder, namely hopelessness (concept of time required) and worthlessness (concept of self-image required), are not yet fully developed at that age. Puberty seems to be an important trigger for psychotic symptoms of bipolar depression, such as delusions and hallucinations, to become a feature of depression. The classification of the different types of depression is still being worked out. At present it is sufficient to understand that depression presents in a number of different forms, all of which need to be taken seriously.

The distinction between distress, depression and despair is an important one. Distressed children are reacting as expected to adverse circumstances or events. Depressed children, on the other hand, experience symptoms that have grown out of proportion to the situation to such an extent that they have a significant adverse effect on the child, interfering with everyday life. Those who reach the point of despair as a result of extreme stress are very much at risk. They have become overwhelmed by their emotions and often present as unusually withdrawn children who fail to thrive. Depressive symptoms frequently accompany other psychiatric disorders, especially conduct disorder and anxiety states. Thus the presence of lowered mood is a relatively non-specific symptom on its own. It is the accompanying pattern of symptoms that give a more accurate indication of the emotional state (Box 28.13).

Diagnosing depression

Many of the biological concomitants of depression found in adults have also been reported in children, including a failure of dexamethasone to inhibit cortisol secretion, lower nocturnal and 24-hour plasma melatonin levels and a reduced REM latency on the sleep EEG in depressed children. Unfortunately the use of psychobiological markers in clinical practice is of limited value since they fail to distinguish

---

> **Box 28.13**
> **Diagnostic features of depression**
>
> - Lowered mood, misery, tearfulness
>   - Persisting for more than 2 weeks
>   - Severe enough to interfere with everyday life
>   - Associated with two or more of the following symptoms:
>   Feelings of worthlessness
>   Sense of hopelessness
>   Disturbed sleep
>   Altered appetite
>   Irritability
> - Anxiety or phobic behaviour
> - Pessimistic and morbid thoughts
> - Suicidal ideas or acts

---

between distress, despair and depressive disorder. Diagnosis will depend on identifying the typical pattern of associated features such as:

- Hopelessness and worthlessness.
- Altered appetite and sleep pattern.
- Irritability and deteriorating relationships.
- Poor concentration and giving up previous interests.
- Altered perception and morbid thoughts.
- Suicidal thoughts or actions.

Children of depressed parents are more likely to suffer from depression themselves and at an earlier age than the children of non-depressed parents. The same group is also at risk of a wide range of health and behaviour problems. This link between depression in children and their parents is a strong one, but complex and interactive in nature. An interesting and frequent finding is that parent's and their children's rating of the child's depression correlate poorly. Parent's ratings are almost always lower than their children's own ratings of depression, confirming the general tendency for adults to underestimate the strength of children's distress.

Deliberate self-harm

Suicidal thoughts occur in a third of depressed children. The frequency increases with age (particularly in girls), but suicide attempts are rare before the age of 11 years. Suicidal children appear to have particular difficulty thinking through the consequences of their actions and in using a problem-solving approach to cope with their feelings of anger and depression. The factors associated with suicide and attempted suicide such as a history of psychiatric disorder in the family or the child, difficulty with relationships, problems with communication and high states of emotional arousal are so frequent in the general population that it makes the prediction of suicide attempts virtually impossible (Box 28.14). High self-esteem and a warm trusting relationship with an adult are strongly protective against deliberate self-harm and other psychiatric disorders.

The management

A diagnosis of depressive disorder during childhood suggests a high level of stress and/or an emotional vulnerability. The first step must therefore be to identify all the sources of stress in the child's life and to deal with them as far as possible. Various forms of counselling, supportive psychotherapy and cognitive therapy may be used to help children to become more resilient and understand why they feel as they do. Family therapy may also be useful where it is thought that family dynamics are a significant factor in causing or maintaining the depression. However, family therapy may actually compound the depression where a parent is also depressed or where there is significant marital disharmony. Parents need to understand that their child is 'ill' in the sense that they should make special allowances for any uncooperative behaviour and at the same time provide additional care and affection. Parents and teachers can play a key role by helping to improve the child's self-esteem.

Treatment with antidepressant medication should be reserved for clinicians with specialised knowledge of child psychiatric disorders as they have not been shown to be particularly effective in children. The assistance of the child psychiatry service should be sought if childhood depression fails to respond to simple treatment or where there is evidence of suicidal or psychotic thoughts.

GENERAL TREATMENT APPROACHES TO EMOTIONAL AND BEHAVIOURAL PROBLEMS

Psychological treatments

This section summarises the main psychological treatment approaches that can be used for childhood psychiatric disorder. A number of treatment strategies for particular disorders have already been outlined. What evidence there is suggests that all the main types of psychological treatments can be effective. What is less clear is how much more successful one approach is over another. The powerful positive effects of kindness and empathic care should not be underestimated. Sympathetic support and understanding is often more appreciated and just as effective as high-powered 'technical' therapeutic procedures.

Family therapy

Family therapy developed as the result of two major impulses. On the one hand psychoanalytic

---

Box 28.14
Main associated features of attempted suicide

- Disturbed or disrupted home life
- Poor functioning at school
- Low self-esteem
- Antisocial and aggressive behaviour
- Poor impulse control
- High levels of dysphoria and depression
- Substance misuse (especially alcohol)
- High frequency of stressful life events in the last year
- Family history of affective disorder
- A friend or relative who has attempted suicide

theory was found lacking in its ability to explain many aspects of child behaviour in a social context and practical treatment approaches did not result from the theory of the unconscious mind. On the other hand, the application of social systems theory to groups of people developed new ways of understanding how organisations worked, in particular how one part of a social system that malfunctions will affect every other part. It is this basic idea that underpins most family therapy, together with the notion that the family also has an unconscious life of its own.

There are many different forms of family therapy, but all methods share the belief that the family can be treated as a single entity and that many of the symptoms of individual members are actually the manifestation of a dysfunctional family. Therefore the family as a whole has to take responsibility for the malfunction of one of its members. This notion does not appeal to some parents and compliance with treatment can be poor. Family therapy is a specialised therapeutic technique that should only be used by experienced therapists in circumstances where there is clear evidence of primary family dysfunction. The use of family therapy for treating individuals in front of the family audience is unhelpful and should not be regarded as family therapy.

Behaviour management

Identifying the factors that have contributed to the behaviour should be the first step in any management programme. Taking a detailed history of the behaviour and gaining relevant background information can be therapeutic in itself. Parents may sometimes gain insight simply from the experience of being able to step back a bit and look objectively at what has been happening. In every case it is helpful to carefully identify the *Antecedents* of the behaviour, details of the *Behaviour* itself and the *Consequences* of that behaviour — the so-called ABC approach.

It is also important to know about the social context in which the behaviour occurs. This means collecting details of family relationships and functioning as well as details about how the child is in school. Knowledge of these complex interactions is important, but at the same time it should be recog-

nised that the full significance of each aetiological factor can only be guessed at. In every case the diagnostic assessment should arrive at a hypothesis to be tested by the outcome of the treatment.

It can be helpful to all concerned if parents keep a record of the behaviour using the ABC method of analysis. The diary of behaviour helps parents to be more objective about their child's behaviour and their own reaction to it. The record also assists in monitoring progress and identifying typical sequences of behaviour. The very act of recording and objectifying the behaviour, together with the support of a sympathetic and understanding clinician, may have a most positive effect.

In much the same way that psychotherapeutic treatments are multiple and highly individual, so too are behavioural methods. These are based on learning theory and include notions of reward and punishment (Box 28.15). Unfortunately the oversimplistic application of behavioural approaches has given them a bad name. Behavioural pro-

---

Box 28.15
General guidelines for behavioural treatments

- First consider methods of prevention
- Identify probable causes and deal with them as far as possible
- Focus on rewarding appropriate behaviour
- Check that any rewards really are desired
- Avoid punishment — it only works in the short term
- Use restitution — making good whatever has been wrong
- Promote behaviour that is incompatible with the unwanted behaviour
- Encourage training by repetition of the desired behaviour
- Set a good example
- Close supervision is often necessary for the child and the parent
- Keep a sense of humour

Emotional and behavioural problems

grammes require careful thought and should be individually and creatively developed for each case as a collaborative effort between parent, child and clinician. Certainly drawing up a simple star reward chart is a complex matter and keeping it going is harder still. Other behavioural approaches include the removal of attention (parent walks away from the child) or isolating the child from attention (child sent to bedroom) contingent on a child's bad behaviour. Alternatively, many parents use sweets or pocket money as a reward for good behaviour. However, when parents seek help, most of these methods have failed. The usual reason for this is that parents have either failed to agree with each other or have not followed through in a consistent and determined way.

Drug treatment

The role of psychopharmacology in the community-based treatment of child psychiatric disorders is very limited. The use of these drugs should therefore be restricted to those with specialist knowledge who prescribe these drugs in routine clinical practice. There are high risks associated with the use of mind-controlling medication in children that relate to the possible long-term consequences and to the potential for parents and children to expect drugs to resolve problems while they remain passive and uninvolved.

If treatment fails (Box 28.16)

If treatment fails to produce the expected result, it should not be immediately discarded as no good. There may be hidden factors that serve to maintain the problem such as:

- bullying
- relationship problems
- parental marital difficulties
- relative academic failure
- abuse of any kind.

Referral to the child and adolescent psychiatry service

Such is the stigma of psychiatry that the decision to refer a child and family to the child and adolescent

---

> **Box 28.16**
> **Checklist for failed treatment**
>
> 1. The parents are uncooperative and have not complied with treatment
> 2. Hidden factors are present that have been missed:
>   a. bullying
>   b. academic failure
>   c. parental relationship problem
>   d. sexual abuse
>   e. problems with peers
> 3. The treatment was too brief or too superficial
> 4. The wrong treatment was used
>
> An explanatory developmental model of enuresis. Any explanatory model of enuresis has to be able to integrate all the research findings and provide a satisfactory explanation for the complex relationship between enuresis and psychosocial stress too

---

mental health service (CAMHS) is often delayed until the disorder is so well established that any change will be difficult to achieve. It is therefore better to refer too early than too late. Most child mental health services provide assessment, consultation and treatment on a multidisciplinary basis, but there is considerable variation in the level of back-up resources in different parts of the country. The CAMHS is finding new ways of working in the community and in supporting other professionals in their work. Consultation can therefore be requested in the first instance and is always better done before referral of the more complex, multi-problem cases, to ensure that the most efficient and effective approach is taken.

Referrals are best made to a named clinician giving details of the problem, the family background and any other agencies involved. Most important of all is the cooperation of the child and parents and good parental motivation to follow things through. These are both greatly influenced by the way the referral is made and the attitude of the referrer. Parental motivation is increased if the

Emotional and behavioural problems

referrer appears to value and have confidence in CAMHS.

Prognosis for emotional and behavioural problems

Follow up of children with mental health problems shows that there is a strong tendency for continuity. Problems that arise in the first 4–5 years usually do not continue, but children who fail to gain reasonable control of their anger and tempers by 5 years are likely to continue to have problems with aggression. In addition, children born with a difficult temperament are more prone to behavioural problems in the early years and these can continue into later life. The mechanism for continuity is complex, but often involves a process of labelling a child as a problem followed by a fixed misperception of the child that can be difficult to change. Eventually the child comes to see himself as a problem and behaves accordingly. A further factor that encourages continuity is the tendency for any repeated behaviour to become set as a habit which can then be difficult to break.

Continuity of aggressive behaviour is strong after the age of 6–7 years. In fact it is almost as stable a characteristic as intelligence. Anxiety and obsessional behaviour also tends to persist, but more as a personality characteristic than as a problem, although any period of stress is likely to bring about a recurrence of the problem. Phobias however are likely to continue if the child is able to avoid the feared situation. Virtually all adult phobias can be traced back to childhood. Depression is also likely to recur if it is not resolved quickly. One reason is that it interferes with children's developmental progress that is then difficult to catch up. Altered relationships may continue and the negative mind set changes the child's view of the world.

Parents, school and peers also influence prognosis. The effect of schools has already been referred to above, but in addition schools also play a major part in children's self-esteem, determined mainly by academic success and status amongst peers. Parental disharmony is a significant factor that tends to maintain problems as is maternal mental illness and general ill health. Poor parental discipline and hostile rejecting attitudes also tends to perpetuate emotional and behavioural problems. It is important to note that almost all these factors can be influenced, given appropriate resources and understanding.

REFERENCES AND FURTHER READING

American Psychiatric Association 1994 Diagnostic and statistical manual of mental disorders, 4th edition (DSM IV) American Psychiatric Association Washington, DC 66–78

Anders T F, Weinstein P 1972 Sleep and its disorders in infants and children: a review. Pediatrics 50:312–324

Angold A 1988 Review: childhood depression. British Journal of Psychiatry 152:601–607

Asperger H 1991 'Autistic Psychopathy' in childhood. (translated by Frith U) In: Frith U (ed) Autism and Asperger syndrome. Cambridge University Press, Cambridge 1991:37–92

Baker L, Cantwel D P 1987 A prospective psychiatric follow-up of children with speech/language disorders. Journal of the American Academy of Child Adolescent Psychiatry 26:546–553

Berg I 1985 Management of school refusal. Archives of Disease in Childhood 60:486–488

Bishop D V M 1987 Causes of specific developmental language disorder. Journal of Child Psychology and Psychiatry 28:1–8

Bohman M, Sigvardsson S 1979 Long term efects of early institutional care. Journal of Child Psychology and Psychiatry 20:111–117

Brooksbank D J 1985 Suicide and parasuicide in childhood and early adolescence. British Journal of Psychiatry 146:459–463

Brunn R D 1984 Gilles de la Tourette's syndrome: an overview of clinical experience. Journal of the American Academy of Child Psychiatry 23:126–133

Campbell M, Spencer M K 1988 Psychopharmacology in child and adolescent psychiatry: a review of the past five years. Journal of the American Academy of Child Psychiatry 27:269–279

Clarke R V G 1985 Delinquency, environment and intervention. Journal of Child Psychology and Psychiatry 26:505–523

Cox A 1975 Assessment of parental behaviour. Journal of Child Psychology and Psychiatry 16:266–270

Cox A, Puckering C, Pound A, Mills M 1987 The impact of maternal depression in young children. Journal of Child Psychology and Psychiatry 28:917–928

Duncan M K 1985 Brief psychotherapy with children and their families: the state of the art. Journal of the American Academy of Child Psyciatry 23:544

Frankel E F 1985 Behavioural treatment approaches to pathological unsocialised physical aggression in young children. Journal of Child Psychology and Psychiatry 26:525–551

Garralda M E, Jameson R A, Reynolds J N, Postlethwaite R P 1988 Psychiatric adjustment in children with chronic renal failure. Journal of Child Psychology and Psychiatry 29:79–90

Gath A 1977 The impact of an abnormal child on the parents. British Journal of Psychiatry 130:405–410

Golombok S, Spencer A, Rutter M 1983 Children in lesbian and single parent households. Psychosexual and psychiatric appraisal. Journal of Child Psychology and Psychiatry 24:551–572

Graham P 1985 Psychology and the health of children. Journal of Child Psychology and Psychiatry 26:333–347

Graham P, Rutter M 1973 Psychiatric disturbance in young adolescents — a follow up study. Proceedings of the Royal Society of Medicine 66:1226–1229

Gratten-Smith P et al 1988 Clinical features of conversion disorder. Archives of Disease in Childhood 63:408–414

Green R et al 1987 Specific cross-gender behaviour in boyhood and later homosexual orientation. British Journal of Psychiatry 151:84–88

Herd D 1987 The relevance of attachment theory to child psychiatric practice: an update. Journal of Child Psychology and Psychiatry 28:25–28

Hetherington E M, Cox M, Cox R 1985 Long-term effects of divorce and remarriage on the adjustment of children. Journal of the American Academy of Child Psychiatry 24:518–530

Hoare P 1984 The development of psychiatric disorder among school children with epilepsy. Developmental Medicine and Child Neurology 26:3–24

Kanner L 1943 Autistic disturbances of affective contact. Nervous Child 2:217–50

Kaszdin A E, Esveldt-Dawson K et al 1987 Problem solving skills training and relationship training in the treatment of anti-social child behaviour. Journal of Consultation and Clinical Psychology 55:76–85

MacFarlane A C, Policansky S, Irwin C P 1987 A longitudinal study of the psychological mobidity in children due to a natural disaster. Psychological Medicine 17:727–738

Macquire J, Richman N 1986 Screening for behavioural problems in nurseries. The reliability and validity of the pre-school behaviour check list. Journal of Child Psychology and Psychiatry 27:7–32

Marks I 1987 The development of normal fear: a review. Journal of Child Psychology and Psychiatry 28:667–697

Matson J L, Benavidez D A, Compton L S, Paclawskyj T, Baglio C 1996 Behavioral treatment of autistic persons: a review of research from 1980 to the present. Research in Developmental Disabilities 17(6):433–65

Nicol A R, Stretch D D, Fundatis T, Smith I, Davison I 1987 The nature of mother and toddler problems. Journal of Child Psychology and Psychiatry 28:739–754

Offord D R 1987 Prevention of behavioural and emotional disorders in children. Journal of Child Psychology and Psychiatry 28:9–19

Patterson G R, Chamberlain T, Reid J P 1982 A comparative evaluation of a parent training programme. Behaviour Therapy 13:638–654

Pfeiffer S I, Norton J, Nelson L, Shott S 1995 Efficacy of vitamin B6 and magnesium in the treatment of autism: a methodology review and summary of outcomes. Journal of Autism & Developmental Disorders 25(5):481–493

Pynoos R S, Frederick C, Nadar K et al 1987 Life threat and post traumatic stress in school age children. Archives of General Psychiatry 44:1057–1063

Rapin I 1997 Autism. New England Journal of Medicine 337(2):97–104

Rapoport J L 1986 Childhood obsessive-compulsion disorder. Journal of Child Psychology and Psychiatry 27:289–295

Russell A B 1990 Attention–deficit hyperactivity disorder: a handbook for diagnosis and treatment. Guilford Press, London

Rutter M 1980 School influences on children's behaviour and development (the 1979 Kenneth Blackfan lecture). Pediatrics 65:208–220

Rutter M, Quinton D 1984 Parental psychiatric disorder: effects on children. Psychological Medicine 14:853–880

Rutter M, Schopler E 1987 Autism and pervasive developmental disorders: concepts and diagnostic issues. Journal of Autism and Developmental Disorders 17:159–186

Sandler A D, Sutton K A, DeWeese J, Girardi M A, Sheppard V, Bodfish J W 1999 Lack of benefit of a single dose of synthetic human secretin in the treatment of autism and pervasive developmental disorder. New England Journal of Medicine 341(24):1801–6, Dec 9

Shafer D 1978 'Soft' neurological signs and later psychiatric disorders in children. Journal of Child Psychology and Psychiatry 19:63–65

Shafer D, Garland A, Gould M, Fisher P, Trautman P 1988 Preventing teenage suicide: a critical review. Journal of the American Academy of Child and Adolescent Psychiatry 27:675–687

Sturge C 1982 Reading retardation and antisocial behaviour. Journal of Clinical Psychology and Psychiatry 23:21–31

Taitz L S, Wales J K, Urwin O M, Molnar D 1986 Factors associated with outcome in management of defaecation disorders. Archives of Disease in Childhood 61:472–477

Thorley G 1986 Hyperkinetic syndrome of childhood: clinical characteristics. British Journal of Psychiatry 144:16–24

Weissman M M, Gammon G D, John K et al 1987 Children of depressed parents: impaired psychopathology and early onset of major depression. Archives of General Psychiatry 43:847–853

Werry J 1988 Behaviour therapy with children and adolescents: a 20 year overview. Journal of the American Academy of Child Psychiatry 28:1–18

Werry J S 1987 Attention deficit, conduct, oppositional and anxiety disorders in children. 1. A review of research on differentiating characteristics. 2. Clinical characteristics. Journal of the American Academy of Child and Adolescent Psychiatry 26:133–143, 144–155

Wing L 1997 The Autistic Spectrum. Lancet 350:1761–1766

Wolkind S, Renton G 1979 Psychiatric disorder in children in long-term residential care: a follow-up study. British Journal of Psychiatry 135:129–135

Woolston J L 1983 Eating disorders in infancy and early childhood. Journal of the American Academy of Child and Adolescent Psychiatry 26:123–126

World Health Organization 1992 The ICD-10 classification of mental and behavioural disorders: clinical descriptions and diagnostic guidelines. World Health Organization. Geneva 252–259

Yates A 1990 Current perspectives on eating disorders: treatment, outcome and research directions. Journal of the American Academy of Child and Adolescent Psychiatry 29:129

29 | Counselling

This chapter aims to provide some basic and practical advice on how to begin to develop a counselling approach in your work. As such it is primarily aimed at developing a style which will make interviewing and short-term involvement with patients and families more productive and satisfying for all concerned. The counselling approach described is applicable to adults and to adolescents. Work with younger children often needs to proceed at a less verbal level using activities like play and painting and is not covered here.

There are many definitions of counselling, but in this context it means talking with people in a way which enables them to express themselves, to help them to understand themselves and their problems better and to develop ways of coping with or ameliorating their difficulties.

Counselling operates on the psychological plane and may at first be thought of as appropriate only for psychological problems, for example anxiety, depression, fears. However it is important to recognise that there is no clear separation between physical and psychological difficulties. A counselling approach to all encounters will enhance the quality and quantity of information you receive and the person is likely to find the encounter to be of positive value to them.

In some cases of physical illness, psychological factors may play a role in their genesis and maintenance. All physical illnesses have a psychological impact and this becomes increasingly important in chronic, incapacitating and life-threatening diseases. People suffering from or caring for those with such diseases often derive considerable benefit from being able to discuss their feelings, fears, practical concerns, etc. with someone who is knowledgeable in the area. As an example, a counselling-type interview with a parent about a child with diabetes may reveal the difficulties which the special diet creates within the family and explain why relatively poor control is being obtained.

LONGER-TERM COUNSELLING

In cases where problems are serious or severe, your role may be to refer on to more specialist services. Such services vary in different parts of the country both in terms of availability and organisation. It would be worth investigating the following services in your locality: clinical psychology (National Health Service (NHS)), educational psychology (local education authority (LEA)), Child and Adolescent Mental Health Service (CAMHS) or social services, self-help groups, voluntary agencies.

If you wish to develop your own counselling work, then training in the first place and supervision in the longer term should be considered as essential. Working with people with psychological problems can be both difficult and emotionally draining and access to an experienced supervisor is necessary in your own and your patient's interest.

BASIC REQUIREMENTS FOR EFFECTIVE COUNSELLING

It is a worthwhile exercise to consider what you, yourself, would be looking for if you were seeking counselling and then to contemplate whether you are able to provide that for those you are seeing. It is also a good idea to think about what you would find aversive and make you disinclined to return for a further session.

Physical surroundings

It is usually helpful to be able to see people in an informal room where it is possible to sit in a relaxed way on comfortable chairs. A counsellor sitting behind a desk instantly produces a formal atmosphere which is not conducive to open discussion. A vital ingredient is that the person who is talking should feel that it is private and that they will not be overheard by those in the room next door or in the corridor. Every attempt needs to be made to avoid interruptions during the session and the setting should be relatively quiet and peaceful.

Whilst these seem like relatively simple arrangements they are very difficult to achieve in many community settings where the rooms which are used are often temporarily made available and have been designed for other functions. In many schools, the medical room has been planned for clinical rather than counselling purposes and a sense of privacy may be very hard to achieve. Depending on the physical siting of the room it is often the case that noises in the corridor, telephone calls and conversations next door intrude on the counselling session and if you can hear them, you assume that they can hear you.

Another major physical constraint is the amount of time which you have available to talk to the person. In a busy clinic schedule with patients every 5 minutes it is not possible to enter into a counselling relationship. A person needs to feel that you do have the time for them and if they are going to talk about matters which have emotional impact they need to be given the time to talk these through. You will not be able to relax and give them this sense of time if you are aware of a lengthening queue developing. Counselling sessions need to be planned accordingly.

Characteristics of the counsellor

Again it is worth considering what you would be looking for yourself. It is likely that you would want to see someone who you felt was genuinely interested in you and cared about your welfare. You would want to be listened to and understood and to have the sense that what you were saying was accepted, not judged to be good/bad, acceptable/unacceptable, sensible/foolish. You would want to be able to talk at your own pace, to have time to think and not be rushed.

You are likely to be assessing the counsellor and judging their reactions to you. If you felt patronised, interrupted, misunderstood or that the counsellor found you boring or irritating, then you would be unlikely to confide in that counsellor.

Rogers (1961) summarised the basic conditions for effective counselling to take place and described the three essential characteristics in a counsellor as empathy, genuineness and unconditional positive regard (Box 29.1). Frank (1973) argues that underlying all effective therapeutic relationships there are the following characteristics: warmth, respect, kindness, hope, understanding and the provision of 'explanation'. When people turn to a counsellor in a time of trouble they are usually unhappy and confused. They tend not to understand the nature of their problems and cannot see ways out of it. Within counselling you are working with the person in a *joint* endeavour to try to understand them and their difficulties — 'to provide explanations' and to work out ways forward.

Box 29.1
Three essentials characteristics in a counsellor

- *Empathy*: This is the ability to be able to see the world from the other person's perspective, to understand the feelings they have and the meanings they ascribe to their experiences. In order to do this you have to develop an understanding of that person in their context — their life experiences, the nature of their relationships, their belief structures

- *Genuineness*: This is about being interested and concerned about the other person

- *Unconditional positive regard*: This is sometimes described in terms of warmth and being non-judgemental, accepting the person as they are and not making value judgements

Characteristics of counselling

When people are asked to consider what they might hope to gain if they sought counselling, the initial answers tend to be in terms of problem solving — yet many people have problems for which there is no straightforward solution. An example of this is in bereavement where the counselling is aimed at helping the person through the grieving process towards long-term adjustment to the bereavement.

The supportive element is vital in any counselling relationship and in many cases may be the only thing you have to offer. Being on the person's side, being willing to care, being available for them to share their problems and helping them to find ways to cope are very valuable.

In many cases you may be working towards helping the person to find a way to deal with their difficulties. On occasion this may be purely practical, for example obtaining rehousing, and you are able to use your knowledge and influence to make things happen. In other cases people simply need a piece of factual information to enable them to sort things out for themselves. Even in such cases, your message is more likely to be heard if you have established a relationship in which the person feels valued as an individual by a counsellor who is genuinely interested in them.

THE FIRST SESSION

When you see someone for the first time it is not possible to know whether this will be a one-off occasion or the beginning of a longer relationship. However, there are certain aspects to a first contact which need to be present as they will lay the basis for longer-term work or permit a single session to proceed and be concluded in a satisfying manner. Three main activities need to take place:

1. Laying the foundation — introductions, explanation.
2. Beginning the exploration of the problems and their context.
3. Beginning the process of developing a therapeutic relationship.

Laying the foundation

It is easy to forget how a person feels when they are coming to see you for the first time to discuss a problem. They are likely to feel anxious and uncertain in what is, for them, an unfamiliar situation. They may not know who they are to see, what will be expected of them, how they will be able to explain their situation. Introducing yourself and explaining how the session will be conducted are useful starting points and every effort should be made to make the situation a comfortable one. You should remember that when people are anxious they are less likely to retain information which is given and failures of communication are a common complaint that people have about their encounters with professionals.

Beginning the exploration of the problems and their context

It is usually helpful to have a flexible structure in which you begin to explore the areas of concern and obtaining a history is a very valuable starting point. The means by which this is done will be covered in more detail later but at this early stage you are trying to develop an understanding of the problems, their history and context. At all stages it is crucial not just to obtain factual information but to explore the person's feelings about events, to understand the meaning that they have for them. It is in this way that you can develop an empathetic relationship and it is at the level of feelings and meanings that counselling should operate. In this process you are not simply recording information but are also looking for clues to help you to develop hypotheses about a person's difficulties. Later you will need to test out your hypotheses.

In any given situation, a person's reaction will be dependent on their past experiences, their present situation and their expectations about the future. Failure to get a job applied for may be a minor setback to someone who has a fairly high level of self-esteem with a history of successful work behind them, but may feel like a major disaster to someone with little self-confidence and a history of rejection in social relationships and who expects to fail to achieve what they want in life.

Counselling

> ### Box 29.2
> **Areas which you should aim to cover for an adolescent**
>
> - *School*: Which ones, experiences at infant, junior, secondary. Favourite and least favourite subjects. Any academic difficulties. Relationships with teachers. Relationships with peer groups. Any social difficulties, e.g. bullying. Plans and expectations for the future. Worries and concerns
>
> - *Family*: Close family, names, ages, occupations, brief descriptions of family members. Who is living at home. In case of separated parents, amounts of contact. Relationships. Extended family, particularly grandparents, including information on those who are deceased
>
> - *Background*: Moves to different houses, schools, changes in family circumstances over time, significant events, e.g. financial problems
>
> - *Social relationships*: Friendships or lack of them. Opposite sex relationships. Nature of any difficulties
>
> - *Leisure*: What the person is interested in. How they spend their free time

It is therefore very important to get to know about a person's life through taking a history (Box 29.2). However, in a first interview only limited information can be obtained and it often takes a considerable length of time before a person can trust you enough to begin to disclose their most sensitive and painful feelings. Thus on a first interview, a person may describe their childhood as wonderful and their family as happy only later beginning to talk about a violent father or a sense of being unloved compared to a sibling.

This first attempt at getting the history should therefore be regarded as a shallow trawl for clues.

Developing a therapeutic relationship

Again, the stress is upon feelings and meanings not just upon events. As an example, a child may tell you that he sees his natural father two or three times a year. The immediate response should be to ask how he feels about that — he may wish to see him more/less/not at all. It may or may not be important.

If you refer back to the important characteristics in a counsellor, it is important to establish yourself in that mode from the beginning: as warm, sympathetic and genuine. In doing this, the way in which you listen to the person and respond to them is crucial and listening is an active not a passive process.

Setting the right atmosphere

Within comfortable physical surroundings you should be aiming to make the person aware that you are concerned and interested and have time for them. You should sit in a relaxed way and maintain normal eye contact even if the person does not appear to be looking at you. An atmosphere of relative stillness is helpful and restlessness, doodling, etc. should be avoided. It is important to allow the person to talk without rushing them or butting in when they may be thinking about what they want to say. Silences are usually helpful — you can use them to give you time to think and decide on your response too.

Taking in what is said

Make sure that you are actually listening rather than thinking about your own concerns, for example what you will say next. It is important to recognise that the ways of talking described here are just as valid in conducting an interview, even one which appears at its outset to be a simple information-gathering session.

Processing the information

In listening to someone's words it is important to be aware of non-verbal communication too and what may not be said. This is part of the looking for clues as you are putting together what is said with other information — non-verbal clues, past statements, putting the current situation into the perspective of the person's past. You should be trying to feel what it would be like to be them and then making hypotheses on the basis of that.

Deciding on your response

You must decide how you are going to respond to what is said. Some ideas are given below on how different types of questions and responses lead to a much fuller understanding.

HOW TO CONDUCT A COUNSELLING SESSION

Open vs. closed questions

A counselling situation is very different from a conventional medical consultation where the initial concern is to narrow the focus of discussion down to a diagnosis. In counselling it is necessary to open out the discussion, to talk about and explore other areas rather than focus on symptoms. In order to do this it is important to ask more open-ended questions. A simple working definition of a closed question is one that can be answered by 'yes' or 'no'. An open-ended question requires the person to think and give you his answer in his own terms.

Boxes 29.3 and 29.4 provide two examples of how a dialogue could progress with two different counsellors; in Box 29.3 only closed questions are asked, whereas Box 29.4 uses only open-ended questions.

In Box 29.3, the counsellor is looking towards finding solutions to the woman's problem and so focuses directly on possible ways of dealing with her situation — the police and a women's refuge. In this type of format Mary is constrained in what she talks about by the counsellor's focus on action rather than feelings and has no opportunity to talk about what actually happened to her. The counsellor has gained a small amount of factual information but has no understanding of how the woman feels or what has led her to reject the possibilities of prosecution or a refuge. The counsellor is proceeding towards problem solving on the basis of his own preconceptions of how to deal with a situation rather than trying to develop an understanding of Mary's perspective. Mary is also likely to feel on the defensive following this interchange, with a sense of being pushed, having to account for herself, not being understood.

In Box 29.4, the counsellor uses open-ended questions to explore what happened and how Mary feels about it, allowing her to talk about it in her own

---

Box 29.3
Dialogue using closed questions

Mary: My husband came home drunk again last night and that's why I've got this black eye.

Counsellor: Did you call the police?

Mary: Yes, or at least my neighbour did.

Counsellor: Are they going to prosecute?

Mary: No, I don't want that to happen.

Counsellor: Have you thought any more about going into a refuge?

Mary: Well, I do think about it but I don't think it would really help.

Box 29.4
Dialogue using open-ended questions

Mary: My husband came home drunk again last night and that's why I've got a black eye.

Counsellor: How did it happen?

Mary: Well, he came in and started shouting that I hadn't got his supper ready. This woke up our son who came down and told his Dad to shut up and his Dad went for him. I tried to stop him hitting Steven and then he started on me. Steven ran next door and the neighbour called the police.

Counsellor: What happened then?

Mary: When they came he calmed down and said he was sorry and everything and begged me not to let them take him.

Counsellor: How did you feel then?

Mary: Well, I always feel sorry for him when he breaks down like that and I know that it's only the drink which makes him aggressive. I just don't know what to do for the best. I don't think he'd ever really hurt me but I'm worried about the effect on the kids. But I don't think he could manage if I left him.

Counselling

way. A considerable increase in the amount of information is noticeable both in terms of the events of the night before and her feelings about it.

In the example using open-ended questions the counsellor has begun to understand the conflict of emotions which is preventing Mary from being able to act to change her situation. She is torn between her husband and her child and is also torn in regard to her fear and pity for her husband. This counsellor is able to see why Mary did not prosecute and does not leave the home and has the basis on which to proceed to help Mary with her difficulties.

Mary is likely to feel positive about this counsellor. She has been allowed to express herself without pressure and would not feel judged on what she has done. She would probably feel that the counsellor is interested in her and understands her.

This is not to say that closed questions do not have a place — at times they may be the most efficient way of gaining a particular piece of information. However, in using a closed question the counsellor is doing the work and the person can simply answer yes or no. An open-ended question means that the person has to think about their feelings or behaviour and put it into words for the counsellor to hear. This should help the counsellor to see the person's perspective, whereas closed questions are more likely to come from the counsellor's own perspective.

Reflection

Reflection is a style of talking in counselling which was developed by Rogers in his client-centred therapy. Rogers focuses on the importance of understanding the person from the person's perspective and grasping the meaning for the individual of his experiences — developing an empathetic understanding of that person.

Reflection is a means by which that process can occur. The counsellor needs to listen to what is said, to try to understand what that feels like and then to put a description of that understanding back to the person. Reflection operates at the level of feelings and meanings.

In the example in Box 29.5, the counsellor is listening to what John has to say, trying to put herself in his place and work out what that place feels like.

Box 29.5
An example of dialogue using reflection of the client's feelings

John: Although I go out quite a lot now, to clubs and things, the people I'm with are really my brother's friends.

They seem to like me and we have a good time but I just get worried that perhaps they're not really my friends at all. Sometimes I think they just feel sorry for me or have me along as a favour to my brother.

Counsellor: So, even though you are now part of a group, you feel very unsure about whether the others really see you as a friend, as part of the group?

John: Yes — I don't really see why they should want me around unless it was a favour to Michael. He is so confident and cheerful and gets on well with people whereas I'm shy and find it hard to talk.

Counsellor: So you feel that, in comparison to your brother, people would not find it easy to get to know you?

John: It's not really that — it's more that I don't think I'm interesting to people anyway. I can't tell jokes and make people laugh, I can't even think of things to say unless I've had a bit to drink.

She then reflects back that feeling — trying to put succinctly the essential aspect which has struck her. This then gives John something to focus his thoughts around — is the counsellor's statement accurate? He then explores the topic further. On the second occasion, the counsellor is somewhat off-beam with the reflection but this serves to get John to analyse and explain what is crucial for him about this uncomfortable situation.

In this way a joint exploration can take place into the underlying causes of John's sense of social unease. Although John knows he is uncomfortable in social situations he does not really understand the reasons for this and the process of counselling is helping to clarify these. He is likely to feel that his counsellor is interested, concerned and understanding following an interchange like this.

Learning to use reflection is often difficult at first as questions tend to leap to mind. It may be helpful to recognise the process by which we arrive at questions. When we listen to someone we are automatically forming an impression of the person and their world. A question will then be based upon that impression which itself remains internal to us. Reflection makes the impression explicit. The counsellor asks herself how the person is feeling/thinking/behaving and then puts the answer back to the person in the form of a reflection.

Summarising

In real-life counselling situations, discussions are usually rather more meandering, confused or ill defined than the examples given so far. It is often helpful for the counsellor to be able to draw together the threads of discussions, to refocus attention on aspects which seem particularly relevant. In this way, the person may become aware of contradictions in their statements which have occurred over a session or realise that there are consistencies in their reactions to several seemingly diverse situations which have been discussed over a few sessions.

Making the generalisations specific

People have a tendency to generalise their experiences and to make global statements, for example 'things always go wrong for me' or 'whenever I sit down to a meal with my parents it always ends up in a row'. Such statements are difficult to work from and it is always important to analyse the actual nature of the situations referred to. Taking the example of the rows with the parents, it is useful to ask for a specific example which can be discussed in more detail and then related to other examples.

In Box 29.6 it can be seen that the counsellor has now begun the process of helping Paul to analyse the arguments with his parents, to look at what triggers them, how each family member contributes, what feelings are evoked. In the end it would be hoped that this understanding of the pattern would enable Paul to change it.

Advice and strategies for change

Many people will come into a counselling session asking for advice but their response to being given

---

Box 29.6
An example of dialogue aimed at drawing out specific information from a client's generalised statements

Paul: Whenever I sit down and have a meal with my parents, it always ends up in a row.

Counsellor: Can you think about the last row like that and describe to me what happened.

Paul: Well, I went to have Sunday lunch and I was determined to avoid the usual topics. It started off OK and we were talking about the holidays. I said that I was going to get a railcard and travel round Europe and that did it. Dad started on his usual thing about how I should get a job for the whole vacation and how was I going to clear the overdraft and on it went.

Counsellor: You seem to be suggesting that the topic of money and your bank balance is something that usually makes your Dad angry.

Paul: Yes — he had to leave school and get a job when he was 16 and he really resents the fact that times have changed and I can do things he never could.

Counsellor: What was your Mum's reaction to this?

Paul: She just got upset and said we were ruining the meal she'd spent all morning preparing.

Counsellor: So how did you feel in all this?

Paul: I just can't help answering back when he starts. I can only take so much of it.

---

it is often negative. There are obviously times when a straightforward piece of advice, an item of knowledge which the counsellor has access to, is useful, but as a general rule it is better for the person to develop their own strategies than to be given them. It is important to discover what types of strategy a person has tried already and what effects they have had. An example is shown in Box 29.7 — a mother is concerned about the fact that her young son has been taking money from her purse. As part of the history-taking the counsellor will wish to know what her past reactions have been.

The counsellor in Box 29.7 is here gaining a clearer idea of the situation — knowing what has

---

Box 29.7

An example of dialogue aimed at discovering the types of strategies a client has tried and the effects they have had

Counsellor: What ways have you tried to deal with the stealing so far?

Mum: Well, at first I couldn't be sure it was really happening so I kept a closer check on my money. When I felt sure it was happening, I was so angry that I stopped all his pocket money as a punishment till he'd paid it back. The trouble is that just made him worse and he stole more.

Counsellor: Have you tried anything else?

Mum: I've tried talking to him but he won't tell me why he does it and I just get so angry when all he says is 'don't know'.

Counsellor: What are you doing at present?

Mum: Well I try to keep all my money locked away. He has no pocket money and I don't let him out in case he starts stealing outside.

Box 29.8

An example of dialogue aimed at discovering a client's own resources and ideas for making change

Counsellor: Once you are into an argument, you seem to reach a point where you feel too angry to be in control of yourself. It is important to find a way to stop arguing before you reach that point. Have you any ideas about how you could break the pattern and calm yourself down?

Michael: The only way is to get away and be on my own. I can't get calm when they're still there and on at me.

Counsellor: How do you think you could organise that?

Michael: Well, it would be best if I went up to my room and put some music on.

Counsellor: How do you think your parents would react to that?

Michael: I'm not sure, I think they might agree if we explained it to them.

---

gone before makes it easier to see where to go to next. It is also useful to tap people's own resources and ideas of making changes. As an example, Box 29.8 shows a counsellor's dialogue with a boy who keeps arguing with his parents and these arguments just build up often ending in physical violence.

Moving towards action

In the discussions so far, the emphasis has been upon understanding the predicament of the person being counselled in a joint endeavour to elucidate its meaning. However, insight by itself changes little and change is usually what is being sought. It is important to be aware of how difficult making changes in our lives can be. A person may be in a very unhappy situation but at least it is familiar, making changes means moving out into uncharted territory, taking risks, dealing with the unknown.

Many people who we see have very little room to manoeuvre in their personal circumstances anyway, being limited by poverty, lack of education or lack of resources. The sources of most people's problems are in the world surrounding them, the relationships they have and the past experiences which lead them to construe their world in their own individual way.

People vary in the amount of power that they have to control their world — children and adolescents being among the most powerless. It may be necessary for adults to bring about the necessary changes to enable them to develop. Whilst it may be possible to produce the necessary changes for someone, for example obtaining a day-nursery place for the child of an oppressed single parent, there are many other social factors which we cannot alter on an individual level. A teenager living in a family in which he is very unhappy, but whose treatment does not constitute sufficient grounds to be taken into care, may have little prospect of change until he is old enough to leave. If the family are unwilling to become involved in the counselling process then supportive work with the teenager may be the only avenue open.

It is sadly the case that it is not possible to be of help to everyone. You may be aware of how unhappy a person is, but you cannot force them to accept your help. Counselling of this type can only take place when voluntarily entered into.

A positive outcome to counselling would be that a person is able to proceed with his life with a greater understanding of himself and his world, having been validated in his views through the counselling process. This greater understanding may lead him to direct his energies towards change, solving a problem or accepting and finding ways to live with the situation.

In doing this, the continued understanding, encouragement and support of the counsellor will be a vital ingredient. This may mean that the person becomes dependent on his counsellor during a very vulnerable period. Counsellors may feel rather anxious about such dependence and need to recognise that it is to be expected.

Working towards ending of counselling is a vital part of the process, enabling the person to consolidate what they have learned and gradually grow from dependence to independence. Counselling should therefore be wound down rather than ended abruptly and proceed at a pace which is appropriate for the person concerned, preferably by agreement with him. At the end of this process, it should be the aim of any counsellor that the person ends with a sense of greater self-efficacy, better equipped to deal with the inevitable future difficulties which will come their way.

REFERENCES AND FURTHER READING

Abrams R 1992 When parents die. Letts, London
Bannister D, Fransella F 1971 Inquiring man. Penguin, Harmondsworth
Bowlby J 1988 A secure base: clinical applications of attachment theory. Tavistock, London
Bradshaw J 1996 The family. Health Communications
Catan L, Dennison C, Coleman J 1996 Getting through: effective communication in the teenage years. Trust for the Study of Adolescents/BT Forum
Crompton M 1992 Children and counselling. Edward Arnold, London
Dunn J, Plomin R (eds) 1990 Separate lives: why siblings are so different. Basic Books, New York
Fenwick E, Smith T 1993 Adolescence: the survival guide for parents and teenagers. Dorling Kindersley, London
Frank J 1973 Persuasion and healing. The Johns Hopkins University Press, Baltimore
Geldard K, Geldard D 1999 Counselling adolescents: the proactive approach. Sage, London
Graham L 1992 Teenagers: a family survival guide. Chatto and Windus, London
Herbert M 1991 Clinical child psychology. John Wiley, Chichester
Hobday A, Ollier K 1998 Creative therapy: activities with children and adolescents. BPS Books, Leicester
Jewett C 1982 Helping children cope with separation and loss. Batsford, London
Kaplan L 1995 Lost children. HarperCollins, London
Keung Ho M 1992 Minority children and adolescents in therapy. Sage, London
Lane D, Miller A (eds) 1992 Child and adolescent therapy. Open University, Milton Keynes
Mabey J, Sorenson B 1995 Counselling for young people. Open University, Milton Keynes
McLeod S 1981 The art of starvation. Virago Press, London
Noonan E 1989 Counselling young people. Tavistock/Routledge, London
Packer A 1992 Bringing up parents: the teenagers handbook. Free Spirit Publishing
Rogers C 1961 On becoming a person. Constable, London
Rogers W S, Hevey D, Roche J, Ash E (eds) 1992 Child abuse and neglect. Open University, Milton Keynes
Smail D J 1978 Psychotherapy: a personal approach. Dent, London
Smail D J 1984 Illusion and reality: the meaning of anxiety. Dent, London
Smith S, Pennells M (eds) 1995 Interventions with bereaved children. Jessica Kingsley, London
Street E 1994 Counselling for family problems. Sage, London
Steinberg L, Levine A 1992 You and your adolescent. Ebury Press, London
Truax C B, Carkhuff R R 1967 Towards effective counselling and psychotherapy: training and practice. Aldine, Chicago

30 | Children with special needs

This chapter considers those children with more long lasting and complex needs. The meaning of the term 'special needs' will be considered, who it applies to and when the child who may have special needs is likely to be recognised.

'Special educational needs' (SEN) is the term used in section 312 of the 1996 Education Act, to describe those children who may have a learning difficulty that calls for special educational provision. The definition of disabled children differs between the Children Act 1989, the Disabled Persons Act 1995 and the definition of SEN in the Education Act. Educational legislation does not differentiate between special educational needs and disability secondary to medical needs.

The Children Act 1989 states a child is disabled if he or she is blind, deaf or dumb or suffers from mental disorder of any kind or is substantially handicapped by illness, injury or deformity. This act then places a duty on local authorities to promote and safeguard the welfare of children in such difficulties. These children are then termed as being 'in need'. ('Children in need may thus include children with SEN and/or disabilities.)

Under the Disabled Persons Act a person has a disability if there is a physical or mental impairment that prevents them going about their day-to-day tasks.

Within the 1996 Education Act there is a clear expectation that children with SEN will be included in mainstream schools. A child will then be considered as having a SEN if their learning and educational opportunity is impaired by:

- A significant difficulty in learning compared to the majority of similarly aged children.

- A disability which either prevents or hinders the child from accessing educational facilities available to that age group.
- Is under 5 years and has the above difficulties.

It is important to appreciate that children who do not have English as a first language do not immediately have a SEN but these children may be particularly at risk from a delay in recognition of a SEN. Similarly the non-English-speaking parent may have difficulties in voicing any parental concern. Where such a difficulty is suspected local education authorities (LEAs) must provide interpreters or signing services.

The medical label that defines the child's condition is not always the most important priority. However for a paediatrician the search for a correct diagnosis is part of his duty to the child or young person. In addition the identification of impairment, disability and handicap as defined by the World Health Organization (WHO) is often as useful in the description and understanding of the effects of disabling conditions. Recognising the disability not only assists in the provision of services but may also help both the affected child and the caring family.

INTERNATIONAL CLASSIFICATION OF FUNCTIONING AND DISABILITY: LINKING OUTCOMES AND INTERVENTIONS

(ICIDH-2, WORLD HEALTH ORGANIZATION 1999) (Fig. 30.1)

- *Body function and structure (impairment).* This is any loss or abnormality of physiological

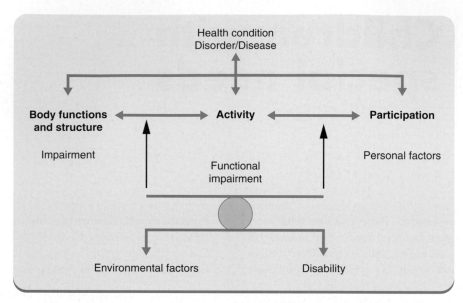

Fig. 30.1 International Classification of Functioning and Disability: linking outcomes and interventions. (From World Health Organization 1999)

body system, for example heart or joint structure.

- *Activity/activity limitation.* This is defined as the performance of a task. Activities are simple or complex. Activities are limited if an individual is restricted from performing an age-appropriate task, for example walking and moving around.
- *Participation (disability)* is an individual's involvement in life. The complex interactions of health, body, physical and social environment, for example participation in social relationships.

Looking at these definitions again reminds us that the same impairment can have a different impact on different individuals, for example if someone breaks a leg this impairment prevents them from walking and that is their disability. The handicap to them which follows from that disability will depend on what they do, it will be different for a secretary or for a professional footballer. Treatment such as the provision of a supporting cast or a pair of crutches will modify the disability. The handicap will depend very much on the availability of support from family and friends. The disability caused by any impairment, and the handicap resulting from that disability can be modified by medical, educational and social interventions. It is

without doubt our continuing duty to continue to develop measures that prevent handicap.

PREVALENCE OF DISABILITY

It has been estimated that 20% of children will have a special educational need at some stage during their school lives. It is also expected that in a given child population approximately 2% of children will have a complex disability requiring consideration of a statement of special educational needs (Table 30.1).

RECOGNITION OF DISABILITY

A disability may be recognised in:

- The *antenatal period*. Babies are increasingly recognised to have disabling conditions in utero during routine antenatal ultrasound scans, for example neural tube defects, cerebral malformation syndromes, heart defects.
- *At birth*, when a disability syndrome or central nervous syndrome abnormality is recognised, or when a baby has such a severe problem that neurological abnormality seems an inevitable consequence. Many other conditions are more likely to

be initially recognised by the hospital paediatric staff, for example Down's syndrome.

- *In the first year* deafness, motor, and profound and severe disability may become apparent. Often it is the parents themselves who first raise the possibility of a problem. A variety of health professionals, family doctor, health visitor or community paediatrician are likely to be consulted.

- *In the pre-school years* moderate or even severe disability, mainly as a result of a language disorder or autism, may become recognised, often not until the child is in the second or third year or later. Parents and close family are usually the first to recognise a problem, though others involved in the care of the child such as health visitors and experienced nursery staff may be the first to question the child's progress.

- *After disasters*, for instance head injury, encephalopathy or other life-threatening illnesses. Parents and healthcare staff alike can be slow to recognise permanent impairment. However such events trigger more detailed assessments (Table 30.2).

Children with special educational needs are therefore identified by a combination of child health promotion contacts, parental referral and in response to concerns from other professionals. All three are important.

REACTION TO DISABILITY

Whether the news of a disability comes suddenly or after a period of anxiety, no parent is really prepared to hear the news that there is something wrong with his or her child. Parents' dreams are shattered and they find it difficult to make sense of

Table 30.1
Prevalence of disability

Handicap	Prevalence (per 1000 children)
Severe learning difficulties	3
Moderate learning difficulties	30
Physical disability	3
Visual handicap	0.3
Severe hearing loss	1
Moderate hearing loss	2
Autism	0.2–2

Table 30.2
Causes of disability

Prenatal	Perinatal	Postnatal
Genetic	Effects of prematurity	Meningitis
Chromosomal	Birth asphyxia Perinatal infection	Other severe illness Head injury
Rubella		
Toxoplasma		
Cytomegalovirus		
Other infections		
Poisons — drugs, smoking, alcohol		

Children with special needs

Table 30.3
Model reaction to disclosure of disability

Parent is told	Manifestations	Needs
Shock phase	Emotional disorganisation, confusion, disbelief	Sympathy and support
Reaction	Sorrow, grief, anxiety, aggression, denial, guilt, defence mechanisms	Listen to parent with sympathy but also honesty
Adaptation	'What can be done?'	Reliable information on medical and educational support and future
Orientation	Parents start to plan and organise future	Provide regular help and guidance

what is happening or to plan the future. Professionals need to understand, not only the classical stages of bereavement reaction, but also the variability of the reaction, from family to family, and from parent to parent. This may vary from day to day and week to week in the same family.

Sharing concerns

The most appropriate method of sharing the news has been the subject of intense debate not only as to how, by whom, where and when, but also in the very terms of the consultation. 'Giving the diagnosis', 'breaking the bad news' are some terms that have been frequently used in the past. However professionals, after many years of experience and listening to parents views who have had such experiences, prefer the term 'sharing concerns'. There are now guidelines of good practice (Lingam & Newton 1996) available to help you try to deliver information in an empathetic, appropriate and accurate manner. The antenatal team as well as the paediatric team should apply such guidelines.

The first reaction of numbed shock may last a few moments or for weeks. Many people take in only a tiny proportion of the first disclosure made to them, but others seek out help and information from the beginning. Following this, parents become overwhelmed with feelings of fear and loss, anger and blame for themselves or others. It is not unusual for parents to want physically to get away from the sit-

uation, and sometimes from the child. Others avoid thinking and talking about it, arguing it must be a mistake. Many parents describe how they hoped their child would not survive. The feeling that 'This isn't happening' has survival value, giving parents space to get thoughts into some sort of order which makes sense to them. Gradually they accept the diagnosis and try to come to terms with it. It is at this stage that many parents seek further information to help them get things into perspective (Table 30.3).

Parents, and other relatives, swing between times of calm when they feel more organised and times of intense sadness. Sometimes their strong feelings of protectiveness cause them to overreact to any hint of criticism about the child by others. Parents can also feel very threatened or even revolted by the thought of handicap or disability. Many describe how they feel confused in themselves between loving the child and hating the diagnosis.

Gradually most families settle down to the reconstruction of their lives, which we call the process of adjustment. On the one hand they may become keen members of a parents' organisation, or throw themselves into a campaign they see as constructive; on the other hand they may integrate the care of their handicapped child into their ordinary family life, and avoid 'special' facilities as much as possible. This variability of parental reaction makes it difficult to give parents the appropriate information at the right time.

However, the majority of studies report that

<hr>

Box 30.1
When and how to tell parents about their child's problem

<hr>

- By a consultant paediatrician (if possible with the health visitor who is to be involved in early intervention present)

- As soon as possible after the birth of the baby

- Both parents being told together

- The information given privately, with no nurses or students present

- With the newborn infant present, unless seriously ill

- The information to be given directly, and the parents given time to ask questions

- The parents are told that the health visitor will see them again soon. They are given adequate privacy immediately after the interview

- 24 hours after disclosure, a further interview is arranged with the consultant paediatrician and the health visitor

<hr>

parents do not wish for any delay in being told of the concerns of those attending their child or of what their child's special needs might be. Cunningham et al (1984) showed that a 'model procedure' for giving parents the information that their child has Down's syndrome led to a much greater rate of parental satisfaction with their care (Box 30.1).

When a disability becomes apparent slowly it is often very difficult for the child, family, friends and carers to come to terms with. When do we share our fears with parents? Sometimes in an effort to be kind, we hold back until we are certain of the diagnosis but, again, retrospectively parents tell us that they would far prefer to be involved from the moment that there are any doubts in the doctor's or therapist's mind.

It is good practice once a firm diagnosis has been made to give parents and carer's written information and in particular make them aware of an appropriate support group. The organisation 'Contact a Family' is particularly helpful here.

MANAGEMENT OF DISABILITY

The practical ways in which help is provided will differ according to the time at which special needs are recognised, whether that recognition is gradual or sudden, and of course the nature of the special need (Fig. 30.2). The role of the community paediatrician in the management of disability in childhood is not only to be involved in the direct provision of services, but also to plan and develop services, and to be responsible for training of future paediatricians who will work with child development teams. A significant amount of the paediatrician's training will need to be in the paediatric neurology clinic. The doctor traditionally finds himself in a central and powerful position coordinating care for disabled children; however much of the practical work is done by other disciplines. To be successful the doctor must understand their contribution to the total management of the child. Paediatricians, in addition to their role in diagnosis, assessment and management, have a duty to provide understanding and continuity of care. The practice of regular review, where a parent may see a different doctor every visit, has little to offer the family or the child with long-term special needs.

Multidisciplinary assessment of the child with special needs

Children with presumed special needs, particularly if they have an educational implication and are preschool, may need an assessment by a multidisciplinary team. Such a team may be found in a child development centre. The constitution of such a team may vary depending on the needs of the child, for example a child with a congenital absence of a hand may be assessed by a paediatric physiotherapist, paediatric occupational therapist and preschool teacher whilst a child with a cerebral palsy would require all of the above and in addition a paediatric speech and language therapist and a paediatric dietician. The paediatrician should take a major coordinating role for the disabled child and their families and provide continuity between assessment and day-to-day management. Assessment units or child development centres are often,

Health services:

Medical diagnosis and treatment, nursing care, physiotherapy,occupational and speech and language therapy

Parent support

Social services:

Child protection, opportunities for nursery care, relief care opportunities, advice about benefits sitting services

Assessment for services needed after leaving school

Education services:

Pre-school home teaching services, educational assessment, nursery schooling

Relief care

Education, whether in mainstream or special schools and colleges

Voluntary bodies:

Parent support, play facilities, educational

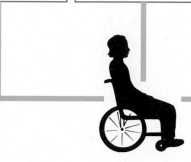

Fig. 30.2 Services provided by different agencies

Box 30.2
The functions of a child development team

1. To provide investigation and assessment of certain individual children with complex disorders and to arrange and coordinate their treatment

2. To provide parents, teachers, child-care staff and others who may be concerned in their care with the professional advice and support that can guide them in their management of the children

3. To encourage and assist professional fieldwork staff in their management and surveillance of these and other disabled children locally, by being available for consultation either in the district child development centre or in other local premises

4. To provide primary and supporting specialist services to special schools in the district

5. To be involved with others at district level in epidemiological surveys of need; to monitor the effectiveness of the district service for disabled children; to present data and suggestions for the development of the service; to maintain the quality of its institutions

6. To act as the source of information within the district about handicap in children and the services available

7. To organise seminars and courses of training for professional staff working in the district

From: Committee on Child Health Services 1976

Table 30.4
Members of the child development team

Team member	%
Paediatricians	100
Nurses	71
Psychologists	64
Social workers	59
Consultant Paediatricians (CCH)	78
Speech therapists	92
Physiotherapists	85
Occupational therapists	85
Teachers	71

From: *Zahir & Bennett 1994*

but not always, on hospital sites. Referrals most frequently come from doctors. Assessment is then usually multidisciplinary involving not only doctors, nurses, psychologists and paediatric therapists but in addition multiagency involving social services and the education authority. However, generally the child development team is usually in service teams classed as a health provision (Box 30.2).

The core staff of the child development team originally planned by the Court Committee (Committee on Child Health Services 1976) consists of a consultant community paediatrician, a paediatric nurse, a specialist social worker, a principal psychologist and a teacher. Ideally there should also be a paediatric physiotherapist, an occupational therapist and a speech and language therapist (Table 30.4). A recent survey has found that most child development centre teams have a paediatric physiotherapist, but fewer have an educational psychologist or social worker. Paediatric occupational therapy, a valuable part of the multidisciplinary team to a child with special needs, is to many alas

a scarce luxury. The input of a visiting paediatric neurologist is extremely helpful and a close working relationship with a child psychiatrist is nearly essential. As investigative and diagnostic ability, demand and knowledge increase, access to both will become essential to provide a quality service.

Studies conducted in the 1980s found that the membership and function of the 'district handicap teams' was very varied. Most teams expected to see children from birth or soon after, but the upper age limit varied from 5 years to well after school leaving age. Some were concerned with children suffering from asthma and cystic fibrosis as well as more usual diagnoses such as cerebral palsy and developmental delay. More recent studies (Zahir & Bennett 1994) have found a similar pattern. More frequently, however, the children presenting to child development teams fall into two broad categories — that of motor problems with an assortment of additional difficulties and those with communication, behaviour, play and social problems. Nowadays children with common paediatric problems are more often managed by the local community paediatric team in partnership with hospital-based colleagues. A recently published Child Development Centre review has attempted to suggest broad recommendation of good practice for child development teams.

Full multidisciplinary assessment is a costly process and may take several weeks. It puts a heavy strain on parents and at its conclusion may still not answer all their questions. Assessment usually consists of examination of the child by several members of the team. The structure and process may vary from centre to centre and there is no accepted consensus of the right way to organise this. What is essential and accepted is that information must then be shared with parents and this is best done initially verbally and in writing. This usually occurs in a coordinating meeting where each involved discipline imparts their observations and care plan.

The questions that seem to remain unanswered often are those of aetiology and, in the early stages, detailed prognosis. The aetiology of many handicapping conditions is becoming more frequently recognised but failure to achieve a diagnostic cause does not necessarily bring with it any lesser chance of improvement. Counselling and parent support is just as important as actions more directly concerned with helping the child.

THE EDUCATIONAL APPROACH

Before the 1974 Education Act children with mental handicaps had been considered 'unsuitable for education in school' and provided for either in long-stay hospitals, or in junior training centres.

The 1981 Education Act brought in terminology that radically changed the concept of assessment and provision for children with handicaps. This in turn has been succeeded by the 1993 Education Act within which a Code of Practice (1996) was issued to all local education authorities and governing bodies of all maintained schools on their responsibilities towards all children with SENs. This Code is now being revised and the revision is expected to take effect from 2001.

Code of Practice (1996)

The fundamental principles of the Code of Practice are:

- The needs of pupils who may have special educational needs are addressed.
- Children with SENs have access to a broad and balanced curriculum.
- The needs of most pupils will be met in mainstream school and without a statutory assessment or statement of SENs.
- Even before a child reaches compulsory school age a child may have SENs and require the intervention of the LEA and health services.
- Parents and child's views are vital.

It is wholeheartedly agreed by all that these SENs need to be addressed as early as possible. The Revised Code (currently undergoing consultation) recommends developing a more inclusive approach to SENs and the general adoption of a graded model of SEN provision. Schools will identify children who are finding difficulty in progressing relative to their peers and will via the school's special educational needs coordinator (SENCO)

take 'Action'. This will entail each child having an Individual Educational Plan. If despite this the child's progress causes concern the school may require outside advice and thereafter 'Action Plus'. The revised framework discusses schools adopting the terminology of School Support and Support Plus. The latter involves outside services delivering more specialist assessment, therapy and teaching targets advice.

Individual Education Plan

This will be reviewed at least twice a year within the school with the parents. Other agencies may be present according to individual need.

The Statement of Special Educational Needs

It is a statutory duty of a district health authority to ensure that their trusts both primary and acute providing child health services inform LEAs of children who they think have special educational needs and provide medical advice to LEAs. The education authority should then consider whether an assessment is necessary with reference to the Code of Practice. Parents may however also ask for an assessment.

There are clear criteria for deciding to make a statutory assessment. A child may have learning difficulties, emotional and behavioural difficulties, physical or sensory (vision and hearing) problems that precipitate the LEA to consider how to meet that child's needs.

For the purpose of a statutory assessment the LEA should seek written:.

- parental advice
- educational advice
- medical advice
- psychological advice
- social services advice
- child's views wherever possible
- other relevant agency.

Assessment under the Education Act includes asking for reports from the child's nursery or school, from social service departments, and from any other professionals known to be involved with the child and also from the parents. This assessment is initiated and coordinated by the education authority. It must include a medical report, which is coordinated by the school health service, who are responsible for collecting reports from therapists and collating medical and nursing advice. The provisional statement drafted by the education authority, after it has gathered advice from all sources, together with all the reports must be seen by the parents before it is passed. Parents have a right of appeal if they are not satisfied.

The LEA makes the decision as to how and where to provide for each child's special needs. No one may pre-empt this decision, and it is very important for doctors not to say in an unguarded moment 'such and such school would be just right for your child'. This can cause parents unnecessary anxiety when teachers and psychologists suggest other schools. Doctors can and should, however, put forward strongly their views on a child's health needs.

Parents, teachers and others (including paediatricians) hold strong views on the merits of mainstream and of specialised schooling (Box 30.3). However it is a clear expectation of the Education Act 1996 that pupils with SENs are included in mainstream schools.

Transition review

The 1996 Education Act also provides that the needs of all *statemented pupils* (a clumsy adjective), whether in special or mainstream school, should be reviewed with their parents annually, and that there is a statutory reassessment of all statemented pupils between the ages of 13 years 6 months and 14 years 6 months (year 9). The process is similar to that of the original assessment and is called the *transition review*. This review should also involve social services staff. Within the revised Code it is planned for there to be a 'connections service' phased in from April 2001. This service will aim to ensure the participation and progression of young people with SENs aged 13–19. A connection personal adviser should be made aware of young people with SEN in year 8 and should attend the year 9 transition review.

Progress towards the integration of pupils into

> Box 30.3
> **Merits of mainstream and special schools**
>
> *Special schools provide:*
> - Teaching in smaller classes
> - Teachers may have more experience of that specific disabling condition
> - Health service support in the form of medical and nursing care, and help for pupils and staff from therapists
>
> *Mainstream schools:*
> - Have comparatively large classes
> - May have much or little extra educational and health service support (usually support from 'outreach' teachers from special schools)
> - Buildings may be poorly adapted
>
> BUT THEY DO PROVIDE:
> — A local environment
> — Normal role models and expectations
> — Local contacts for parents

mainstream schools has been uneven in different localities, depending on political will and on the finances available. The 1989 Education Reform Act has provided that all pupils shall have access to the national curriculum, and great efforts have been made to adapt the different strands of the curriculum to pupils' needs.

SOCIAL SERVICES

Under the Children Act 1989, social service departments are expected to identify 'children in need' in their area. Children who are, or may be, disabled are included in the definition of 'children in need', and departments are expected to keep a register of such children. Social services departments are expected to be aware of other bodies providing services for children in need, and have a duty themselves to provide a range of services (Box 30.4).

The Children Act gives social service departments an increased statutory responsibility for pro-

> **Box 30.4**
> **Services to be provided for disabled children by social service departments**
>
> - A named person who is to act as assessment officer, and to be the first contact within the department
> - Help with day care including day nursery provision
> - Respite care facilities
> - Help in the home
> - Advice about benefits

viding services to children with special needs from an early age.

Disabled Persons Act 1986, Disability Discrimination Act 1995 and the disabled school leaver

The definition of disability is the outdated one used in the 1948 National Assistance Act: 'Persons who are blind, deaf, or dumb, or who suffer from mental disorder of any description, and other persons who are substantially or permanently handicapped by illness, injury, or congenital deformity.' Local authorities have added their own guidelines to this definition; most refer to the wishes of the young person and their carers, and to the likelihood that the young person will have a need for locally provided services.

The social service department must make its assessment of needs for statutory services under section 5 and 6 of the Disabled Persons Act when informed of the young person's school leaving date. They should also give advice about the welfare of the disabled person, and their family, and make a referral to other agencies regarding employment, education, health care and benefits.

The health advice should contain a description of the young person in broad terms including the medical cause of disability if known, together with an account of medical care needed in adult life

including important causes of concern. The report should make clear who is to provide health care, whether the family doctor or specialised adult services. The report should also contain the date and result of latest hearing and vision tests, and advice about future surveillance.

Many working parties have been set up to consider the problems of transfer of care from paediatric to adult services. There is no clear agreement about the age of transfer, the best way to approach the transfer, nor the type of service which should be provided for adolescents. Paediatric services for the child with a handicap and their family are best described as holistic, because many paediatricians caring for children with long-term conditions are basically general paediatricians who also have a special interest. Adult services are far more specialised, for example, the psychiatrist in mental handicap caring for a person with multiple handicaps would not expect to be asked to give an opinion about the state of the patient's hips. Children and young people in schools receive much of their treatment in the school setting, and are reviewed regularly by their school doctor. There are few corresponding adult services in only a few areas, and opinions differ as to whether adults with handicap should use services different from those available to the general population. Current legislation surrounding community care for people with disabilities may help to bring added urgency to this debate.

EQUIPMENT

Equipment for children with a disability may be needed in a variety of locations and this will mean that more than one set may be required, for example at home and at school. Some equipment may be very expensive, for example computers, wheelchairs, stairlifts, high-tech hearing aids. However, walking aids and magnifiers, are relatively cheap and effective. Funding may be difficult and voluntary bodies and charities often prove useful. The Disabled Living Foundation is a national charity that promotes 'independence through information' for people of any age with a disability.

VOLUNTARY AGENCIES
(See Chapter 19 and Appendix 1)

A number of voluntary agencies are concerned with the welfare of children with special needs and their families. Some are large national agencies with numerous local branches; others are smaller groups concerned with a local issue, or with a single diagnosis. Such bodies are usually readily available for consultation from parents, children or young people or other interested individuals. Voluntary bodies have an important part to play in the dissemination of information, in parent support, and in the setting up of both local and national services. By their nature they are able to set up innovative services in areas of need, and to adapt themselves to changing situations and changing priorities. The Contact-a-Family Directory is an important reference book to direct a professional or carer to the existence of a support group.

MULTIDISCIPLINARY AND MULTIAGENCY SERVICE

Any account of provision for children with special needs demonstrates the complexity of the services provided. Voluntary agencies, health, education and social services each provide services, each with a somewhat different agenda. Despite, or perhaps because of, the bewildering array of professionals involved, some families miss out on services which would have been invaluable to them, while others can barely call their time their own.

A truly multiprofessional service needs to be conceived at three levels: at the political level, where legislation and the organisation of funding should recognise the interaction of statutory services; at the management level, where service heads should sit down together to integrate their policies rather than sending one another ready-made policy documents for comment and thirdly at casework level, where the needs and wishes of families should as far as practicable mould the service they receive.

SPECIAL NEEDS REGISTERS

The Court Report recommended that every health district should maintain a register of children with

> **Box 30.5**
> **The purposes of registers are**
>
> - To improve and coordinate the care of individual children
> - To facilitate planning of services
> - To provide epidemiological data

handicap (Box 30.5). Previously many areas had run 'Observation' registers of categories of children thought to be at high risk of handicap; these had proved cumbersome and of limited value. There has been no uniform format for what have been called special needs or special conditions registers and districts have developed their own models. Some (Colver & Robinson 1989) have been developed on microcomputer systems, and others (Woodruffe & Abra 1991) linked to district child health systems.

All schemes register those children who have a statement of educational needs and those with serious disabling conditions. Difficulties arise in the definition of 'seriously disabling condition'. Epilepsy, asthma, congenital heart disease can be seriously disabling to one sufferer but in others can only have a minor impact on a child's education and life. It is even more difficult to decide inclusive criteria for young pre-school children who have developmental delay without reverting to the observation register of former times. It has been suggested that those children requiring either (a) above average input from one or more services involved with the professional care of the child, i.e. health, education, social services (excluding cases of child abuse), or (b) prolonged specialist treatment or supervision should be included.

Problems of registers

The upkeep of a special needs register is an onerous task, for field workers, clerical staff and for the paediatrician in charge of the register, especially if large amounts of data are entered (Box 30.6). Unless a

Box 30.6
The special needs register

Inputs to special needs register include:
- Registration and demographic data

- Diagnoses using ICD 11 or Reed Codes, and associated local codes for disability and aids to daily living

- Listing of health service personnel involved

- Current educational provision including whether the child is statemented

- Social service involvement

Outputs from a register
Regular reports required for the management of children on the register, for example:

- Data sorted by GP or hospital paediatrician to enable joint discussion of cases and coordination of medical care

- Sorted by school to facilitate school-based reviews: by health visitor to help enable both the health visitor and the community paediatrician to target individual children needing help, and to alert the schools of pre-school children with special needs

- Sorted by disability, to help plan adaptations to homes and schools; by diagnosis, to look at the trends over time and over geographical areas

- For processing of ad hoc enquiries of varying complexity. A researcher may wish to look at the different ages at which a specific condition was diagnosed before carrying out a detailed study about how the diagnosis was made. Educational authorities may wish to enquire how many children in certain schools require extra help with various aspects of daily living

Resources
The resources that should be provided for children with special needs and their families divide into a series of 'menus':

- People and skills

- Places where those skills are delivered

- Equipment

- Financial help (benefits)

The resources may be needed for medical diagnosis and treatment, education, recreation and family support. The latter two are important for quality of life for the child and his family. The limits of provision are determined by funding (contracts), local policy both within and between agencies, access which may be limited by geography, transport and mobility and of course the wishes of the child and family. The possible combinations of people and places is very large and a district service often develops as a series of best buys rather than an ideal that provides a made to measure service for every child. There are sadly always children for whom the off-the-peg service is not adequate. Under the 1989 Children Act, the local authority now has the duty to identify need and provide services for all children in need, including those with disabilities

register is seen to be a useful tool then it will not be valued and will become unreliable.

It has been suggested that registers should be shared between health, education and social service departments. However there are problems, not only of confidentiality, but also of the rather different requirements of the different professions. Health authority registers contain many diagnoses irrelevant to educational provision; social service registers of disabled children are to be based on the

Box 30.7
Investigation of children showing delayed development

Principles:
- There is no standard investigation list
- Investigations depend on the child's problem and the degree of the problem

History:
- It is essential to take a two-generation family history. Specifically enquire is there a history of learning difficulties, reading, writing problems; vision, hearing problems; epilepsy or fits?
- The finding of a positive history will be relevant to the investigations you plan
- The history should certainly enquire as to whether there is any developmental regression. If there is, the investigations will need to be precise as to the nature of the problem and be carried out in collaboration with the paediatric neurology service and the regional metabolic laboratory

Clinical examination:
- Examine the child, particularly not neglecting to measure and plot head circumference on an appropriate chart
- A full system examination is essential. Particularly look for cutaneous markers of neurocutaneous disease
- Visual and hearing tests are mandatory
- Consider the need for specialist audiological and ophthalmic opinions. A cataract or retinal abnormality will give you further directional clues regarding investigation and differential diagnosis
- Search for an examination lead — you are more likely to find a cause, e.g. it is easier to investigate short stature and developmental delay
- Prepare parents and carers with the information that in at least 25% of children with significant developmental delay no cause will be found

Commonly carried out investigations are:
- FBC and ferritin (There is well-documented evidence that iron deficiency anaemia is common in our pre-school children; an association with developmental delay has been made)
- Chromosomes analysis with fragile X (increasingly non-dysmorphic children with developmental difficulties are found to have a chromosomal abnormality.) Consider recognised syndromes, e.g. CATCH 22 — developmental difficulties and congenital heart disease
- Creatinine kinase (particularly in boys less than four with falling, motor and speech delay)
- Urinary organic and amino acids, GAGs (glycosaminoglycans) (cheap, low yield, easy, foolish to miss)
- Cranial imaging, particularly if head size is inappropriately big or small and there is developmental delay
- EEG often very useful, certainly if suggestion of epilepsy, but also can be an aid to diagnosis, e.g. Angelman's syndrome
- Genetic opinion after appropriate investigations have been completed

The complete list of biochemical investigations is exhaustive. Refer to a textbook. Be intelligent with your choice. Ask for advice.

Children with special needs

prediction of 'Substantial and permanent disability' and will exclude many children with medical and educational special needs.

AUDIT

Evidence-based medicine is just as important in the provision of services to children with special needs as to coronary artery surgery. Our treatments and outcome data are however more difficult to evaluate and many accepted models of therapy have little research-based evidence of efficacy.

Bower has recently conducted many elegant studies evaluating the value of physiotherapy as treatment in children with cerebral palsy. This research has been long awaited. However, there are increasing numbers of studies that are using the Gross Motor Function Measurement (GMFM) index as a measure of activity and activity limitation. In addition the Paediatric Evaluation of Disability Inventory (PEDI) is a method that can measure levels of participation (disability).

There is a desperate need for us to monitor and evaluate our methods. To date there is no ideal tool available. There are some pilot studies looking at the effect of various therapies on children in term of their outcomes in relation to degree of handicap, impairment, disability and well being (Box 30.7). We wait for results of these studies. In the mean time it is essential we monitor our services particularly in relation to patient and family satisfaction.

REFERENCES AND FURTHER READING

Bower E, Mchellan D, Arney J, Campbell M 1996 A randomised control trial of different intensities of physiotherapy and different goal setting procedures in 44 children with cerebral palsy. Developmental Medicine and Child Neurology 38:226–238

British Association of Community Child Health 2001 Standards for child development services, April. British Association of Community Child Health, London

Cass H D, Kugler B T 1993 Evaluation and audit in a paediatric disability service. Archives of Disease in Childhood 68:379–383

Colver A F, Robinson A 1989 Establishing a register of children with special needs. Archives of Disease in Childhood 64:1200–1203

Committee on Child Health Services (Chairman Court D) 1976 Fit for the future. HMSO, London

Contact a Family. On line. Available: http://www.caf.org.uk

Cunningham C C, Morgan P, McGucken R B 1984 Down's syndrome, is dissatisfaction with disclosure of diagnosis inevitable? Developmental Medicine and Child Neurology 26:33–39

Hall D 1997 Child development teams:are they fulfilling their purpose? Child:Care, Health and Development 23:87–99

Hayley S M 1992 Pediatric evaluation of disability inventory. New England Medical Centre Hospitals and PEDI Research Group, Boston

Jones K L 1996 Smith's recognisable patterns of human malformation. WB Saunders, Philadelphia

Lingam S, Newton R 1996 Right from the start. British Paediatric Association Guidelines PPG/96/02. BPA, London

McConachie H R et al 1999 How do child development teams work? Findings from a UK nation survey. Child:Care, Health and Development 25:157–168

Palasion R J 2000 Conceptual framework for evaluation of intervention. European Academy of Childhood Disability, Tubingen

Russell D, Rosenbaum P L, Cadman D T, Gowland L, Hardy S, Jarvis S 1989 Gross motor function measure:a means to evaluate the effects of physical therapy. Developmental Medicine and Child Neurology 31:341–352

Stephenson J B P, King M D 1989 Handbook of neurological investigations in children. Wright, London

Woodruffe C, Abra A 1991 A special conditions register. Archives of Disease in Childhood 66:927–930

World Health Organization 1999 International Classification of Functioning and Disability: linking outcomes and interventions, ICIDH-2. WHO, Geneva

Zahir M, Bennett S 1994 Review of child development teams. Archives of Disease in Childhood 70:224–228

31 | Physical disability

Young people with a severe physical disability will need the lifelong involvement of many professional services (Fig. 31.1). They also need continuous support from parents, family, friends and their local community. The transition into adulthood will not be smooth without a considerable amount of motivation and hard work on the part of all involved, not least the young person himself. The aim of management during childhood and adolescence is to enable the child to develop into an adult who can be as physically independent as possible, within the limitations of their disability, and who has the emotional independence to enjoy adulthood. They should leave the paediatric services with a full knowledge of their disability and should be familiar with the services they should be requesting and how to seek them.

Whilst there are many causes of physical disability, the principles of management are similar whatever the cause. In many children the medical problems are manifest at birth or within the first few months of life, for example, spina bifida, whilst others have an acquired disability. The acquired handicaps may be static as a result of a traumatic or infective incident or progressive such as with a neurodegenerative or inflammatory condition.

Children whose diagnosis has been made during their early life are likely to have a multidisciplinary assessment in the context of their local child development team. Those with acquired problems may not have such well organised management plans. The parents of children with cerebral palsy and spina bifida often have intense support and counselling at the time of diagnosis. The infant is too young to be involved in this and without positive efforts to counsel them as they mature, it is easy for them to reach adolescence without knowledge of their condition or involvement in their management decisions. Children whose diagnoses become manifest during their childhood are more likely to be involved in discussions about their illness from the outset, so hopefully will be better informed and more able to be involved in planning their management from the start.

The emotional aspects of progressive disorders need to be considered, not only for the young person, but also for their families and carers. Many conditions have a genetic component and more than one member of the family may be affected. The younger children sometimes have to cope with the death of their siblings or peers knowing that their life is following the same course. The community paediatrician certainly needs to be supported by a large group of people around them. Parents, siblings, extended family, therapy staff, teachers and leisure staff are usually involved but school transport staff, dinner ladies and teachers of the unhappy brothers and sisters must not be forgotten.

EPIDEMIOLOGY

The prevalence of physical and multiple disability amongst school children is approximately 10–20 per thousand. There are few epidemiological studies looking at the prevalence or changing prevalence of physical disability in childhood. The numbers of children with profound and multiple handicaps with high nursing and dependency needs are increasing. Hopefully special needs registers will be able to provide information on the prevalence of such disability.

The commonest cause of physical handicap is cerebral palsy with an incidence of 2.5 per 1000 live births. Neuromuscular disorders including

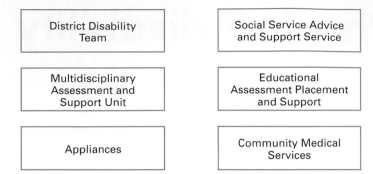

Fig. 31.1 Agencies involved in the care and support of a physically disabled child

Duchenne muscular dystrophy are less common (0.3 per 1000 male live births). The incidence of spina bifida has fallen significantly because of peri-conceptual folic acid supplementation, antenatal screening and unexplained reduction in natural incidence. Arthritis is more successfully treated and less disabling. Rare disorders when considered as a group account for a significant proportion of disability. These include skeletal dysplasias, arthrogryposis, degenerative neurometabolic conditions and neurological tumours.

EDUCATION

Until recently many, if not most, children with a physical disability would have attended a special school. With inclusion policies children are more often attending their local school. Some authorities have focus schools with enhanced provision for the disabled student (staff and equipment). Schools for children with physical disability now have much smaller numbers and consist almost entirely of children with profound and multiple disability, or neurodegenerative problems. Outreach support may be provided for children in their local or focus school. Inclusion or integration offers a broader based curriculum with their able-bodied peers. The educational, social, medical and nursing needs of a student must be considered within the context of available resources (Fig. 31.2). Access to the school building, toileting provision, communication expertise and staffing needs to be addressed. Work has to be done within the school to ensure that pupils are fully included with their peers in all aspects of school life. The children who are most likely to succeed in their local school are those who are self motivated, without learning problems, with outgoing personalities and where the school and parents are committed to integration. Difficulties tend to arise with children who have communication and continence problems and those with poor self-esteem.

Children in mainstream schools could in theory be deprived of the services, facilities and expertise which special schools have developed, in particular opportunities for regular therapy, independence training and sport and leisure facilities. There are however many local initiatives endeavouring to use examples of good practice to support the placement of children with special needs in mainstream placements. Expertise needs to be shared in information technology, management of specific learning difficulties and counselling both for pupils and their carers. Some children will have split placements so that they can benefit from each school. However this can be time consuming for both the therapy and support services duplicating support at each type of school. Many schools will have just one child with a physical disability and this can give rise to feelings of isolation for pupils, parents and staff.

ASSESSMENT AND MANAGEMENT

All children with a physical disability will need repeated assessment and appraisal of their needs so that a management plan can be initiated. The most important people to consider are the young persons

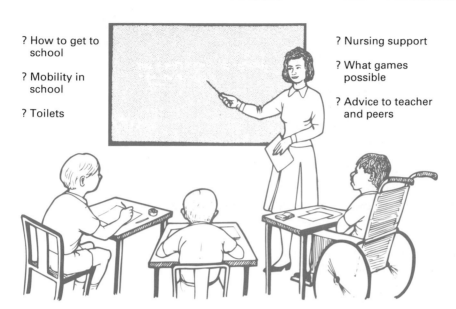

? How to get to school

? Mobility in school

? Toilets

? Nursing support

? What games possible

? Advice to teacher and peers

Fig. 31.2 Integration into schools

themselves, along with their parents and family. Many professionals are likely to be involved even if the physical handicap is not complicated by sensory impairment, learning difficulties or other medical problems. It is important that these professionals liase not only with each other but also with the family. A multidisciplinary case review should occur repeatedly and especially at key times such as initial diagnosis, pre-school needs assessment, school entry, transfer to secondary schooling, planning for school leaving and at the time of transfer to higher education, employment or day care (Box 31.1).

It is useful at review meetings for everybody involved in the care of the child to produce current status reports so that written plans can be produced for circulation to all those involved. Nowadays, parents invariably participate in such review meetings and often the young people themselves. The review meetings are best held at the place where the child has most involvement, which may be at the hospital, the child development centre, the nursery, the local health centre or the school. In some areas child development centres and schools for physically disabled children are working as places of excellence from which the resources, both staffing and equipment, are then disseminated into

---

Box 31.1
Review of personnel involved with a child with a physical disability

Doctors: general practitioner, hospital paediatrician, community paediatrician, specialists

Paramedical staff: occupational therapist, physiotherapist, speech therapist, health visitor, school nurse

Educational: parent, teacher, counsellor, educational psychologist, teacher for the visually impaired

Social: social worker, local authority occupational therapist, voluntary society social worker, link family

Family: grandparents, aunties, uncles, step families

Friends: neighbours, support groups, leisure clubs

---

the community with day-to-day management based within a more personal and local setting.

Role of the community paediatrician

The role of the community paediatrician will vary, depending upon the strengths of the other staff involved in the care of the child. Many would perceive the task as being that of coordinating the medical care, identifying and reviewing the child's multiple needs, in association with other members of the team. In reality, few teams are fully staffed since the turnover of personnel is high and there are frequent vacant positions. At a medical review, there are three aspects to be considered: identification of personnel involved with the family, consideration of medical needs and review of the child's activities of daily living. The emphasis placed on different aspects will depend upon the skills of others within the team. If there is no occupational therapist actively involved then the latter needs to be discussed so that appropriate referral is made.

Involvement of other team members

It is important to identify everybody involved with the family, not only the professionals. In some families a grandparent may be the key person in the family dynamics, whilst in others lack of family support may be a real problem. Some families will have an abundance of professionals involved and restricting these to those most essential at any one point in time may make a family feel more in control of their own life, and not 'swamped' by time-consuming appointments. Other families may not have been in contact with an important agency and since a maturing child's needs vary, services develop and family needs change, the contacts have to be repeatedly appraised. Parents can obtain considerable support from workers employed by voluntary societies or other families in support groups. They should be welcomed as part of the team sharing information depending upon the family's wishes.

MEDICAL REVIEW
Mobility

The child's mobility will not only depend upon their functional ability, but also upon the environment in which they are living and the appliances with which they are equipped. The physiotherapist will be promoting motor development as well as encouraging functional development at the same time as trying to prevent deformities. The latter will occur more frequently when there is neuromuscular imbalance.

Hand function

A child's hand function is assessed by an occupational therapist who can help with the provision of appropriate equipment. Prior to this, a child's seating has to be optimal so that they can see, reach and interact with their environment so that play and learning can begin. Older children may need assessment for accessing assisted technology with specialist keyboards or touch controls.

Growth, nutrition and oral hygiene

Many children with a physical disability will have restricted growth. This may be the main functional problem such as in achondroplasia. The occupational therapist may need to provide suitable equipment for height access. It is equally important to assess the symmetry of growth, muscle imbalance, immobility and posture, all of which can contribute to the problems of kyphoscoliosis or hip subluxation.

A balanced diet should be offered to prevent nutritional deficiencies. The appropriate consistency of food should be given to ensure the correct amount can be swallowed. A high-fibre diet may be needed to overcome problems of constipation which may result from the child's immobility or neuromuscular problems in the bowel. The speech therapist can help with oral desensitisation programmes for children with cerebral palsy and can improve upon dribbling. Children with progressive bulbar problems, i.e. progressive spastic paraparesis, can find these aspects of their disease quite distressing. Children with a physical handicap need regular dental review. Oral hygiene can be poor and regular brushing difficult either by the child or carer. Electric toothbrushes can be very helpful. Fluoride coating and fissure sealing is sometimes advised. Abnormal dentition and malocclusion can occur as part of the primary diagnosis, for example in osteogenesis imperfecta and juvenile arthritis.

The development of obesity may turn a walking child into a wheelchair user. Transfers will become difficult, skin care will become harder, personal hygiene poorer and self-catheterisation in those children with a neurogenic bladder may become impossible. Some children, for example with cerebral palsy, may have problems with their body awareness and may ignore their ill-functioning limbs. Their body image can be distorted along with their ideas of self-esteem. Anxieties about puberty and sexuality frequently occur in parents and young people and early open discussion can minimise fears. Advising on methods of menstrual control in girls can often allow anticipated problems to be dispelled.

Vision

The testing of visual acuity can be difficult especially in the young child with a physical disability who has additional learning or communication problems. Many children with spina bifida and cerebral palsy will have perceptual and visuospatial problems, some of which only become apparent as the child grows older and can more easily be tested. Awareness of these problems is important but planning ways of overcoming them is very difficult. Some children will have problems with scanning and initiating gaze movements like those with nystagmus. In the case of nystagmus, although a child may have normal visual acuity, the use of vision may still be difficult. If in doubt ask for an assessment from the outreach support teacher service for the child with visual difficulty. In some areas this may be called the peripatetic teacher service.

Hearing

As with visual testing, assessment of hearing with audiometry can be equally difficult in these children. Sensorineural deafness may be present from diagnosis, as occurs with cerebral palsy, or may develop later, for example following mumps. Cochlear implants are appropriate for a few children. Conductive deafness needs to be managed promptly to maximise the child's sensory input.

Table 31.1
Medical review of child with a physical handicap

Every occasion	Sometimes
Vision	Immunisations
Communication	Genetics
Hearing	
Oral problems	
Growth	
Sleep	
Continence	
Behaviour	

Associated balance disorders such as may occur in cerebral palsy can be detrimental to mobility.

Table 31.1 summarises the aspects that should be considered in a medical review of a disabled child.

Communication

Delay in the development of language and communication skills is a critical problem in the care of the handicapped child. Lack of understanding of expressive language raises barriers to further learning with immense frustration for both parents and children.

Speech and communication problems can be difficult to assess in the young multiply handicapped child who may also have various general or specific learning problems. Children with progressive bulbar involvement have equally difficult but different problems. Significant communication problems can lead to serious frustration, behaviour problems, social isolation and underestimation of intellectual function. Simultaneous problems with hand function, such as in the child with athetoid type cerebral palsy, may mean that a communication signing system like Makaton is inappropriate.

A manual board with symbols or words which can be pointed at may be the most functional form of communication. The board can be personalised for the child and the child's vision and hand control can dictate the picture size. The combined assessment by the speech and language therapist, occupational therapist and teacher is important.

Language development programmes demand careful assessment of the child to record current abilities. This means paying attention not only to comprehension, expression and articulation but also to other more basic skills of symbolic understanding and attention control. From these initial observations an individual language programme can be constructed, based on the child's ability. Each step in the programme is structured so that the progress of the child can be easily monitored. Opportunities to acquire language skills should be available throughout the day as well as concentrated in therapy spells. The use of carefully chosen toys to encourage growth of attention and symbolic understanding is most useful.

Speech and language therapy

The specialised speech and language therapist is essential to the team assessment of the child and in directing therapy. They must be involved early and not just as an afterthought because speech has failed to develop. The speech therapist has a number of roles, the first begins very early in the disabled child's life. In their initial assessment they evaluate tongue, palate and mouth movements and advise over feeding problems. At a slightly later age they can assess the child's inner language, the essential prerequisite to expressive language. They will see what concepts of language have developed and how this development can be enhanced through play. The therapist will not be confined to verbal communication but will concentrate on functional communication by all means so that the child's needs can be met. In the pre-school years, the therapist works with and through the parents and carers of the child (e.g. nursery nurses in a day nursery). As in physical development, the development of communication may not be automatic. Often a considerable amount of therapy through play is necessary. Hence it is doubly important that parents and carers understand concepts of early

language development and enact the development programmes themselves. Once at school the child's communication therapy is again more likely to be directed by the speech therapist via the work of teachers and parents than given directly. The therapist will advise on alternative communication systems. Throughout the child's life the therapist and community paediatrician will ensure that hearing is checked.

Communication systems

Communication problems can result in frustration, social withdrawal and underestimation of a child's abilities. Physically handicapped children also can have problems if their speech or hand function is affected. An alternative means of communication may therefore be necessary. A communication signing-system such as Makaton, or communication equipment such as a voice output communication aid may be used. Parents are often afraid that using such a device may inhibit normal speech development and as a result they tend to be introduced too late rather than too early. On the whole, alternative systems and equipment encourage rather than inhibit language development. Sometimes they are used at a young age and abandoned later as natural communication takes over. In practice such devices are only helpful in a minority of multiply disabled children. It is not easy to decide which children will benefit. Three questions should be asked:

1. *What is the child's ability and motivation?* The child needs to want to communicate and to have a cognitive ability of at least 12 months, preferably 18 months. Sometimes verbal comprehension is the only means by which one can assess the child's cognition. If the child has severe learning difficulties, chronological age is rarely important.
2. *How is the child communicating?* If the child is already communicating all his needs as much as he apparently wants, a device will not be successful. However, if he is not, the type of communication he and his parents are using will give a clue to what sort of equipment is appropriate. Is the child using any speech and if so, how much? Is he using direct pointing or associative

pointing (that is pointing directly to food or to plate meaning 'I'm hungry')? Is the child using symbols like pictures in a book? Can the child cope with delay in communication? Is he using gesture or mime?

3. *What are the limitations for the parents/carers/ school?* For any device to work, both the parents and the school have to be committed to it. If a family takes on an alternative system all or almost all those dealing with the child have to use it, which can be a considerable strain. Families often cope very well but schools and other institutions have problems if only one or two children are using a particular sign system.

Types of communication systems

Sign languages
These have the advantage over other systems in that they are immediate in their communication. Their disadvantages are that they demand a lot of effort from both the parents and school staff and require a certain level of hand function in the child.

British sign language for the deaf
This was developed from spontaneous gestures into a formal language. The gestures are equivalent to ideas rather than spoken language and it has its own grammar. There is a finger-spelling supplement and communication is aided by facial expression and body language. It is rarely suited to the multiple disabled because it needs good cognition and reasonable two-handed function. Details are available from the RNID, 105 Grosvenor Street, London WC1E 6AH.

Makaton vocabulary
This takes 350 of the most useful and easier hand signs from the British sign language. It was developed for the deaf and severely mentally handicapped and is now used widely by severely disabled children and adults in schools and adult training centres. Parents and carers talk while they sign. It is possible to start with a few basic signs and build up to a larger collection. Makaton is less successful for children with severe motor problems and two-handedness is needed.

Paget–Gorman
This needs more cognition than Makaton and the hand movements are complex. Parents often find it hard because of its complexity. It is a translation of spoken English and you talk as you sign. Hence it is much used in schools for the speech impaired.

Total communication
This is a manual, auditory and oral system of communication, recognising signs as an essential reinforcement to oral and auditory aspects of communication for deaf persons. While it is rarely formally used for multiply disabled children, many parents are naturally using all these modalities of communication.

Non-sign languages

Direct pointing picture or word boards
The BLISS symbol board was developed in Canada and uses a mixture of pictograms, abstract symbols and ideograms each representing an idea or concept rather than a 'word'. Arrays of symbols are displayed on a board or TV screen for children to point to. The English equivalent words are displayed above each symbol so parental/carer training is less necessary. Details of courses are available via BLISS Symbolics Communications Resource Centre (UK). Children need only limited motor skills for this system. It is rather laboured for the parents and the child needs cognition above a 2.5-year level.

Physical devices
There are a variety of these being developed in parallel with advances in computing technology, but as yet few are available widely. There are 'direct accessing' devices, for example head-pointing apparatus for those with poor hand function and specialised keyboards for those with limited but usable hand function. 'Indirect accessing' equipment such as scanning devices which run a pointer or light over a list of letters, symbols or words with the child halting the scanner when he chooses, are also being developed. Voice output communication aids (VOCA) are becoming a reality for some of our young patients.

Many of these devices are heavy and are often only usable in one place, thus a child using a com-

Physical disability

puter can only communicate where that equipment is located. There are currently problems in getting this equipment supplied and paid for. However, portable communication aids with computer links and voice synthesizers are a rapidly improving field. These aids are either based on prerecorded speech with limited output or on simulated speech with endless combinations produced. The user needs to be highly motivated in communication, to have adequate manual dexterity and to have receptive listeners.

Continence

The development of a regular bowel regimen should be started early. Whilst immobility of a child with a physical handicap may lead to constipation, neurouromuscular problems and a low-fibre diet also contribute. Bulking agents and bowel stimulants often have to be used together; for emotional reasons suppositories and enemas should be avoided if possible. Urinary continence is often easier to achieve than bowel control. Constipation in itself can often lead to poor bladder function so both aspects have to be managed together. Children with a neuropathic bowel and bladder need a clear regimen which is rigidly adhered to. Intermittent clean catheterisation can be commenced with babies. Children with good hand function, motivation and support can learn to do this alone at a young age.

Children with a physical handicap may wet because of problems with communicating their toiletting needs to their carers or because of delay in physically reaching the toilet. These should be clearly separated from the problem of lack of sensation or control. Some children wet or soil as part of their behavioural problems associated with their physical handicap.

Behaviour

Physical handicap can lead to frustration, isolation and unhappiness. The problems can be different for the child with an acquired handicap who has lost his previous skills whilst the child who has never known normality has missed many early experiences and may have been treated as 'being handi-

capped' all their lives. The children with progressive conditions may see their hard-earned skills lost as they deteriorate, in spite of much work to retain their functional abilities. The prospect of early death may also have to be faced, as in the child with progressive muscular dystrophy.

The children's reaction to their physical condition will be coloured by their family's response to their disability. A supportive environment with positive encouragement can lead to healthy emotional development rather than a multiply handicapped child and family.

Behaviour problems may be compounded by central neurological involvement, for example head injury or encephalopathy. These in turn may be worsened by uncontrolled epilepsy. The side effects of some medication can also lead to mood changes.

Immunisations

In addition to all routine immunisations children with a physical handicap should be considered for pneumococcal vaccine and annual influenza vaccine if their disability makes them more liable to chest infections (scoliosis) or neuromuscular disease.

Genetics

The need for genetic counselling has to be repeatedly re-assessed. This can be directed to the child with the handicap, the parents or the siblings. Part of the role of the medical review will always be to ensure if there is a specific diagnosis, it is made. Is the diagnosis correct, is there any new investigation available? A re-appraisal of the diagnosis may mean a genetic cause has become apparent, like a progressive spastic paraparesis from a previous diagnosis of cerebral palsy. Constantly look for clues, for example loss of motor skills would warrant a review of the child with cerebral palsy; looking for an underlying metabolic or structural cause. Often a new diagnosis does not mean a change in treatment but it may have major implications for the immediate family including the need for genetic counselling. Change in family circumstances with either parent acquiring a different partner may mean that the new couple need counselling.

Advances in medical knowledge need to be relayed on to families so that they are aware of new genetic tests.

Older children may need the opportunity to discuss their sibling's diagnosis. Many parents find it hard to discuss objectively their child's handicap with their able-bodied offspring. The siblings may have distorted views of the genetic implications for themselves, which simple counselling can easily dispel.

Play and leisure

Normally children acquire fine and gross motor skills and knowledge of the world around through play. The child learns through imitation and imaginary play, and with other children learns to socialise. Although play is primarily for pleasure, children learn considerably from their experiences. Those with physical handicap should be encouraged to play, not only for enjoyment but also for the education. Suitable play equipment needs to be provided and many child development centres have toy libraries which will lend out not only small items but also larger equipment.

All children should be encouraged to enjoy leisure activities. These may involve joining local or specialist clubs. Many cub or brownie packs will welcome children with varying handicaps. There are an increasing number of sports groups aimed at the physically disabled such that most activities can be appropriately adapted. These can include swimming, horse riding, angling, archery, table tennis and, for the more adventurous, outdoor pursuit centres will teach wheelchair abseiling and yachting. Involvements in such activities can not only give pleasure, but also a feeling of achievement and increasing self-confidence. Many people however do not like joining group activities and individual hobbies should be encouraged. However, it is very easy for a physically handicapped child to be offered the 'company' of a television, video or computer games, without considering that most leisure pursuits can be modified if the interest is there. A normal part of adolescence is 'kicking over the traces' of adult control, like sneaking into an 'X' film. This is much harder to do in a wheelchair and can lead to a lot of frustration. Some carers have found ingenious ways around this.

EQUIPMENT FOR THE PHYSICALLY DISABLED CHILD

When considering equipment for a child with a physical disability, the requirements not only of the family, therapists and teachers but also those of the child must be considered. Supplying something which a child does not want is of no value, it will not be used and will be a wasted expense. Some splints, supports and seating can worsen a handicap so that a child's total requirements need to be assessed *before* providing any gadgets. Resource centres increasingly allow equipment to be tried before being purchased. When equipment is ordered, it should arrive promptly for a child to achieve maximum benefit, as otherwise the needs may be outgrown before it arrives. Sadly this is often a frustrating problem and increasingly so as budgets become tight.

Equipment to prevent deformities and allow development

Seating

Correct seating can both open up the disabled child's world and prevent deformity (Fig. 31.3). For the multiply or physically handicapped child very soft seating such as bean-bags are contraindicated as they lead to contractures. Seating must be firm and promote an upright posture. Some useful seats are: corner seats, moulded seats, activities tables with inset, saddle seating for adductor spasms, self-propelled chairs and Matrix body supports.

Prolonged sitting keeps a child's hips flexed for too long a period. Some time spent standing is useful and is achievable in all but the most handicapped child by the use of a standing frame.

It would however be wrong simply to select a chair from the above 'shopping list'. Each child needs individual assessment by a therapist. When placing a child in a seat his posture must be con-

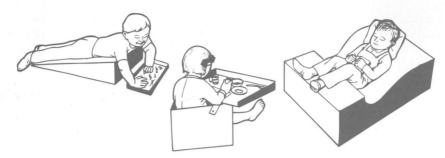

Fig. 31.3 Equipment used to help in posture

sidered critically, particularly that of the hips and spine. A fixed deformity may need surgical intervention before adequate seating is achievable.

Splints and supports

Ankle–foot (AFOs) and knee–ankle–foot orthoses (KAFOs) are useful in holding joints in positions which are not possible naturally due to spasticity or weakness. Although they appear simple in design, their use is a highly specialised subject. Most centres are now using rigid plastic orthoses which are cosmetically much preferable to the older metal braces. Much more straightforward are gaiters which will keep arms, legs or bodies straight; they are especially useful for arms that insist on flexing back towards the child.

Wedges and rolls

These are excellent in helping the floppy child develop spinal and head control.

Mobility equipment

The disabled child's world opens up when he becomes mobile (Fig. 31.4). Some useful appliances are: Orlau walkers, rollators and prone boards (for very floppy children).

Equipment that helps with skills

Wheelchairs

There is no perfect buggy or wheelchair, again individual assessment by a therapist is essential. Wheelchairs are either for being pushed or for self-propulsion. Lightweight or sports chairs can be more mobile. Powered wheelchairs are available for indoor or outdoor use. Transporting wheelchairs is easier particularly with people carrier cars but if the child is to be seated in it during travel there must be good fixation and harnessing.

Feeding

There are lots of children's equipment easily available nowadays including dishes, cutlery and beakers. These can be useful for older children with poor motor skills. Dycem mats (sticky mats that stop plates sliding about), heated dishes and suction bowls can be extremely useful.

Bathing

Bathing a child with disability can be helped by equipment some of which is easily available. Non-slip bathmats increase safety as can bath inserts. Bath chairs can enable children to have showers. Hoists are needed for heavier children and tracked systems from bedroom to bathroom can help.

Toiletting

For any success at toiletting it is essential that the child feels secure on the toilet. A number of devices are available including potties with sides or insert seats for the family toilet. Most mobile physically disabled children of school age will need substantial home alterations including a toilet with handrails or the provision for a wheelchair transfer. Children requiring intermittent catheterisation will need hand-washing facilities, a chair or variable height couch and an accessible work surface. There needs to be a lot of forward planning with therapists and parents and social services. Toilets incor-

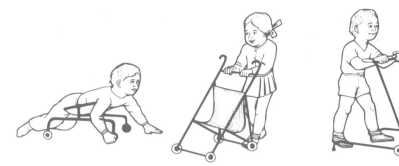

Fig. 31.4 Equipment used to help with mobility

porating a bidet and dryer are useful for the independent older child. Clearly this is an important issue in relation to the child with a disability in school.

How to obtain equipment

Usually the therapists are aware of statutory and voluntary sources of funding. Where to apply and who pays will depend on the equipment, the age of the child and where it is to be used. For the more expensive items a number of options often have to be explored.

- *Department of Health*. The Department has rulings over the substantial items it will and will not supply.
- *Disability centres* often have a certain number of items for loaning out, especially if they have a resource centre.
- *Social services departments* will provide many home and personal appliances. Contact the social services department's occupational therapists who also can advise on home alterations.
- *Local education authorities* will provide equipment for educational purposes. Some districts have negotiated combined budgets for equipment, particularly high-cost items such as communication devices.
- *Local charities* if approached will sometimes pay for equipment.
- *Businesses* sometimes will loan out equipment on a short- or long-term basis.
- The *Family Fund* (a government-financed agency)

can help out for items that are not the responsibility of other agencies.
- The *employment agency* can sometimes provide equipment (e.g. a word processor) if it will enable a person to gain employment. Enquiries should be made to a disablement resettlement officer.
- *The family*. Parents and extended family members can be very resourceful in providing home-made equipment. This is to be encouraged as they know their child's needs best. However, they should not be expected to pay out large amounts as the financial burden of a handicapped child is considerable.

CEREBRAL PALSY

Cerebral palsy is an umbrella term covering a group of non-progressive but often changing motor impairment syndromes secondary to an anomaly of the developing brain often arising in early brain development. It is by far the commonest cause of physical handicap in childhood. As well as the motor disability, children have many associated problems which include epilepsy, visual disorders or hearing loss (both conductive or sensorineural). There is enormous individual variation in the pattern of disability and multiple handicaps frequently occur.

Early diagnosis is not always easy since there is such a wide variation in normal motor development. It is important not to rush into an early, incorrect diagnosis in children with transient neurological abnormalities in the neonatal period.

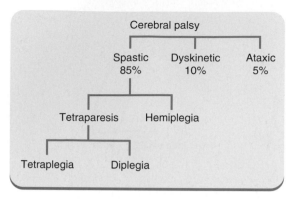

Fig. 31.5 Classification of cerebral palsy

However persistent problems with failure of developmental progress should be appropriately assessed. Cerebral palsy may present in infancy as feeding difficulties, crying or unsettled behaviour. Appropriate multidisciplinary assessment and management needs to be initiated in any child where there is a concern that their developmental progress is abnormal.

Patterns of involvement

Cerebral palsy may be classified according to neuromuscular tone: spastic, dyskinetic or ataxic (Fig. 31.5). It can also be grouped according to the pattern of the limbs affected: hemiplegia, diplegia, quadriplegia (tetraplegia). There have been changes in the relative incidences of these subgroups over the years, for example the increasing frequency of spastic diplegias and the decreasing frequency of ataxic cerebral palsy. In the 1970s and 1980s cerebral palsy rates increased among low birthweight babies, latterly this trend has not been as clear but the severity of the cerebral palsy does seem to be increasing among the low birthweight survivors. It is important to realise that these patterns are not static and that during the course of neurological maturation children may go from a hypotonic phase through a dystonic phase to a spastic phase. However, as a general rule, those with total body involvement will tend to present earlier in the first year of life than children with a diplegic cerebral palsy.

Initial assessment

Clues about aetiology may be obtained from the antenatal, perinatal and postnatal history. A family history can also be relevant, for example familial spastic paraparesis. Physical examination will show delay in motor development. Motility assessment is also an important part of the neurological assessment of the young baby. Prechtel considers that observation of the pattern of movement of a baby particularly between 3 and 5 months can give useful information with regard to the possibility of the child developing a cerebral palsy syndrome.

Tone may be increased or decreased according to the patterns described above and primitive reflexes may be unduly persistent. Tendon reflexes are often very brisk and increase or imbalance in muscle tone may cause abnormal posture or deformity. Voluntary movements are poor and lack precision. Where the cause is not obvious, further investigation should be considered. This may include investigations for congenital infection (rubella, cytomegalovirus, toxoplasma, herpes simplex), amino acid chromotography and metabolic studies, skull X-ray, neuroimaging and chromosomal analysis. A detailed examination of the eyes and hearing is essential not only for assessing the presence of visual or hearing problem but also to exclude markers of an underlying illness.

Management problems

Feeding and eating problems
These problems often require a multidisciplinary approach. Poor weight gain is a recurrent problem in children with cerebral palsy often of a multifactorial nature. Dietetic advice is essential and often after detailed assessment in children with more severe cerebral palsy a gastrostomy may be required. This in itself can revolutionise the child's and family's life.

Motor and movement problems
Physiotherapy is the mainstay of treatment. There are many different therapy models, for example Bobath, Peto (conductive education), Vojta, each having evolved from different philosophies and each requiring specific training to carry out. The majority of paediatric physiotherapists will use an

eclectic approach in their management of the child with cerebral palsy.

Persisting primitive reflexes

Persisting primitive reflexes, particularly the asymmetrical tonic neck reflex and the tonic labyrinthine reflexes, may interfere with postural reactions and the development of voluntary hand movements. Central head positioning is vital in inhibiting those reflexes.

Deformities

Deformities are common but are often preventable when they result from muscle imbalance, immobility and incorrect positioning. Management will largely be to prevent this occurring using footwear, orthoses, suitable buggies and chairs. Paediatric orthopaedic surgeons have a large role here and like to see a child with cerebral palsy early in the child's life — not to plan an operation but to assess the child over time. Children with cerebral palsy are particularly at risk from hip problems and it is current recommended practice that children with spasticity should have a hip X-ray at around 30 months to look for hip dysplasia. The hip dysplasia may not be directly related to the severity of the cerebral palsy. Newer treatments, for example the use of botulinum toxin injection, should be considered to improve the quality of gait in some of the ambulant children with cerebral palsy. Other surgical treatments are still being evaluated (e.g. intrathecal baclofen).

Communication difficulties

These difficulties often the result of the motor disorder and not necessarily secondary to a learning difficulty per se. Alternative and augmentative communication devices are increasingly available, each tailored to the individual needs. A multidisciplinary approach to assessment and management is essential. Early speech and language therapist involvement, a low index of suspicion of bulbar involvement in the cerebral palsy (drooling and feeding difficulties) and early introduction of augmented and alternative communication systems (note this will not prevent speech development) are all essential. Total communication systems are increasingly adopted by children with cerebral palsy where speech, signing, symbols, gesture and voice output systems enable an individual who otherwise may have 'no say' to become an effective communicator.

Continence

Continence can usually be achieved. Firm, comfortable seating in which the child feels secure is vital as training is easily upset by anxiety. Behavioural approaches are often useful.

Perceptual problems

Perceptual problems relating to the identification of shapes, directions in space and body image, produce practical difficulties in self-help such as undressing and in acquiring reading and writing skills. In some intellectually able children, these problems may only become apparent when they are struggling with mathematical concepts such as the conversion of a table of numbers into a linear graph or pie chart or in geography with the conversion of a flat map into a three-dimensional picture.

Deafness

Deafness is common, both conductive and sensorineural. The latter is particularly frequent with high-tone loss in children with athetosis.

Vision

Vision may be affected in a variety of ways. There may be refractive errors, a squint, hemianopia and other field defects. The latter may impair left–right sequencing in reading or writing.

Circulation

Circulation to arms and legs is sometimes poor, making them susceptible to cold injury. Advice on warm clothing can be helpful.

Children with cerebral palsy can usually cope in their local school if the problems of mobility can be overcome. The child with spastic quadriplegia often has more complex needs both in terms of therapy, posturing and learning problems. The greatest challenge to education is often the child an athetosis who may have a combination of communication difficulties and involuntary movements but who may also have the intellectual ability to greatly benefit from advanced and complex electronic equipment.

MUSCULAR DYSTROPHY

Muscular dystrophy is a generic term covering a variety of types of muscle disorder. The most common form is Duchenne muscular dystrophy (incidence 0.3:1000 boys). The condition should be suspected in any boy with delayed or progressive difficulty in walking. Prominent hypertrophied but weak calf muscles are an important sign. Associated learning difficulties are common and may even be the presenting problem. The diagnosis is initially considered when a raised creatinine phosphokinase is found in blood. Molecular genetics studies can confirm the diagnosis, occasionally proceeding to a muscle biopsy. Even allowing for individual variation, the disease is relentless progressive loss of motor skills. The boys often not walking unaided beyond 10 years old. Spinal fixation can help posture and delay cardiorespiratory failure. Oxygen supplementation by night or day may improve well being terminally. Further therapeutic interventions continue to be researched and are currently being evaluated, for example the use of steroids. Currently however death usually occurs in early adult life.

Inheritance is by an X-linked recessive gene with a considerable number of spontaneous mutations. Carrier mothers, aunties and sisters can be detected once a case is identified. Genetic counselling for all the family should be offered as antenatal diagnosis is available with the option of termination of an affected fetus.

Educational implications

Most boys start at their local school, but as they get older and the handicap progresses, more help is needed with toiletting, dressing and mobility. Some boys become depressed or angry as their disability increases and this may be expressed in many ways. Their increasing dependency and associated learning difficulties, coupled with the implications of a life-limiting condition, mean that many boys choose to transfer to a special school. In the special school the child will meet others with the same condition which will make them more aware of their long-term prognosis, particularly when one dies. Expertise in handling this is greater in a school that experiences it more often.

This disease has such a predictable course that it should be easy to anticipate the future needs of the boys and their families. It is vital for professionals and parents to help plan for these needs (house conversions, ramps for wheelchairs, adjustable beds for night-turning, toileting aids, lifting facilities), so that facilities are provided for when they are needed.

HYDROCEPHALUS AND NEUROPATHIC BOWEL AND BLADDER

The number of infants with severe handicap due to spina bifida has fallen significantly. Hydrocephalus occurs more often now with other conditions, (for example cerebral palsy). Similarly neuropathic bladder occurs in a variety of diseases, for example sacral agenesis or spinal tumours. Multidisciplinary working with neurosurgeons, orthopaedic surgeons, paediatricians and paediatric surgeons is still important to retain the expertise originally gained from the management of the spina bifida children.

Management problems

Urinary continence

In some children there is a flaccid paralysis of the bladder and in others there are strong uncoordinated bladder contractions likely to produce back pressure vesicoureteric reflex and kidney damage. Bladder pressure studies can help decide on the appropriate regimen for each individual child. Possible approaches include the use of simple toilet training regimens, drugs, intermittent catheterisation, bladder manual expression, penile appliances, ureterostomies and ileal loop diversions.

Hydrocephalus and shunt

Shunts may become infected or blocked with serious implications. These problems may present with drowsiness, pyrexia, personality or visual changes. Prompt neurosurgical review is therefore essential.

Puberty and adolescence

Menarche is often early in girls with hydrocephalus. A combination of immobility, incontinence and menstruation can cause considerable distress. Anxieties about sex and fertility are common and counselling needs to cover not only these aspects, but also any genetic aspects to their condition.

Educational problems

Learning difficulties are common in children with hydrocephalus. Characteristically, many of the children have 'cocktail party' speech in which the child has deceptively precocious expressive language with very poor comprehension. There may also be significant fine motor problems and visuo-spatial difficulties. Careers have to be chosen with these problems in mind.

EPILEPSY

This is one of the commoner handicapping conditions of childhood. The prevalence in the population as a whole is 0.5–1%. However in children with a tetraplegic form of cerebral palsy it occurs in 50–90% and in those with severe learning difficulties 60%. It is not too surprising that the epilepsy may contribute to learning, and behaviour problems.

A multidisciplinary team is needed, comprising the paediatric neurologist (available in specialist centres for the more complex patient), a paediatrician, preferably based in the community, and in addition a psychologist, social worker, epilepsy liaison paediatric nurse and strong educational links, which are all essential to optimise management of the young person.

ACQUIRED BRAIN INJURY

Traumatic brain injury is the most common cause of acquired brain damage in childhood (~180 per 100 000). Three thousand children a year acquire a significant neurological or cognitive disability from a traumatic brain injury. Other non-traumatic causes of brain injury are a brain tumour or an infection or inflammation often called an encephalitis (~64 per 100 000). In the UK half a million children and young people with traumatic brain injury attend our casulty units per year. Central nervous system (CNS) tumours affect 450 children per year in the UK. Both of these groups of children may have long-term consequences not only in relation to potential physical handicap but cognitive and behavioural consequences as well. Often it is difficult to determine the degree of long-term difficulty a person will suffer immediately after the brain injury. In addition those children with brain tumours and leukaemia may have additional CNS damage as a result of the treatment, i.e. chemotherapy and radiotherapy. Increased survival has occurred as a result of our treatment techniques but the cost may be late cognitive impairments as a result of adjuvant radiotherapy and CNS-directed radiotherapy.

It is essential that this group of children is managed by a coordinated multidisciplinary rehabilitation team involving health, education and social services. Unfortunately this objective in many areas is proving difficult to achieve.

ARTHRITIS

Advances in the management of juvenile idiopathic arthritis mean that fewer children will have long-term disability. Many children with this and other inflammatory conditions (i.e. dermatomyositis) are having weekly community administration of parenteral methotrexate. The supply of long-life preloaded syringes means that children can self-inject with monthly drug monitoring. The control of the extra-articular features of systemic arthritis is still difficult. Functional outcome measures such as the CHAQ (Child Health Assessment Questionnaire) are increasingly being used for drug studies and audit purposes.

REFERENCES AND FURTHER READING

Aicardi J, Bax M 1998 Cerebral palsy. In: Aicardi J (ed) Diseases of the nervous system in childhood, 2nd edn. MacKeith Press, Cambridge
Bax M, Tydeman C 2000 The European Cerebral Palsy

Physical disability

study; initial results of the physical examination of children at two years and upwards. European Academy of Disability, Tubingen

Carr LJ, Cosgrave AP, Gringras P, Neville BGR 1998 Position paper on the use of botulinum toxin in cerebral palsy. Archives of Disease in Childhood 79:271–273

Crouchman M 1990 Children with head injuries. British Medical Journal 301:1289–1290

Dubowitz V 1995 Muscle disorders in childhood, 2nd edn. WB Saunders, London

Finnie N 1997 Handling the young cerebral palsied child at home, 3rd edn. Butterworth-Heinemann, London

Glennen SI 1997 Handbook of augmentative and alternative communication. Crocus Books, London

Hagberg B, Hagberg G 1996 The changing panorama of cerebral palsy — bilateral spastic forms in particular. Acta Pediatrica International Journal of Paediatrics 85:954–960

Hall DMB, Hill PD 1996 The child with a disability, 2nd edn. Blackwell Science, Oxford

Jeffree DM, McConkey R, Hewson S 1985 Let me play. Souvenir Press, London

Levitt S 1995 Cerebral palsy and therapy, 3rd edn. Treatment of cerebral palsy and motor delay. Blackwell Scientific, Oxford

Mutch L, Alberman E, Hagberg B, Kodama K, Perat MV 1992 Cerebral palsy epidemiology: where are we now and where are we going? Developmental Medicine and Child Neurology 34:547–555

Neville B 2000 Paediatric epilepsy management as part of a comprehensive disability service. (Proceedings of meeting.) EACD Tubingen

O'Donohoe N 1985 Epilepsies of childhood, 2nd edn. Butterworths, London

Pharoah POD, Cooke T, Cooke RW, Rosenbloom L 1990 Birthweight specific trends in cerebral palsy. Archives of Disease in Childhood 65:602–606

Prechtel HFR, Einspieler C, Cioni G, Bos AF, Ferrari F, Sontheimer D 1997 An early marker for neurological deficits after perinatal brain lesions. Lancet 349:1360–1363

Riddick B 1982 Toys and play for the handicapped child. Routledge, London

Scrutton D, Baird G 1997 Surveillance measures of the hips of children with bilateral cerebral palsy. Archives Disease in Childhood 56:381–384

Smith D 1997 Recognisable patterns of human malformation, 5th edn. WB Saunders, London

Thomas AP 1989 The health and social needs of young adults with physical disabilities. MacKeith Press, Oxford

32 | Learning and health

Educational medicine is concerned with the different ways that health and education interact. In its crudest sense, it involves the general fitness of children to receive education and in its more sophisticated sense, it is concerned with the ways particular health problems or disabilities produce learning difficulties. Achievement or failure to achieve results from a complex mix of individual, medical, social and educational factors. No one professional group has the monopoly of knowledge and no one group can function effectively without an understanding of these multidisciplinary aspects. Paediatricians, teachers, educational psychologists and social workers are all experts on children, but see childhood from different perspectives. It is important to understand these differing professional views, but also to resist straying too far into areas where we lack training and authority.

The presence of learning difficulties and their implications also have large emotional overlay for parents and children. The involvement of the community paediatrician may raise expectations from parents, children and teachers that we may be unable to meet. Parents may look for a medical cause and also a medical cure; teachers may be looking for practical medical advice; children may just want to feel better about themselves as they become conscious of their learning difficulties. Involvement of the paediatrician should, therefore, start with a discussion of the 'problem' as perceived by parents, children and teachers, their expectations of the paediatrician (and of the child) and of their feelings about the learning difficulties.

This chapter will discuss four aspects of educational medicine:

- General factors affecting learning.
- The effects of illness on learning.
- Specific learning disorders.
- Assessment of the child with learning difficulties.

FACTORS AFFECTING LEARNING
The school

Children spend at least 10 years of their life at school and it would be surprising if the quality and content of this experience did not have some, if not a major effect upon their behaviour, academic attainment and success in adult life. Rutter (1979) in '15 000 hours' studied the intake of 12 London comprehensive schools in 1970, comparing assessments at age 10 in primary school with those at age 14 and examination results at age 16. They showed that children did much better in some schools than in others, and that these differences could not be explained by differences in their intake. For example, the intake of one school contained 31% of children with behavioural problems, which was reduced to 10% by the age of 14. In another school the intake contained 34% of children with behavioural problems, which had risen to 48% by the age of 14. The type of school that produced the best results largely followed the model of firm and consistent discipline, high academic standards, homework, school uniform and a wide range of extracurricular activities in which children could engage and take responsibility. Other characteristics such as modern buildings and facilities were not shown to be important factors.

The pastoral side of education in both primary and secondary schools can do much to compensate for adverse social circumstances and to supplement the positive influences of family life. Indeed the hallmark of many successful schools is that they not only influence their children, but that they also

Learning and health

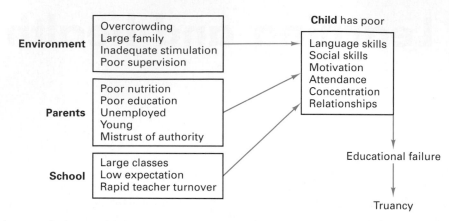

Fig. 32.1 The roots of educational failure

influence parents and the surrounding community. In return, parents and community can make a great contribution towards the life of the school. The strength of such feeling becomes very evident when the school is deprived of resources or threatened with closure.

Social life

The ability of a child to succeed in school is determined by a mixture of inhibitory and facilitating factors (Fig. 32.1). They may compensate one another and include such factors as opportunity to receive education, intelligence, temperament, health, disability, social disadvantage or advantage, and quality of teaching. These factors are also not independent of one another so that, for example, social disadvantage may have a negative effect upon health.

Although the quality of education has an important influence upon educational attainment, social inequality has a very large effect as shown by data from the National Child Development Study (Wedge & Prosser 1973, Wedge & Essen 1982) (Fig 32.2). The reasons for this are diverse and complex, but include such elements as material resources (housing, nutrition), pre-school opportunities for learning, parental and teacher expectations, and parental interest and involvement in their child's education. Among the parents of 11 years olds followed in the National Child Development Study (Wedge & Prosser 1973), neither mother nor father

had visited the school of three in every five children in the previous 12 months in the disadvantaged group, compared to only one in three of the other children.

The consequences of early sensory, social and emotional deprivation have been extensively studied. Children brought up in institutions which provided material care, but where emotional needs and stimulation were not provided, were found to have poor language development, poor school attainment and an impaired ability to form emotional attachments. The newborn infant fixes on a human face, and, under normal circumstances, this will be reinforced by the mother and thus the child is encouraged to take greater and greater interest. The neglected child becomes apathetic and does not learn the joy of taking an interest in his surroundings. Others will find the world a hostile place and learn to react negatively to contact. Lack of early linguistic stimulation will impair the development of language. Restricted language in turn delays the development of basic reading and writing skills. Such children often become more aggressive and impulsive and are less able to rationalise and think through conflicts because of lack of inner language. Knowledge of shape, colour, size, texture is needed as a basis for early education and this need may not be met if the child is reared in dull surroundings. Neglected, suppressed children may, at school entry, have little understanding about the sea, mountains, farms, animals that is assumed in some teaching materials designed for children of this age.

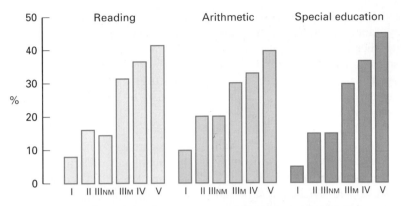

Fig. 32.2 Educational attainment and social disadvantage: National Child Development Study

Health and well being

For some children with obvious physical, mental or sensory disability, their learning problems can be explained by a medical diagnosis. However, using the framework of impairment (the medical 'lesion'), disability (the functional consequence of the impairment) and handicap (the limitations in lifestyle and activity that stem from the disability), we can see that like impairments do not produce like disabilities and handicaps. Two children may have identical levels of visual impairment or hearing loss and similar intelligence, yet one may be functioning at the top end of a mainstream school and another may be lacking in basic skills. The importance of the medical diagnosis must not be allowed to hide other factors, which have led to a much greater disability arising from a similar level of impairment. Other social and environmental factors may act to prevent, minimise or increase the disability.

For most children with learning problems in mainstream schools or children with moderate learning difficulties in special schools, there is no medical diagnosis, but up to 50% may be found to have a medical condition or risk factors which have contributed towards the learning problem (Lamont & Dennis 1988). For some this may be a single problem such as fragile X, or a conductive hearing loss; for others it may relate to past medical history, which led to a prolonged period of ill health and poor school attendance; and for others, it is a combination of problems that might be minor individually, but which collectively are important (Box

---

Box 32.1
Risk factors in children with moderate learning difficulties. After Lamont & Dennis (1988)

- No medical risk factors   58%

- Definite medical risk factors   42%
  Prenatal   13%
  Perinatal   24%
  Postnatal   5%

- Possible risk factors   37%

- Family history of learning problems (both parents)   51%

32.1). Other factors affecting school performance are discussed later in this chapter.

LONGSTANDING ILLNESS

About 10% of children have some form of longstanding illness that may affect school progress through a variety of mechanisms (Bolton 1997, Biser 1989, Larcombe 1995, Lightfoot 2001).

Absence from school

This may be because the child is ill at home or requires frequent hospital outpatient or inpatient attendances. There are obvious conflicts between the demands of treatment and education, though clearly they are interdependent. School doctors may be asked by education authorities for their opinions as to whether a certain degree of non-attendance is reasonable on medical grounds. These are difficult issues. It is important that the doctor is not seen by the child and parents as an inquisitor whose job it is to establish innocence or guilt. The doctor's task is to see how a particular child's medical management might be structured so that his educational needs can be more adequately met. Examples might relate to the scheduling of appointments in relation to school holidays and timetables or by the school health team taking a greater role in day-to-day medical management.

Non-treatment absences

These may be common in children with chronic illnesses where school absence is greater than can be explained by the child's illness or disability. Important factors may be parental anxiety, combined with a desire to protect against actual or potential adverse factors, for example bad weather or a minimal upper respiratory infection. Parents may also be trying to make some sort of compensation for the loss of quality of life caused by the illness or simply, and understandably, are adopting a softer approach. The child may, through anxiety or intent, exaggerate the effects of symptoms. There may also be a degree of collusion between parents and children. The doctor's role is to understand the underlying factors, to provide reassurance and support and to explain the importance for the child's future in keeping up with schoolwork.

Other children may be withheld from school, whilst in very good health, under the pretext of illness, but with the intention of helping mother look after the house, a younger child or an elderly relative. There are often very real difficulties at home and a sympathetic and helpful attitude mobilising services through the general practitioner and health visitor may be more successful than a critical approach.

Present but ill

In some cases the child is present at school, but is receiving treatment that does not adequately control their symptoms. Examples would include children whose activity is limited due to asthma, who are distracted by itching from their eczema or whose attention span is interrupted by petit mal attacks. The underlying problem may be inadequate treatment being prescribed, poor compliance or real difficulties in providing an effective therapeutic regimen. Compliance may be poor because parents do not understand the treatment or the techniques of administration, for example of inhalers. On others occasions, families may not be sufficiently well organised to ensure that they have a continuous supply of medicine, although they might recognise the need. Occasionally, parents may deny the existence of a specific diagnosis and therefore withhold treatment. The child may be reluctant to accept the discipline of regular medication, even when it is successful in controlling symptoms. This is often a problem among adolescents, for example those with diabetes, who may attempt to manipulate or sabotage the effects of treatment.

A thorough review of treatment and compliance is often needed in order to optimise control of symptoms. School health services can have an important role in the day-to-day monitoring of medication and its effectiveness. For a few children, treatment results in some improvement, but, in spite of an optimal regime, there is still significant disability. In this instance, awareness and understanding of the disability and the provision of additional educational resources can serve to minimise the child's educational difficulties.

Treatment is interfering with the ability to learn

Learning difficulties as a side effect of drug treatment are rare, but do need to be considered in children with learning problems who are on long-term medication. Medicines that may cause drowsiness such as some of the older antihistamines and anticonvulsants should be considered in this context. Excessive use of salbutamol and resultant hyperactivity has been described as an example.

The child's reaction to his illness

Some children in response to chronic ill health will adopt a 'sick role' in which their conception of disability is generalised into many other fields of activity in which it does not apply. Fortunately, most children will rise to the challenges faced by ill health, but a few use it to shield themselves from other demands, such as education. Parents and teachers may, to some extent, collude with this, by regarding the child as 'delicate' and decrease pressure on and expectations of him. In the real world, children with a disability will need more education and not less if they are to compete for jobs when they leave school. Children should therefore be encouraged to take a positive attitude to their health problems and may sometimes require a fairly firm approach to their school work. Parents and teachers will need support in this as they often find it difficult to apply pressure and standards to children with disabilities. Occasionally, the sick role is part of a much deeper and more generalised depression. In these circumstances, discussion with the child and family therapy team or liaison psychiatrists may be needed.

The reaction of other children

Successful integration of a child with special needs requires careful consideration of the possible attitudes or reactions of other children. Minor features that draw attention to a child as being different, for example wearing glasses, may provoke comments from class members that might add to the misery of a child who is already feeling sensitive about his altered appearance. Peer group reactions or pressure may have an adverse effect upon the use of glasses, other aids or appliances or the use of medication in school. Children may be amused by the abnormal gait of a child with cerebral palsy or the language difficulties of a child with a stammer. Children may also be frightened of a child with a disfigurement. It is easy to see how a child with a disability can become isolated and unhappy and, as a consequence, work poorly in school.

Managing these problems in the classroom may prove to be extremely difficult. They first of all need to be recognised. Many children will choose to suffer in silence as peer group pressure dictates that you do not tell the teacher. Other children have personalities that do not succumb to this type of treatment and will not fit into the role of victim. It is certainly a valuable experience for a class of children to gain understanding about disability and learn to overcome the fear and prejudice that can be a common reaction. One should not underestimate the skills required of a teacher to do this and too often the solution is to remove the victim to more secure surroundings. To some extent, problems can be prevented through the promotion of self-esteem from an early age and by providing support and an open channel for communication of hurt feelings. Education also has the challenge of reversing the attitudes to disability that children too often acquire from their families and the local community.

On occasions, the opposite problem is seen in which classmates become overprotective and provide too much assistance, inhibiting the development of self-help skills.

Unnecessary restrictions

Teachers in mainstream education have probably received little or no instruction about childhood illnesses. They will inevitably have to deal with the common health problems that will affect the children in their charge particularly with more mainstream integration. Without proper information, teachers are unlikely to wish to take responsibility for activities, which they may regard as involving extra risk. Thus a child may be excluded for incorrect reasons from lessons such as PE, chemistry or metalwork and might be sent to the medical room or indeed home as a strategy for dealing with all medical concerns. The loss in education may be very significant. It is the role of the school medical team, with parental permission, to explain to the teacher the nature and consequences of the child's problems. Usually, there would be no limitations: a negative statement about lack of limitations is as important as a positive statement imposing restrictions. The school medical team must be willing to accept responsibility for the advice that they have given the school. The 1996 Education Act, with its emphasis on the integration of children with special needs, broadens the role of teachers in the care of children with disabilities.

SENSORY AND COMMUNICATION
(see also Chapters 33–35)

Problems with hearing and vision need to be considered in every child with learning difficulties or poor academic progress. In the past, they were sometimes missed (hopefully now a very rare event), particularly where testing is difficult.

Vision?

What is the near and distant visual acuity? Are the visual fields full? Assessment of visual fields is not routinely required, though it is important in children with neurological defects, for example cerebral palsy, where a hemiplegia may be associated with a homonymous hemianopia. The hemianopia, if unrecognised, may inhibit the development of reading and writing skills. In any report written for teachers, it is important to remember that their training does not include the ability to understand medical shorthand, so telling a teacher that a child's visual acuity is 6/12 is usually not helpful. The teacher in a special school for visually handicapped children will understand this, but most children with impaired vision will be in ordinary school. What the teachers really want to know is a practical application of the child's visual ability, that is the size of print that the child can read easily in a book or on the board. Information in this form is a good starting point for sorting out a child's individual needs.

Hearing?

Hearing losses of as little as 20 db or common fluctuating hearing losses can impair schoolwork and lead to behavioural problems in individual children. Fluctuating hearing loss in early and middle childhood should be suspected where there is a history of recurrent ear infections. Children should never be labelled as uncooperative in hearing tests, as this avoids making a diagnosis of deafness, a behaviour problem or a degree of learning disability, which renders the child unable to perform that

particular test which is appropriate to his chronological age. The effect of any level of hearing loss depends upon a range of factors including concentration, intellect, level of stimulation at home and the need to learn a second language on starting school. Teachers need practical advice on the level and frequencies of hearing loss, the effects of that hearing loss in the classroom and playground and how they can help, for example by appropriate position of the child's seat in the classroom.

Language

A child's language development is the most reliable predictor of educational progress. Time and skill are therefore required to make a proper assessment of language and the child's linguistic background. Assessment of expression, comprehension and articulation is important using information obtained from parents and teachers as well as personal observations. Minor problems of articulation are of little significance, but other concerns, particularly about comprehension, may indicate the need for assessment by a speech and language therapist. Specific language difficulties, in the absence of other developmental problems, are uncommon. Diagnosis may be difficult and incorrect labels such as learning disability or behavioural problems made instead of expressive or receptive language problems. Clear understanding of the specific difficulties can make a significant difference to professionals teaching these children.

It may, on the surface, seem easy to identify children who are non-English speakers. However, unless we ourselves are also fluent in Hindi, Urdu or any other language that the child may speak, we will fail to identify the child who may have considerable delay in his own language. The parents are also likely to speak little English, adding to our difficulties in making a proper assessment. This challenge is one which needs to be taken up earlier rather than later in the child's school career and, hopefully, long before school entry. Investments in time, patience, an interpreter or, better still, a multilingual speech therapist are essential.

More commonly children enter school who speak English as a second language, but whose skills in English are not as well developed as those of the language in use at home. Most young children will rapidly expand their English vocabulary with appropriate help in school, for example by 'English as a second language' teachers in primary schools or through special units for children of secondary school age. However, a superficial examination may fail to reveal the depth of individual children's difficulty in English and their comprehension may be inadequate for educational purposes. Combinations of factors should be recognised such as a minor hearing loss, which may assume much greater significance in a non-English-speaking child.

A second language should not be regarded as a problem, but as a potential asset in the international community. The child who is bilingual requires to have this advantage valued rather than ignored. Language is an important part of cultural identity as well as simply a means of communication.

Dialect problems such as a strong regional accent may produce temporary difficulties in understanding. Learning difficulties that in the past have been ascribed to this cause, for example in children of West Indian origin, are more likely to be due to other factors such as preschool experience or differences in the cultural setting between home and school.

Other perceptual difficulties

Other perceptual difficulties including disorders of visual perception, auditory perception, body image and coordination can be associated with learning difficulties. It is estimated that 5–15% of children may fit into this category of the 'clumsy child'.

PHYSICAL WELL BEING
Lack of sleep

Children who are tired, for whatever reason, are likely to perform poorly at school. Lack of sleep may be caused by the failure to apply an appropriate (or in some cases any) bedtime. Noise and overcrowding and bedroom television may also be contributing factors. It is accepted that the amount of sleep that children require in order to not feel tired the next morning varies very widely. A survey

of television programmes that children claim to watch often provides a good indication of bedtime, provided that the paediatrician is also suitably informed. Many children who cannot tell the time appear to have a built-in clock, which tells them precisely when a particular programme is on. Older children may be tired because they are out late at night. Children who are tired often present with behavioural problems, which include short attention span, hyperactivity, frustration and general argumentative behaviour, and unlike adults they are frequently not obviously tired. Paediatricians may need both to advise on bedtimes and on methods of implementation. (The management of sleep problems is discussed in Chapter 28.)

Lack of food

Not all children will want or eat breakfast; however, among 15 000 ten year olds studied from the 1970 birth cohort, 2.6% never ate breakfast and 18.9% had breakfast 'sometimes', this being a more common occurrence in manual social classes (Haslam et al 1984). There appears to be a 'no breakfast syndrome' in which the child often appears tired and unwell at school. He may be seen by child health services because he has fainted or referred with abdominal pain. A noticeable improvement is seen after a mid-morning snack or dinner at midday. This child, in practice, has often gone for 18 hours without a meal, so these symptoms are not surprising. This is a sensitive area and needs to be taken up with some tact, promoting better eating patterns, without being openly critical (Fig. 32.3).

The role of poor diet as a cause of developmental delay is discussed in Chapter 23. There is a strong association between failure to thrive, iron deficiency and learning problems and convincing evidence that nutritional supplementation results in improvement (Grantham-MacGregor et al 1991, Lozoff et al 2000). Careful assessment of nutritional status is therefore an important part of the medical examination. Long-term learning problems may result from prolonged poor nutrition over the first 2 years of life when brain growth is rapid. There is little evidence to support the case for additional vitamins and minerals in children who are not clinically deficient.

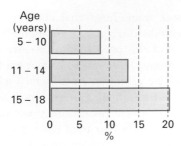

Fig. 32.3 Percentage of children in different age groups missing breakfast

Overworked?

The situation of a child being tired and unable to benefit from schooling because of excessive hours of work outside of school is largely historical as the hours and ages and suitability of paid work undertaken by children is strictly regulated. A paper round or a Saturday job may be regarded as good work experience. However, there are instances where children are given excessive burdens in housework, in a family business or are set by their parents unreasonable amounts of extra school-type work at home with the aim of improving their attainments. These situations are fortunately rare, but can usually be identified by asking the child to take you through what they do in a typical day. Advice to parents or the help of the education welfare service, one of whose roles is to regulate employment of children, may be needed.

The most common problem in this category is impaired development due to a lack of early childhood experience, which may be coupled with lack of parental support for child and teachers resulting in limited contact between parents and school and little encouragement to do well. Neither the parents nor the child expect success. Although prevention is the best strategy, improvements at any stage can come about through changes in opportunity, experience and home life (Rutter 1979).

Problems at home

Many children are able to dissociate themselves in school from disruption and turmoil at home, and find there a 'haven' in which they can thrive. More commonly, family disharmony may present in school life as aggressive behaviour, lack of work coupled with poor attainment, excessive anxiety or depression and withdrawal. Children who manifest emotional and behavioural problems are more likely to come to the attention of professionals, whereas those who come from difficult home circumstances but who thrive at school are less likely to be recognised. Violence at home, lack of continuity of parenting and rules, episodes of reception into care, many moves of house and school provide an unstable and unpredictable background from which it is difficult to make educational progress. Anxiety and aggressive feelings arising from the home situation are displayed in the school setting.

General approaches must include obtaining a full social history, seeing the child and family over a period of time, discussions with teachers with pastoral care responsibility, the primary health care team, clinical psychologists, child and family therapy services, education welfare officers and social workers. Notes often record the families as 'difficult to engage' which usually means they do not come to appointments and have a profound mistrust of the services, keeping us at arm's length.

Behavioural problems

School refusal

This is a fairly frequent problem encountered by the school health services. It is discussed more fully in Chapter 28. A wide range of contributory factors need to be explored including anxiety about separation from parents, relationships with other children, particular lessons, changing for PE or use of school toilets. An early return to school is essential before a pattern of non-attendance becomes too firmly established and before the continuity of school work and relationships is severely disrupted. Education welfare officers may be useful in these circumstances but are not employed by all UK schools.

Conduct disorders

Truancy from school and/or the presentation of behavioural problems within the classroom are a frequent cause for consultation between teachers and the school health team. The outcome may often be poor in terms of educational attainment and adjustment in adult life. The keys to management in school are a warm caring attitude, firm consistent discipline, counselling, stimulating lessons and improvements in self-image. Quality teaching and continuity of adult–child relationships are essential components. The school health team may become involved in a counselling role or because of wider associated health or family problems.

Depression

Depression is commonly seen in the upper age groups in the secondary school. It is often described as 'boredom' with general withdrawal and inactivity. The child may be very easily upset or cry for reasons that cannot be explained. Although this may be transient, it often coincides with times when there is increased pressure from examinations and the need to formulate plans for the future. Counselling is needed for some and a few suffer serious depression with suicidal thoughts. Exploration of the depth as well as possible causes always needs to be made.

Poor attention control

Children with a limited attention span, poor concentration and who fidget (hyperactivity) are going to have difficulty in the learning situation. They often have problems with impulsivity and no sense of danger. These children often perform worst at school where there are many distractions as compared to doing their homework one to one with a parent. Children who go unrecognised often tend to be punished for their inattention leading to a difficult cycle of negativity with potentially the child developing an aversion to the school environment. Underlying and associated problems include hearing difficulties, sleep difficulties, effects of medicines, solvent misuse, family difficulties, learning difficulties or neurological disorders, for example petit mal.

Solvent misuse

Solvent misuse often goes unrecognised. However, up to 14% of children admit to knowing someone who misuses drugs of some kind. Teachers may notice impairment of concentration, deterioration in behaviour with swings in mood. Solvent misuse may be suspected from the smell of the breath, spilt solvent on the clothes or a perioral rash. Management involves control of access, explanation of risk and exploration of underlying factors. Misuse of other substances should be considered in all children with unexplained behavioural problems.

Child abuse

Deterioration in schoolwork or change in behaviour may present as a feature of child abuse. Children with learning difficulties, particularly those from deprived backgrounds, are much more vulnerable to sexual abuse than other children (McCormack 1991).

Psychotic disorders

These are extremely uncommon, and perhaps as a consequence of their rarity are not correctly diagnosed for some time. For example, a secondary school girl's written work was described as 'lively and imaginative' without the recognition that her essay revealed elements of delusion and thought disorder. She fatally stabbed a teacher the following week.

Differences in culture

Cultural differences in outlook, behaviour and social norms as well as in clothing and language may cause difficulties in adjustment to the school environment. Children may 'adapt' by staying within their racial group or schools may recognise the diversity of their catchment population and modify their own institution to reflect the needs of the community. Conflicts can, however, develop between standards and patterns of behaviour expected at home and at school. Pupils may find that many of their peer group have different freedoms at home. In order to appreciate the importance of these issues, the teachers and school medical team need to acquire information about the cultural backgrounds of the families whose children attend the school. Useful sources of information are 'Asian Patients in Hospital and at Home'

(Henley 1979) and 'Child Health in a Multicultural Society' (Black 1990).

POOR SCHOOL PROGRESS

The following scheme is offered as a framework for the medical assessment of children who have been referred because of poor progress in class. The policy of mainstream integration and education has meant that many teachers are now responsible for children with complex health and psychological problems and learning difficulties not previously seen outside special schools. The success of the integration process depends on detailed knowledge of the child's strengths and difficulties and ways in which that child may be taught to achieve their potential in the community.

Poor educational achievement does not always indicate poor educational potential. However, where teachers' and educational psychologists' assessments indicate that one basis is limited intelligence rather than limited opportunity, the paediatrician has a role in its investigation. Errors, of course, can be made and the danger of a medical label that lowers expectations and changes expectations into self-fulfilling predictions must always be borne in mind. Parents may have differing views to those of teachers and psychologists and may have information on their child's strengths and areas of achievement that have not been observed in school, for example in elective mutism. The following questions should be asked.

Is there a specific condition or syndrome associated with handicap?

Fragile X would be an important example, affecting 1 in 10 of boys and 1 in 22 of girls with moderate learning difficulties. Diagnosis of specific conditions may be helped by the careful recording of a family tree and physical examination for dysmorphic features. Positive identification of a named condition will help in establishing a prognosis, alerts one to look for known associated impairments, provides an explanation for parents and teachers, gives access to medical literature on management and should indicate the often neglected need for genetic counselling. It is easy with such a diagnosis for the child to 'become the syndrome'.

The child is *an individual with the syndrome* and we need to remember the large range of individuality in appearance, personality and attainment.

Are there any events in the past medical history which may be the cause of handicap?

Some events may be relatively straightforward in providing an explanation, for example a history of congenital infection or head injury. In other cases, it may be much more difficult: for example birth asphyxia may be cited as a cause of cerebral palsy, whereas antenatal and genetic factors are much more likely, perinatal factors accounting for only 8% of cases (Hall 1989).

What is the difficulty? Is it general or specific in nature?

A detailed assessment of strengths and difficulties is needed to understand the child's abilities and how best to be able to assist the child to achieve his full potential. This is often most easily accomplished within the context of multidisciplinary teams including expert teachers, educational psychologists, clinical psychologists, speech and language therapists, occupational therapists, physiotherapists, paediatricians, audiologists and others.

Format of assessment and reports

A paediatric assessment may be carried out formally under the 1996 Education Act, as part of a full assessment in the child development centre or within a consultation or series of consultations in a paediatric clinic or at school. The consultation is dissimilar to most in paediatrics in that the results are intended for use by the education authority as well as for the parents and child. There should not usually be any conflict of interest here, but the paediatrician must be aware of the different nuances in a consultation where a child is seen at the request of the education authority rather than the parents. The parents must not feel sidelined in this situation and the philosophy should be to address the consultation and its findings to the parents first and to regard the transfer of information to the education authority as a secondary activity following full discussion with the parents and child. The child is the subject of this assessment and, like his parents, must feel in control and informed. Children are anxious about changes in their school, teacher or content of lessons, as these activities take up the major part of their waking life. They are aware of their successes and failures and of their achievements relative to their peers. The consultation must, therefore, focus on the child's strengths as well as his weaknesses. The approach, too often seen in the past, of listing 'defects' only serves to reinforce poor self-esteem. Lack of self-esteem is often an important factor in maintaining low levels of attainment. Until a child can feel good about himself, it is difficult for him to face school tasks with confidence.

Report

The report should be written in plain English as it is intended to be understood by parents and teachers. If medical terms are used, then they should be explained. The report starts with a description of the child. This must include strengths as well as weaknesses and relevant past medical history. The description of a medical condition must include an interpretation of the effects of that condition upon the child's daily life and activities at school, for example with regard to mobility, self-help, hearing in the classroom or ability to read normal size print. The need for medical management and follow-up at home and at school should be described in terms of medication, therapy (e.g. physiotherapy, speech therapy), aids, appliances and adaptations or special transportation to school. Advice from others, for example speech and language therapist or child psychiatrist, may be required to incorporate into the report or to be sent separately. Negative as well as positive findings must be included, for example normal vision and hearing. The report should be comprehensive, covering physical health, development, mobility, hearing, language, vision, behaviour, feelings, social skills, interests and accomplishments.

Bright children

Very intelligent children can make poor school progress if their special needs are unrecognised or unmet (Lobascher & Cavanagh 1977). In some instances, this may result from boredom because the educational programme is not sufficiently challenging. Others may present with psychosomatic symptoms, behavioural problems or feelings of isolation from their peer group. Some may have high levels of anxiety about failure and this may impair their ability to concentrate. Parental expectations may also be high and children may be put under great pressure resulting in a lifestyle that lacks a reasonable balance between utilising obvious talents and enjoying leisure pursuits. Children may derive from this situation high self-expectations in which it is not permissible to fail or be anything but best or top all the time. Management involves encouragement of relaxation and honest communication, and an acceptance of the child as a person unqualified by demands for success. Failure should explicitly be allowed so that the child does not have to convert such fears into physical symptoms or open revolt. A sense of humour is an asset to be treasured in an intelligent and serious mind, and can become an essential survival aid.

Clumsy children

Clumsy children are those showing difficulties in motor coordination which is more poorly developed than their other abilities (Gordon & McKinlay 1980). Various estimates of from 5% to 15% of school children have been made. Boys are affected more often than girls. The clumsiness may be associated with learning problems or with emotional problems. The latter may well be as much a reaction to how adults respond to their difficulties as to their own frustration. The label has become a popular one and should not hide children with specific neurological disorders such as cerebral palsy, cerebellar ataxia or lower motor neurone disorders. For this reason, a careful neurological examination should always be carried out. 'Clumsiness' is sometimes quite a difficult term for the paediatrician to understand as it represents the rare use of an ordinary English word to describe a medical 'condition'. In the Oxford Dictionary it means 'awkward in movement'; in medical literature, it becomes ennobled to 'a deficit in the acquisition of skills requiring fluent coordinated movement, not explicable by general retardation or demonstrable neurological disease'. Management has been described, perhaps unfairly, as finding out what the child cannot do, and then making him practice it over and over again.

Aetiology

Much of what is said about the aetiology of clumsiness is speculative. The children probably form the lower part of the normal distribution of gross and fine motor skills rather than having a discrete disorder (Hall 1988a). It may also represent a delay in achieving neuro-maturational skills. Genetic factors may also be important. It is, however, difficult to separate these out from environmental factors, in that parents with high degrees of fine and gross motor skills tend to provide opportunities and encouragement of their children to develop these skills from an early age. Some children go through a transient stage of clumsiness during periods of rapid growth such as in adolescence, when their perception of body image does not keep pace with changes in body size. Organic factors that are insufficient to cause gross neurological impairment may contribute towards later clumsiness, but it is difficult to provide convincing evidence for this in individual children.

Although clumsy children are frequently slow to develop laterality, the suggested association of handedness with neurological or perceptual deficits cannot be supported. Those 'left handers' who do have difficulties are usually those who have some dysfunction of the preferred side and hence transfer to the non-preferred side (Bishop 1983). Likewise, a number of 'right handers' have difficulty with functioning on the left and have hence transferred to the right. As the right-handed group is much larger than the left-handed group, incorrect conclusions can be drawn about the significance of left-handedness unless the function of the non-preferred hand is examined. Further examination of the phenomenon of crossed laterality (differences in the side of dominance of eye and hand) has established that this too is unimportant as a reason for poor gross motor or fine motor functioning.

Natural history

Anecdotal evidence suggests that clumsiness improves with maturation either during the first 2 years of schooling between 5 and 7 years of age or at adolescence. However, Losse et al (1991) in a follow-up study of children at age 15–17 years, who were first seen when they were six, found that the majority of children still had motor difficulties, poor self-concept and poor academic attainment.

Presentation

Clumsiness may present with difficulties or delays in developing self-help skills such as dressing. The child may have difficulty with fastening buttons or shoes, assembling a zip and some children may almost strangle themselves whilst attempting to put on or take off a jumper. The child may be very poor or untidy at feeding himself, either missing the target area of the mouth or being unable to capture the food on the plate with a spoon or transfer it to the mouth without spillage. In play, the child may have trouble with such materials as jigsaws, building blocks or with drawing. Climbing through a hoop may turn out to be an impossible task where the child is unable to work out the correct sequence of movements. Some children may present with the problem of frequent falls. Older children may be referred because of associated learning difficulties, particularly poor handwriting. Others will come to attention because of extremely poor performance in physical education. Such skills are important within their peer group and a noticeable lack of skill may result in social isolation. It is not unusual for emotional problems to be the main cause for referral. Improper understanding by teachers or parents may result in a child's difficulties being attributed to laziness or naughtiness, thus adding to the child's feeling of frustration.

Examination

There are standardised tests of motor performance, using scores based on activities such as pencil control, cutting with scissors, catching in one hand or balancing on a board, for example TOMI (Test of Motor Impairment — Stott et al 1984, Movement ABC — Leemrijse C et al 1999). However, for most clinical purposes, simple observation of appropriate tasks is usually adequate, followed by a detailed assessment by an occupational therapist and physiotherapist where there is a significant disability (Fig. 32.4).

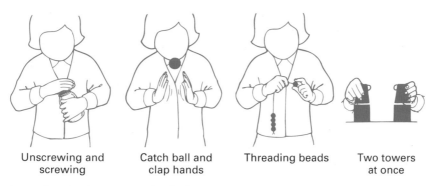

Unscrewing and   Catch ball and   Threading beads   Two towers
screwing   clap hands   at once

Fig. 32.4 Simple tests for school entrants to identify clumsiness

Fine motor skills

The clumsy child may have difficulty in building a tower of bricks, in repetitive fast tapping, pronation and supination movements or finger–thumb opposition sequences. The movements are jerky and imprecise. Drawing may be difficult and such exercises as tracing or colouring within lines may demonstrate the child's difficulties in classroom activities. Threading beads, a discipline which involves accurate eye–hand coordination, is a useful test. It should be remembered that repeated activities that focus on the child's difficulties may be a distressing experience and the child may 'refuse to cooperate'. Observation of the emotional reaction or interaction with parents is often as important as the motor difficulties themselves.

Gross motor skills

The child usually has problems with such exercises as standing on one leg, hopping, skipping, kicking a ball or heel–toe walking. Most 5 year olds should be proficient in these skills. In the older primary school child, the clap-catch test, in which the child is required to throw a ball into the air, clap the hands and then catch the ball, may be quite impossible. Walking on the lateral aspects of the feet is another useful test. Associated movements of the upper limbs as a sign of neuromaturation is seen normally in younger children, but persists after the age of ten in clumsy children.

Mouth coordination

The difficulties with motor coordination may sometimes be demonstrated in the muscles of the face. There may be difficulty with exercises such as blowing, whistling, tongue protrusion, licking, clenching the teeth or rapid in-and-out or side-to-side movements of the tongue.

Management

Management involves the practice of appropriate tasks in order to improve skills in those areas which the child finds difficult. These tasks start within their own level of ability so that confidence can be boosted and success ensured. Specific measures aimed at relieving tension or anxiety within the child or family may be needed. Remedial teaching at school and sympathetic encouragement may be required to help the child overcome associated learning difficulties. A detailed assessment by an occupational therapist, physiotherapist and educational psychologist will determine the level and nature of difficulty. Without this, a blind attempt at improving motor function may involve the child in attempting tasks which are quite impossible for him and where success, even if obtained, will not generalise into other areas such as writing. There are specific general programmes designed to assist children, which can be instituted within school PE sessions, for example perceptual motor programmes.

Activities may be centred around awareness of body image, for example drawing around the whole body, identifying parts, or in singing games, which involve imitation of posture or gesture. Other activities can introduce awareness of rhythm such as dance. Swimming may be useful to develop coordination, though confidence in the water is a

Learning and health

prerequisite. Eye–hand coordination can be developed through such activities as drawing, tracing and work with scissors. Practical training in self-help skills in eating and dressing is often useful. The development of skills often results in improvements in confidence and self-esteem. Sometimes the emotional problems need to be tackled in a more direct way when they block progress in other programmes or in schoolwork.

PROBLEMS WITH READING AND WRITING

In general, problems with reading and writing are the professional concern of teachers rather than doctors. However, medical, developmental or behavioural problems may be associated with learning difficulties and, in practice, it is important to identify or exclude these. It is also desirable for two professions who work exclusively with children to share some understanding of their work.

General reading difficulties

It is estimated that approximately two million adults in the UK, comprising 6% of the adult population, are illiterate. Twenty-five per cent of children leaving the infant school at age 7 have significant reading difficulties and 10% of those transferring to the secondary school at age 11 have persisting problems. In many, the problem is part of a general learning difficulty, which depresses achievement and understanding in all areas of the curriculum. In others, there is a specific difficulty confined to reading, with much better results in other areas. However, educational opinion is quite divided on the issue of whether within the spectrum of children with difficulty learning to read, there is a special group called specific reading difficulties or dyslexia, which is quite distinct from the rest. Dyslexia has different meanings to different groups of professionals and the child with reading problems needs a full assessment to define these difficulties and to enable understanding of the child's process of learning, thereby allowing appropriate assistance to be given. Reading difficulties are likely to give rise to parental anxiety and in the child loss of confidence, a sense of failure and emotional problems. Reading is an essential skill in most school subjects and many jobs in adult life (Box 32.2). A third of children with conduct disorders are described as having reading difficulties. Which is cause and which is effect may not always be clear; however the strong association is well recognised. It has been proposed that early identification of children with potential reading problems, coupled with appropriate teaching, will do much to prevent the establishment of these difficulties (Lansdown 1978).

Reading, writing and spelling problems are often related, but not rigidly so. Some children are able to read words which they cannot spell, and others can spell words which they are unable to read. Reading difficulties are more common in manual social classes and with ascending birth order. They are increased in schools with a high rate of teacher and pupil turnover. Unfortunately, these educational disadvantages often go together.

Assessment

Some reading tests, for example the Schonell Test, scores the ability to read individual words graded by difficulty. They are not tests of 'real' reading in that the words are presented as lists out of context. Speed in reading is obtained by scanning the text rather than by the recognition and interpretation of individual letters. The Neale Reading Test involves recording errors accumulated whilst reading a particular passage. A more detailed assessment may be required to understand higher order processing which may explain the difficulties.

Remedial help

Systems have been devised which concentrate upon the analysis of presumed basic problems, such as visuo-motor difficulties and the introduction of programmes designed to improve these skills. However, they often improve these 'underlying skills' but not reading. Early identification and individualised help are important, before secondary emotional and other problems become established. The teacher must gain the child's confidence and interest and the programme should be designed to achieve early success which is recognised and rewarded by parents and teachers.

> ### Box 32.2
> **Skills required for reading**
>
> - The ability to understand and use spoken language. A delay in speech and language development is often found in the history of children who are later found to have reading problems and may alert teachers to the need for careful early assessment of any difficulties
>
> - The ability to recognise visual symbols. Visuo-motor problems are regarded as much less significant than language in the causation of reading difficulties. However, the task of sorting out similar letters such as p's, b's, d's and q's, differentiating the m from the w and correctly orientating letters such as s may give rise to difficulties in writing as well as in reading. Children with visuo-spatial problems may also have sequencing difficulties. They may be unable to remember a telephone number or the order of the months of the year. They may have important spelling problems, having difficulty with the order of letters
>
> - They must have normal sound perception and discrimination. Children who have difficulties in reliably classifying speech sounds and in producing rhymes often go on to have reading problems (Bryant & Bradley 1985)
>
> - They must be able to relate written symbols to oral sounds and to relate words and spaces in print to words and phrases in speech
>
> - They require a well-established lateral preference. This does not mean that left handedness or crossed laterality causes problems in reading or writing, but confusion over laterality does. Children require a 'directional' approach to print in order to be able to read
>
> - Normal emotional development is needed. Defects in concentration, and impulsive behaviour are found more commonly among children who have difficulty in reading
>
> - They require normal memory

Specific reading difficulties

Specific reading retardation (sometimes called dyslexia) occurs in some 4–10% of junior school children. This term defines those children whose reading problems cannot be explained by low intellect. The term 'dyslexia' is a descriptive term for children with specific reading difficulty: it is not a 'disease' for which one can imply a common aetiology and regarding it in the framework of a medical model is generally regarded as unhelpful. It is more commonly seen in boys (ratio of 3 or 4 to 1) and there are frequently others in the family with reading problems. Language difficulty is frequently found at earlier stages of development. The children may also have trouble with writing and sometimes arithmetic. Many features of their writing simply resemble those of younger children, such as reversal of pqbd, but others are quite different as shown in bizarre spelling or mirror writing (Fig. 32.5). Left/right confusion (which is distinct from crossed laterality) is common and the children show difficulty in sequencing from left to right, this

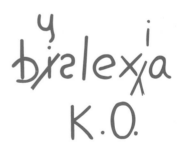

Fig. 32.5 Example of dyslexia

being a necessary skill for reading and writing in English. The sequencing difficulties affect order as well as direction, producing difficulties in memorising tables or other sequences such as the days of the week. Handwriting is often very poor and becomes even more untidy through alterations and indecision. Misuse of grammar is also seen.

Secondary problems may arise if the child's intrinsic reading difficulties are not appreciated. Pressure, criticism or even punishment may be applied when an obviously intelligent child is failing to progress as expected. The child's reaction may set up emotional barriers, which may themselves present formidable barriers to progress.

Aetiology

A large amount of educational and psychological research has been carried out on the complex skill of reading and on children with reading difficulties. The result has been a series of associations, the most important of which is with language problems, but it has not been possible to isolate factors that can be successfully harnessed into a remedial programme. For example, visual problems were thought to be important and children were treated with tinted lenses or monocular occlusion, however the claims of benefit from this form of management have not been substantiated (Hall 1988b).

There may be coding/decoding difficulties, but this perhaps represents a description of the problem rather than a formulation of a cause. Neurological causes have been proposed particularly with regard to left or right cerebral hemisphere location of function. Visuo-perceptual problems have been proposed because of the incorrect orientation of the letters p, b, q, d, though this is a normal feature of younger children. The ability to retrieve visual or auditory information from the short-term memory may be lacking. Others have stressed the importance of integration of senses, vision, fine touch and spatial awareness. These facets need to be understood in children with any specific learning difficulty.

Management

Management of complex problems of reading difficulties is clearly the role of the teacher and advice given by the paediatrician through ignorance is not likely to be warmly received. All approaches depend upon detailed analysis of the child's individual ability and difficulties rather than in broad terms, which may have different meanings for different people. They build upon the child's strengths and use these to develop those areas where difficulty exists. It is often necessary to begin with tasks that he can be expected to achieve. This is impor-

tant, as many children have lost confidence by the time that they start to receive extra help. They need to find again the pleasure that reading and writing can give. Detection and intervention at the earliest stages of learning to read may prevent greater problems developing. This model of secondary prevention certainly fits with the professional strategies of community paediatrics.

REFERENCES AND FURTHER READING

Bishop D V M 1983 How sinister is sinstrality? Journal of the Royal College of Physicians 17:161–171

Biser C, Zoum C 1987 Teachers concerns about chronically sick children: implications for Paediatricians. Child Neurology 29:56–63

Black J 1990 Child health in a multicultural society. BMJ Books, London

Bolton A 1997 Losing the thread, pupils' and parents' voices about education for sick children. National Association for the Education of Sick Children, London

Bryant P E, Bradley L 1985 Children's reading problems. Blackwell Scientific, Oxford

Gordon N, McKinlay I 1980 Helping clumsy children. Churchill Livingstone, Edinburgh

Grantham-MacGregor S M, Powell C A, Walker S P, Himes J H 1991 Nutritional supplementation and mental development of stunted children: the Jamaican study. Lancet 338:1–5

Hall D M B 1988a Clumsy children. British Medical Journal 296:375–376

Hall D M B 1989 Birth asphyxia and cerebral palsy. British Medical Journal 299:279–282

Hall M 1988b Dyslexia. Not one condition but many. British Medical Journal 297:501–502

Haslam M, Morris A, Golding J 1984 What do our ten year old children eat? Health Visitor 57:178–179

Henley A 1979 Asian patients at home and at hospital. The King's Fund, London

Idjradinta P, Pollitt E 1993 Reversal of developmental delays in iron-deficient anaemic infants treated with iron. Lancet 341:1–4

Lamont M A, Dennis N R 1988 Aetiology of mild mental retardation. Archives of Disease in Childhood 63:1032–1038

Lansdown R 1978 The learning-disabled child: early detection and prevention. Developmental Medicine and Child Neurology 20:496–497

Larcombe I 1995 Reintegration into School after Hospital Treatment. Aldershot, Avebury

Leemrijse C, Meijer O G, Vermeer A, Lambregts B, Alder H J 1999 Detecting the individual change in children with mild to moderate motor impairment: the standard error of measurement of the movement ABC. Clinical Rehabilitation 13:420–429

Lightfoot J, et al 2001 Supporting Pupils with special

health needs in mainstream schools: policy and practice. Children Advisor 15:57–69

Lobascher M E, Cavanagh N P C 1977 The other handicap: brightness. British Medical Journal 2:1269–1271

Losse A, Henderson S, Elliman D, Hall D, Knight E, Jongmans M 1991 Clumsiness in children — do they grow out of it? A 10 year follow-up study. Developmental Medicine and Child Neurology 33:55–68

Lozoff B, Jimenez E, Hagen J, Mollen E, Wolf A 2000 Poorer behavioral and developmental outcome more than 10 years after treatment for iron deficiency in infancy. Pediatrics Electronic Pages 105(4) (Part 1 of 2):852

McCormack B 1991 Sexual abuse and learning difficulties. British Medical Journal 303:143–144

National Dairy Council 1981 Nothing for breakfast. Taylor Nelson, London

Rutter M 1979 The long-term effects of early experience. Developmental Medicine and Child Neurology 22:800–815

Stott D H, Moyess F A, Henderson S E 1984 The Henderson revision of the test of motor impairment. Psychological Corporation, San Antonio, Texas

Wedge P, Essen J 1982 Children in adversity. Pan Books, London

Wedge P, Prosser J 1973 Born to fail? Arrow Books, London

33 | Vision

Vision is a complex process involving the interpretation of images received by the brain, transmitted via visual pathways and sent on by the optic nerve from the back of the eye. There are therefore numerous lesions which may affect the final image seen, problems with the eye itself, lesions of the visual pathways or visual cortex lesions.

DEFINITIONS

A child with a visual impairment has corrected vision sufficiently abnormal to interfere with development or to have ongoing educational implications; in cases where visual acuity can be measured and is relevant this equates to a visual acuity of 6/18 (Snellen) or worse in the better eye.

The definition recognises that some children are difficult to assess because of motor impairment or severe learning difficulties. In this group measurement of distance visual acuity is a challenge.

Registration of children as blind or partially sighted is not a reliable guide to severity as some families may choose not to have their children registered, or because the ophthalmologist has not wished to raise the issue of registration.

Recently, a working party looking at definitions of disability has further detailed the degrees of visual impairment into mild, moderate and severe (Table 33.1). Where it is possible to measure, visual acuity is the gold standard for defining visual loss and also has the benefit of being more easily understood by professionals. However it is essential to recognise that visual field defects alone can have disabling effects on vision without central visual acuity being severely affected.

INCIDENCE OF VISUAL IMPAIRMENT

The global picture

Of the 30 million blind people in the world, 6 million live in Africa, 20 million live in Asia and nearly 2 million live in Latin America. The prevalence of blindness increases with age in all parts of the world, with the risk of blindness in people over the age of 60 years being 20–100 times that of children (Fig. 33.1).

Causes of visual loss in childhood depend upon the place of birth. In the developing world there are over a million blind children due to measles infection and subsequent vitamin A deficiency. The figures would be higher but up to 75% of blinded children die within a few months of the measles infection from secondary respiratory infections or the malnutrition associated with the vitamin A deficiency (Fig. 33.2).

Vitamin A deficiency

Breast feeding is protective against vitamin A deficiency; those babies not breast fed in Asian countries have a sixfold increased risk of blindness following measles. Infant feeding practices are also very important. In some of the Asian high-risk countries, children lose their sight even though locally available foods containing vitamin A could have saved them. Vitamin A is obtained from two sources: the first source is fat-soluble vitamin A in milk, eggs, butter and fish liver oils; the second source is as the precursor betacarotene in dark green leafy vegetables, red palm oil, and in red- or orange-coloured fruits such as mango, papaya, carrots and sweet potato. Community interventions

Table 33.1
Definitions of visual impairment (British Association for Community Child Health and the Department of Health 1994): these codings depend upon the child's ability to function independently, the use of aids, educational needs or visual acuity

Code	Function
Mild	Able to function independently VA 6/6–6/18 corrected in better eye Severe or profound problem with one eye only, other eye normal Partial or less visual field loss
Moderate	Enough awareness for normal mobility Able to read print with simple aids and/or educational assistance VA6/24–6/36 in better eye Defect in at least half visual field VA may be normal May be eligible as partially sighted
Severe	Mobility restricted without special provision Unable to read large print without educational assistance or sophisticated aids VA 6/60–3/60 in the better eye Severe visual field defect with impaired visual acuity Eligible for registration as blind or partially sighted
Profound	Mobility restricted without special provision Requires education by non-sighted methods Very little useful vision VA <3/60, i.e. counting fingers, hand movements, light perception or less Eligible for registration as blind
VA = visual acuity	

that have been proposed to prevent vitamin A blindness are to educate parents to provide a diet rich in vitamin A or betacarotene. Home growing of foods or local cooperatives may be encouraged where suitable food is not available locally. Other interventions are to provide expensive vitamin A supplements or to fortify the staple foodstuffs within a country. The last strategy has been shown to be successful, however it is difficult to maintain in the long term.

Cataract

The second major cause of childhood blindness in developing countries is cataract, due to prenatal infections or postnatal acquired causes such as malnutrition, measles and herpes simplex infections or bacterial infections. Blindness due to cataract is curable but is dependent upon early surgery. Therefore reduction in the numbers of children affected worldwide depends upon the availability of eye services.

Infectious causes of blindness

River blindness (onchocerciasis) is now treatable with ivermectin. Trachoma infection is still causing blindness; this infection starts in childhood as a chronic infection that gradually scars the eyes during life leading eventually to blindness. It is treatable with tetracycline eye ointment.

The challenges for countries with poorly developed health services are to finance the drugs, to diagnose the conditions and to distribute the treatments. Health promotion also has an important role in reducing infections that may lead to poor vision.

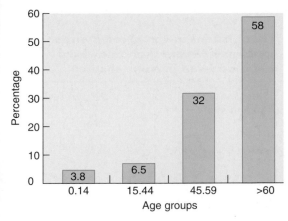

Fig. 33.1 Global distribution of blindness by age

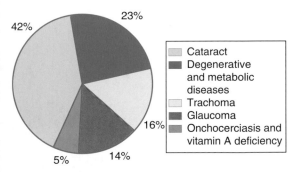

Fig. 33.2 Major causes of bilateral blindness in children in developing countries. From Thylefors et al (1995)

Genetic causes are accountable for relatively few cases of blindness in these populations.

The UK picture

Accurate prevalence figures for childhood visual impairment in the UK have been difficult to obtain because of the variability in definitions used in the past and the problems of assessing multiply disabled youngsters. Blindness registration statistics have been found to be seriously underreported; Goggin & O'Keefe (1992), in their community survey in the Republic of Ireland, found that 108 out of 172 blind children had not been registered.

A distinction must be drawn between mild visual defects and more severe ones that have a greater impact on development. It has been estimated that 9% of 4 year olds have a visual deficit (Kohler & Stigmar 1973). An Oxford study in 1978–79 found that 4% of children have a manifest squint, 3% a refractive error and 1% a latent squint. Hence mild visual problems are common.

By contrast, severe visual impairment is a condition with a low incidence. An estimated prevalence of severe visual impairment (blind vision <3/60 in the better eye) is 1.5 per 10 000 children, 0–15 years old.

Low vision <6/18 in the better eye is even more difficult to estimate accurately as more children are being identified within the multiply disabled group. A survey of a special school for children with profound disabilities within Salford (K M Holt & S A Cannor, unpublished data, 1995) found that about 66% had some form of visual deficit. Although the visual loss was not the main disability affecting the child, it still had implications for learning. Recognition can be very helpful in the development of an individual educational programme.

Michael Rogers looked at the prevalence of visual impairment in Liverpool and found an estimated prevalence of both low vision and severe visual impairment of 18.1 per 10 000 population aged 0–15 years (approx. 2 per 1000) (Rogers 1996). This is an important figure to guide the development of services, as vision below a level of 6/18 is likely to impact upon development and learning. Rogers found a figure of 3–4 per 10 000 for severe visual impairment.

THE AETIOLOGY OF SEVERE VISUAL IMPAIRMENT IN THE UK

When referrals to district disability teams are analysed, there appear to be two groups of children with moderate to severe visual problems. Approximately one-third of children fall into a group labelled uncomplicated visual impairment (Fig. 33.3). Two-thirds have visual impairment with additional pathology.

Two-thirds of children with uncomplicated visual impairment have a genetic cause (Table 33.2). There is a constant trend during this century away from infectious causes towards genetic and acquired causes. The prevention of blindness in

Vision

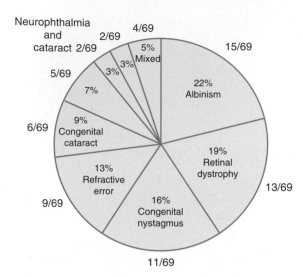

Fig. 33.3 Causes of uncomplicated visual impairment in 69 children: Liverpool data. From Rogers (1996)

Table 33.2 **Visual lesions in complicated visual impairment: more than one visual lesion occurred in some children.**		
Cortical visual impairment	**Visual lesion**	
	No.	**%**
Nystagmus	29	22
Refractive error	28	22
Optic atrophy	27	21
Squint	23	18
Visual field defect	13	10
Retinopathy	6	5
Cataract	6	5
Amblyopia	5	4
Retinopathy of prematurity	5	4
Optic nerve hypoplasia	4	3
Tumour	4	3
Anophthalmia/microphthalmia	3	2
Ptosis	3	2
Coloboma	2	1.5
Various	4	3
From Rogers (1996)		

this country partly depends upon genetic counselling wherever there is a known risk to a family or by antenatal diagnostic testing where testing is possible.

About half of all visually impaired children have learning difficulties. About half of all visually impaired children have multiple disabilities. Children with cerebral palsy commonly have a visual deficit and a number of these will also have seizures. Where a cortical lesion is the underlying cause of the physical impairment a degree of cortical visual impairment may also be present (Table 33.3).

Cortical visual impairment

Cortical visual impairment is now the commonest cause of visual disability in the UK. The commonest cause is perinatal hypoxia/ischaemia. Congenital infections, congenital cerebral defects and hydrocephalus also occur frequently. All of the cortically visually impaired group in Rogers' study had at least one additional impairment, some as many as four or five (Rogers 1996). Most will have a leaning difficulty. Some children will have evidence of a deficit in the anterior visual pathway, for example retinopathy of prematurity.

There are no eye signs in a child with cortical visual impairment. The eyes appear normal, the pupil responses are normal and examination of the retina is normal, unless there is additional anterior pathology.

Commonly the child may appear to have fluctuations in visual perception; the child may respond better to brightly coloured toys than to black and white ones. The peripheral visual field may be better preserved as this is represented in the anterior part of the visual cortex. It may be noticed that the child turns his head to look at something with

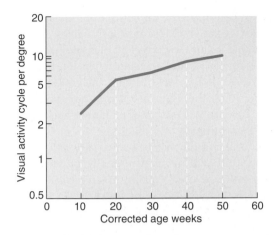

Fig. 33.4 The development of visual acuity as measured using preferential looking (mean values). From Atkinson & Hof-van Duin (1993)

Table 33.3 **Causes of severe visual impairment: Oxford register of early childhood impairment 1998.**	
Impairment	% a moderately to severely visually impaired cohort 1984–88, 0–4 years
Cortical visual impairment	36
Optic atrophy	5
Cataract	22
Nystagmus	13
Retinal dystrophy	14
Retinopathy of prematurity	6
After Crofts et al (1998)	

side vision. Neuroimaging may reveal infarction of the cortex, hydrocephalus or periventricular leucomalacia. The visual prognosis is variable: there can be considerable improvement in vision in the early years; the prognosis is poorest where there is periventricular leucomalacia.

Retinopathy of prematurity

Progressive retinopathy of prematurity can lead to blindness. The incidence has been declining with improved perinatal care, but there are still cases that arise. Originally it was believed that the cause of retinopathy of prematurity (ROP) was high oxygen concentrations administered in the neonatal period; however it is now thought to be multifactorial in origin.

The onset of retinopathy is most likely between the gestational ages 28 and 45 weeks. Infants below 28 weeks are rarely affected. ROP is unusual in babies with a birthweight higher than 1500 g. ROP is unlikely where inspired oxygen does not exceed a concentration of 40%. Other associated risk factors for ROP include twin pregnancies, high CO_2 concentrations, intraventricular haemorrhage, repeated bradycardias, recurrent apnoeas, respiratory distress syndrome, relative vitamin E deficiency and exchange transfusions.

Genetic causes of severe visual impairment

There are numerous inherited causes of visual impairment. Where vision is the prime impairment, the defect may lie in the lens, retina, optic nerve or visual cortex. The exact cause can take a long time to diagnose and investigation includes electrophysiological testing and detailed eye examination. Consultation with a neurologist and geneticist is often necessary.

NORMAL VISUAL DEVELOPMENT

The visual systems of the newborn infant are not like the adult. Both the eye and the neural pathways undergo anatomical and physiological changes during the early years. Using preferential looking techniques it is possible to measure visual acuity in babies and this research has shown that there is rapid development of visual acuity during the first year, due to maturation in the visual pathways (Fig. 33.4). Clinically paediatricians assess the visual acuity using behavioural assessments of vision.

In the newborn visual attention can be assessed when the child is in an alert and quiet state. Babies will usually fixate on an object from the age of 33 weeks' gestation. Most newborn babies fix their gaze and follow an object if it is moved slowly horizontally. Vertical tracking is usually first seen between 4 and 8 weeks of age. The easiest way to demonstrate this is to use a red 'pom-pom' suspended in front of the baby and moved horizontally and then vertically.

Binocular vision may be seen as early as 2 months of age and will develop normally provided that both eyes are used equally to give clear images that are aligned and can be fused. In the newborn the attention of the infant is held mainly within a short distance of around 20 cm from the child's face. During development, the child becomes aware of the wider and wider sphere of visual material being extended to around 1 m at four months and 2 m at 5 months. In order to do this the eyes must develop the abilities of accommodation and convergence by which visual information is taken in at an increasing variety of distances. Growth of the eye will result in changes in the refractive properties of the eye and hence there needs to be a continuum of adjustment in the control of the eyes if normal vision is to be maintained. Adult colour vision is probably obtained by the age of 5 months.

Clinical aspects of visual development

During the first year of life the baby is observed to develop visually directed behaviour if the visual system is intact. In the first year of life concerns about visual impairment will arise where visual behaviour is abnormal, and paediatric assessment will include tests of visual behaviour.

Table 33.4 shows the development of visually directed behaviour.

Clinical signs of severe visual impairment

- Visual behaviour is delayed.
- Pupil examination — pupil reactivity:
  - sluggish may reflect an anterior visual pathway defect
  - normal may be a posterior pathway defect.
- Nystagmus:
  - if present will probably indicate vision loss, but not necessarily so.
- Ophthalmoscopic examination:
  - careful inspection using a 3+ lens from a distance of 10 cm should detect a cataract as a silhouette against the red reflex.

Table 33.4
Development of visually directed behaviour

Looks at face	0–6 weeks begins
Follows large objects to midline	2 weeks to 2 months
Follows large objects beyond midiline	2–3 months
Follows large objects over 180 degrees	3–5 months
Fixates on small sized objects	4–6 months
Takes small sized objects	6–7 months
Grasps small sized objects	8 months onwards
Note: Tests of early visual behaviour are crude and only exclude severe visual impairment	

NOTE: Any parental concerns about delayed visual development needs urgent referral to an ophthalmologist as early diagnosis and treatment may significantly improve the visual outcome.

THE IMPACT OF SEVERE VISUAL LOSS UPON DEVELOPMENT

Vision has a coordinating role in early development. It can be helpful to think about early development as occurring in two phases: the global and the integrative phase.

The global phase

The global phase spans the first 4 months during which the baby becomes aware of 'self'. A baby's interest in the surrounding world becomes awakened. This is usually a very visual phase. Newborns are unable to reach out or move towards objects, hence they need to use their senses in order to begin to understand the environment. Early interaction with caregivers is visual. Positive feedback from caregivers motivates a baby to learn more; this is called drive. Healthy babies develop an inner drive to learn. Visual drive is very important for the development of motor skills. Parents play a key role in facilitating this phase of development. Parents are saddened and can find it difficult to interact with a visually impaired baby; blind babies are characteristically passive, and may be alarmed and cry when handled and cuddled because of their difficulty in knowing what is happening about them. When a sighted baby is held by his mother he will gaze up at her face, encouraging her to look back and to develop a strong bond with the baby. Smiles gradually emerge and the beginnings of turn taking in communication. A blind baby gives no feedback to the mother, in terms of eye contact or smiles, and the interaction between mother and baby can become non-communicative episodes of feeding and changing without the warmth that usually develops between mothers and their newborn infants. This early phase needs to be helped along by developmental counselling and emotional support to the parents. Hence blind babies can fail to develop 'drive', it is a developmental emergency.

If a blind baby's motivation to learn is not awakened by a few months of age, then subsequently it can be a struggle to awaken it at a later stage.

During the global phase a baby will learn about himself; he will learn that he has hands and arms, that they exist in space. Seeing babies start to use their hands by about 10 to 11 weeks of age, initially for grasping and then for transferring objects, at 20–24 weeks.

In order to grasp and reach, the baby must perceive the need to do so. Both blind and partially sighted children can lag behind the seeing children in the development of fine motor skills. Fraiberg (1968) found that at 22 weeks of age his study group only showed chance midline hand encounters and no coordinated hand activity until some months later. Norris et al (1957) found that at 24 weeks, less than half of visually impaired babies were able to transfer but by 36 weeks, 75% were transferring. However they were looking at an ex-preterm group of babies, many of whom if their age was corrected for gestation would have been demonstrating normal age-appropriate hand function. Reaching for objects is another developmental stage which can be delayed. The data on this is mixed. It is suggested that visually impaired babies with some light perception are at an advantage to those with none. Therefore with a visually impaired baby each developmental skill needs to be assessed individually; where it does not exist the aim is to promote the skill.

The integrative phase

The integrative phase is concerned with bringing together the senses and motor skills. It can be summarised as 'How I work', and 'How the world works'. Vision acts as a tutor of the other senses, enabling the baby to learn about the permanence of objects, locating sound, the nature of objects, and the relationships of people and objects within the environment. A seeing baby will use his vision to locate the position of an object and then move to collect it. If the baby hears a noise it will turn to see what it is or to confirm what it is and then move towards it. This emphasises the integration of the senses with motor development. As described above a blind baby will not automatically realise that his hands are there, that objects can be transferred between them and that he can reach out to grasp objects; all this needs to be taught. Normally by 5 months auditory and visual impulses have been integrated, so that a sound becomes to mean an object or person; integration takes a lot longer in a visually impaired child. A seeing baby on hearing a rattle will turn to see it, then may reach out for it, realising that he has the capacity to grasp the object. In a blind baby the noise will have no meaning until someone has taken his hand to the noise and demonstrated what the rattle is. Environmental noises similarly will have no meaning for a blind baby until he has been shown or at a later age explained to. Doors banging, dogs barking, the telephone are all noises that a seeing baby would be able to make some sense of using vision. Not so the blind baby. Hence this phase of development generally needs some facilitation by the caregivers of a blind baby.

Specific developmental skills

Language development

There are qualitative differences between totally blind children's language development and that of sighted children. There are two ways language development may occur. Firstly some blind children are expressive ahead of their sighted counterparts and ahead of their comprehension of language. When words start to represent true object labels, the blind children start to lag behind. The other group of blind children is delayed in expressive language in relation to their sighted counterparts; the first clear words may not emerge until 2 years. The developmental outcome for this group of children is mixed. Within this group there are some children who later turn out to have learning difficulties.

Gross motor development

Gross motor development describes the beginnings of movement of a baby in relation to his environment. The development of movement depends upon muscular effort not being motivated by visual stimulation or attraction so that the onset of crawling and walking will be delayed even when physi-

cal development is normal. Children move in order to achieve a goal. Sighted babies walk at a mean age of 13 months; there is evidence to show that visually impaired babies begin to walk at a mean age of 15.3 months (range 11.5–19 months). Some blind babies can learn to move as early as their sighted counterparts, so there are clearly numerous variables involved in this stage of development. The recurring problem with the study of a series of visually impaired babies is that they form a heterogeneous group — some are ex-preterm babies; many have additional disabilities which may only come to light with ongoing assessment.

Cognitive development

There is little information about early cognitive development in the visually impaired. Tests of cognitive function often involve visually based tasks, clearly more of a challenge for the visually impaired. What can be said is that it is possible for visually impaired children with no additional disabilities to achieve high academic standards — GCSE, A level and university. Along the way there are many obstacles and challenges which can be overcome where emotional, educational and community support is maximal.

Social and emotional development

The family is a social unit where children spend most of their early years and therefore the parenting style and relationships that exist within the unit are going to impact upon the developing child. The existence of some vision may be partially protective. If there are severe or multiple disabilities and neurological abnormalities the outlook is poorer. Where parents have adjusted well to the visual impairment and allow learning experiences for their child, this allows the child to develop autonomy. There is a risk that a blind baby can become passive; being fed rather than feeding himself, being poorly motivated to explore or becoming trapped within an understimulating environment. Where parents have an inability to accept the visual impairment this will impede the child's development because of the lack of appropriate responses by the family. Parents can be helped by providing emotional support during the early years. If parents are well supported then they will be more likely to be able to offer emotional support and advice to their children. Redhill Royal National Institute for the Blind, (RNIB) College studied a group of visually impaired young adults and found that many do have problems with self-esteem; however it is possible for visually impaired young people to adjust well.

Problem behaviours

Specific behaviours that can develop in visually impaired children, such as stereotypies, occur where the child remains internalised and lacking in drive. Developmental arrest can occur following a period of encouraging development during the second year of life. There may be an association with emotionally stressful family or health related episodes. The second year is a vulnerable time for a visually impaired child.

COORDINATING SERVICES FOR CHILDREN WITH VISUAL IMPAIRMENT

Each child is unique and the level of support required to develop their individual abilities and care for their medical needs depends upon the severity and combination of these additional impairments.

Professionals who will need to be involved early on with a visually impaired child are: ophthalmologist, developmental paediatrician with experience of visual impairment, specialist teacher for the visually impaired and a representative from a local support group coordinating with social services (Fig. 33.5). Paediatric neurologists, geneticists, therapists and health visitors may also have an important role depending upon the individual child's needs. As many of these children have multiple disabilities it seems appropriate that their assessment and follow-up should be based within a district's developmental services. These vary but may often include a child development team. The RNIB, in a policy document about children's services, emphasised the need for children's services to promote equal opportunities. For a service to do this, they need to have a clear understanding about the impact of disability on the child and family. The impact is unique to each family; a pre-prescribed package of care will not suit all. Within the system there needs to be flexibility. Some families will need

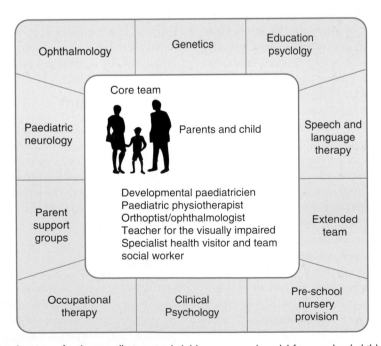

Fig. 33.5 Coordinated services for the visually impaired child — proposed model for preschool children

regular home visiting by the teachers early on, others will find that intrusive. Joint assessment and care planning in partnership with the family is an ideal that child development teams increasingly aspire to. Continuity of care is highly appreciated by the families and important for team learning.

The author's experience of working within a team of professionals dedicated to the care of pre-school visually impaired children was evaluated (I A McKinlay & R Moody, unpublished, 1997). Parents reported a high degree of satisfaction with the team. At one visit the family would meet with a specialist teacher, paediatrician, orthoptist and, if relevant, a physiotherapist. Joint assessment and care planning prevented unnecessary duplication. Some joint working took place within the family home; concerns raised by the teachers were quickly responded to by the team. Joint working also allows for discussion of challenging problems, such as developmental arrest where one person is unlikely to have the answers or where solutions lie in the interagency arena. The paediatrician provides an overview of the child's health and development. Associated disabilities may only gradually become apparent and the paediatrician will have to share this with parents and arrange any necessary further investigations or opinions. In relation to emotional support for the parents, the teachers and therapists were present at the time of disclosure of the disabilities and were able to repeat what was said or come back to other team members for further clarification. Representatives from parent support groups can be contacted if necessary. The orthoptist was able to carry out a detailed visual assessment and also have a direct contact with the ophthalmologist where necessary. The physiotherapist was very useful in the early evaluation of co-existing physical disabilities and in the planning of the intervention programme. Teachers for the visually impaired are responsible for the facilitation of early development and promotion of residual vision. They also have a liaison role with education, facilitating the educational placements of the children in schools best suited to their needs. In totally blind children the early intervention will also consider the tactile skills necessary for learning Braille.

Education of a visually impaired child

The education of a visually impaired child needs to take proper account of the abilities and disabilities of each individual. Educational planning should occur in partnership with parents and seamlessly follow on from the early assessments. Increasingly children of all abilities are being educated within their local schools with resources gradually shifting from the special school sector into local schools, a policy supported by the RNIB. There needs to be ongoing support for visually impaired children in school from the specialist teachers. Access to the curriculum may only be possible with the use of low-vision aids, magnification of the written word, individual support for the child and mobility training. In the school-aged child the lead comes from education but there can be ongoing medical and social needs that need addressing and close co-operation between the agencies will ensure that all the needs are met.

SQUINTS, AMBLYOPIA AND REFRACTIVE ERRORS

Mild visual problems are common. Nine percent of 4 year olds are estimated to have less than perfect vision, 4% have a manifest squint, 1% a latent squint and 3% a refractive error.

Manifest squint

A manifest squint occurs when one or other of the visual axes is not directed towards the fixation point. The presence of a manifest squint can lead to suppression of the image from the squinting eye. The brain will ignore the image from the squinting eye to prevent seeing double. If this persists then amblyopia will develop.

Amblyopia

Amblyopia is the commonest visual disability affecting the UK population, estimated as 2–5% of the population. It is defined as a reduction in the visual acuity measured using a Snellen chart or equivalent of one or more lines, in the absence of any ocular pathology or refractive error. Where a refractive error is responsible for a squint then the management would be to prescribe corrective glasses and not to patch. The natural history of amblyopia and the merits of treatment remain controversial, with some workers highlighting the psychological ill effects of patching and others claiming therapeutic success.

Development of binocular vision

Binocular vision gives the advantage of distance judgement and the slightly enlarged visual field. In order for this to develop three criteria must be met: both eyes must be looking at the same object; both images must be clear; and the brain must be able to join these images to produce one visual impression (sensory fusion). From around 6 weeks of age the eyes begin to fix on the same object and normal binocular vision can be established. If the eyes are not both fixated at the same point then a double image will result. However, feedback of the double image will cause the extraocular muscles to realign and hence fuse again into a single image. This process is called motor fusion and the range of angles over which it is possible to maintain normal binocular function is called the fusion range. If the tendency for the eyes to turn out of alignment is greater than the central nervous system's ability to control it, then a squint will develop. Thus the tendency for an eye to turn in becomes a convergent squint (esotropia). If the tendency for the eye to turn can be controlled by motor fusion then there is a latent squint; if it cannot, then a manifest squint will occur.

Causes of manifest squint

This is a congenital inability to fuse the images from both eyes — often seen in children with a family history of squint. Children with congenital squints do not develop normal binocular function even with optimal treatment.

Opacities or a unilateral refractive error lead to a blurred image in one eye, because the information from this eye is not clear the brain finds it difficult to know where to point the eye and as a result the eye often becomes convergent. Hence one may often see convergent eyes in severely visually impaired children because the blind eye is not providing sufficient information to the brain.

In other children there are abnormalities in the control mechanism for the extraocular muscles by the cranial nerves, resulting in their inability to move together within the exacting limits required for fusion. Neurogenic lesions account for the majority of palsies, with the sixth, fourth and third cranial nerves being affected. Most congenital palsies occur in children who are otherwise healthy but there can be associations with severe developmental deficits. Acquired nerve palsies can affect the nerve anywhere along its course. Paralytic squints due to mechanical restriction are caused by factors that interfere with muscle contraction or relaxation or otherwise prevent free movement of the globe. Myogenic palsies are those which directly affect the muscles but these are rare in children.

Hypermetropia (longsight) is the commonest cause of an acquired squint. Children with unequal refraction in the two eyes (anisometropia) do not always develop a squint and may appear to have two normal eyes. However on testing the eyes separately it is found that one eye is weaker than the other but has become amblyopic.

Latent squint

A latent squint is one which is not apparent until the cover test reveals it.

Ocular motor examination

Assessment of ocular alignment in primary gaze is the first step in examining the ocular motor system. In babies this may be done by looking at the corneal light reflex and checking for symmetry. The cover test allows for a more accurate test of ocular alignment (Fig. 33.6). Orthoptists are also trained to carry out more specialist tests of ocular alignment such as the 4D base-out prism test.

Management of squint

The aim of treatment of squint is to prevent amblyopia. The mainstay of treatment is occlusion of the

Vision

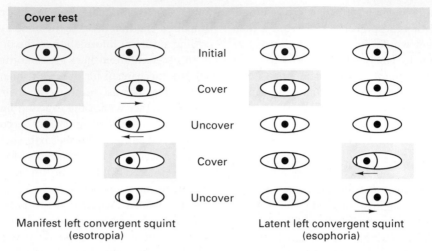

Fig. 33.6 The cover test

non-squinting eye which forces the squinting eye to fixate. However the treatment can be difficult as some children resist occlusion. There is disagreement about the effectiveness of treatments, fuelling the debate on vision screening and the potential to prevent amblyopia. If the cause of squint results from a refractive error then glasses may be all that is necessary. Surgery may be necessary in some children for cosmetic reasons.

Acceptance of glasses

Children frequently do not wear the glasses that have been prescribed for them. A few of these may have been prescribed for minor defects but there are still a significant group of children for whom the wearing of spectacles for near or distant work is important. In these cases close cooperation from doctors, parents, teachers and the children themselves is required. Attempts at educating all children about the value of spectacles will probably be more successful than putting pressure on individual children.

Abnormalities of refraction

Hypermetropia

In hypermetropia the eyeball is slightly shorter than normal so that parallel rays of light are brought

to focus behind the retina (Fig. 33.7). This is the normal state in the infant and diminishes with growth. Minor degrees are overcome by the normal powers of accommodation but difficulty will be experienced in more pronounced cases when distance vision is tested. In severe hypermetropia, near vision is usually quite good though the child may need to bring his eye very close to the object he is looking at. Distant vision is impaired. Hypermetropia may produce frontal headache or convergent squint. It may be associated with astigmatism. It is treated with glasses using convex lenses to aid convergence of the light source.

Myopia

In myopia the eye is marginally too long and parallel rays of light are brought to focus in front of the retina (Fig. 33.7). The myopic child has difficulty with distant vision. Myopia usually develops between the ages of 5 and 15 due to excessive growth of the eye. There is often a family history. The condition is treated with glasses and the defect is corrected by concave lenses. Rarely congenital myopia occurs and may be associated with retinal detachment.

Astigmatism

This arises when the curvature of the cornea and lens is different in the horizontal and vertical

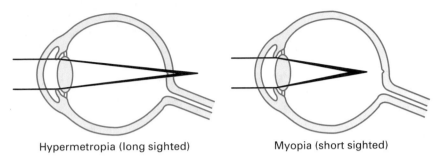

Hypermetropia (long sighted)   Myopia (short sighted)

Fig. 33.7 Hypermetropia and myopia

planes. Minor degrees of astigmatism have no significance but greater degrees produce difficulties in focusing horizontally and vertically simultaneously and will give rise to difficulties in reading and a dislike of prolonged close work. Some children screw up their eyes in an attempt to improve acuity.

Refractive error

For most of the defects in visual acuity it is necessary to measure the degree of refractive error causing that diminution in acuity in order to apply appropriate correction. In young children this is generally done by retinoscopy following the use of drops to dilate the pupil and paralyse accommodation. With the eye in this condition the underlying properties of the lens may be determined. If there is no error of refraction, parallel light entering the eye will emerge as parallel light. If the eye is hypermetropic the rays are divergent, if the eye is myopic the rays are convergent and if the eyes are astigmatic the rays emerge in a band. Trial lenses are then applied in front of the eye until the rays emerge parallel, indicating that refractive error has been corrected. This method is generally used for children under the age of six. Older children may be assessed using a trial frame and a chart. The strength of lenses is measured in dioptres: convex lenses have positive values, concave lenses have negative values.

COLOUR VISION

Problems with colour discrimination are found in 8% of boys and 0.5% of girls. The importance of a colour vision defect is that it can lead to difficulties in carrying out some occupations. Those whose career may be affected by colour vision defects should be advised to see an optometrist for an assessment. It is not clear whether a screen of the whole school population for colour vision defects is beneficial. For further information see the Polnay report on school health (Polnay 1995).

Box 33.1 shows careers where defective colour vision would be a handicap.

VISION SCREENING

Child health screening focuses on the early detection of childhood disorders in order to reduce disability.

Although the effects of mild visual deficits in childhood is difficult to assess, the experience in adults is that it is worthwhile correcting the vision at a level of 6/12 or worse. It is extremely difficult to measure this in children below the age of 3 years but from the age of three most children are testable. Achieving a high coverage at age three is difficult unless all children are in nursery places. At 5 years of age it is easier to achieve a universal screen because children are seen in school. For screening to be justifiable the treatment offered should be safe, acceptable and effective. For amblyopia there

Vision

> **Box 33.1**
> ## Careers where colour vision needs to be perfect
>
> - Armed Forces certain grades
> - Civil aviation
> - Colour matcher in dyeing textiles, paints, inks, coloured ceramics, cosmetics
> - Carpet darner/inspector, spinner, weaver, bobbin winder
> - Electrical work — electrician, electronics, colour TV mechanic, motor mechanic, telephone installer
> - Navigation — pilot, fisherman, railways
> - Police — certain grades
> - Radio — telegraphy

are difficulties in assessing the impact of treatment as the natural history is not known. There have been various attempts to demonstrate that vision improves with treatment but it is not known what the psychological impact of treatment might be. The present recommendations are that all children should have a vision test at school entry with referral on to an optician where the acuity is 6/12 or 6/9 if there are other concerns. An ophthalmological assessment is recommended where there is assymetry of the acuity or the vision is 6/12 or worse. The importance of detecting potentially treatable conditions should be recognised.

Detection of moderate and severe visual impairment

Most cases of severe visual loss will be detectable by parents. Where a parent raises a concern about vision it is recommended that the child should be seen by an orthoptist or an ophthalmologist as soon as possible. Sometimes an appointment with an orthoptist can be obtained at a community clinic

Table 33.5
Vision screening recommendations (Hall 1996)

Age	
Infants screened <31 weeks' gestation; <1500 gr	Ophthalmologist examination at 5–7 weeks' postnatal age
Neonatal screen	GP or paediatrician eye examination for opacities
6 weeks' postnatal age corrected	GP or community child health examination of eyes for opacities and assessment of early visual behaviour
All ages	Secondary screen by orthoptist/ophthalmologists of high-risk infants or where parents are concerned. Professionals have noted abnormal visual behaviour
School entry	Visual acuity measure by the school nurse; checking each eye separately
Ages 8, 11 and 14	Visual acuity measure by the school nurse. The value of universal screening after the age of five is being challenged, though practice may vary from district to district
Age 11	Colour vision screen using City Plates or Ishihara test. (Ishihara is very sensitive and will pick up children with trivial defects who will pass the City Plates)
School acuity test is likely to be replaced by a preschool orthoptic appointment	

within a day, or it may be possible to arrange an ophthalmology appointment quicker than one at a child health clinic. Some conditions such as cataract, retinoblastoma or congenital glaucoma are treatable, others have genetic implications. It is important for parents to receive developmental guidance as early as possible. Signs such as progressive failure or squint can be part of a neuro-degenerative condition and consultation with a paediatric neurologist may be advised.

Some children at high risk of vision problems may require special attention. These include pre-term babies who have received intensive care, children where there is a family history of squint, amblyopia or visual impairment and children with other disabilities, for example cerebral palsy, where there is a much higher incidence of eye problems.

Vision testing programme

This is part of the child health promotion programme (see Chapter 8). In young children the important elements are parental observation, supplemented by experienced professional observation of visually directed behaviour and observation of the eyes. In the older age group tests for visual acuity can be applied; they require cooperation, concentration and the ability to match symbols. For these children the use of linear charts is preferable to the matching of single letters as the latter can overestimate visual acuity by as much as two or three lines compared to a standard chart. This is known as the crowding phenomenon in which single letters are seen more easily than those in rows of letters.

A systematic review of the literature on preschool vision screening by Stewart-Brown & Snowden (1997) revealed no clear evidence that screening was beneficial. However, where children have developmental problems, or learning difficulties, vision should always be assessed. This may need to be done in difficult cases by a specialist team. In adults there is also a need for an increased awareness of the possibility of visual deficits coexisting with other disabilities.

Table 33.5 summarises the vision screening programme according to Hall (1996).

REFERENCES AND FURTHER READING

Atkinson J, Hof-van Duin J V 1993 The management of visual impairment in childhood. Childhood Clinics in Developmental Medicine no 128

Baird G, Moore A T 1993 Epidemiology of childhood blindness. In: Fielder A R (ed) The management of visual impairment in childhood. MacKeith Press, Cambridge, pp 1–8

British Association for Community Child Health and the Department of Health 1994 Disability in childhood. Towards nationally useful definitions. BACCH, London

Crofts B, King R, Johnson A 1998 The contribution of low birth weight to severe vision loss in a geographically defined population. British Journal of Ophthalmology 82:9–15

Fraiberg S 1968 Parallel and divergent patterns in blind and sighted infants. Psychoanalytic Study of the Child 23:264–300

Gardiner P A 1982 The development of vision. MTP Lancaster

Goggin M, O'keepe M 1991 Childhood blindness in the Republic of Ireland: a national survey. British Journal of Ophthalmology 75:425–429

Hall D 1996 Health for all children, 3rd edn. Oxford University Press, Oxford

Ingram R M 1979 Amblyopia: the need for a new approach. British Journal of Ophthalmology 63:236–237

Kochler L, Stigmar G 1973 Vision screening of four-year-old children. Acta Paediatrica Scandinavica 62:17–27

McConachie H 1990 Early language development and severe visual impairment. Child: Care, Health and Development 16:55–61

Moore B D 1994 Pediatric cataracts — diagnosis and treatment [review]. Optometry and Vision Science 71:168–173

Norris M, Spaulding P J, Brodie F H 1957 Blindness in children. University of Chicago Press, Chicago, IL

Polnay L 1995 Health needs of school age children. British Paediatric Association, London, pp 49–50

Reynell J, Zinkin P 1981 Reynell-Zinkin development scales for visually handicapped children. Manual. NFER Nelson, Windsor

RNIB 1990 New directions: towards a better future for multihandicapped visually impaired children and young people. RNIB, London

RNIB 1997 Policy document, planning quality services 2. RNIB, London

RNIB 1997 An introduction to the multiple disability team. RNIB Multiple Disability Services, London

Rogers M 1996 Vision impairment in Liverpool: prevalence and morbidity. Archives of Disease in Childhood 74:299–303

Sonksen P M 1983 Vision and early development. In: Wybar K, Taylor D (eds), Paediatric ophthalmology. Current aspects. Marcel Dekker, New York, pp 85–95

Sonksen P, Levitt S, Kitsinger M 1984 Identification of constraints acting on motor development in young visually disabled children and principles of

Vision

remediation. Child: Care, Health and Development 10:273–286

Sonkson P, Petrie A, Drew K J 1991 Promotion of visual development of severely visually impaired babies: evaluation of a developmentally based programme. Developmental Medicine and Child Neurology 33:320–335

Stewart-Brown S, Snowden S 1997 Preschool vision screening, NHS R&D. In: Health technology assessment vol 1, no 8. NHS Centre for Reviews and Dissemination, York

Stewart-Brown S, Haslam M N, Howett B 1988 Preschool vision screening: a service in need of

rationalisation. Archives of Disease in Childhood 63:356–359

Taylor D, Hoyt C 1997 Practical paediatric ophthalmology. Blackwell Science, Oxford

Thylefors B 1992 Present challenges in the prevention of blindness. Australian and New Zealand Journal of Ophthalmology 20:89–94

Thylefors B et al 1995 Global data on blindness. Bulletin of the World Health Organization 73:115–121

Warren D 1994 Blindness and children: an individual differences approach. Cambridge University Press, Cambridge

34 | Hearing

INTRODUCTION

The early detection of hearing problems in childhood is vital in the interest of the child's social, emotional, linguistic and educational development. Even slight degrees of hearing difficulty can influence these areas of development and undetected severe or profound hearing losses can prevent the child from developing spoken language and have other permanent detrimental effects if appropriate support is not provided in the first weeks or months of the child's life. Yoshinaga-Itano et al (1998) has shown in a large case study that deaf children fitted with hearing aids before 6 months of age outperform those fitted after six months in measures of expressive and receptive language development.

Approximately 1 child per 1000 (840 babies per year in England and Wales) will be born with a sufficient degree of hearing loss to require special support in the form of hearing aid provision, and between one-quarter and one-third of these children (210–280 per year) will subsequently benefit from cochlear implants.

Some parents may chose to use a manual (signing) system of communication, such as British Sign Language, rather than adopt one based on the utilization of spoken language. Very early hearing aid provision or cochlear implantation can, however, help profoundly deaf children to acquire spoken language as their dominant means of communication. Prior to the introduction of the technique of cochlear implantation many profoundly deaf children did not have a sufficient degree of residual hearing to develop spoken language, even with the provision of the most powerful hearing aids and the use of lip reading, and in these cases sign language became their dominant means of communication.

Now that cochlear implants are available it can be anticipated that the number of children who need signing as their primary means of communication will reduce quite significantly in the future. This is something that concerns the deaf community, some of whose members believe that the surgical intervention of cochlear implantation deprives children of their cultural identity as deaf individuals. Ninety per cent of deaf children are, however, born to hearing parents and it is understandable that these parents will want their children to develop spoken language if at all possible.

Sign language skills can be developed at any time and many aural deaf children will wish to become proficient with this method of communication as a second language as they grow up. There are, as we have seen, periods of maximum sensitivity for the development of a spoken language approach and these may be within the first months but are certainly within the first year or so of life. If there is no effective stimulation of the neural pathways for hearing and speech within these early sensitive stages then the ability to develop an effective spoken language approach may be lost forever.

TYPES AND DEGREES OF HEARING PROBLEMS

Hearing problems may be classified as conductive, sensorineural or a mixture of both. The hearing losses may be permanent or temporary. The prevalence of permanent childhood hearing loss (PCHL) is very small but the prevalence of temporary fluctuating conductive hearing loss, associated with glue ear, is high and 1 in 10 children under the age of 5 years will have middle ear effusion at any one time. Children with PCHL are just as likely as children with normal hearing to develop a temporary conductive hearing loss associated with middle ear effusion and glue ear and this could prevent the child from hearing speech through their hearing aids. All children with PCHL should remain under surveillance at a paediatric audiology department to ensure that they are receiving appropriate amplification from their hearing aids.

The classification of degrees of hearing loss relates to the audiogram where the hearing level for sounds is recorded in decibels (dBHL, that is decibels hearing level). The audiogram records the threshold level, that is the quietest intensity (loudness) at which the child responds to pure tone sounds of differing frequency (pitch) in the speech frequency range from 250 Hz up to 8000 Hz. Hearing problems are classified by taking the average of the thresholds at 500 Hz, 1 kHz, 2 kHz and 4 kHz and the categories are typically:

- Mild (20–39 dBHL).
- Moderate (40–69 dBHL).
- Severe (70–89 dBHL).
- Profound (90 dBHL or more).

Figure 34.1 shows an air conduction audiogram chart with illustrations of the sound levels of everyday sounds superimposed. Air conduction audiometric thresholds are recorded using headphones and are plotted as circles for the right ear and crosses for the left ear. Bone conduction thresholds are also shown in Fig. 34.1 as triangular symbols. These are recorded by placing a vibrator on the mastoid to transmit the pure tone signal directly to the cochlea by bone/tissue conduction. In this case the middle ear is bypassed and so any conductive hearing loss will not elevate the bone conduction thresholds. The bone conduction thresholds will be increased only if a sensorineural hearing loss is present. A difference of 10 dB or more between the air conduction and bone conduction thresholds (that is an air–bone gap of at least 10 dB) will indicate the presence of a conductive hearing loss. The most common form of hearing problems is temporary and fluctuating conductive hearing losses resulting from the presence of fluid in the middle

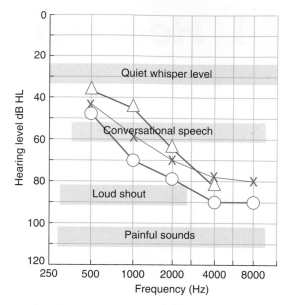

Fig. 34.1 Audiogram with typical everyday sounds superimposed

ear (otitis media with effusion or OME or 'glue ear') which impedes the conduction of sound across the middle ear A typical range of hearing losses resulting from this condition is shown in the audiogram in Fig. 34.2. During the early stage of the disease the hearing thresholds for low-frequency sounds are most affected but as the fluid thickens the hearing thresholds for the high and then middle frequencies will be affected and the loss will then be relatively flat in nature.

Conductive hearing losses may be caused by any abnormalities of the pinna, external auditory meatus, tympanic membrane, ossicular chain or stapes footplate. The absence of a pinna may lead to a 20-dB hearing loss because the funnel effect will be lost. With the absence of the tympanic membrane or ossicular chain the conductive loss will not be greater than 60 dB. This is because the sound pressure wave can still impinge on the oval window thus transmitting a pressure wave along the fluid-filled cochlea. The normal mechanical transfer function of the middle ear will be lost in such an extreme case. In cases with total atresia (without any external auditory meatus) the conductive hearing loss does not exceed 70 dB.

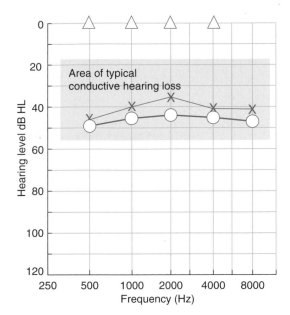

Fig. 34.2 Conductive hearing loss

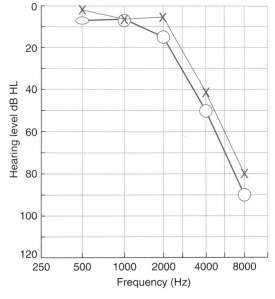

Fig. 34.3 High tone hearing loss

The term sensorineural hearing loss embraces any condition in which the lesion is within the sensory organ (cochlea) or within the auditory nerve. In 95% of sensorineural hearing loss the lesion is within the cochlea. Unlike conductive hearing loss sensorineural losses tend to show a greater effect in the high-frequency region and in some cases the low-frequency hearing thresholds may be nearly normal.

An example of a high tone hearing loss is shown in Figure 34.3. These 'ski slope' high frequency hearing losses can easily be missed in very young children if they are not tested carefully with specific high-frequency stimuli. Most sounds in the environment contain energy in the low-frequency region and children may respond to these without necessarily being able to hear intelligible speech. Poor speech production and delayed language development with absence of any suspicions of hearing problems are classic signs of high tone hearing loss and children with this condition have sometimes been misdiagnosed as slow learners.

The above example is of the extreme case of a sensorineural hearing loss and it is much more common to have a more gradually sloping loss with a reduction in hearing thresholds at all frequencies.

Sensorineural losses with flat audiometric configurations are possible and will be associated with aetiologies which affect the cochlear uniformly throughout its length (e.g. rubella or anoxia). As a general rule any hearing loss in excess of 55 dB will be sufficient to prevent a child from hearing conversational speech and this will impose an obvious barrier to the development of spoken language.

Figure 34.4 shows a severe hearing loss which can be alleviated to a considerable degree by the use of hearing aids. Hearing aids act as acoustic amplifiers and they increase the pressure of the air-borne vibrations so that the oval window transmits a more forceful vibration to the cochlear. The effects of an appropriate hearing aid fitting on the hearing thresholds for the previous example is shown in Fig. 34.5, and it can be seen that this amplification has improved the hearing and made normal conversational speech audible.

By contrast, Fig. 34.6 shows a profound hearing loss with very limited potential to benefit from acoustic amplification. The improvement in the hearing thresholds provided by the most powerful hearing aid available is shown in Fig. 34.7 and it can be seen that speech is not audible. Such a case would be an ideal candidate to consider for a

Hearing

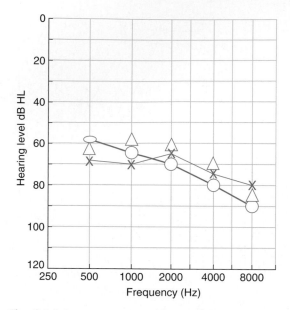

Fig. 34.4 Severe sensorineural hearing loss

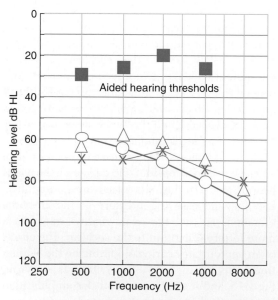

Fig. 34.5 Severe sensorineural hearing loss with aided hearing thresholds plotted on the audiogram

cochlear implant because this system provides direct electrical stimulation of the auditory nerve pathway beyond (and therefore bypassing) the hair cells (Fig. 34.7). This is achieved by means of an implanted electrode array and associated circuitry

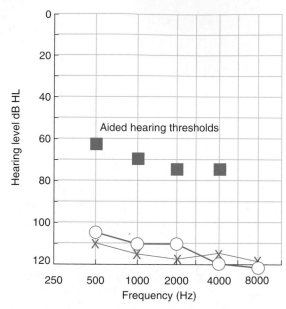

Fig. 34.6 Profound sensorineural hearing loss with aided hearing thresholds shown

for stimulating the auditory nerve directly with a series of digitally generated pulses.

The electrical pulses convey a pattern of stimulation to the auditory nerve which faithfully follows the pattern of the acoustic signals detected in the environment by the implant's microphone. When using cochlear implants children will normally have hearing thresholds in the region of 25–45 dB across a wide frequency range spanning 250 Hz to 8 kHz or above. They can therefore hear even quiet conversational speech.

METHODS OF SCREENING FOR HEARING IMPAIRMENTS

Universal hearing screening utilizing the health visitor distraction test (HVDT) has been a feature of the UK health service for more than 30 years. Two health visitors or a health visitor and a healthcare assistant perform the distraction test. One attracts and controls the baby's attention at the front with the baby sitting on the parent's knee, and the other remains out of vision and presents a series of very quiet sounds (35–50 dB) of varying and known fre-

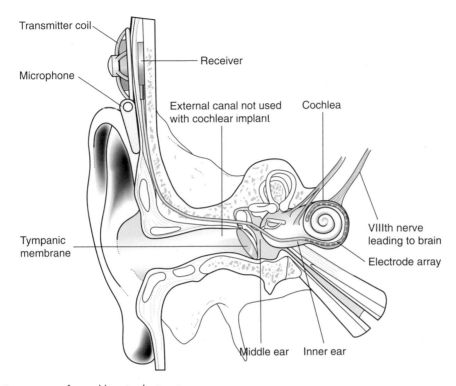

Fig. 34.7 Components of a cochlear implant system

quency content. The sounds may be low- and high-frequency warble tones or other sounds of discrete frequency content, for example a special high-frequency rattle, a quiet hum, or the repetition of the /s/ consonant. The baby passes the test if full 90 degree head turns are elicited, on two out of three presentations of low- and of high-frequency sounds, when the baby is judged to be in an appropriate state of attention. Silent 'observation' periods are needed at various intervals during the test to ensure that the baby's attention state is appropriate and that the head turns are not just random checks. When sufficient attention is paid to these details this test has been shown to be extremely effective (McCormick 1991). Unfortunately the general quality of the test has not been good (Scanlon & Bamford 1990) and even in areas with a history of good practice the standards can easily slip if insufficient refresher courses are maintained for health visitors.

An alternative approach has been piloted in one district in the UK with health visitor 'surveillance'

replacing 'screening'. Unfortunately the surveillance method proved to be no more effective than the HVDT test in that area (Sutton & Scanlon 1999). The performance of both methods in that district produced a disappointing sensitivity of less than 50% and this did not approach that of better performing districts. Davis & Wood (1992) reported a sensitivity for the distraction test of 88% in the Nottingham district over the same period.

Considerable effort is required to maintain a satisfactory level of performance for a community hearing screen utilizing the distraction test, and even in the Nottingham district there have been temporary periods when the sensitivity fell below 50% (Wood et al 1997).

Unfortunately the majority of services have been unable to devote the time and effort needed to maintain a consistently good hearing screening service in the community and hence the general results nationwide have been very disappointing. This finding, and the desire to detect hearing problems as early as possible, prompted a move towards

Hearing

the introduction of hearing screening techniques which could be applied at an earlier age.

Neonatal hearing screening

Techniques for screening the hearing of newborn babies have been developed and piloted mostly with special care babies. Approximately 7% of births fall within this category and by testing this relatively small subpopulation it should be possible to detect over 40% of congenital deafness. Three screening techniques are in common use:

- The *portable auditory response cradle* (PARC) which utilises micro-chip technology and sensors to record the baby's behavioural responses to intense sounds (Bhattacharya et al 1984).
- The *auditory brain stem response* (ABR) method records sound-induced electrical activity in the brain utilising surface-mounted electrodes positioned on the scalp. This technique has the advantage that it enables hearing to be screened at any chosen level (mostly 40 dBnHL or 50 dBnHL). The disadvantages are that it does not test the entire auditory pathway and the baby has to be in a calm state for 20 minutes or more to obtain satisfactory recordings.
- The *otoacoustic emissions* (OAE) method uses a single soft-tipped probe which is placed in the external auditory meatus to record acoustic signals which are generated by a normally functioning cochlea. The test has the advantage that it is very quick and it requires minimal contact with the baby. This makes it an attractive test and most programmes adopt this as the first choice for neonatal hearing screening. It has the disadvantage that it does not test the integrity of the hearing system above the level of the cochlea.

Pilot studies using the above techniques for Universal Neonatal Hearing Screening (UNHS) have met with considerable success and have achieved respectable levels of sensitivity (>85%) and specificity (>90%). In a report produced for the Health Technology Assessment Programme in the UK, Davis et al (1997) have recommended the cautious introduction of such programmes, concluding that a system based on UNHS followed at 7 months by a targetted infant distraction test is the most equitable and responsive, and gives best value for money. It will take several years for these recommendations to be taken up by most health authorities and in the meantime we can expect to see a range of screening systems being deployed at different stages.

Two of the hearing screening methods described above (ABR and OAE) can be used at any age but if UNHS replaces the HVDT there will be a long gap of 4 or 5 years before the child has another universal hearing screen on school entry. At this time the Sweep Screen Pure Tone Audiometry test will be undertaken. This simplified version of audiometry typically checks that the child can hear at least four frequencies (500 Hz, 1000 Hz, 2000 Hz and 4000 Hz) as they are swept through at a constant level of, say, 25 dBHL. Roughly 6% of children tested during their first year at school will fail this test.

Parental suspicion

If parents suspect the presence of deafness in their children there is a 90% chance that they are correct. The parental handout form shown in Figure 34.8 can be used to support such suspicions. McCormick (1988) and Watkins et al (1990) showed, however, that only one in five families detect the signs of deafness and so the method cannot be used as the sole indicator of deafness in childhood. No detection system should be based on surveillance techniques alone in the absence of tests which sample the child's response to different frequencies.

DIAGNOSTIC HEARING TESTS

Diagnostic hearing tests may be termed objective (e.g. ABR) or behavioural (e.g. pure tone audiometry). Objective tests are reserved for the very young or for children who are very difficult to test by normal behavioural means. Diagnostic ABR investigations can help to give estimates of the child's hearing acuity mostly at high frequencies but they cannot provide full audiometric data. The information obtained from objective tests compliments but does not replace the more detailed information obtainable from behavioural tests.

Hints for Parents

Can your baby hear you?

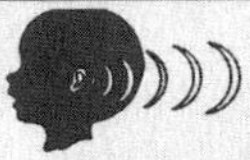

Here is a checklist of some of the general signs you can look for in your baby's first year: YES/NO

Shortly after birth
Your baby should be startled by a sudden loud noise such as a hand clap or a door slamming and should blink or open his eyes widely to such sounds.

By 1 Month
Your baby should be beginning to notice sudden prolonged sounds like the noise of a vacuum cleaner and she should pause and listen to them when they begin.

By 4 Months
He should quieten or smile to the sound of your voice even when he cannot see you. He may also turn his head or eyes toward you if you come up from behind and speak to him from the side.

By 7 Months
She should turn immediately to your voice across the room or to very quiet noises made on each side if she is not too occupied with other things.

By 9 Months
He should listen attentively to familiar everyday sounds and search for very quiet sounds made out of sight. He should also show pleasure in babbling loudly and tunefully.

By 12 Months
She should show some response to her own name and to other familiar words. She may also respond when you say 'no' and 'bye bye' even when she cannot see any accompanying gesture.

Your health visitor will perform a routine hearing screening test on your baby between six and eight months of age. She will be able to help and advise you at any time before or after this test if you are concerned about your baby and his development. If you suspect that your baby is not hearing normally, either because you cannot answer yes to the items above or for some other reason, then seek advice from your health visitor.

©
Produced by Dr. Barry McCormick
Children's Hearing Assessment Centre, Nottingham

Fig. 34.8 Leaflet providing checklist of general hearing signs in the first year

Tympanometry

Tympanometry is sometimes considered to be an objective test of hearing but this is an incorrect interpretation of the situation. The tympanogram provides information about the middle ear pressure and about the mechanical properties of the middle ear system, most notably the mobility of the tympanic membrane and ossicular chain (Cottingham 1995). Reduced middle ear pressure or reduced middle ear mobility will be associated with conductive hearing loss but hearing levels are not actually recorded. Sometimes the technique is extended to include the recording of stapedial reflex activity and this does offer an opportunity to sample an aspect of hearing function for high levels of sound. When intense sounds are presented to the ear these cause the stapedial muscle to contract thus increasing the stiffness of the ossicular chain. This change

in stiffness is easily recordable by tempanometry and the effect is greater for more intense sounds.

The *diagnostic application of ABR* to record hearing thresholds under sedation is invaluable if the child is difficult to test by other means, either because of developmental factors or because of poor cooperation. Such testing can give an indication of hearing thresholds mostly in the middle- to high-frequency region and to some degree also in the low-frequency region (with modification of the technique) but the reliability is poorer for low frequencies.

Steady state evoked potential

Another electrophysiological test known as steady state evoked potential (SSEP) recording is showing some promise for predicting the audiometric thresholds across a wide frequency range and this is likely to gain in popularity over the next decade.

Modified OAE methods may have some potential in the future for predicting actual hearing thresholds, but so far the reliability for indicating anything other than the presence or absence of deafness is questionable.

The distraction test

This test can be used at a diagnostic level as well as at the screening level. The major difference will be that a wider range of frequency-specific stimuli will be used and the hearing thresholds at which the child first responds to each sound will be assessed. A particular virtue of this form of testing is that the child's responsiveness to sound stimulation, to visual stimulation and to tactile stimulation, can be checked. If there is no response to sound an object can be brought into the visual field from the side to see if there is a quick response to vision, and if there is still no response the child can be touched on the ear to see if this elicits a response. This will inform the testers about the child's general state of attention. If the child fails to respond to the sound but is quick to respond to the other modalities this will indicate a significant problem with hearing. If the child is generally unresponsive to all three modalities then the test technique is clearly inappropriate either because the child is not developmentally ready for the test or because the attention state is not optimal on the day (the child may be unwell or too tired). Great care must be taken to ensure that the child is responding to the sound stimuli rather than any inadvertent clue and the use of 'no sound' or observation trials are essential for this purpose. These trials should be included at frequent intervals during the test to check for searching behaviour and to assess the difference in nature between a genuine response to sound and a random turn. Skilled application of the distraction test can provide very useful information about the hearing of babies from approximately 6 months of age until well into the second year of life.

Visual reinforcement audiometry

This is an extremely useful technique for application at the diagnostic level. Sound stimuli are presented through a calibrated loudspeaker system and the child's head turn responses are rewarded with a visual display (e.g. an illuminated puppet) which is usually located adjacent to the speaker. The use of ear insert 'tube phones' to replace the speaker permits the recording of hearing thresholds for each ear separately and the technique can also be extended to include the use of a bone conduction vibrator. Visual reinforcement audiometry (VRA) techniques can be used from the latter half of the first year of life through to 4 or 5 years of age. Some clinicians use the technique routinely to replace the distraction test but in some cases it is useful to apply both techniques. They both have advantages: the distraction test enables a better assessment to be made of the infant's general state of attention, the VRA technique can give hearing thresholds which can be a few decibels more precise because of the well-calibrated system employed.

Performance test

When the child has reached a mental age of $2^{1}/_{2}$ years it should be possible to undertake a performance test of hearing. For this the child is conditioned to wait for a sound stimulus and then to respond with a simple play activity (e.g. placing a peg in a board). It is important to vary the delay between sound presentations to avoid establishing a predictable response pattern and the sounds must be presented without any visual clues. Sounds of different frequencies spanning the speech range can be presented from speakers (sound field) or from headphones or insert phones, in which case this can represent the first attempt at *pure tone audiometry*. Full pure tone audiometry can normally be performed by a skilled clinician with children of 3 years of age and above. There are set rules for performing audiometry: the threshold recorded for each frequency is the quietest level at which the child responds to the tone on at least 50% of ascending presentations as the signals are decreased in increments of 10 dB and increased in 5-dB steps. If there is the possibility of a difference of 40 dB or more between the air conduction thresholds for each ear it will be necessary to present a masking signal to the better ear to prevent the signals from crossing over the head and being heard in that ear. The level of the masking signal must be very carefully controlled to ensure that enough masking is presented but not too much otherwise the masking sound could also cross the head. The situation becomes more complex with bone conduction testing because it must be assumed that no matter where the bone vibrator is positioned on the skull the signal will be received equally at each cochlea by bone and tissue transmission across the skull. Thus masking will always be needed to enable a correct interpretation to be made of the air and bone conduction configuration on the audiogram: the only exception will be when the true hearing thresholds are equal in both ears. An excellent training guide for audiometry is given by Wood (1993).

Speech discrimination

So far the discussion has concentrated on the measurement of hearing acuity. A second aspect of audiological measurement is concerned with the actual ability to understand speech, hence the term speech audiometry. For very young children measuring the ability to understand single words at known listening levels is the most direct and accessible technique available. The *McCormick Toy Discrimination Test* (McCormick 1977) is the most widely used test of this nature in the UK. This test can be used as a screening test, if the speech is presented at a fixed presentation level of 40 dB(A)*, and as a diagnostic test if the level is varied at measured intervals. The test consists of seven pairs of toy items, which have been carefully chosen: (a) to be within the vocabulary of a child with a mental age of 2 years, and (b) to sound similar when spoken at quiet levels (e.g. plate, plane). The child is asked to point to the toys and will pass a screening test if four out of five names are heard correctly (80% score) at a listening level of 40 dB(A) in a typical community clinic setting. In a well-treated audiology clinic the levels can be varied from 15 dB(A) up to 80 dB(A) or more and an accurate measure of speech discrimination ability can be documented. When administering the test it is important to ensure that there are no visible

clues (lip reading or signing) if the auditory discrimination ability is being measured. With deaf children it can be useful to extend the test to include these other clues if they are unable to perform the test with listening alone and, of course, the child's ability to perform the test with hearing aids or cochlear implants can provide useful information. Interesting automated versions of this test using digital recording technology have appeared in the field, for example, the *Institute of Hearing Research/ McCormick Automated Toy Discrimination Test* and *The Parrot* manufactured by Soundbyte Solutions. These add extra precision to the test by standardizing the presentation at well calibrated levels and by the introduction of automatic scoring.

AETIOLOGY AND EPIDEMIOLOGY OF PERMANENT HEARING LOSS

Two major studies by Das (1988) in Greater Manchester and by Fortnum & Davis (1997) in the Trent region have provided valuable information about the presence and causation of PCHL in the UK (Box 34.1).

The Manchester study was prospective finding a total of 164 children with bilateral sensorineural hearing loss (SNHL) of 30 dB or more from 36 000 births over a 5-year period between 1981 and 1984, thus giving a prevalence of 1 per 1000 live births. This study did not include children born with a permanent conductive loss. All children in the study underwent day-case admission for investigation of the possible cause of their SNHL: a full family

---

* dB(A) is a scale used to measure sounds with a sound level metre in a typical room setting rather than through headphones as in audiometry. The dB(A) and dBHL scales differ by about 2 dB in the speech frequency region.

> Box 34.1
> **Permanent childhood hearing loss: key facts**
>
> - Genetic causes are probably present in half of all cases of PCHL
> - 20–30% of childhood deafness is syndromic
> - 70–80% of childhood deafness is non-syndromic
> - Meningitis is the most common single cause of acquired PCHL

Hearing

history was obtained and parents and siblings were examined for hearing impairment.

Following investigation 36.5% of the children could not be ascribed a cause for their SNHL. A positive family history for congenital hearing loss was found in 20.1% of the children, and 3.7% of children had a syndromic genetic cause with 3.7% of children having a chromosomal cause for their hearing impairment. In a further 14.6% the SNHL was attributed to adverse perinatal factors including prematurity. A congenital infection (rubella, cytomegalovirus (CMV) or toxoplasmosis) was found in 9.8% of the children, and 6.1% of the total number of children acquired a SNHL following bacterial meningitis. There was an additional 5.5% whose cause of SNHL was ascribed as miscellaneous.

Thus in conclusion just over 60% of cases had a cause identified for their SNHL with 30% having a genetic cause.

The Trent Ascertainment Study analysed 8 years of retrospective data from children in the Trent region covering the period 1985–93. All cases of PCHL (i.e. sensorineural and conductive) with better ear thresholds of 40 dB or more were included.

The prevalence figures quoted were 133 per 100 000 live births (1.3 per 1000), with 16% of the total being acquired causes (postnatal, late-onset or progressive). One-third of these occurred following meningitis. Fifty-nine per cent of the children had a stated cause for their PCHL and 41% had an unknown cause.

Forty-one per cent of children were quoted as having a genetic cause for their PCHL (syndromal, non-syndromal and craniofacial abnormalities were included in this group) and 30% of cases had a family history of hearing loss. This study also identified other problems and it is particularly important to note that 40% of the children with PCHL had other clinical or developmental problems.

Although there are slight differences in the two populations in these studies, there is general consensus that within the population of children with PCHL, at least 30% of cases have an unknown cause and between 30% and 40% have genetic causes (either syndromal or non-syndromal). Acquired

losses following meningitis represents around 5–6% of PCHL.

CLASSIFICATION AND CAUSATION OF HEARING LOSS IN CHILDHOOD

Hearing loss may be congenital or acquired and the causation may be within the prenatal, perinatal or postnatal periods. The summary of the classification in Box 34.2 is illustrative rather than exhaustive within the context of this chapter.

A description of all syndromes associated with permanent hearing loss is not the remit of this chapter since other genetic and paediatric texts can supply more detail. However the reader in community paediatrics is recommended to have a particular knowledge of those syndromes where there is multisystem involvement, for example Alport's syndrome, branch-oto-renal (BOR) syndrome, Usher's syndrome types 1–4, Marshall–Stickler syndrome and Pendred's syndrome, as participation with other specialists, for example in renal medicine, ophthalmology and endocrinology, will necessarily be part of these children's continuing medical care.

Research continues into genetic causes of permanent hearing loss and to date the chromosomal location of more than 60 genes, and six on the X chromosome, have been identified as being implicated in hearing impairment deletions in the PAX3 gene located on chromosome 2 is responsible for de Waardenburg's syndrome type 1 (Tassabehji et al 1992). Mutations in one gene, GJB2, encoding the connexin 26 molecule, have been found to be a very common cause of non-syndromic childhood deafness, and may account for up to half of all such cases (see Chapter 6).

Bacterial meningitis remains the most common cause for an acquired hearing loss with 1 in 10 children surviving meningitis developing a permanent bilateral sensorineural loss (Fortnum & Davis 1993).

Causation of sensorineural hearing loss
Pre-natal
- Genetic — see Chapter 6

- Intrauterine infections — rubella, CMV, toxoplasmosis, syphilis

- Ototoxic drugs — antimalarials (e.g. quinine), aminoglycosides, diuretics (e.g. loop diuretics)

- Metabolic — congenital hypothyroidism

- Unknown — probably genetic (mainly autosomal recessive)

Perinatal
- Prematurity — hypoxia, hyperbilirubinaemia, ototoxic drugs (e.g. aminoglycosides)

Postnatal
- Infection — meningitis bacterial (e.g. *Meningococcus, Pneumococcus, Haemophilus*), measles, mumps, other viruses (adeno, EB, rhino)

- Trauma — head injury (transverse fractures), noise (exposure to loud music)

- Ototoxic drugs — streptomycin, desferrioxamine, cytotoxic drugs

Causation of permanent conductive hearing loss
Prenatal
- Genetic, syndromal — autosomal dominant (Treacher–Collins, Crouzon's, Apert's, otosclerosis, osteogenesis imperfecta), autosomal recessive (mucopolysaccharidoses), X-linked (Hunter's)

- Chromosomal — Down's

- Genetic, sporadic — Wildervanke's, Goldenhar's, Pierre Robin

Postnatal
- Trauma — head injury — (longitudinal fracture, ossicular dislocation), explosion (perforated tympanic membrane)

INVESTIGATING A PERMANENT HEARING LOSS

It can be seen, from the epidemiological and aetiological studies outlined above, that medical investigations to establish a cause for a permanent hearing loss can only lead to positive findings in 50–60% of cases and all parents should be counselled regarding this before embarking on the various tests. Parents may find this process extremely beneficial if it answers their questions and gives a 'reason' for their child's hearing loss. It may identify a genetic cause and consequently genetic counselling may be advised for the family. Alternatively a condition requiring treatment may be diagnosed, for example Jervell–Lange syndrome, Alport's syndrome, BOR syndrome and hypothyroidism.

In some cases there remain great difficulties in establishing a cause for a PCHL. The late diagnosis of a congenital loss may mean that exclusion of congenital infections as a cause (particularly cytomegalovirus and rubella) may be difficult or indeed impossible since IgG antibodies may exist due to intercurrent infection and immunisation and confound the diagnosis. In some areas there are limited resources for genetic investigation and consequent genetic counselling, so that a proportion of certain genetic causes may remain unidentified.

Often the diagnosis is retrospective and there may be more than one potential cause for a hearing loss with each having an additive effect. In a small retrospective study it has been found that in prematurity, the presence of hyperbilirubinaemia at the same time as acidosis, or the presence of hyperbilirubinaemia and the use of netilmicin (aminoglycoside) were associated with SNHL whereas these factors were not associated alone (Marlow, Hunt & Marlow, 2000).

Vision care and investigation is extremely important for deaf children because of their reliance on lip-reading and the use of sign language to compensate for the loss of hearing in adverse communication situations. Forty-five per cent of deaf children have some visual problem and there are more than 30 syndromes with vision and hearing associations with Usher's syndrome accounting for

50%. In Usher's type 1 the child is born with severe/profound hearing loss and vision deteriorates at a later age, typically after the age of 7 years. In Usher's type 2 there is a progressive moderate/severe deafness with later deterioration in vision.

Recommended medical investigations

Investigation of the possible cause of hearing loss is complex but important. Investigation should include the following:

General:
1. Full physical and neurological examination.
2. General ophthalmic examination and assessment of visual acuity.
3. Examination of the child's birth and paediatric records to assess perinatal adverse factors and infections.
4. Audiological examination of parents, siblings and if indicated other hearing-impaired relatives.

Specific:
1. Virological examination — rubella, toxoplasma and mumps antibodies (prior to MMR); toxoplasma antibodies (post MMR).
2. Three consecutive urines sent for CMV analysis.
3. Urinalysis for protein, blood and full metabolic screen (to exclude Alport's syndrome and mucopolysaccharide disease).
4. Blood for urea and creatinine estimation (to exclude renal disease in Alport's syndrome or BOR syndrome).
5. ECG (to exclude a prolonged QT interval present in Jervell–Lange syndrome).
6. Thyroid function tests (to exclude hypothyroidism).
7. Lateral skull X-ray (to exclude congenital infection when calcification over the mastoid is often seen).

Further investigations:
1. Chromosomal studies if dysmorphic features found on physical examination.
2. CT scans of the cochleae if a profound or progressive hearing loss exists or X-linked hearing loss is suspected — a profound loss may be associated with absent cochleae, a progressive loss with a dilated vestibular aqueduct syndrome and an X-linked loss with a dilated internal auditory meatus.
3. Renal ultrasound if external ear abnormality or pits exist to exclude brachio-oto-renal (BOR) syndrome.
4. If Pendred's syndrome is suspected CT scans should be performed. The Mondini defect (blind ending) of the cochlea is associated with Pendred's syndrome. A perchlorate test can then be used to confirm the diagnosis.

ORGANISATION OF SERVICES

Services vary widely, but in general children who have failed audiological screening tests are referred to community audiological clinics. If further assessment is required or if a permanent hearing loss is suspected, children are referred to the children's hearing assessment centre, the ENT department or the audiological medicine department, depending upon local arrangements. These centres have access to a wider range of testing facilities and to ENT and speech and language therapy advice.

The local education department should become involved at a very early stage, usually at the time of diagnosis of a permanent hearing loss. Preschool children are seen regularly at home by the peripatetic teacher of the hearing impaired who will advise the family on hearing aid use, listening and communication skills and sign language.

Children with a significant degree of hearing loss are usually assessed by the education authority to ensure that their special needs are met in nursery and primary school. Equipment for use in school, for example radio aids or group aids, are usually provided by the education authority.

Peripatetic teachers continue to provide advice throughout the child's school career, which is now usually provided within hearing-impaired units or mainstream school rather than in special schools.

REFERENCES AND FURTHER READING

Bhattacharya J, Bennett M J, Tucker S 1984 Long term follow-up of newborns tested with the Auditory

Response Cradle. Archives of Disease in Childhood 59:504–511

Cottingham C 1995 Middle-ear measurements. In: McCormick B (ed) The medical practitioner's guide to paediatric audiology. Cambridge University Press, Cambridge, ch 6, p 65

Das V K 1988 Aetiology of bilateral sensorineural deafness in children. Journal of Laryngology and Otology 102:975–980

Davis A, Wood S 1992 The epidemiology of childhood hearing impairment: factors relevant to planning of services. British Journal of Audiology 26:77–90

Davis A, Bamford J, Wilson I, Ramkalawan T, Forshaw M, Wright S A 1997 Critical review of the role of neonatal hearing screening in the detection of congenital hearing impairment. Health Technology Assessment 1(10):97–102

Fortnum H, Davis A C 1993 Hearing impairment in children after bacterial meningitis: incidence of and resource implications. British Journal of Audiology 27:43–52

Fortnum H, Davis A C 1997 Epidemiology of permanent childhood hearing impairment in the Trent Region, 1985–1993. British Journal of Audiology 31:409–446

Marlow E, Hunt L, Marlow N 2000 Sensorineural hearing loss and prematurity. Archives of Disease in Childhood, Fetal Neonatal Edition 82:141–144

Martini A, Read A, Stephens D 1996 Genetics and hearing impairment. Whurr, London

McCormick B 1977 The Toy Discrimination Test: an aid for screening the hearing of children above a mental age of two years. Public Health 91:67–73

McCormick B 1991 Screening for hearing-impairment in young children. Whurr Publishers, London

McCormick B (ed) 1993 Paediatric audiology 0–5 years. Whurr, London

McCormick B (ed) 1995 The medical practitioner's guide to paediatric audiology. Cambridge University Press, Cambridge

Scanlon P E, Bamford J M 1990 Early detection of hearing loss: screening and surveillance methods. Archives of Disease in Childhood 65:479–484

Sutton G J, Scanlon P E 1999 Health visitor screening versus vigilance: outcomes of programmes for detecting permanent childhood hearing loss in West Berkshire. British Journal of Audiology 33:145–156

Tassabehji M, Read A P, Newton V E et al 1992 Waardenburg's syndrome patients have mutations in the human homologue of the PAX-3 paired box gene. Nature 355:635–636

Watkins P M, Baldwin M, Laoide S 1990 Parental suspicion and identification of hearing-impairment. Archives of Disease in Childhood 65:846–850

Wood S 1993 Pure tone audiometry. In: McCormick B (ed) Paediatric audiology 0–5 years. Whurr, London, ch 6, p 155

Wood S, Davis A C, McCormick B 1997 Changing yield of the health visitor distraction test when targeted neonatal screening is introduced into a health district. British Journal of Audiology 31:55–61

Yoshinaga-Itano C, Sedey A L, Coulter D K, Mehl A L 1998 Language of early and later identified children with hearing loss. Pediatrics 102:1161–1171

35 | Speech and language

This chapter is written from the perspective of a community paediatrician. The acquisition and the aetiology and classification of disorders in speech and language will be discussed but should the reader require more detail on intervention and rehabilitation, speech and language therapy texts should be consulted.

The community paediatrician is frequently asked by other healthcare professionals to assess a child with delayed speech and language. Their investigations must always include accurate hearing assessment (to exclude permanent and temporary hearing losses) and full developmental assessment. Speech and language delay is frequently seen as part of a more global developmental delay and, if found, medical examination to exclude known syndromes and conditions associated with developmental delay should be performed. Advice regarding diagnosis, intervention, treatment and likely outcome is gathered from a multidisciplinary team including speech and language therapist, audiologists, educational psychologists, clinical psychologists, paediatric neurologists and others.

THE ACQUISITION OF LANGUAGE

Within a very few years the human child develops the most complex cognitive function known to man, that is the acquisition of a spoken language.

In recent years most research has proposed that the child is 'pre-programmed' to comprehend and to develop such a system. It seems that a child inherits a 'language processor' which enables the child to develop and to refine a linguistic apparatus and that we cannot explain the acquisition of language by imitation alone.

The development of language is an individual process with universal trends. It is a gradual process continuing well into primary school years and even then it cannot be said to be complete, for modification and acquisition of higher and more complex language takes place in teenage and adult years.

The acquisition of a spoken language is an interactive process, depending upon active conversational practise with parents, siblings and others and is not based on imitation alone, although it does have a role, with some children imitating more than others. It seems that the active participation of the child, 'trying out' new vocabulary and 'testing out' new conversational rules, is the key to the successful acquisition of language.

The human baby develops pre-linguistic skills in the first year of life. He is born with a very mobile tongue and sophisticated vocal organs to allow vocalisation and soon after birth he becomes a highly sociable being, initiating two-way interactions with his carers by looking, smiling, cooing and crying.

A neonate also has sophisticated auditory perceptual skills and is capable of distinguishing individual speech sounds (e.g. 'p' and 'b'). This has been shown by analysis of changes in amplitude of sucking pressures on an artificial nipple, in response to tape-recorded speech sounds.

In addition the human baby has the ability to develop symbolic systems and seems to be 'pre-programmed' to comprehend and develop grammatical patterns.

All of these factors have particular relevance to pre-lingually hearing impaired children and to those with conditions of defective social interaction such as autism.

At 3–6 months babies start to vocalise developing babble patterns, containing consonant and vowel sounds (e.g. 'ba' and 'da'). At around 6–12 months babble then becomes repetitional (e.g. 'ba-ba' and 'da-da') and also becomes more speech like. Babble then drifts towards the child's own language, for instance a Chinese baby's babble by 9 months of age may sound quite different to that of an English baby of a similar age. Distinct words then gradually emerge from babble patterns and can initially be quite difficult to distinguish.

At around 12 months of age the child acquires his first word which is individual to that child; indeed the author's own four children each had a different first word — 'food', 'Dad', 'train' and 'bed'. First words may not have a specific syntactic role, 'drink' for instance may be used as a noun for a cup, as a subject for fruit squash or as a verb for the act of drinking.

Throughout his first year, the child's motivation to communicate advances as does his attentional and listening skills.

At around 12–14 months the child develops referencing. The child is able to filter out of a spoken sentence an object name and understands what that object is by looking (e.g. 'that's a cat over there'). At the same time meaningful pointing begins, when the child looks and points to an object (e.g. a cup) and then turns to look to the parent and back to the object as if to say 'I know that you know, that I would like a drink!'

When a child has acquired around 30 words in his vocabulary there tends to be a rapid spurt in further acquisition and vocabulary tends to become more adult like. When the child has developed a vocabulary of around 50 words, a child starts to combine words into phrases. Typically a child uses two-word utterances for naming (e.g. 'that car'), for possession (e.g. 'baby book'), description (e.g. 'pretty bird') or plurality (e.g. 'two dog'). This trend appears to be universal across languages (and indeed across manual signing systems).

At around 2 years a child tends to develop early grammar, for example 'daddy sleep' (object and verb). Some language produced at around this age may appear to be grammatical but on further analysis seems to be the addition of little chunks on to some already learned grammar, for example, 'that's mine — sweetie'. Grammar continues to develop by the child actively participating in conversation to trial their use of grammar. Clark long ago in 1974–76 coined the phrase 'talking to learn rather than learning to talk'.

A child tends to acquire a grammatical system between the age of 2 years and 4 years 6 months. There is great individual variation but there does appear to be some universal ordering. Most children develop the use of 'ing', i.e. 'he is running', before the correct use of past tense. Three-word phrases tend to appear from the age of 2 years through to the age of 2 years 6 months with four- and five-word sentences appearing around 3 years of age to 3 years 6 months. A general maturation of language and grammatical skills takes place from the age of around 3 years 6 months for a further year when syntactical development is usually complete. Language continues to develop stylistically from around school entry age and can be used creatively to express ideas and thoughts and to direct activity.

Throughout the process of acquiring grammar and sentence structure, a child practises his conversational skills constantly, with parents and carers providing interaction, feedback and correction by indirect means. Parents do not normally provide absolute correction of grammatical mistakes but do offer indirect correction in the form of contingent questioning. For example:

Child: He runned in a race
Parent: When did he run the race?
Child: Yesterday
Parent: Yes he ran the race yesterday

Nature or nurture?

Undoubtedly the development of an effective spoken language will depend upon the conversational environment in which a child is reared and those children deprived of conversational input frequently develop deviant language.

Nature does play a part and it has been known for some time that communication difficulties run in families. Recently strong evidence has been provided by Dale et al (1998) in the Twins Early Development Study that heritability is stronger amongst those with the poorest language skills. There is also evidence of a genotype for specific language impairment, which may explain the language delay for some children growing up in a rich conversational atmosphere.

Can the way parents speak to a young child enhance development of an effective spoken language system? This aspect is relatively under-researched but certainly many cultures use 'child-directed speech' as a way of interacting with their children before they are able to keep pace with adult conversation. This type of speech has differing sound features to that of an adult. The pitch is higher, the intonation is more exaggerated and the tempo is slower. This appears to capture and maintain the child's attention and makes it clear that the parent is talking to the child and no one else. The utterances are predominantly short, only two to three words longer than the child's own utterances, and well formed. This enables the child with a shorter attention span to follow the whole sentence. In child-directed speech there are fewer false starts and hesitations and fewer complex sentences and subordinate clauses. It is highly repititious and uses recasts and reformulations, providing correct 'models of speech'.

As the child becomes more linguistically competent parents tend to use more questions rather than imperatives. A younger child would probably be directed (imperative) to 'Give Mummy the cup' but an older child (though still acquiring language and grammatical skills) might be asked the closed question 'Are you going to give me that cup?' Open questions are more usually employed when the child has developed a competent language and grammatical system.

By looking in detail at the process of acquisition of spoken language it can be seen that those children with permanent (or temporary) hearing loss, those with global developmental delay, those with social and emotional developmental delay and those with social deprivation are likely to have significant difficulty and therefore delay in acquiring an effective spoken language system (Table 35.1).

PREVALENCE OF SPEECH AND LANGUAGE DISORDERS

Silva et al (1987) found in his review of prevalence studies for speech and language disorders that prevalence ranges from 3% to 15% with a median of 6–8%. There is considerable variation due to differences in definition of language impairment and sample numbers of children included in the studies. However most researchers agreed on a prevalence rate of around 1% for severe language impairment. Prevalence rates are generally higher for boys than girls (by a factor of two) and for lower socio-economic groups.

It has also been shown that low IQ scores are more common among children with language disorder than among the general population. Twenty-five per cent of 7 year olds with any language disorder had a low general IQ with 13% having a low IQ in a total sample of 7 year olds. In the same study (Silva et al 1983) 40% of children with language impairment affecting both expressive and receptive abilities had low IQ scores.

In the Dundee study, Drillien & Drummond (1983) showed that 26% of pre-school children having language disorders also displayed behaviour difficulties including hyperactivity, poor concentration, attention-seeking behaviour, tantrums and aggressive and disruptive behaviour, compared to an estimated frequency of 5.4% for a total pre-school population. Subsequently, Silva et al (1984) found behavioural problems occurred more frequently in those children who had a low IQ and language impairment.

CAUSES OF LANGUAGE DELAY

Distinction must be made between speech and language delay which is associated with developmental delay in other areas and specific language disorders where development in other areas is essentially normal.

Bishop & Rosenbloom (1987) have produced a medical model for classification of speech and language impairments by the supposed aetiology. They have identified seven groups which are detailed in Box 35.1.

Table 35.1
The typical pattern of language acquisition over time

Age level (months)	Language development	Grammatical structures	Sound system
9–18	First words	Noun-like: cup Verb-like: gone Other: bye bye	p/b/t/d/w/m/n final consonant — missing Reduplication: gee-gee
18–24	Two-word phrases	SV: Daddy kick SO: Mummy shoe VO: kick ball	As above
24–30	Three-word phrases	SVO: daddy kick ball Use of: the/is/a Word endings: ing/ed Plural: s	Above and k/g/ng/h Final consonant may be missing still
30–36	Four-word phrases	SVAA: me go in kitchen in a minute Have been + could have er/est/s/	Above and f/s/l/y Clusters may appear Final consonants present
36–42	Five-word phrases	More complex sentences Use of because Me becomes I Tenses appear	As above
42–54	Maturation of language skills	Correct past tense I goed = I went Sheeps = sheep Plurals	As above and v/z/sh/ch/j/r
54 onwards	Creative language to express ideas and thoughts	Syntactic development complete	Mature sound system b but may still be w for r and th for f

S = subject; V = verb; O = object; A = adverb

LINGUISTIC ELEMENTS OF SPEECH AND LANGUAGE

Figure 35.1 illustrates the link between the auditory–perceptual pathway, higher brain functioning and the expression of oral language.

Various linguistic terms are attached to elements within spoken language. Phonology is the study of the sound system of language, with phonetics being the study of the production of single speech sounds. The grammatical system is divided linguistically into morphology, the study of the internal structure of words (e.g. kicked versus kicking), and syntax, the study of sentence structure. Semantics is the study of the way meaning is organised within language and pragmatics is the study of the factors that govern our choice of language in social interaction.

Linguistic classification of speech and language impairments

Speech and language disorders can be categorised into expressive or receptive impairments, which can then be subdivided linguistically into four areas of difficulty, relating to the level of language system that is impaired. If both receptive and expressive functions are affected the language disorder is then redefined as a general language impairment.

Phonological problems occur when the child has difficulty producing and/or perceiving contrasts between speech sounds, for example p and b. Syntactic problems are difficulties with expression or comprehension of grammar and semantic problems are present when the child is unable to express or understand the meaning of individual words and sentences. Pragmatic disorders prevent the child using language to communicate correctly or to recognise the communicative intent of the speaker. A child with a pragmatic disorder may repeat a speaker's question instead of formulating an answer.

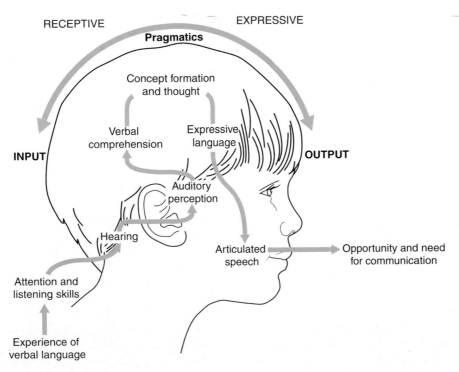

Fig. 35.1 Pathway from 'sound to speech'.

Speech and language

> ### Box 35.2
> ## Classification of language disorders
>
> 1. Speech limited in quality/quantity but other language skills normal
> 2. Generalised delay of language development
> 3. Specific problems with syntax and phonology
> 4. Specific problems with semantics and pragmatics
> 5. Poor understanding and limited verbal expression
> 6. Severe impairment of non-verbal as well as verbal communication

Language disorders can be broadly classified into six groups to include both immature and disordered patterns. Box 35.2 gives details of this classification.

SPECIFIC LANGUAGE DISORDERS

A child has a specific speech and language disorder when difficulties exist in the language area while other areas of development are essentially normal. Speech and language problems associated with autism, hearing loss, cerebral palsy and general learning difficulties, for example, are therefore excluded from this group.

The most common of the specific language disorders is the phonological-syntactic syndrome which falls into the third group of linguistic classification outlined above. These children have difficulty mastering the expressive sound system and grammar of language. They may have mild comprehension difficulties which show up on formal testing but these are much less severe than their expressive difficulties. They use a very restricted range of speech sounds which renders their speech unintelligible to the unfamiliar listener. This disorder ranges in severity and some children do well with formal speech and language therapy but others will need input from a speech and language programme in school or from specialised language units. Many children make good progress but may have later educational problems with the language disorder transferring to difficulties with reading and spelling.

Developmental vebal dyspraxia is less common than the syndrome described above and is also a disorder of phonology and syntax. The child does not have difficulty in producing individual sounds but does have difficulty in accurately programming a rapid sequence of sounds. The aetiology is controversial and there is debate as to whether the disorder is a sensory-motor disorder of the speech apparatus or is part of a more general problem of motor speech planning. Some of these children have other problems, for example abnormal EEG, non-speech apraxias or other motor disorders.

The semantic-pragmatic disorder of speech and language is rarely seen and on first hearing, the child's speech may appear normal, as the child's grasp of phonology and syntax is well developed. Yet conversation is extremely hard work as the child may conduct a monologue including irrelevant detail whilst omitting important points. Communication may break down as the usual sequence of turn taking is not followed. Non-verbal aspects of communication such as eye contact and facial expression are not used in the normal manner. Understanding of sentence structure may be normal but comprehension is 'concrete' in nature and the child is not aware of alternative meanings of words and phrases and cannot interpret the tone of the conversation. Unlike autistic children they do have a desire to communicate and are very much aware of their failure to interact with their carers and peers.

Auditory verbal agnosia, seen in the very rare Landau–Klefner syndrome, is a severe example of a language disorder in the category of poor understanding and limited verbal expression. The primary problem is one of comprehension leading to severely restrictive expression. Indeed the child is often thought to be deaf. The child starts to develop language early which then regresses with the onset of EEG abnormalities and seizures. These children may depend on visual cues, for example lipreading and signing to understand language. If a sign system is used in intervention and remediation it is usually the Paget–Gorman sign system, which includes signs to indicate grammatical inflections unlike other sign systems. Understanding of written language may also be affected.

SPEECH AND LANGUAGE DISORDERS ASSOCIATED WITH OTHER DEVELOPMENTAL DELAY

Hearing impairment

The development of an effective spoken language is unusual in those who have a severe to profound permanent hearing loss (85 dBHL or greater), even with amplification. Those with a moderate to severe loss (50–70 dBHL) tend to develop an effective and oral language once adequately amplified.

However there are exceptions to this rule and the potential to develop spoken language cannot be accurately predicted from the audiogram alone. A manual signing system employed alongside spoken language by carers is now often recommended at diagnosis of a severe to profound hearing loss to allow both systems to develop to full potential in a bilingual approach. The education of hearing-impaired children in the UK is varied and may follow a bilingual approach (oral and written English plus British Sign Language), a total communication approach (using spoken and signed English, lipreading and gesture) or an oral-aural approach depending on the county's policy.

The earlier a child is amplified the greater the potential for spoken language, and recently Yoshinaga-Itano et al (1998) has shown in a large study that children adequately aided before the age of 6 months have significantly better oral language skills than those who were amplified after the age of 6 months (whether or not they were exposed to signing systems). This has led to the drive for universal neonatal hearing screening programmes in the UK.

Acquisition of language in hearing-impaired children

Hearing-impaired children do develop babble but at a later age (15 months rather than 7 months in a hearing child) and their babble has a different quality having more glides and glottal stops. The consonant types decrease with age in hearing-impaired children whereas in hearing children consonant types increase in number as babble drifts into speech. Eventually babble ceases in hearing-impaired children unless they are effectively aided.

Acquisition of spoken language in hearing-impaired children seems to follow the same pattern as in hearing children but at a much later age, even if appropriately aided. The first word may only be achieved by the age of 3 years and a 5-year-old hearing-impaired child in school may still be in the 'acquisition of language' stage, when child-directed speech and closed questions in conversation might still be appropriate. His teacher's conversation and language may be 'out of his reach' and beyond his capabilities to comprehend.

Hearing-impaired children relying only on auditory input, develop 'referencing' much later than hearing children. Parental use of conversation with a hearing-impaired child may be much curtailed if they cannot play an interactive role, leading to less practice of coversation. Hearing-impaired children have great difficulty acquiring the semantics of words and grammatical meanings. In English some words have different meanings in different contexts, for example give me a hand. An 8 year old hearing-impaired boy in school is asked to paint a picture — he loads a paint brush with green paint and paints a magazine cover green.

A hearing-impaired child does not go through the stages of semantic invention, that hearing children do, when taught formally at later stages. At 2 years 3 months a hearing child may well exclaim 'Mummy trousers me' when talking about being dressed. Hearing-impaired children tend not to develop such inventions.

Hearing-impaired children are not good at developing contingent questions and this stage appears much later. In order to develop conversational skills, hearing children develop contingent queries at around 3–4 years, for example Mummy: 'Put the dolly on the table', Child: 'Which dolly?' In addition hearing-impaired children tend not to provide information as a speaker thus limiting conversational skills. They are not able to 'talk to learn' as do hearing children.

Incidental listening (the overhearing of the conversation of others) is much curtailed in hearing-impaired children. At first language is learned in a one to one situation but is later greatly extended by overhearing other adults' and children's speech.

It is interesting to note that hearing-impaired children born into hearing-impaired and signing families tend to develop signing language skills over a similar time scale and at similar (or even earlier) ages to hearing children developing spoken language.

Temporary hearing loss associated with secretory otitis media (glue ear) may lead to significant speech and language delay, depending on the degree and the duration of hearing loss and on the stage of language acquisition. Once the diagnosis is made and grommets or hearing aids are employed to restore hearing to normal levels then the language delay tends to resolve rapidly. Maw (1999) has shown that after 18 months of normal hearing there are no significant residual language deficits.

Social deprivation

Referring back to the process of acquisition of speech, it is easy to see how social deprivation and therefore lack of language input and conversational experience may lead to delay in acquisition of speech and language. This delay often resolves rapidly if a change to a conversationally rich atmosphere takes place. This is frequently seen in cases of fostered or adopted children who have been emotionally or socially deprived.

Delayed global development

In syndromes or conditions of delayed global development, speech and language skills reflect the degree of developmental delay. Many of the genetic or chromosomal syndromes involving developmental delay also have associated hearing impairment (e.g. Down's syndrome) and speech and language may be further delayed than the general developmental level. Speech and language thera-

pists will often use manual signing systems (e.g. Makaton) with such children to enhance communicative ability. Makaton borrows some signs from British Signed Language (BSL) but the individual signs are generally easier to comprehend and to execute, thereby matching the child's developmental level.

Elective mutism

This condition is a rare emotional disorder, where a child is reported to speak and to use sentence structure in one environment (usually the home) but to be completely silent in other situations of their choosing (school, shops or anywhere outside the home). It can be very difficult to treat and may require sensitive handling and psychological support. More often than not speech and language skills are within normal limits when eventually demonstrated.

Autistic disorders

Delayed or disordered communicative development is one of the defining characteristics of autism. Other characteristics are impaired social development, ritualistic or repetitive behaviours and onset of symptoms before the age of 30 months.

Speech and language skills may never develop normally or may appear to develop normally at first but are then lost (before the age of 30 months). Rutter & Lord (1987) reported that 70–80% of autistic children also have severe learning difficulties and that about 50% of autistic children (the majority of which also have severe learning difficulties) never develop functional speech.

A very wide range of linguistic abilities exist within the complete autistic spectrum. At one extreme a child diagnosed as autistic may be completely mute and another autistic child may score within average range on verbal tests by teenage years. However even those with better speech and language skills tend to have deficits in the semantic and pragmatic aspects of language. Rapin & Allen (1987) found in a group of autistic children a range of linguistic problems similar to that shown by a group of children with specific language disorders, but semantic/pragmatic problems were more frequent in the autistic group. Autistic children also have difficulties with non-linguistic aspects of communication which link with semantics and pragmatics, such as difficulties in producing and understanding gesture, facial expressions and intonation.

A common characteristic of autstic language is the use of echolalia. These children tend to build up stock phrases which seem superficially accurate but are often used in inappropriate situations. There is debate as to whether autistic children use echolalia with communicative intent.

INTERVENTION AND TREATMENT

Formal speech and language therapy is provided to enhance and improve communicative ability in developmental speech and language disorders and to remediate those linguistic areas affected in specific speech and language disorders. This is performed in a variety of ways by speech and language therapists specialising in childhood disorders. Individual therapy in the clinic, combined with 'homework' performed by parents, may result in considerable improvement in the milder developmental disorders. In more severe disorders, group therapy (in the clinic or opportunity groups) to provide more intensive conversational experience may be combined with higher levels of individual work.

At school entry, speech and language programmes provided by educational assistants and monitored by speech and language therapists may be necessary for those with moderate to severe disorders, and these children may enter the statementing process for those with special educational needs. More severely affected children may require intensive remediation in language units within schools, where speech and language therapists and specialised teachers are on the staff.

PROGNOSIS FOR SPEECH AND LANGUAGE DISORDER

The prognosis for general language impairment is less good compared to specific language impairments, which do not persist for so long. Silva et al (1983) found in a longitudinal study that 40% of children who had any language impairment at 3 years still showed impairments at 5 years, and that 31% of children who had a language impairment at 5 years still had impaired language at 7 years. Of those who had a general language impairment at 3 years, 79% still had a general impairment at 5 years and of those children with general language impairments at age 5 years, 53% had a persisting impairment at age 7 years.

Speech and language problems may also persist into adolescence as Sheridan & Peckham (1978) showed in the National Child Development Study. At 16 years 51% of children who had speech and language problems at 7 years still had some persisting language difficulties. So far few longitudinal studies have carried on until adult years but there is an indication that severe and specific language disorders may persist to some degree even into adult life.

Bishop & Edmundson (1987) found that speech and language therapists can by assessment predict with a 90% accuracy whether or not speech and language disorders in 4-year-old children will resolve within an 18-month period of time. Those children at 4 years with the most severe and the most general speech and language impairments (assessed by a battery of linguistic and non-linguistic tests) were the least likely to recover.

Prognosis for reading abilities

It has been generally understood that children with speech and language impairments in pre-school years often have difficulties later with acquiring literacy. Bishop & Adams (1990) followed children with language disorder from 4 years to 8 years 6 months and found that it was only those children who had persistent disordered spoken language that had difficulties with acquiring literacy. If the spoken language difficulties had resolved by the age of 5 years 6 months the children had no more difficulty than others with no history of language problems in learning to read and write.

CONCLUSIONS

The community paediatrician has a vital role to play in the full developmental assessment of a child with speech and language disorders in order that the correct aetiology is assumed and that appropriate therapy and interventions can be planned and instituted.

The community paediatrician will also be closely involved with alerting educational authorities to the child's special educational needs in respect of their communication difficulties. In the most severe cases children will benefit from special educational programmes and continuing therapy and medical care.

REFERENCES AND FURTHER READING

Bamford J, Saunders E 1992 Hearing impairment, auditory perception and language disability. Whurr, London

Bishop D, Adams C 1990 A prospective study of the relationship between specific language impairment, phonological disorders and reading retardation. Journal of Child Psychology and Psychiatry 31:1027–1050

Bishop D, Edmundson A 1987 Language — impaired 4-year olds: distinguishing transient from persistent impairment. Journal of Speech and Hearing Disorders 52:156–173

Bishop D, Rosenblam L 1987 Classification of childhood language disorder. In: Yule W, Rutter M (eds) Language development and disorders. MacKeith Press/Blackwell, Oxford

Crystal D, Varley R 1993 Introduction to language pathology. Whurr, London

Dale PS, Simonoff E, Bishop DV et al 1998 Genetic influence on language delay in two-year-old children. Nature Neuroscience 1:324–328

Donaldson ML 1995 Children with language impairments. Jessica Kingsley, London

Drillien C, Drummond M 1983 Developmental screening and the child with special needs. Heinemann Medical, London

Law J, Parkinson A, Tamhne R 2000 Communication difficulties in childhood. Radcliffe Medical Press, Oxford

Maw AR 1999 Early surgery with watchful waiting for glue ear and effect on language development on spre-school children: a randomised trial Lancet 353(9157):960–963

Rapin I, Allen D 1987 Developmental dysphasia and autism in preschool children: characteristics and subtypes. In: Proceedings of the First International Symposium on Specific Speech and Language Disorders in Children. AFASIC, University of Reading

Rutter M, Lord C 1987 Language disorders associated with psychiatric disturbance. Language Development and Disorders: MacKeith Press/Blackwell, Oxford

Sheridan M, Peckham C 1978 Follow-up to 16 years of school children who had marked speech defects at 7 years. Child: Care, Health and Development 4:145–157

Silva PA, McGee R, Williams SM 1983 Developmental language delay from three to seven years and its significance for low intelligence and reading difficulties at age seven. Developmental Medicine and Child Neurology 25:783–793

Silva PA, Justin C, McGee R, Williams SM 1984 Some developmental and behavioural characteristics of seven year old children with delayed speech development. British Journal of Disorders of Communication 19:147–154

Silva PA, Williams SM, McGee R 1987 A longitudinal study of children with developmental language delay at age three: later intelligence, reading and behaviour problems. Developmental Medicine and Child Neurology 29:630–640

Yoshinaga-Itano C, Sedey AL, Coulter DK, Mchl AL 1998 Language of early and later identified children with hearing loss. Pediatrics 102:1161–1171

36 | Learning disability

TERMINOLOGY

The term learning disability is generally accepted by professionals and carers in the UK, and those with a learning disability themselves, as the most appropriate term to describe people who have a reduced ability to understand new or complex information, to learn new skills and to cope independently, which started before adulthood, and with a lasting effect on development (Department of Health 1995).

Over the years, many other terms have been used, and some still are in different organisations and cultures. For instance, 'mental retardation' is commonly used in the USA, and many English language medical textbooks refer to 'mental handicap'. Some terms are, at best, old fashioned and inaccurate. They may also be viewed as negative and patronising, and can cause offence.

Clear terminology is important for a variety of reasons, not least in providing an easily understood 'shorthand' when communicating with others. It is essential that we ensure that the terminology we use is acceptable to others, by checking we have a shared understanding of the meaning, and that we do not offend.

The terms used may illustrate society's, or an individual's, attitude to people with learning disability. Terms that may be acceptable at one time, come to be used inappropriately, sometimes completely out of context as a derogatory term, and therefore become unacceptable, even when used as originally intended. Changes in terminology are therefore likely to continue (Table 36.1). They should not be 'written off' as 'political correctness' without careful thought, and the new terminology should be welcomed and incorporated into everyday language.

Confusion may still exist with the various terms currently used by different organisations or cultures, or in other languages or countries. The reader should be aware of the different way in which the term 'learning disability' is used in the USA. The term 'mental retardation' is still used where we would use 'learning disability'. Learning disability is used in the USA to describe where the child does not have a global impairment of intellect and functioning but has difficulties with specific areas of learning, for example reading (dyslexia) or motor coordination (clumsiness). On this side of the Atlantic, we describe these problems as specific learning difficulties or disabilities (see Further discussion in Chapter 32).

Traditionally, measured IQ has been used to subdivide people with learning disability according to their level of functioning. In the UK, formal IQ testing is not commonly carried out, partly because of its limitations, but mainly because of the value of concentrating on an individual's strengths and needs, rather than 'pigeon-holing' them into an IQ group.

Medical classification, on the one hand, as in the International Classification of Diseases (ICD 10) (Table 36.2), does subdivide into four categories on the basis of IQ. Educational terminology, on the other hand, has concentrated on two groups — those with severe learning disability (SLD), with an IQ less than 50, and those with moderate learning disability (MLD) with an IQ of 50–70. There is of course no distinct cut-off point between any of these groups, and it is always wise to be wary of overgeneralisation, but broadly speaking these two

Table 36.1
Historical use of terminology to describe learning disability

Approx IQ	Prior to 1959	1959 Mental Health Act	1968 World Health Organization	Pre- 1971 Education Act	1971 Education Act	1981 Education Act
0–20	Idiot		Profound mental handicap			
20–35	Imbecile	Severely subnormal	Severe mental handicap	Ineducable	ESN (S)	SLD
35–50			Moderate mental handicap			
50–70	Feeble minded	Subnormal	Mild mental handicap	Educationally subnormal (ESN)	ESN (M)	MLD

Table 36.2
Classification of learning disability according to ICD 10

Degree of learning disability	IQ	Approximate mental age likely to be achieved as adult in years
Mild	50–69	9–11
Moderate	32–49	6–8
Severe	20–34	3–5
Profound	<20	<3

groups do have different characteristics as shown in Table 36.3. For the purposes of the remainder of this chapter, SLD will be used to describe those with an IQ less than 50, and MLD with an IQ greater than 50, rather than the ICD classification.

HOW MANY CHILDREN HAVE LEARNING DISABILITY?

The number of children who are said to have a learning disability will vary depending on the definition used as discussed above, and the methods used to identify affected children within a popula-

tion. Furthermore, differences in rates in different studies may reflect genuine variation in prevalence between communities and countries. In general, those with severe disability are more likely to be identified, as their needs are greater and therefore more obvious. Most studies suggest that 3–4 children per 1000 live births will have severe learning disability (IQ < 50), and about ten times that number moderate learning disability (IQ 50–70) (Roelveld et al 1997). Many children with learning disability also have another disability. Table 36.4 shows an estimate of numbers of children with learning disability and various other conditions likely to be found within a typical health district of 250 000 people.

CAUSES OF LEARNING DISABILITY

The likelihood of finding a biological explanation for a child's learning disability increases with the degree of disability (Fig. 36.1). For children with SLD, an explanation should be available for the majority. Swedish studies suggest that only 18% of those with an IQ less than 50 will not have an identifiable cause, whereas for those with MLD, an IQ in the range 50–70, 55% have no known cause (Hagberg & Kyllerman 1983).

With developments in technology, including new imaging techniques and advances in molecular

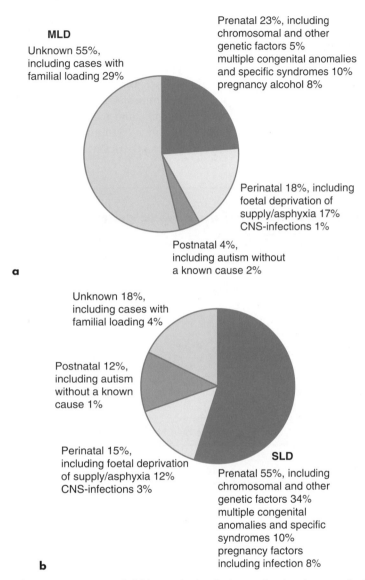

MLD

Unknown 55%, including cases with familial loading 29%

Prenatal 23%, including chromosomal and other genetic factors 5% multiple congenital anomalies and specific syndromes 10% pregnancy alcohol 8%

Perinatal 18%, including foetal deprivation of supply/asphyxia 17% CNS-infections 1%

Postnatal 4%, including autism without a known cause 2%

a

Unknown 18%, including cases with familial loading 4%

Postnatal 12%, including autism without a known cause 1%

Perinatal 15%, including foetal deprivation of supply/asphyxia 12% CNS-infections 3%

SLD

Prenatal 55%, including chromosomal and other genetic factors 34% multiple congenital anomalies and specific syndromes 10% pregnancy factors including infection 8%

b

Fig. 36.1 Pie charts indicating proportions of children with identified cause for their learning disability. From Gillberg (1995). (**a**) Moderate learning difficulties. (**b**) Severe learning difficulties

genetics, it is likely that a biological explanation will be found for a greater proportion of the children in the future. Table 36.5 suggests a classification of recognised causes of learning disability. In addition, the glossary at the end of this chapter shows the range of syndromes related to learning disability.

ASSESSMENT AND MANAGEMENT OF CHILDREN WITH LEARNING DISABILITY

The general approach to assessment and management of a child with a learning disability will be similar to that for other children with special needs.

Learning disability

This has been covered in more detail in Chapter 30. This chapter looks particularly at adapting the approach for the child with learning disability.

Who should assess and manage the child with learning disability?

A number of different professionals are likely to be involved in the care of a child with a learning dis-ability, from different disciplines within the health services, as well as from other agencies, for example education, social services and the voluntary sector. For children identified prenatally or in infancy (see below), their initial presentation is likely to be to health professionals. They are likely to see their GP initially, and may be referred to a general paediatrician, a community paediatrician, a developmental paediatrician or a paediatric neurologist. This

Table 36.3		
Differences in characteristics between groups of people with SLD and MLD		
Characteristic	**SLD**	**MLD**
Organic cause	Likely	Unlikely to be found
Associated disabilities and medical problems	Likely	Unlikely
Family history of learning disability	Unlikely	Likely
Social class distribution	Typical of population	Skewed towards lower socio-economic groups
Independence as an adult	Unlikely to be achieved	Quite likely

Table 36.4		
Prevalence and incidence of learning disability and associated conditions per health district of 250 000.		
Type/degree	**Children (no.)**	**Incidence per annum**
SLD	200	15–20
MLD	400	30–40
SLD + cerebral palsy	40	3–4
SLD + epilepsy	80	6–8
SLD + psychiatric problems	125	10–20
SLD + autism	20	1–2
SLD + visual impairment	40	3–4
SLD + hearing impairment	40	3–4
Adapted from British Paediatric Association (1994)		

Table 36.5
A classification of recognised causes of learning disability

Cause of learning disability	Example
Genetic	
Chromosomal aneuploidy	
Autosomal	Down's syndrome — Trisomy 21
Sex chromosomes	47XXX, 47XXY, 47XYY
Single gene	Turner's syndrome 45XO
Autosomal	Tuberous sclerosis
	Neurofibromatosis
	Angelman's
	Prader–Willi
	William's
	Amino acid disorders, e.g. phenylketonuria
	Mucopolysaccharidoses, e.g. Sanfilippo
X-linked	Duchenne muscular dystrophy
	Fragile X syndrome
Intrauterine	
Congenital infection	Rubella, toxoplasmosis, cytomegalovirus
Drugs in pregnancy	Alcohol
	Phenytoin
Cerebral malformations	Anencephaly
	Porencephaly
Perinatal	
Disorders of pregnancy	Pregnancy-induced hypertension
	Premature labour
Problems of labour and delivery	Birth asphyxia
	Trauma
	Prolonged labour
	Fetal distress
Neonatal problems	Hypoglycaemia
	Jaundice
	Meningitis
	Intravantricular haemorrhage
Postnatal	
Trauma	Accidents and non-accidental injury
Infection	Meningitis
	Encephalitis
Anoxia	Asphyxia
	Status epilepticus
Metabolic	Hypoglycaemia
	Hyponatraemia
Endocrine	Hypothyroidism
Poisoning	Lead

Box 36.1
Tasks for the paediatrician in managing a child with learning disability

- Identification of learning disability
- Assessment of nature of learning disability
- Assessment of associated problems
- Search for cause of the disability
- Explanation and information for the parents
- Support for the family
- Treatment of specific conditions
- Management of associated problems
- Coordination with other agencies
- Transition to adult care

---

service may be offered in a local health centre, a hospital or a child development centre, depending on how services are organised in that district. For older children the presentation may not be to health professionals, but via education. In some cases where the child's needs appear to be entirely related to learning, the medical assessment may be overlooked, or even thought inappropriate. However, it is important that the child has a comprehensive paediatric assessment for the many reasons summarised in Box 36.1, and expanded in the subsequent text.

Wherever the child is seen, the approach needs to be multidisciplinary. The doctor is just one player amongst the team of professionals. The tasks involve much coordination across agencies. The community-based paediatrician is likely to be in a good position to undertake this role.

IDENTIFICATION

Learning disability may be first suspected or identified in a child at any time from fetal life onward. The way in which the problems present will vary according to a number of factors, including the nature and severity of the disability, associated

problems, the environment in which the child lives, the astuteness of the carers and any health/developmental surveillance programmes in operation. Particular types of problems are however likely to present at particular times.

Prenatal

Sometimes, and increasingly frequently, a diagnosis that is likely to lead to learning disability is made during pregnancy. This may arise from findings on a routine scan, or from more specific testing, for example amniocentesis. In some cases the condition suspected is well understood (e.g. Down's syndrome), and the parents can be given information about the problems the child is likely to face. Often however an anomaly is picked up on scan, the nature of which is not entirely clear, but which is considered to be a 'marker' of a syndrome associated with learning disability. For example, choroid plexus cysts are associated with a number of chromosomal anomalies, but in many cases appear to have no significance, and occur in fetuses that have no subsequent problems.

The paediatrician, if invited by obstetric colleagues, may become involved at this stage, to give the prospective parents information about the condition suspected. In some circumstances, this information may lead to the parents not proceeding with the pregnancy. Unfortunately some parents complain of feeling pressurised into making such a decision, and that they are made to feel socially irresponsible if they allow their disabled child to be born. It is unacceptable for professionals to make parents feel like this. It is vital that accurate information is given honestly and sympathetically, in a non-judgemental and a non-directive manner. The final, often harrowing, choice lies with the parents. Their choice must be respected and supported whatever decision they reach. Where the pregnancy proceeds, the paediatrician may have an important role in providing information, which may help the family adjust to the diagnosis before the birth, and plan their child's future care.

Perinatal

Learning disability is often first considered in the perinatal period, either because the baby is noted at birth, or soon after, to have a syndrome associated with learning disability (e.g. Down's syndrome, Prader–Willi syndrome), or because the child has perinatal complications likely to cause brain damage, and subsequent learning disability (e.g. birth asphyxia, neonatal meningitis, intraventricular haemorrhage, extreme prematurity). In some babies, the suspicion of future learning disability will be high from the outset because of abnormal neurological behaviour in the neonatal period. In other cases, there may be no such indicator, but a high degree of suspicion because of the severity of the insult. All these 'high-risk' babies should have a special programme of follow-up so that subsequent problems can be identified early.

Infancy

Children with the most severe learning disability may present with difficulties with feeding and subsequent failure to thrive. Those with Prader–Willi syndrome often suck poorly, and feed very slowly. Children with cerebral palsy may have difficulty coordinating sucking and swallowing. Otherwise, the first concerns are usually about delay in reaching developmental milestones. At this stage, the concerns are around motor milestones, such as poor head control and delayed sitting. Sometimes the parents worry that the child cannot see or hear. In some cases, this will be because the child does indeed have an associated sensory impairment. Commonly, however, the infant appears to have a hearing or vision problem because of its global developmental delay.

Within this age group the parents usually raise the concerns, but delay may first be identified during routine child health surveillance in the primary care setting.

Early childhood

In young pre-school children the concern is usually because of delay in reaching milestones, most commonly with delayed language development. In children with moderate learning difficulties, early motor milestones may have been reached at the appropriate times, but they then show marked speech delay. Behavioural problems are also particularly common in this age group, and although the majority of troublesome toddlers have entirely normal development, it is always worth considering that the behavioural difficulties may be secondary to previously unrecognised developmental problems. Behavioural difficulties are commonly the presenting problem in children who are subsequently found to have a diagnosis within the autistic spectrum.

Later childhood

The majority of children with significant learning disability should be identified in infancy or early childhood, and well before school entry. Occasionally children 'slip through the net', and are only recognised once they start school. This may represent a failure of the child health surveillance system, though generally this relies heavily on parental report. Some parents are not able to see, or may be unwilling to acknowledge, problems that become obvious when the child is in the classroom environment. Children with less severe learning disability may well go unnoticed, until they are confronted with the greater demands of school. In some cases the parents may have noted their child as being different, but are so in tune with them, understanding them, and anticipating their every need that it is only when they go into a strange environment that the problems become apparent. This is often true for children with autistic spectrum disorders. Children with specific learning difficulties are unlikely to present until well into their schooldays, but this is beyond the scope of this chapter.

Acquired disability

A small number of children will acquire a learning disability following an episode of illness or trauma, or will have a deteriorating neurological condition. Sometimes these events are dramatic with severe consequences, of which learning disability is just a part, and the child's changed needs are obvious. They do however present major challenges to the families in coming to terms with the disability, and to the statutory agencies in making adequate provision. In some circumstances, for example moderately severe or even minor head injury, the child may be assumed to have made a full recovery, but has been left with a more subtle learning disability that requires careful evaluation.

ASSESSING THE LEARNING DISABILITY

The first task is to establish that the child does have a global learning disability, and the nature and extent of the difficulties. The paediatrician starts by taking a detailed medical, family and developmental history, together with an account of the child's current skills. Armed with this information the clinician can then plan the rest of the assessment. For an experienced paediatrician, a good evaluation of the child's development can be made by observing the child in the clinic, interacting with its parents and playing with simple toys. However, it is usual to go on to do a more detailed assessment using norm-referenced tools. This may be a screening type of test, for example Schedule of Growing Skills, Denver Developmental Screening Test, or a more detailed assessment such as the Griffiths Scales of Mental Development (see Chapter 5 for more details of developmental assessment). This is usually appropriate for the young preschool child.

For older children formal psychometric assessment by a clinical or educational psychologist may be preferable. Direct assessment in a clinical setting needs to be supplemented by observations of the child in other settings. Observational reports from playgroups, nurseries and schools are extremely valuable, and staff there will often have already prepared their own detailed developmental profile.

The developmental profile will identify the child's areas of strength and weakness in the different parameters of development. At this point, the clinician should be able to make a judgement as to whether the child does indeed have a global learning difficulty or whether there is any other explanation for the child's developmental difficulties (Table 36.6). Some of the conditions that can masquerade as learning disability will only become apparent with further assessment, for example a hearing assessment. The developmental profile should help decide what further assessment is necessary.

Table 36.6

Conditions that may be confused with learning disability — comparison of developmental profiles

	Motor	Language	Eye/hand co-ordination	Performance	Social
Severe learning disability	N/M	S	M/S	S	M/S
Moderate learning disability	N	M/S	N/M	M	N/M
Hearing impairment	N	M/S	N	N	N/M
Visual impairment	N/M	N	M	N	N/M
Autism (without significant cognitive impairment)	N	M/S	N/M	N	S
Specific language disorder	N	M/S	N	N	M/S
Environmental deprivation	N	M	N	N	N/M
Cerebral palsy	M/S	N/M/S	M/S	N/M	N/M
Specific learning difficulty — reading	N	N	N	N	N
Specific learning difficulty — motor	M/S	N	M/S	N	N

N = Normal; M = mild/moderate difficulty; S = severe difficulty

For children who are confirmed as having a learning disability this part of the assessment is important for a number of reasons. Firstly, knowing the degree of disability will be helpful in giving the parents an idea of the child's prognosis. There has been some debate about the predictive value of developmental assessment (Pollak 1993). In infancy, the correlation between test results and subsequent development is poor. It improves with age and over the age of three, developmental assessment scores do seem to correlate with subsequent development. Some parameters of development, namely language and performance or adaptive scales, give better predictions than others do, i.e. motor and social scales. The association between early assessment results and later development is also greatest for those with more severe disability, and more unreliable for those with borderline difficulties. The clinician needs to be aware of the limitations of developmental assessment. However with experience, and when the results are considered alongside the history, medical examination (see below) and reports from elsewhere, a much more accurate picture can be built. This will enable the paediatrician to discuss with the family the child's expected developmental progress, therapy and support they may need, and the degree of independence they are likely to achieve.

Investigation of cause

One of the most important tasks involved in assessing the child with a learning disability is to look for a biological explanation for the problem. As discussed earlier, this is likely to be possible for the majority of children with SLD, but the minority of those with MLD. Judgement is needed for any particular child as to how vigorously to investigate. Before embarking on invasive, unpleasant or even costly tests careful thought needs to be given to the likelihood of making a specific diagnosis, as well as the potential benefit to the child and family of making such a diagnosis. Only rarely will a diagnosis explaining the learning disability lead to a specific treatment. However there are a number of other reasons why a diagnosis may be of benefit (Box 36.2). A specific diagnosis may help with prognosis, particularly where the disease is degenera-

> **Box 36.2**
> **Why try to make a diagnosis**
>
> - Prognosis
> - Specific treatment
> - Appropriate management
> - Genetic counselling
> - Benefit of 'having an explanation'
> - Support groups

tive. In some cases, a diagnosis will be of a condition with particular associated medical and behavioural problems. Diagnosis of the underlying cause may therefore be critical in formulating an appropriate plan of management. Examples of this are tuberous sclerosis, fragile X, Prader–Willi syndrome and Down's syndrome. The latter will be discussed towards the end of this chapter. If the aetiology is genetic, a precise diagnosis will allow discussion of recurrence risks for the parents, siblings, the wider family and even the child. Having an appropriate 'label' will allow the parents to access relevant support groups. Lastly, the importance to the family of simply having an explanation should not be underestimated.

Physical examination

The physical examination is an important part of the assessment, and the approach is the same as for any child. However as well as considering the child's general health, the paediatrician needs to look for features that may lead to a specific diagnosis. General physical examination may reveal, for instance, a heart defect that has not had a significant impact on the child's health, but is associated with a specific diagnosis, for example aortic stenosis in Williams' syndrome. There may be signs of a metabolic disease, such as hepatosplenomegaly. Neurological examination may pick up evidence of cerebral palsy or a neurodegenerative condition. Growth assessment and a careful look at the skin, facial features, hands and genitalia may give clues to diagnosis. Some examples of such features are given in Table 36.7. It must be remembered that

Table 36.7
Physical features in learning disability

Physical feature	Syndrome
Growth	
Short stature	Chromosomal e.g. Down's Turner's
Tall stature	Sotos, fragile X
Obesity	Prader–Willi
Skin	
Café-au-lait spots, neurofibromas, axillary freckling	Neurofibromatosis
Depigmented patches, adenoma sebaceum	Tuberous sclerosis
Facial port wine stain	Sturge–Weber
Head	
Large	Fragile X, Sotos,
Small	Smith–Lemli–Opitz, Down's
Face	
Eyes	
Stellate iris	William's
Brushfield spots, up slanting	Down's
Down slanting	Noonan's
Nose Upturned	William's, fetal alcohol
Ears	
Large	Fragile X
Small	Down's
Low set	Seckel, Noonan's
Lips	
Prominent	William's
Teeth	
Wide spaced or bowed	Angelman's
Palate	
Clefts	Smith–Lemli–Opitz
High arched	Sotos
Hair	
Hypopigmentation	Prader–Willi
Thin	Down's
Hands	
Size	
Small	Prader–Willi
Dermatoglyphics	
Single palmar crease	Down's
Genitalia	
Small penis	Prader–Willi
Large testes	Fragile X

many of these features may also be found in the general population, and are not of diagnostic value if considered in isolation. A useful text to refer to is 'Smith's Recognisable Patterns of Human Malformation' (Jones 1997).

Investigations

There are many investigations that may be done in children with learning disability. There is no consensus in the medical literature or amongst paediatricians as to how the child with a learning disability should be investigated (Gringras 1998). Judgement is required in deciding which children should be investigated, and how extensively. The decision should be based on the likelihood of finding a diagnosis (Fig. 36.1) and the benefit of a diagnosis to the child and family. The paediatrician must also consider any risks or unpleasantness for the child that may be involved in the investigation. For instance, a CT scan involves a considerable amount of radiation, and may require a general anaesthetic. Lastly, in a service of limited resources, some consideration must be given to cost.

There have been huge advances in technology in recent years and parents often expect us to be able to find an explanation for their child's disability. The parents must be included in discussions when planning how to investigate, and be given an explanation of the likelihood of finding a specific cause, together with the risks and benefits of investigations. A list of some of the investigations that may be considered is given in Box 36.3.

As well as the factors discussed above, the paediatrician may be guided by the history and findings when deciding which if any of these investigations to perform. Sometimes a decision will be made not to investigate, particularly if the child has moderate learning disability, and has no abnormalities on physical examination. It is often said that such children should only be investigated if their level of ability is significantly below that which would be expected after considering their parents' ability and their environment. However, it may be that both parents and child have the same diagnosis, and therefore should be appropriately investigated.

Although no recommendation of routine investigations is being made, it is worth considering which

> **Box 36.3**
> **Investigations to consider in a child with learning disability**
>
> *Commonly carried out:*
> - Full blood count and iron
> - Chromosomes — cytogenetic
> - Molecular genetics for fragile X
> - Creatine phosphokinase
> - Thyroid function
> - Urinary metabolic screen — organic acids, amino acids, mucopolysaccharides
>
> *Other tests to consider:*
> - Serum amino acids
> - Liver function tests
> - Calcium, phosphate
> - Lead, copper
> - White blood cell enzymes
> - Very long chain fatty acids
> - Serology — cytomegalovirus, toxoplasmosis, rubella
> - Skull X-ray
> - Cranial CT scan
> - Cranial MRI scan
> - EEG
> - Nerve conduction studies
> - ERG
> - Biopsy — muscle, skin, nerve

tests are commonly done, and most likely to be useful. Chromosome analysis and a test for fragile X using molecular genetic techniques are probably the most commonly carried out. Advances in technology within this field have been so rapid that it is worth considering repeating these tests in children who had 'normal' results in the past, but in whom there is a high degree of suspicion of a chromosomal anomaly. It is likely that many diagnoses of fragile X were missed in the past on cytogenetic analysis alone (Gringras & Barnicoat 1998). Creatine kinase estimation is worth doing in boys with motor delay as part of the picture because of the frequency of learning disability in muscular dystrophy. It is usually worth checking haemoglobin and iron, as iron deficiency is common in any group of children, and is known to impair learning. Thyroid function is also often performed, although hypothyroidism is most likely to be suspected from other aspects of history or examination. Lastly, a urinary metabolic screen is often requested, probably in part because it is relatively inexpensive and non-invasive. Important diagnoses, such as mucopolysaccharidoses, may be picked up before other characteristics of the condition are noted.

Parents will frequently request a 'brain scan', believing that if there is something 'wrong' with the child's brain, then you should be able to see it. For children with significant disability, or abnormal neurological findings, a CT scan may be useful, though some would now consider a magnetic resonance imaging (MRI) scan preferable in the investigation of learning disability. Imaging techniques are becoming increasingly sophisticated, and it is now not unusual to discover abnormalities in scans of children with moderate learning disability who we would not have even considered scanning a decade ago. It is likely that in the future it will be appropriate to investigate a much larger proportion of children with learning disability with some sort of neuroimaging technique.

Hearing and vision assessment

Whilst other parts of the assessment may be discretionary, an assessment of hearing and vision is mandatory for every child with a suspected learning disability. Occasionally the child may turn out not to have a learning disability, but the sensory difficulties are the primary problem. More commonly, the sensory impairment is not the cause of the learning disability, but is a significant associated factor. Many syndromes associated with learning disability also have hearing or vision problems as part of the constellation of signs and symptoms, for example Down's syndrome. This will often be associated with a congenital anomaly of the ear or the eye. For children who have a learning disability as a result of a cerebral 'insult', i.e. infection, asphyxia or trauma, damage may also have occurred to the neural pathways for hearing or vision. In many cases, the visual or hearing impairment is not directly connected to the learning disability, but the child coincidentally has the type of problem that occurs commonly in any child, such as 'glue ear' or a refractive error.

Whatever the cause of the problem it is essential that the sensory impairment is not overlooked, and is managed appropriately. Uncorrected visual or hearing impairment can be a cause of considerable secondary handicap to the learning disabled child. A bright child with a hearing loss is likely to recognise it themselves and seek appropriate help, to make allowances for their difficulty by sitting near the teacher, or asking friends to speak up, and often rapidly learn to lipread. The learning disabled child may depend on others to notice their difficulty. All too often it is overlooked, and any apparent problems dismissed as 'just part of the syndrome'. They are less likely to be able to work out their own strategies to minimise the problem.

An aggressive approach to diagnosis and treatment of sensory impairment is therefore justified. Details of methods of assessment and treatment are given in Chapters 33 and 34. Assessing a child with learning disability however can be a quite a challenge, and for some children considerable expertise and patience are needed. Sometimes children with learning disability miss the screening opportunities offered to all children because of these difficulties. Usually it will be necessary to arrange specialist assessment at a secondary or tertiary level. With this expertise, assessment is possible for most children using standard methods, but perhaps employing methods usually used for younger children. Occasionally the child will not be able to cooperate with testing, and electrophysiological tests will be required. This should be considered in the initial assessment of any child where the severity of learning disability makes testing difficult. It is probably not justifiable to do such tests repeatedly, particularly as sedation may be required, for example for brain stem evoked responses. However, as for all children, some sort of screening programme should be in place to detect sensory impairment arising after initial assessment. For the most disabled children where cooperative testing is not possible, it may be appropriate to rely on the observations and

Learning disability

opinions of the parents, teachers and other carers. Given the level of close individual attention this group of children require, such opinions are likely to be reliable. For the majority of children with learning disability who can be tested using standard or adapted cooperative methods, a proper screening programme should be in place. At a minimum, this should be the same as for any child, but for some groups the nature of sensory problems in that group may necessitate a more intensive programme (see below for recommendations in children with Down's syndrome).

MANAGEMENT OF ASSOCIATED MEDICAL PROBLEMS

After the initial assessment, one of the paediatrician's main roles is to identify and treat medical problems that may be associated with the disability. Children do not always spontaneously present with these problems, and part of the paediatrician's expertise is to know the range of problems likely to occur, ask the right questions in the history, and to pick up clues on examination.

Growth

Disorders of growth are common in children with learning disability. This may be a feature of the underlying syndrome, for example short stature in William's, Turner's, Seckel's and Smith–Lemli–Opitz syndromes, tall stature in fragile X and Sotos' syndrome. The paediatrician should however be cautious about accepting abnormal growth as part of the syndrome without considering that the child may be growing poorly, because of a coincidental health problem, growth disorder or poor nutrition. Growth assessment should therefore be part of the medical review, as for any other child. For some syndromes specialist growth charts are available reflecting the different patterns of growth (e.g. Down's and Turner's syndromes).

Obesity is associated with Prader–Willi syndrome where overeating seems to be due to a central problem with appetite regulation. Careful control of calorie intake and behavioural techniques can be successful. A tendency to obesity is common in many other syndromes, particular Down's syndrome where it is often assumed that it is an inevitable part of the syndrome. There is no real evidence to prove this. Rather, it seems that the obesity is a consequence of allowing inappropriate calorie intake for size and levels of activity, as is true for any individual. The health risks of obesity are the same as for the rest of the population, and possibly greater for children with associated cardiac or orthopaedic problems, and obesity should never be accepted without considering possible medical cause (e.g. hypothyroidism) and offering advice about diet and exercise.

Nutrition

The importance of good nutrition is covered elsewhere in this text (see Chapter 7). However ensuring an adequate nutritional intake can be difficult in the child with learning disability. In children with cerebral palsy, there may be difficulties with a number of different aspects of feeding, including chewing and coordination of swallowing. Children with neurological problems may not be able to swallow safely, and may choke and aspirate food leading to respiratory problems. Gastro-oesophageal reflux is also common in this group and may exacerbate the problem. The child with a learning disability may not acquire the skills to feed independently, especially if he has an associated physical disability. Parents and carers often spend several hours each day feeding their child, and become extremely skilled at doing so. Often the child still gains weight poorly despite the parents' best efforts.

A coordinated approach from the multidisciplinary team can help overcome many of these problems. This may be best offered from a specialist feeding clinic. An assessment of oromotor function by the speech and language therapist can help define the nature of the difficulty, sometimes with the assistance of videofluoroscopy. This advice may lead to altering the textures or thickness of food and drink, or feeding the child in a different position.

The occupational therapist can help with appropriate seating and special utensils. The dietician can advice on suitable foods with appropriate texture and nutritional supplements. Sometimes a decision will be made that oral feeding is not the most appropriate way to feed the child, and a gastrostomy suggested. Parents often see this as a drastic measure and are reluctant to consider it. However, the decrease in the amount of time spent feeding, and reduction in stress around mealtimes can improve the family's quality of life considerably. This together with improvements in the child's nutrition and subsequent health often justify the use of a gastrostomy.

Nutritional problems in learning disability are not always due to neurological problems. Many children with learning disability are poor eaters or have faddy diets. This is particularly true for children with autistic spectrum disorders who often have very restricted diets. Although the diet may be bizarre, it may not be nutritionally inadequate. The paediatrician should assess the child's nutritional status clinically and ask a dietician to assess the content of the diet. Where there are deficiencies (commonly iron and calcium), supplements may be given. It may be necessary to supplement the energy intake, and the dietician can advice the family on how they can do this within the range of foods the child will accept. In children in whom nutrition seems adequate, the parents can be largely reassured from a health point of view. However, they may still require referral to a clinical psychologist for advice about how to extend the range of foods accepted, and how to encourage appropriate mealtime behaviour.

Ear, nose and throat problems

Hearing problems are commonly associated with learning disability. The importance of diagnosis and treatment has been discussed. Managing the hearing impairment once diagnosed may also present challenges. In some circumstances, the management may not be the same as it would be for a child without learning disability. For instance in a child with learning disability the decision to treat glue ear, rather than waiting to see if it resolves, may be taken earlier both because of the child's difficulties in compensating for his hearing loss, and because the natural history may differ from that in other children. For instance in Down's syndrome, where the majority of children have glue ear, the 'glue' is thicker, the tendency for spontaneous resolution with age is less, and surgery is technically more difficult because of the small size of the external auditory meatus and the middle ear.

The treatment of choice may therefore not be to insert grommets, but to provide hearing aids.

Encouraging a child with learning disability to wear hearing aids may also be difficult, and specialist advice from teachers of the deaf can be invaluable.

Other ENT problems common in children with learning disabilities include obstructive sleep apnoea, particularly in children with Sanfilipo's syndrome, Down's syndrome, and other syndromes with midfacial anomalies. Symptoms of disturbed sleep and daytime drowsiness are often dismissed as being part of the learning disability and the diagnosis missed. In general, the treatment is adenotonsillectomy, but for the child with midfacial anomalies this may not be the answer, and other measures including palatal surgery may need to be considered.

Vision

Many children with learning disabilities have associated visual problems. Squints are extremely common and often associated with refractive errors. Examination of the eye, including the fundus, will be important in identifying problems and prescribing treatment but may also give valuable clues to diagnosis. In congenital rubella, there are a number of different eye problems that may affect vision, including microphthalmia, squint, cataracts and chorioretinitis. Some degenerative conditions may first present with failing vision, for example Batten's disease. Optic atrophy is commonly associated with cerebral palsy, hydrocephalus, microcephaly and storage diseases. The phenomenon of delayed visual maturation, where the child does not appear to see in the first few months of life, may also be associated with learning disability. Whilst some of these children do have recognisable ophthalmologic pathology, in others, examination and electrophysiological tests are normal, and vision subsequently improves spontaneously. In these cases it seems that the 'late seeing' is part of their overall developmental delay.

Children with learning disabilities should have their visual problems treated as for any child. For some, the impairment may not be amenable to any medical treatment or spectacles, but a description of their visual difficulties and abilities will help specialist teachers plan appropriate educational approaches. Many children with learning disabilities do benefit from spectacles. As for hearing aids, some skill may be required to encourage the child to wear them initially. Consideration should also be given to providing extra pairs of spectacles as the child with a learning disability may be less able to care for them, and they may be frequently lost or broken.

Sometimes, however, with relatively minor refractive errors it may be felt that the learning disabled child is not going to benefit greatly from a small increase in visual acuity, such as that which may be provided by spectacles to enable them to read the blackboard, because their developmental ability is such that they are unlikely to learn to read. Such a course of action or lack of action may be appropriate, but should not be made by the doctor using his own assumptions of what the child may or may not need to see, but after careful consideration and discussion with parents and teachers.

Continence

Children with learning disability commonly have problems with urinary and faecal incontinence. For the majority there is no pathological reason for this. Consideration of the approximate age level at which the child functions in other areas of development may be helpful in assessing whether in fact the child is developmentally ready to be toilet trained. Children with severe or profound disability may never reach a level where independent toiletting is achieved. For the remainder, methods of toilet training, and management of enuresis or soiling are much the same as for any child. Structured behavioural programmes including star charts and pads and buzzers can be very successful. Flexibility and imagination may be needed in planning a programme that is appropriate for the child's developmental rather than chronological age, and takes into account any relevant associated disabilities, for example physical disability causing problems with access to toilets or undressing, or communication problems that prevent the child making their toilet needs known.

Although most children have no underlying pathology to account for the continence problem, the paediatrician should be aware of medical prob-

lems that may occur in association with learning disability that can lead to incontinence. Children with learning disability often suffer from constipation, and faecal soiling occurs as a result of overflow. Usually the constipation is due to a number of factors including poor diet, inadequate fluid intake and immobility. Hypothyroidism, however, could also be the cause and is relatively common in Down's and Turner's syndromes. Secondary enuresis, particularly nocturnal, may be the result of undiagnosed epilepsy.

Epilepsy

A high proportion of children with learning disabilities will develop epilepsy. The diagnosis may not be obvious and some types of fits are quite subtle, for example complex partial seizures may be mistaken for odd behaviour or temper tantrums. Epilepsy may be the primary cause of the learning disability. The epilepsy may be difficult to control, and require more than one anticonvulsant. The child may frequently require emergency treatment to curtail prolonged fits, for example rectal diazepam or paraldehyde. The community paediatrician may have an important role in advising the education authority so that provision for emergency treatment can be made in school. The paediatrician should also be familiar with the side effects of anticonvulsant drugs, and the effects that such medication may have on the child's health, learning and behaviour (Trimble & Thompson 1985).

Challenging behaviour

Many children with learning disability will have behavioural difficulties. The term 'challenging behaviour' is now commonly used and is defined by the Mental Health Foundation (1997) in their report 'Don't Forget Us':

Severe challenging behaviour refers to behaviour of such an intensity, frequency or duration that the physical safety of the person or others is likely to be placed in serious jeopardy, or behaviour which is likely to seriously limit or deny access to and use of ordinary community facilities, or behaviour which is likely to impair a child's personal growth, development and family life and which represents a challenge to services,

> Box 36.4
> **Types of challenging behaviour in children with learning disability**
>
> - Physical aggression
> - Destructiveness
> - Self-injury
> - Overactivity
> - Running off
> - Faecal smearing
> - Sexually inappropriate behaviour
> - Sleep disturbance

to families and to the children themselves, however caused.

The number of children defined as having challenging behaviour will depend on definitions used, and to some extent services available. Kiernan & Quereshi (1993) estimate that there will be 25 children with severe challenging behaviour and learning disability in a typical health district population of 250 000 people. Although these may not be vast numbers, the severity of some of the problems, the challenges they pose to all the involved parties, the amount of professional time involved in managing the difficulties and the cost involved in the child's care make them a significant concern to the health authority, and to the paediatrician.

The types of behaviour that come within this definition are wide ranging, and not necessarily specific to children with learning disability. Some of the problems encountered are listed in Box 36.4.

There are many reasons why a child with learning disability may show challenging behaviour. One of the simplest explanations is that the behaviour displayed would be accepted as normal for a much younger child, and it is the persistence of the problem, or its very existence in an older, larger, and often stronger child which makes it challenging. For instance, temper tantrums involving kicking and screaming are daily events in the lives of many toddlers, but may be extremely frightening in a 70-kg young man. Physical affection to a teacher may be regarded as cute in a nursery-aged child, but may be sexually intimidating to the carers of a young adult. In many families, the mother is the main carer and copes well with her son's challenging behaviour for much of childhood, but things breakdown when the son becomes larger than the mother and she can no longer physically cope with him.

For some children with learning disability, the challenging behaviour seems to be another manifestation of the underlying brain dysfunction. Many children with organic brain syndromes are overactive, for example in the early stages of Sanfilippo's syndrome. Behavioural problems are commonly associated with epilepsy, particular in Lennox–Gastaut syndrome. In children with epilepsy, it is also important to remember that difficult behaviour may be related to antiepileptic drugs. Other drugs (e.g. benzodiazepines used for night sedation) may themselves be in part responsible for difficult behaviour.

Sometimes the behaviour serves a function for the child. For a child with limited communication skills it may be communicative. The behaviour may be rewarded by attention from carers. Some behaviours such as head banging or masturbation may be self-stimulatory or used to relieve boredom. Self-injurious behaviour may release endorphins in the brain, with a pleasurable effect. Children with autistic spectrum disorders may engage in stereotyped activities to try to maintain 'sameness' around them. Often the behaviours will be a manifestation of a child's distress. This may be because the child is in pain or feeling unwell because of an unrecognised medical problem or injury. The child may be unhappy about something in his environment that he cannot explain. This may be separation from a parent or favourite carer, or sadly that they are being physically, emotionally or sexually abused.

Whatever the explanation for the behaviour the child and his family are likely to need a great deal of support. An assessment by the paediatrician, and discussion with the entire team involved with the child, should take place to try to arrive at an explanation for the behaviour that will lead to an appropriate plan of management. The team may involve a child psychologist or psychiatrist to try to tease out the issues.

Sometimes an understanding of the problem is all that is required to help the family deal with it. Putting the behaviour into a developmental context may help the family. Assessment may identify a medical problem or environmental issue that can be put right. A structured behaviour programme, under the supervision of experienced staff can be very useful. Occasionally drug treatment will be indicated. In the past, drug treatment in this group of children has received bad press, being simply used to sedate without looking at other issues. Used in the correct way, some drugs can be very helpful including anti-psychotic drugs, carbamezepine (used as a mood stabiliser) and stimulant medication. There is a lot of interest in other drugs including naltrexone (an opioid blocking drug to treat self-injury) and fluoxetine (a selective serotonin re-uptake inhibitor used as an antidepressant and in obsessive behaviour). Unfortunately there is little good quality research on the effects of psychotropic medication specifically in learning disabled children. They should therefore only be used with caution, as part of a comprehensive programme of assessment, treatment, including behavioural methods where appropriate, with close monitoring and review.

SUPPORT FOR THE CHILD AND HIS FAMILY

Some of the tasks involved in caring for the child with a learning disability are essentially medical in nature and clearly the province of the paediatrician. Many other tasks involved in supporting the child and family are much less clearly defined and support is likely to come from a number of different sources. This may be largely from within the family, friends and the local community. Voluntary organisations and statutory organisations will vary in their support role depending on the specific needs of the child and family, the nature of the disability, and within any one family the involvement will vary through different stages of the child's life. For tasks that are not strictly medical, the paediatrician and child health team may still be the most appropriate service to offer support and advice, and where they are not they may be involved in ensuring that support is available from another source.

Talking to parents

One of the first tasks involved in supporting the child and family is in talking to the parents. The issue of how to break the news of a child's disability is discussed in Chapter 30. The importance of this task cannot be overemphasised, as it may influence the way the parents adjust to their child's disability, as well as influence their relationships with professionals in the future. Where the diagnosis is of learning disability, particular care needs to be taken over the language used as discussed at the beginning of this chapter. Understanding of how families react to such news is also important when working with them in the future.

Information

The type and amount of information required by families will vary enormously. Most families will want information about the nature of the child's disability, its cause and recurrence risks, possible treatments and prognosis. It is advisable to offer information in a variety of ways, including face-to-face contact and written information. Providing such information in an appropriate way for the family can be challenging. On the one hand, some parents of learning disabled children will have a learning disability themselves, may be unable to read, or do so only with difficulty. Increased use of information on video or audiotape may be helpful. For families from different cultures where English is not the first language, it is not simply a matter of arranging for interpreting services. The paediatrician should also try to gain some insight into how learning disability is viewed in the different cultures. On the other hand, many parents are very able and highly motivated to seek out information themselves. It is not unusual for parents to hand the doctor large quantities of information from the Internet. This can be difficult for the paediatrician who may well not be as up to date as the parents. It is usually best to be honest about the limitations of one's knowledge, but at the same time be prepared to listen to, and discuss with the parents the information they have found.

Another way of providing information for parents is via the personal child health record (PCHR). Several districts have developed additional pages for children with special needs in their area. The Down's Syndrome Medical Interest Group (Down's Syndrome Medical Interest Group 1998) has produced an insert for the PCHR, which is being distributed nationally.

Respite care

The provision of respite care is well recognised as being helpful in supporting families in caring for their disabled child. Benefits to the family include giving the parents a break, particularly where the child requires a lot of physical care, or where the child's behaviour is challenging, so that they can pursue ordinary family activities that are not possible with the disabled child, and spend more time with their other children. Parents are often reluctant to take up respite care. This may be because they feel guilty about wishing to send the child away. They may be helped by pointing out possible benefits to the child in spending time away from the family in achieving greater independence and experiencing different lifestyles. Children without disabilities often have opportunities to do this by overnight stays with friends, or going away with groups. The learning disabled child may be less likely to develop such relationships, and respite care offers a way of creating a similar experience for them. In many families, respite will be available from within their circle of family and friends. However, for some this is not possible, particularly where the child has severe medical problems or challenging behaviour. Services should then be available from health and social services, ideally in partnership. The concept of respite should be viewed widely and should include babysitting schemes, play schemes, care within the child's home and family-based respite, as well as the more traditional concept of 'institutionalised' respite in a health facility or a children's home.

Siblings

Families can be helped by providing support for the siblings of the disabled child. In the initial phases parents may welcome advice about explaining the child's disability to brothers and sisters. They may appreciate an offer of a health professional speaking to the siblings on their behalf. There are some good books that have been written for children that may help (Cairo et al 1985).

Some organisations have set up support groups for siblings. This can give them the opportunity to meet other young people who have a learning disability, compare notes, and offer mutual support.

Home adaptations and equipment

There may be a need for specialist equipment and adaptations within the home. This will be particularly true for children with associated physical disability (see Chapter 31), but there may be important adaptations for the active child with learning disability and challenging behaviour, largely on safety grounds. Such adaptations may include window locks and toughened glass in the bedroom, provision of a safe space in the home, a secure garden for an overactive child to let off steam, or special locks on food cupboards and refrigerators for those with obsessional overeating. Such adaptations should be available via the social services occupational therapy service, but often a supporting letter from the paediatrician will be required. Outside the home provision of a buggy may be indicated for children who are physically able to walk, but whose behaviour is such that trips out are difficult and dangerous without some restraint in a buggy. Seat restraints in cars may be necessary for safety of overactive learning disabled children once they are too large for standard child restraints.

Specialist clothing may be required with simple fastenings to support independence. Children who smear faeces may be discouraged from doing so by wearing all-in-one boiler suits and nightclothes.

Financial support

Children with learning disability may be entitled to a variety of benefits as discussed in Chapter 17. The eligibility for the care component of Disability Living Allowance (DLA) may be obvious, but consideration should also be given to the mobility component. The child may also be eligible for this even if they are independently mobile, on the grounds that the child's mobility is restricted by behavioural difficulties. This is commonly the case for children with autism, but they may well require the support of health professionals in their application to the Benefits Agency.

Support groups

There are many support groups that may be appropriate for the learning disabled child and their family, some of which are listed in Appendix 1. Their functions include providing general support, contact with other families and advice on a range of issues, including health, educational, legal and welfare matters. Some also offer more specialised services including fieldworkers to work directly with families, or may have resources, ranging from babysitting schemes to schools and residential provision. Increasingly, organisations are becoming involved with advocacy and working with the disabled people themselves.

ACCESSING HEALTH CARE

Children with learning disability may have many special health needs, some of which have been discussed above. They also have the same basic health needs that any child has and should have access to a similar range of services. Special thought and flexibility may well be required by services to make sure this is the case.

Primary care

Parent's often complain that their GP and health visitor seem to 'avoid' their child, or exclude them from routine surveillance programmes, assuming that they get their care from specialist services. However, some parent's find inclusion in the routine programmes inappropriate and demoralising, as the child seems to 'fail' all the assessments. Parents also often find that their GP and health visitor know much less about the child's condition than they do. Visits to the GP for minor illness or immunisation are often very stressful. Long waits in crowded waiting rooms may be difficult with overactive children with difficult behaviour. The GP and health visitor should try to ensure that they are informed about conditions their patients may have, recognising that the family may become experts, and that a lot can be learnt from them. They should discuss with families what is the right level of provision for them, and liaise with other service providers. Simple measures, such as arranging appointments at the beginning or end of a session, or visiting the family at home can be very helpful.

Specialist health care

Children with special needs may require specialist health care, other than that directly relating to their disability. This may be because of medical problems associated with the disability, for example leukaemia or congenital heart disease in Down's syndrome, or coincidental health problems. Parents often worry that their child will be treated less favourably because of their learning disability — that their child's life will in some way be considered less worthwhile than others (Down's Syndrome Association 1999). This may be of particular concern where the treatment is expensive, or resources are limited (e.g. on a transplant list). Discrimination on the grounds of disability is unacceptable and should be challenged wherever it is suspected. In some cases there may be solid medical reasons for treating a child with a disability differently. For instance, in the past few decades, not offering surgery for some types of congenital heart disease in Down's syndrome may not have been discriminatory, but based on the fact that the heart defects in those with Down's syndrome were more complex, and operative morbidity and mortality higher than in others. (Happily, advances in surgical technique means that nowadays the majority of children with Down's syndrome and heart disease do have successful surgery.) Parents should always be made to feel that their child's condition has been assessed and managed with the same care and respect as for any child. Where there is concern that this may not be the case, the parents should be offered a further opinion.

Transition to adult care

Transition from child into adult services can be a particularly difficult time for the young person with a learning disability. After years of involvement with child health services during which time strong relationships and sources of support have been built, the young person is to be passed onto the unknown. At the same time the child is also moving on from school, and may be changing social workers and respite care facilities. There is a common perception that resources for adults with learning disability are very sparse. There is generally no equivalent for adults, of a community paediatric service taking an overview of the person's health (Howells 1996). The GP may be best placed to offer an ongoing service, but may not have the specialist knowledge. Psychiatrists specialising in learning disability and their teams are primarily concerned with mental health and social adjustment and may not look at other health needs. The young person with multiple problems may end up being referred from one paediatrician to a number of different specialists, one for each associated problem.

The process of transition can be eased by the paediatrician together with the multidisciplinary team starting to plan well in advance. Ideally, this should start at the 14+ educational or transition review. The concept of a transition manager to see the family through the process is a useful one. Where Disabled Persons Act workers are available they may fulfil this role. Within the last few years of school, the paediatrician should undertake a comprehensive review of the young person's health, and the health care they have received up to that point. They should consult with other health professionals involved and ask them to do the same. Ongoing health-care needs should be identified and a plan drawn up suggesting how these needs will be met. Where referrals to specialist adult services are appropriate, they should be made in plenty of time. A face-to-face handover appointment with staff from child and adult services present can be very effective and often reassuring for the family. When the young person leaves children's services the information gathered and the plans for future provision should be compiled in a written report. This should be discussed in detail with the young person and the family to ensure they understand and agree with the plans. Copies of the report should always be given to the family and the GP as well as other involved parties.

SPECIAL PROGRAMMES OF HEALTH SURVEILLANCE — DOWN'S SYNDROME AS A MODEL

Health surveillance programmes are based on knowledge of problems that are common within a community, which are amenable to treatment with a positive health outcome. Within the population of learning disabled children there are groups of chil-dren who have medical problems associated with their diagnosis that warrants a specialised health surveillance programme tailored to their needs.

Down's syndrome (trisomy 21) is the commonest identifiable cause of learning disability, with a current incidence in the UK of around 0.9 per 1000 live births. A wide range of health problems is known to be associated with the syndrome (Marder & Dennis 2000) (Box 36.5). In the past some of these problems were left untreated because they were regarded as an inevitable part of the syndrome. As a result, some children's progress was hampered by secondary handicap, for example untreated hearing loss or hypothyroidism. To avoid this, children with Down's syndrome should be offered regular paediatric review paying particular attention to easily identifiable, remediable problems. In the UK a group of doctors with expertise in Down's syndrome (Down's Syndrome Medical Interest Group — DSMIG) have recently developed 'Basic medical surveillance essentials for people with Down's syndrome' (Down's Syndrome Medical Interest Group 2000). These include recommendations for identification of heart disease, thyroid disorder, hearing impairment and ophthalmic problems, and the appropriate monitoring of growth. They also include information on the complex issues around cervical spine instability.

In parallel with the guidelines, the group has produced the insert for the personal child health record referred to above (Down's Syndrome Medical Interest Group 2000). Recommendations from the guidelines have been used to compile the suggested schedule of health checks shown below (Fig. 36.2). The overall aim of the guidelines is to help ensure equitable provision of basic medical surveillance for all children with Down's syndrome in the UK. Such an approach could be useful in providing optimal health care for other children with other specific disorders which give rise to learning disability.

GLOSSARY: SYNDROMES REFERRED TO IN TEXT

Angelman's syndrome: Characteristic facial appearance, severe learning difficulties, absent or minimal speech, jerky movements, paroxysms of unprovoked laughter (previously

Box 36.5
Specific medical problems that occur more frequently in people with Down's syndrome

Cardiac:
- Congenital malformation
- Cor pulmonale
- Acquired valvular dysfunction

Orthopaedic:
- Cervical spine instability
- Hip subluxation / dislocation
- Patellar instability
- Scoliosis
- Metatarsus varus
- Pes planus

ENT:
- Conductive hearing loss
- Sensorineural hearing loss
- Upper airway obstruction
- Chronic catarrh

Ophthalmic:
- Refractive errors
- Blepharitis
- Nasolacrimal obstruction
- Cataracts
- Glaucoma
- Nystagmus
- Squint
- Keratoconus

Gastrointestinal:
- Congenital malformations
- Feeding difficulties

- Gastro-oesophageal reflux
- Hirschprung's disease
- Coeliac disease

Endocrine:
- Growth retardation
- Hypothyroidism
- Hyperthyroidism
- Diabetes

Immunological:
- Immunodeficiency
- Autoimmune diseases, e.g. arthropathy, vitiligo, alopecia

Haematological:
- Transient neonatal myeloproliferative states
- Leukaemia
- Neonatal polycythaemia
- Neonatal thrombocytopenia

Dermatological:
- Dry skin
- Folliculitis
- Vitiligo
- Alopecia

Neuropsychiatric:
- Infantile spasms and other myoclonic epilepsies
- Autism
- Depressive illness
- Dementia (adults only)

known as happy puppet syndrome). Typical EEG abnormality, seizures. Majority have deletion on maternally derived chromosome 15 (15q11–13)

Autistic spectrum disorder: Spectrum of developmental disorders characterised by triad of impairments, i.e. impaired social interaction, communication and imagination, together with a rigid and repetitive pattern of behaviour and interests. Commonly, but not invariably, associated with learning disability

Batten's disease: Neuronal ceroid lipofuscinosis.

DOWN'S SYDROME

DOWN'S SYNDROME - SUGGESTED SCHEDULE OF HEALTH CHECKS

The following are suggested ages for health checks. Check at any other time if there are parental or other concerns

	Birth to 6 weeks	7- 9 months	12 months	18 months to 2½ years	3- 3½ years	4 - 4½ years
Thyroid blood tests	Routine Guthrie test		Thyroid blood tests including antibodies		Thyroid blood tests including antibodies	
Growth monitoring	Length and weight should be checked frequently, using Down's syndrome growth charts from age 3 months. Head circumference should be checked at each routine medical check			Length and weight should be checked at least annually using both Down's syndrome and standard charts		
Eye check	Visual behaviour. Exclude congenital cataract	Visual behaviour. Exclude squint	Visual behaviour. Exclude squint	Orthoptic examination, refraction and ophthalmic examination		Visual acuity, refraction and ophthalmic examination
Hearing check	Neonatal screening, if locally available	Community hearing screening		Audiological clinic review	Audiological clinic review	Audiological clinic review
Heart check and other advice	Echocardiogram 0-6 weeks **or** chest X Ray & ECG at birth **and** 6 weeks			dental advice		

	FROM AGE 5 TO 19 YEARS
Paediatric review	Annually
Audiological review	2 yearly
Vision / Orthoptic check	2 yearly
Thyroid blood tests	At age 5 years. Every 2 years afterwards. At least annually for people with thyroid antibodies.

Detailed recommendations for Medical Surveillance Essentials for children with Down's syndrome are available.
For further information contact your local community paediatrician.

DS 6   **Down's syndrome insert © DSMIG 1998**

Fig. 36.2 Down's syndrome — suggested schedule of health checks. Special insert for the Personal Child Health Record Book. Reproduced with permission from the Down's Syndrome Medical Interest Group (DSMIG) 1998

Storage disease characterized by physical and mental regression, progressive visual loss and seizures

Down's syndrome: Trisomy 21. Typical facial features associated with learning disability, congenital anomalies, including congenital heart disease and bowel disorders, short stature, sensory impairment and increased incidence of a range of other medical problems. (See Box 36.5)

Duchenne muscular dystrophy: X-linked hereditary muscular dystrophy, progressive muscle degeneration starting in early childhood, and usually leading to death in early adult life from respiratory or cardiac complications. Associated with mild learning disability

Foetal alcohol syndrome: Prenatal growth retardation, microcephaly. Characteristic facial appearance (short palpebral fissures, thin upper lip with smooth philtrum, maxillary hypoplasia). Moderate learning disability with clumsiness and hyperactivity

Fragile X: X-linked syndrome usually causing moderate to severe learning disability in males. Can also cause learning disability in carrier females. Characteristic facial appearance with long face, prominent jaw and ears, and large testes. Behavioural characteristics include poor eye contact, social impairment and attentional difficulties. A small proportion fulfil diagnostic criteria for autistic spectrum disorder

Mucopolysaccharidoses: Group of storage disorders including three (Hunter's, Hurler's and Sanfilippo's syndromes) that are associated with significant learning disability. Onset usually in early childhood. Features vary with each syndrome, but include coarsening of features, developmental regression, and joint contractures. Autosomal recessive inheritance, except Hunter's (X-linked)

Neurofibromatosis: Neurocutaneous syndrome of multiple café-au-lait patches, neurofibromas, inguinal freckling and Lisch nodules in eyes. Small percentage have severe learning difficulties but about half have specific learning problems, hyperactivity or speech problems. Autosomal dominant inheritance with variable expression. Common subtype, NFI, caused by deletion on chromosome 17. NF2 has a gene locus on chromosome 22, and is strongly associated with acoustic neuroma

Noonan's syndrome: Short stature, characteristic facial appearance, short webbed neck, and congenital heart disease — commonly pulmonary stenosis. Learning disability in about 25%

Prader–Willi syndrome: Characteristic facial appearance (almond-shaped eyes, small mouth, narrow face), narrow hands and feet, hypogonadism, hypotonia and poor feeding in neonatal period, followed by obesity beginning in early childhood. Characteristic behaviour with obsessive food seeking, tantrums and skin picking. Moderate learning disability is usual. Majority have deletion on paternally derived chromosome 15 (same site as Angelman's syndrome, 15q11–13)

Sanfilippo's syndrome: See Mucopolysaccharidoses. Sanfilippo syndrome is characterised by slower physical regression, but often with significant hyperactivity and behavioural difficulties

Seckel's syndrome: Marked growth deficiency, microcephaly, beaked nose, micrognathia and severe learning disability. Autosomal recessive inheritance

Smith — Lemli — Opitz: Short stature, characteristic facial appearance (microcephaly, anteverted nostrils, low-set ears, ptosis), syndactyly of second and third toes, hypospadias and cryptorchidism in boys. Moderate to severe learning disability. Autosomal recessive. Thought to be due to defect in cholesterol synthesis

Sotos' syndrome: Excessive growth of prenatal origin, advanced bone age, large hands and feet, microcephaly. Moderate learning disability and clumsiness, often with behavioural difficulties

Sturge — Weber syndrome: Facial haemangioma, with corresponding central nervous system haemangioma, and cerebral cortical atrophy. Seizures, paresis and learning disability are common. May also involve the eye with buphthalmos and glaucoma

Tuberose sclerosis: Skin lesions (including adenoma sebaceum, hypomelanotic patches, shagreen patches and ungual fibromas), cerebral, cardiac and renal tumours, seizures, including infantile spasms and learning disabilities. Commonly fulfill criteria for autistic spectrum disorder. Inheritance is autosomal dominant with variable penetrance and high rate of new mutations

Turner's syndrome: XO syndrome. Small stature, ovarian dysgenesis. Physical features include webbed neck, widely spaced nipples and narrow palate. Associated with horseshoe kidney and cardiac anomalies. Majority do not have generalised learning disability, but specific difficulties, particularly with visuospatial skills are common

Williams' syndrome: Characteristic 'elfin' facies (full lips and cheeks, wide mouth, upturned nose, long smooth philtrum), feeding difficulties in infancy, infantile hypercalcaemia, cardiac anomalies (supravalvular aortic stenosis or peripheral pulmonary stenosis). Moderate learning disability usual with superficially good conversational skills and sociability. Behavioural characteristics include hypersensitivity to sound, obsessions, anxiety and hyperactivity. Microdeletion on chromosome 7 (7q11.23)

REFERENCES AND FURTHER READING

British Paediatric Association 1994 Services for children and adolescents with learning disability (mental handicap). BPA, London
Cairo S, Cairo J, Cairo T 1985 Our brother has Down's syndrome. An introduction for children. Annick Press, Toronto

Learning disability

Department of Health 1995 The health of the nation: a strategy for people with learning disabilities. DoH, London

Down's Syndrome Association 1999 He'll never join the army. A report on a survey into attitudes to people with Down's syndrome amongst medical professionals. Down's Syndrome Association, London

Down's Syndrome Medical Interest Group 2000 Insert for personal child health record for babies born with Down's syndrome. 2nd edition. DSMIC. Harlow Printing, Nottingham

Down's Syndrome Medical Interest Group 2000 Basic medical surveillance essentials for people with Down's syndrome. DSMIG. (Available from DSMIG, Children's Centre, City Hospital, Nottingham *www.dsmig.org.uk*) Harlow Printing, Nottingham

Gillberg C 1995 Clinical child neuropsychiatry. Cambridge University Press, Cambridge

Gringras, P 1998 Choice of medical investigations for developmental delay: a questionnaire survey. Child: Care, Health and Development 24:267–276

Gringras P, Barnicoat A 1998 Retesting for fragile X syndrome in cytogenetically normal males. Developmental Medicine and Child Neurology 40: 62–64

Hagberg B, Kyllerman M 1983 Epidemiology of mental retardation — a Swedish survey. Brain and Development 5: 441–449

Hall DMB, Hill, PD 1996 The child with a disability. Blackwell Science, Oxford

Howells G 1996 Situations vacant: doctors required to provide care for people with learning disability. British Journal of General Practice 46:60–61

Jones KL 1997 Smiths recognisable patterns of human malformation. WB Saunders, Philadelphia

Kiernan C, Quereshi H 1993 Challenging behaviour. In: Kiernan C (ed) Research to practice? Implications of research on the challenging behaviour of people with learning disabilities. British Institute of Learning Disabilities (BILD publications), Kidderminster

Lunt PW 1994 Diagnosis of developmental delay: the geneticists approach. Current Paediatrics 4:222–226

Marder E, Dennis J 1997 Medical management of children with Down's syndrome. Current Paediatrics 7:1–7

The Mental Health Foundation 1997 Don't forget us. Children with learning disabilities and severe challenging behaviour. Report of a committee. The Mental Health Foundation, London

Pollak M 1993 Textbook of developmental paediatrics. Churchill Livingstone, Edinburgh

Roelvald N, Zielhhuis GA, Gabreels F 1997 The prevalence of mental retardation: a critical review of recent literature. Developmental Medicine and Child Neurology 39:125–132

Trimble MR, Thompson PJ 1985 Anticonvulsant drugs, cognitive function and behaviour. In: Ross E, Reynolds E (ed) Paediatric perspectives on epilepsy. Wiley, Chichester, ch 17, p 141

World Health Organization 1992 The ICD 10 classification of mental and behavioural disorders. WHO, Geneva

Appendix 1
Support organisations

These are only some of the many national and local organisations concerned with child health:

Action for Sick Children, 300 Kingston Road, Wimbledon Chase, London SW20 8LX. Helpline: 0800 0744519. *www.actionforsickchildren.org*

ADD/ADHD Family Support Group, 1a High Street, Dilton Marsh, Westbury, Wiltshire BA13 4DL. Tel. 01373 826045

AFASIC, 69–85 Old Street, London, EC1V 9HX 020 Tel. 7490 9410. Helpline: 08453 55 55 77. *www.afasic.org.uk*

Aid for Children with Tracheostomies, 72 Oakridge, Thornhill, Cardiff CF14 9BQ. Tel. 029 2075 5932

Association for Children with Life-threatening Conditions, Orchard House, Orchard Lane, Bristol B51 5DT. Tel. 0117 922 1556

Association for Glycogen Storage Diseases, 9 Lindop Road, Hale, Altrincham, Cheshire WA15 9DZ. Tel. 0161 980 7303. *www.agsd.org.uk*

Association for Spina Bifida & Hydrocephalus, Asbah House, 42 Park Road, Peterborough, Cambridgeshire, PE1 2UQ. 01733 555988. *www.asbah.org*

Ataxia, 10 Winchester House, Kennington Park, Cranmer Road, London SW9 6EJ. Helpline: 020 7582 1444. *www.ataxia.org.uk*

Barnardos, Tanners Lane, Barkingside, Ilford, Essex 1G6 1QG. Tel. 020 8550 8822. *www.barnardos.org.uk*

Bobath Centre for Children with Cerebral Palsy, Bradbury House, 250 East End Road, London, N2 8AU 020. Tel. 8444 3355. *www.bobath.org.uk*

British Agencies for Adoption and Fostering, Skyline House, 200 Union St, London SE1 0LX. Tel. 020 7593 2000. *www.baaf.org.uk*

Diabetes UK, 10 Queen Anne Street, London W1G 9LH. Tel. 020 7323 1531. *www.diabetes.org.uk*

British Dyslexia Association, 98 London Road, Reading, Berkshire RG1 5AU. Tel. 0118 966 2677. Helplines: 0118 966 8271. *www.bda-dyslexia.org.uk*

British Epilepsy Association, New Anstey House, Gate Way Drive, Yeadon, Leeds LS19 7XY. Tel. 0113210 8800. Helpline: 0808 800 5050. *www.epilepsy.org.uk*

British Institute for Brain-Injured Children, Knowle Hall, Knowle, Bridgwater, Somerset TA7 8PJ. Tel. 01278 684060. *www.bibic.org.uk*

Cancer & Leukaemia in Childhood, CLIC Headquarters, 12–13 King Square, Bristol, Avon BS2 8JH. Tel. 0117 924 8844

Carers UK 20/25 Glasshouse Yard, London EC1A 4JT. CarersLine: 0808 808 7777. *www.carersuk.demon.co.uk*

Centre for Evidence Based Child Health, Department of Paediatric Epidemiology and Biostatistics, Institute of Child Health, 30 Guilford Street, London WC1N 1EH. Tel. 020 7905 2606. *www.ich.bpmf.ac.uk/ebm/ebm.htm*

Child Accident Prevention Trust, 4th Floor, Clerks Court, 18–20 Farringdon Lane, London EC1R 3HA. Tel. 020 7608 3828. *www.capt.org.uk*

Child Bereavement Trust, Aston House, West Wycombe, High Wycombe, Bucks HP14 3AG. Tel. 0 1494 446648

Child Growth Foundation, 2 Mayfield Avenue, Chiswick, London W4 1PW. Tel. 020 8995 0257. *www.cgf.org.uk*

Child Poverty Action Group, 94 White Lion Street, London N1 9PF. Tel. 020 7837 7979. *www.epag.org.uk*

Children's Heart Federation, 52 Kennington Oval, London SE11 5SW. Helpline: 0808 808 5000. *www.childrens-heart-fed.org.uk*

Children's Legal Centre, University of Essex, Wivenhoe Park, Colchester Essex CO4 3SQ. Tel. 01206 872466. Advice: 01206 873820. *www2.essex.ac.uk/clc/*

Children's Liver Disease Foundation, 36 Great Charles Street, Queensway, Birmingham B3 3JY. Tel. 0121 212 3839. *www.childliverdisease.org*

Cleft Lip & Palate Association (CLAPA), 235–237 Finchley Road, London NW3 6LS. Tel. 020 7431 0033. *www.clapa.mcmail.com*

Climb (formerly the Research Trust for Metabolic Diseases in Children), The Quadrangle, Crewe Hall, Weston Road, Crewe, Cheshire CW1 6UR. Tel. 0870 770326. *www.climb.org.uk*

Coeliac Society, PO Box 220, High Wycombe, Bucks HP11 2HY. 01494 437278. *www.coeliac.co.uk*

Contact a Family, 209-211 City Road, London. EC1V 1JN. Tel. 0808 808 3555. *www.cafamily.org.uk*

Crohn's in Childhood Research Association, Park-gate House, 356 West Barnes Lane, Motspur Park, Surrey KT3 6NB. Tel. 020 8949 6209

Cystic Fibrosis Trust, 11 London Road, Bromley, Kent BR1 1BY. Tel. 020 8464 7211. *www.cftrust.org.uk*

Disability Information Trust, Mary Marlborough Centre, Nuffield Orthopaedic Centre, Heading-ton, Oxford OX3 7LD. Tel. 01865 227592

Down's Heart Group, 17 Cantilupe Close, Eaton Bray, Dunstable, Bedfordshire LU6 2EA. Tel. 01525 220379. *www.downs-heart.downsnet.org*

Down's Syndrome Association, 155 Mitcham Road, London SW17 9PG Tel. 020 8682 4001. *www.dsa-uk.com*

Down's Syndrome Medical Information Service, The Children's Centre, City Hospital Campus, Hucknall Road, Nottingham NG5 1PB. Tel. 0115 962 7658 ext. 45667. *www.dsmig.org.uk*

Drug Scope (formed from merger of the Institute for the Study of Drug Dependence, and Standing Conference on Drug Abuse), Waterbridge House, 32–36 Loman St, London SE1 0EE. Tel. 020 7928 1211. *www.drugscope.org.uk*

Dyspraxia Foundation, 8 West Alley, Hitchin, Hert-fordshire SG5 1EG. Helpline: 01462 454986. *www.dyspraxiafoundation.org.uk*

Enuresis Resource & Information Centre — ERIC, 34 Old School House, Britannia Road, Kingswood, Bristol BS15 8DB. Tel. 0117 960 3060. *www.enuresis.org.uk*

Family Fund Trust, PO Box 50, York YO1 9ZX. Tel. 01904 621115. *www.familyfundtrust.org.uk*

Family Welfare Association, 501–505 Kingsland Road, London E8 4AU. 020 7254 6251

Foundation for the Study of Infant Deaths, Artillery House, 11–19 Artillery Row, London SW1P 1RT Helpline: 020 7233 2090 *www.sids.org.uk*

Fragile X Society, 53 Winchelsea Lane, Hastings, East Sussex TN35 4LG. Tel. 01424 813147. *www.fragilex.org.uk*

Friends For Young Deaf People (FYD), East Court Mansion, College Lane, East Grinstead, West Sussex RH19 3LT. Voice: 01342 323444. Minicom: 01342 312639. *www.fyd.org.uk*

FSH Muscular Dystrophy Support Group, 8 Caldercot Gardens, Bushey Heath Herts, WD2 3RA. Tel. 020 8950 7500. *www.fsh-group.org*

Gingerbread, 7 Sovereign Close, Sovereign Court, London E1W 3HW. Tel. 0800 018 4318. *www.gingerbread.org.uk*

Haemophilia Society, Chesterfield House, 385 Euston Road, London NW1 3AU. Tel. 020 7380 0600. Helpline: 0800 018 6068. *www.haemophilia.org.uk*

Heartline Association, Rossmore House, 26 Park Street, Camberley, Surrey GU15 3PL. Tel. 01276 675655

Hemi-Help, Bedford House, 215 Balham High Road, London SW17 7BQ. Tel. 020 8672 3179. *www.hemihelp.org.uk*

Hyperactive Children's Support Group, 71 Whyke Lane, Chichester, West Sussex PO19 2LD. Tel. 01243 551313. *www.hacsg.org.uk*

In Touch Trust, 10 Norman Road, Sale, Cheshire, M33 3DF. Tel. 0161 905 2440

IPSEA (Independent Panel for Special Education Advice), 6 Carlow Mews, Woodbridge, Suffolk IP12 1DH. Tel. 01394 382814 Advice: 0800 018 4016. *www.ipsea.org.uk*

Jennifer Trust for Spinal Muscular Atrophy, Elta House, Birmingham Road, Stratford upon Avon, Warwickshire CV37 0AQ. Tel. 01789 267520. Families: 0800 975 3100. *www.jtsma.demon.co.uk*

Kidscape, 2 Grosvenor Gardens, London SW1W 0DH. Tel. 020 7730 3300. *www.kidscape.org.uk*

Lady Hoare Trust For Physically Disabled Children, 1st Floor, 89 Albert Embankment, London SE1 7TP. Tel. 020 7820 9998

Leukaemia Research Fund, 43 Great Ormond Street, London, WC1N 3JJ. 020 7405 0101. *www.lrf.org.uk*

Lifeline: Manchester Drugs Prevention Initiative. Tel. 0161 839 205

Makaton Vocabulary Development Project, 31 Firwood Drive, Camberley, Surrey GU15 3QD. Tel. 01276 681390. *www.makaton.org*

Mencap, 123 Golden Lane, London EC1Y 0RT. Tel. 020 7454 0454. *www.mencap.org.uk*

Muscular Dystrophy Campaign, 7–11 Prescott Place, London, SW4 6BS. 020 7720 8055. *www.muscular-dystrophy.org*

Myotonic Dystrophy Group, 175a Carlton Hill, Carlton, Nottingham NG4 1GZ. Tel. 0115 987 0080. *www.comcom.org/mdsg*

NASPCS: The Charity For Incontinent & Stoma Children, 51 Anderson Drive, Valley View Park, Darvel, Ayrshire KA17 0DE. Tel. 01560 322024

National Association for the Education of Sick Children, 18 Victoria Park Square, London E2 9PF. Tel. 020 8980 8523. *www.sickchildren.org.uk*

National Asthma Campaign, Providence House, Providence Place, London N1 0NT. Tel. 0207226 2260. Helpline: 0845 701 0203. *www.asthma.org.uk*

National Autistic Society, 393 City Road, London EC1V 1NG. 020 7833 2299. Helpline: 0870 600 8585. *www.nas.org.uk*

National Children's Bureau, 8 Wakley Street, Islington, London, EC1V 7QE. Tel. 020 7843 6000. *www.ncb.org.uk*

National Council for One Parent Families, 255 Kentish Town Road, London NW5 2LX. 0800 018 5026. Enquiries: Tel. 020 7428 5400. *www.ncopf.org.uk*

National Deaf Children's Society, 15 Dufferin Street, London EC1Y 8UR. Tel. 020 7490 8656. Helpline: 020 7250 0123. *www.ndcs.org.uk*

National Eczema Society, 163 Eversholt Street, London NW1 1BU. Tel. 020 7388 4097. Info: 0870 241 3604. *www.eczema.org*

National Foster Care Association, 87 Blackfriars Road, London SE1 8HA. Tel. 020 7620 6400

National Meningitis Trust, Fern House, Bath Road, Stroud, Gloucestershire GL5 3TJ Tel. 01453 768000. Helpline: 0845 6000 800. *www.meningitis-trust.org.uk*

National Portage Association, 127 Monks Dale, Yeovil, Somerset BA21 3JE. Tel. 01935 471641

National Society for Epilepsy, Chesham Lane, Chalfont St Peter, Buckinghamshire SL9 0RJ. Tel. 01494 601300. Helpline: 01494 601400. *www.epilepsynse.org.uk*

NCH Action for Children, 85 Highbury Park, London N5 1UD. Tel. 020 7226 2033 *www.nchafc.org.uk*

(NSPCC) National Society for the Prevention of Cruelty to Children, 42 Curtain Road, London EC2A 3NH. Helpline: 0800 800 500. *www.nspcc.org.uk*

Office for National Statistics, 1 Drummond Gate, London SW1V 2QQ. Tel. 0845 601 3034. *www.statistics.gov.uk*

Parentline, Endway House, The Endway, Hadleigh, Essex SS7 2AN. 01702 554782. Helpline: 0808 800 2222

Perthes Association, 15 Recreation Road, Guildford, Surrey GU1 1HE. Tel. 01483 306637. *www.perthes.org.uk*

Playmatters: National Association of Toy and Leisure Libraries, 68 Churchway, London NW1 1LT. 020 7387 9592. *www.charitynet.org/~NATLL*

Prader Willi Syndrome Association, 33 Leopold Street, Derby DE1 2HF. 01332 365676. *www.pwsa.co.uk*

RADAR (Royal Association for Disability and Rehabilitation), 12 City Forum, 250 City Road, London EC1V 8AF. 020 7250 3222. *www.radar.org.uk*

Rathbone, Churchgate House, 56 Oxford Street, Manchester M1 6EU. Special education advice line: 0800 917 6790

REACH (The Association for Children with Hand or Arm Deficiency), 25 High Street, Wellingborough, Northamptonshire NN8 4JZ. Tel. 01933 274126. *www.reach.org.uk*

Restricted Growth Association, PO Box 4744 Dorchester DT2 9FA. Tel. 01308 898445. *www.rgaonline.org.uk*

Royal National Institute for the Blind, 224 Great Portland Street, London W1N 6AA. 020 7388 1266. Helpline: 0845 766 99 99. *www.rnib.org.uk*

Royal Society for the Prevention of Accidents (ROSPA), 353 Bristol Road, Birmingham B5 7ST. Tel. 0121 248 2000. *www.rospa.co.uk*

Scoliosis Association, 2 Ivebury Court, 325 Latimer Road, London W10 6RA. Tel. 020 8964 5343 Helpline: 020 8964 1166. *www.sauk.org.uk*

Scope, 6–10 Market Road, London, N7 9PW. Tel. 020 7619 7100. Helpline: 0808 800 3333. *www.scope.org.uk*

Syndromes Without a Name — SWAN, 16 Achilles Close, Great Wyrley, Walsall, West Midlands WS6 6JW. Tel. 01922 701234: *www.undiagnosed.clara.net*

Tracheo-Oesophageal Fistula Support Group (TOFS), St George's Centre, 91 Victoria Road, Netherfield, Nottingham NG4 2NN. 0115 961 3092. *www.tofs.org.uk*

The Trust for the Study of Adolescence, 23 New Road, Brighton BN1 1WZ. Tel. 01273 693311. *www.tsa.uk.com*

Tuberous Sclerosis Association, PO Box 9644, Bromsgrove B61 OFP. 01527 871898. *www.tuberous-sclerosis.org*

Unique, Rare Chromosome Disorder Support Group, PO Box 2189, Caterham CR3 5GN. Tel. 01883 330766. *http://members.aol.com/rarechromo*

Young Minds, 102–108 Clerkenwell Road, London, EC1M 5SA. 020 7336 8445. Information: 0800 018 2138. *www.youngminds.org.uk*

Appendix 2
Sources of information

Some of the resources available which include statistics on child health:

Abortion Statistics 2000. Office for National Statistics. Annual. September 2001. ISBN 0 11 621474 0

Birth Statistics in England and Wales 1999. Office for National Statistics. Annual December 2000. ISBN 0 11 621381 7

Births in Scotland 1999–2000. Information and Statistics Division, NHS in Scotland. 2001

Cancer Survival Trends in England and Wales 1971–95: deprivation and NHS region. Office for National Statistics, London School of Hygiene and Tropical Medicine and Cancer Research Campaign. Ad hoc. May 1999. ISBN 0 11 621031 1

Child Protection Register: Statistics for Wales, 1998. The National Assembly for Wales. Annual. 1999. ISBN 0 7504 2324

Children and Young Persons on Child Protection Registers. 2000–2001 Department of Health. Annual. ISBN 1 84182 4372

Children Looked After by Local Authorities. 2000–2001 Department of Health. Annual ISBN 1 84182 4402

Children's day care facilities at 31st March 2001 England. Department for Education and Employment. Annual

Congenital Anomaly Statistics 2000. Office for National Statistics. Annual. December 2001. ISBN 1 85774 4608

Drug Use, Smoking and Drinking Among Young People 2000. Office for National Statistics 2001. ISBN 0 11 3225628

Health Inequalities Decennial Supplement. Office for National Statistics. Decennial. September 1997. ISBN 0 11 620942 9

The Health of our Children. Office for National Statistics. Decennial. September 1995. ISBN 0 11 691643 5

Health Statistics Quarterly. Office for National Statistics. Quarterly. ISBN 1465 1645

Infant Feeding in 1995. Office for National Statistics on behalf of the four UK health departments. May 1997. ISBN 0 11 620918 6

Infant Feeding in Asian Families. Department of Health. Ad hoc February 1997. ISBN 0 11 691693 1

Key Population and Vital Statistics. 1999 Office for National Statistics. Annual. May 2001. ISBN 0 11 6213876

Mortality Statistics: childhood infant and perinatal 1999. Office for National Statistics. Annual. March 2001. ISBN 0 11 6214619

Mortality Statistics: injury and poisoning 1999. Office for National Statistics. Annual June 2001. ISBN 0 11 6214686

Smoking Among Secondary School Children in England 1996. Office for National Statistics on behalf of the Department of Health. October 1997. ISBN 0 11 620945 3

Smoking Among Secondary School Children in Scotland 1996. Office for National Statistics on behalf of the Scottish Health Department. Ad hoc. October 1997. ISBN 0 11 620944 5

Social Focus on Children. Office for National Statistics. Ad hoc. August 1994. ISBN 0 11 620655 1

Vital Statistical Tables on Disk and CD-ROM. Office for National Statistics. Annual

Young Carers and Their Families. Office for National Statistics on behalf of the Department of Health. November 1996. ISBN 0 11 691685 0

Young Teenages and Smoking in 1998. Office for National Statistics on behalf of the Health Education Authority. Occasional. December 1999. ISBN 1 85774 361 X

Websites that include statistical information:

Department of Health. *http://www.doh.gov.uk/public/stats1.htm*

National Statistics. *http://www.statistics.gov.uk*

Public Health Laboratory Service (PHLS). *http://www.phls.co.uk/facts/index.htm*

World Health Organization Statistical Information System (WHOSIS). *http://www.who.int/whosis/*

Organisations that compile statistical information:

Department for Education and Skills (DFES). Tel. 0870 000 2888

Department of Health Statistics Division (Looked After Children) Tel. 020-7972-5799

Information and Statistics Division (NHS Scotland). Tel. 0131 551 8899

National Assembly for Wales. Tel. 029 20 825080

Office for National Statistics. Tel. 0845 601 3034

Stationery Office Publications Centre. Tel. 0870 600 5522

Index

A
A Place to Call Our Own
    (APTCOO), 267
Abdomen
    recurrent pain, 408
    tuberculosis, 304
Abortion (therapeutic termination),
    394
    condition leading to learning
        difficulty, 572
Abuse, see Child abuse
Accident(s) (unintentional injuries),
    309–21
    at home, see Home
    prevention, 160–5, 279, 314–19
        active vs passive, 315
        effectiveness, see Effectiveness
        government strategy (in
            reducing death rate from
            accidents), 273, 314, 319
        health visitors and, 209
        opportunities for, 315–19
        support organisations, 591, 594
    size and nature of problem,
        309–14
Accident and Emergency (casualty;
    A&E), 196–7
    accidental injury treatment in (in
        Nottingham Safe at Home
        Project), 161, 162
    death from, 309
    referral clinics (from primary
        care), 183
Acheson Report, 323–4
Act(s) (of law), see Legislation and
    specific Acts
Activity/activity limitation in
    ICIDH-2, 480
Administrative staff, general
    practice, 195
Admission to hospital, see Hospital
Adolescents/teenagers, 381–400, see
    also Age; Puberty
    educational institutes, 220
    health needs, see Needs
    homelessness, 328, 390–1
    hydrocephalus, 507
    nutrition, 115–18, 384
    offending behaviour, 391–2

poverty, 390–1
primary care, 200–1
    confidentiality issues, 198,
        394–5
    psychiatry service referral, 464–5
    risk-related behaviour, see Risk-
        taking
    school non-attendance, 391–2,
        456–7, 511, 516–17
    services for, 394–8
    sexual health, 392–4
    smoking, 7, 12, 385–6
    social/behavioural development,
        61, 384
    speech and language problems
        persisting in, 565
    suicide, 462
    support organisation, 594
    transition to adulthood (and
        adult services), 397
        disabilities and, 488, 585–6
        government strategy
            concerning, 273
Adopted children
    psychiatric disorders, 431
    support organisation, 591
Adoption orders, 236
Adrenarche, 138
    premature, 148
Adulthood and adult care,
        transition to, see Adolescents
Advisory Committee on Borderline
        Substances, 120
Advisory and inspection services,
    224
Advocacy
    community paediatricians, 12
    school nursing, 212
    voluntary organisations, 264
    young carers projects, 339
Affection, nurture and, and forming
        of attachments, 330, 428–9
Afro-Caribbean origin, Sickle Cell
        Society, 266
Age, see also Adolescents; Infants;
        Neonates; Preschool children;
        School-age children
    accident prevention advice and,
        318

adolescents, legal issues
    rights, 395
    sexual intercourse, 395
anxiety/fear/emotional distress
        and, 432
Child Benefit and, 243
infection and
    immunisation for, 295
    occurrence of, 290
language acquisition and, 560
psychiatric disorders and, 425
vision screening and, 540
Air pollution and asthma, 402
Airway disorders
    lower, see Asthma
    upper, 406
Alcohol, 385, see also Foetal alcohol
        syndrome
Alimentary problems, see
        Gastrointestinal problems
Allele, 69
Allergy, food
    behaviour and, 442
    peanuts, 111–12, 411
Allocative efficiency, 156
Alport's syndrome, 78
Alternative medicine, 187
Amblyopia, 536–7
    prevention, 537–8
Ambulatory paediatrics, 182–4
Amphetamines
    abuse, 388
    in attention deficit and
        hyperactivity disorder, 450–1
Anaemia, iron-deficiency, 110, 410
Analytical epidemiological studies,
    12–14
Androgens, 138, 139
Aneuploidy, 68, 70
    congenital heart malformations
        and, 81
Angelman's syndrome, 76, 77,
    586–7
Anger, 432–3, 459–60, see also
        Temper
Annual business plan, 174–5
Anorexia nervosa, 441
Antenatal period, see Foetus
Antibiotics, preventive use, 293

Anticholinergics, asthma, 405
Anti-inflammatory agents, asthma, 405
Antisocial behaviour, 453–4
    poor outcome, factors associated with, 455
    school and, 455
Anus and perianal region, sexual abuse and, 363–5, 365–6
Anxiety, 432, 457–8
    infantile realism and, 63
Appointments, capacity management, 168
APTCOO (A Place to Call Our Own), 267
Area child protection committees, 368–9
Armstrong, George, 3
Arthritis, 507
Asian communities, child abuse, 378
Aspirin and Reye's syndrome, 13–14
Asthma, 401–6
    epidemiology, 401–2
        impact of studies, 14–15, 16
    support organisation, 593
Astigmatism, 538–9
Asymmetrical tonic neck reflex, 50–1
Attention deficit and hyperactivity disorder (ADHD) and limited attention span, 448–51, 517
    support organisations, 591, 592
Attention-seeking behaviour, 455
Audiometry, 543–6
    in glue ear, 420
    visual reinforcement, 550
Audit, 175
    services for special needs children, 492
Audit Commission report 1994 (Seen but not Heard), 179, 180
Auditory brainstem response (ABR), 548, 549
Auditory–perceptual pathway linking expressive sound to speech production, 560, 561
Autism (and autistic spectrum disorders), 451, 564–5, 587
    genetic factors, 82
    support organisation, 593
Autosomal diseases
    dominant, 70
    recessive, 71–2

B
Bacillus Calmette–Guerin, 304–5
Bacterial vaginosis, 368
'Balance of Good Health', 116
Balance reactions, 51
Barbiturates, 388

Barium swallow, asthma, 403
Bathing equipment, 502
Batten's disease, 587–8
Battered child syndrome, 197
Bayes' theorem, 88, 90
BCG, 304–5
Beckwith–Wiedemann syndrome, 147
Bedwetting (nocturnal enuresis), 414, 445, see also Enuresis
Behaviour (child's/individual's)
    attention-seeking, 455
    autistic child, 451
    development of, 59–60, 279
        adolescents, 61, 384
        Erikson's theories, 60–2
    difficulties/problems in, see Difficult and/or disobedient child; Emotional and behavioural difficulties
    food and, 112, 442
    health-related, 18
        changes, models/theories, 125–8
        international monitoring, 132–3
    indicators of serious disturbance, 437–8
    in local authority care, initiatives influencing, 345
    physically-disabled child, 500
    visually-directed behaviour in infants, 532
Behaviour (health professionals), stress affecting, 32
Behavioural support teachers, 224
Behavioural treatments, 463–4
Benefits (in economic evaluation), 157, 159, see also Cost–benefit analysis
Benefits (social security), 241–52
    learning-disabled child, 584
Benefits Agency website, 252
Bereaved children
    grief, 433–4
    parental loss, 429
    support organisation, 591
Beveridge Report (1942), 5
Bias, 15–16
Bicycle accidents, 312
Binocular vision, development, 532, 537
Birth, see also Foetus; Perinatal period
    disability recognition, 480–1, 572–3
    impact on family, 430–1
Birth records, 17
Birthweight, low, see Low birthweight babies
Bites, human, 359
Biting nails, 439
Black people, see Ethnic groups
Black Report (1980), 43

Bladder
    neuropathic, 414, 506–7
    training, 448
Blindness (and severe/profound visual impairment), see also Vision
    causes
        infectious (developing countries), 528–9
        UK, 531
    detection, 540–1
    developmental impact, 533–5
    registration as blind, 527
    support organisation, 594
BLISS symbol board, 499
Blood pressure, raised, 413
Body function and structure in ICIDH-2, 479–80
Body mass index (BMI), 137, 140
    obesity and, 137, 150
Bonding/attachments, 330, 428–9
Bone
    fracture, see Fractures
    tuberculosis, 303
Bordetella pertussis infection, see Whooping cough
Bottle feeding, see Formula feeds/milks
Bowel, neuropathic, 506–7
Boys, see also Gender; Siblings
    genital anomalies, 415, 415–16
    puberty, 382
Brain damage/injury
    acquired, 507
        non-accidental, 360
    support organisation, 591
Brain dysfunction in learning-disabled child, behavioural problems due to, 582
Brain scan, learning disability, 578
Branchio-oto-renal syndrome, 78
Breakfast, school-age child, 112–13, 515
Breast development, see Thelarche
Breast feeding, 96–8
    gastroenteritis and, 106
    promotion, 97
    reasons for planning, 98
    reasons for stopping, 98, 99
    successful, facilitation, 98
Breast milk, composition, 97
Bright children, poor school progress, 519
Bristol Programme, 333
British sign language for the deaf, 499
Brittle bone disease, 359
Bronchodilators, asthma, 405
Bruises, 357–8
Bullying, 456
Burn(s), 318
    non-accidental, 359

Burnley, Pendle and Rossendale Language programme, 334
Business plan, annual, 174–5

C
Calcium and vegetarianism, 114
Cancer, government strategy of reducing death rate, 273
Cannabis, 387, 388
Capacity management, appointments, 168
Car, Mobility Component of Disability Living Allowance, 246
Carbohydrate, dietary, preschool child, 107
Cardiac disease, see Heart disease
Cardiovascular disease, 412–13, see also Circulation
   adult, and childhood diet, 117
Care Component of Disability Living Allowance, 243–5
Care of the Next Infant programme, 210
Care proceedings, 259–60
Carers (incl. family), see also Family; Professionals
   communication problems and, 499
   of disabled children, benefits, 241, 248–50, 250–1, 251–2
   of looked-after children
      consultation to, 345
      training, 346
   support organisation, 591
   young (= children), 334–41
      assessment, 338–9
      characteristics, 335–6
      definitions, 335, 340
      health inequalities for, tackling, 339–41
      needs, 337, 338
      numbers, 335
      outcomes, 336–7
      rights, 337
      specialist projects, 339
      tasks, 335, 335–6
Carers Act (1995), 337–8
Caries, tooth, sugars and, 107
Carrier status (genetic disorder), testing, 86, 88
Case-control studies, 13
Case finding and screening, distinction, 26
Case management, 170–1
   health visitors, 207–8
Caseload management, 170
Casualty, see Accident and Emergency
Cataract, 528
CATCH phenotype, 74–5
Causality, assessing, 17
Census, 17

Central nervous system tumours, 507
Cerebral palsy, 503–5
   support organisation, 591
Cervical tuberculous lymphadenopathy, 304
Chadwick, Edwin, 3
Chairs, disabled child, 501–2
Chance (in epidemiological studies), 15
Change
   drivers for, 182
   surviving/managing, 173
Charcot–Marie–Tooth disease, 76
Charitable organisations, see Voluntary organisations
Chest X-ray, asthma, 403
Child abuse, 197, 349–80, see also Emotional abuse; Neglect; Physical abuse; Protection; Sexual abuse
   causation theory, 353–7
   definitions, 351–3
   enquiries, 351
   global view, 350–1
   history, 349
   institutional (in local authority care), 234
   mistaken diagnosis/mimicking conditions, 358–9, 360
   organised/multiple, 350
   paediatrician role, 375–6
   recognition/detection/diagnosis, 357–60
   schoolwork and, 517
   support organisation, 349, 593
Child and adolescent psychiatry service (CAMHS), 464–5
Child Benefit, 242
Child Development Programme, 209
Child development team, 483–6
Child-friendliness, general practice, 198–9
Child Health and Education Study, 331
Child Health Informatics Consortium, 277
Child Health Promotion Programme, 278–86
Child Poverty Action Group, 252, 591
Child protection, see Protection
'Child Protection — messages from research, 369
Child sex rings, 353
Childminders, 235
Children Act (1989), 230, 231, 255, 337
   care proceedings, 259–60
   child abuse and, 369
      Section 17, 325–6, 337, 352, 371
      Section 47, 352, 369, 371, 372
      significant harm concept, 352

parental responsibility and, 257, 258
   special needs, 479, 487–8
   young carers, 337
'Children looked After by Local Authority', 344
Children's homes, 231–2, 235, see also Local authorities, looking after child
Chlamydia trachomatis, 367
Choice (in health economics), 155, 156
Chromosomes, 67–8
   abnormalities, 68
      congenital heart malformations and, 81
      learning disability and, 578
      numerical, see Aneuploidy
      short stature and, 143–4
      structural, 68, 70, 74–6
      support organisation, 593
      tall stature and, 143–4, 147
   nomenclature, 67–8
Chronic/long-standing disease
   adults, childhood factors, 116–17
   prenatal/infant birth weight/growth/nutrition and, 14, 116–17, 136
   children
      health visitors and, 209–10
      learning and, 511–14
Cigarette burns, non-accidental, 359, see also Smoking
Circular reactions, Piaget's, 62
Circulation in cerebral palsy, 505–6, see also Cardiovascular disease
Cities, inner city areas, disadvantages, 329
Citizen's Advice Bureau website, 252
Classroom, health promotion, 132
Clinic(s)
   child health
      emergency referral clinics, 183
      in general practice (Nottingham), 198–9
      failure to thrive managed in, 149–50
      health promotion, 275
      teenage health, 396
Clinical diagnosis and management, community paediatrician in, 1
Clinical governance, 186
Clinical guidelines, 175
Clinical Standards Advisory Group, 181
Clostridium tetani, 305
Clumsy children, 519–22
Cocaine, 388
Cochlear implants, 543, 546, 547
Cochrane Library, website, 22

Code of Practice (1996) in Education Acts, 486
Coeliac disease (gluten-sensitive enteropathy), 406–7
    support organisation, 592
Cognition/cognitive skills
    autism, 451–2
    development
        Piaget's observations, 62–3
        visual loss and, 534
Cohort studies, 13, 114
Colic, 106
Colour vision defects, 285, 539
    careers affected, 540
Commission for Health Improvement, 186
Communication between parents and professionals, learning disability and, 583
Communication between staff, 34–5
    child abuse, 378–9
    local authority care, staff and carer consultation, 345
    in primary care
        health visitor–GP, 195–6
        with other services/organisations, 196
Communication problems (child), 427, 497–500, see also Hearing loss; Speech
    autism, see Autism
    physically disabled child, 497–500
        assessment for, 497–8
        cerebral palsy, 505
        management, 498–500
Community, see also Neighbourhood
    concept, 41
    in health promotion
        participation, 128–31, 132
        school links, 132
Community Care Grants, 250
Community paediatric nurses, specialist, 183–4, 184–5
Community paediatrician
    psychological needs, 29–37
    roles, 1–2, 12
        child abuse, 375–6
        travel, 169–70
Community paediatrics, defining, 1
Complaints, 173
Complementary medicine, 187
Concrete operation, 63
Conduct disorders, see Difficult and/or disobedient child
Conductive hearing loss, 544
    causes, 553
Confidence intervals, 15
Confidentiality, 259, 394–5
    adolescents, 198, 394–5
    child protection and, 377
Confounding, 16–17
Congenital deafness, see Hearing loss

Congenital disorders, see also Genetic disorders
    hypothyroidism, 23, 411
    learning disability with, 571
    malformations/anomalies
        head shape/size, see Head
        heart, see Heart disease
        organic solvents and, 16
Connexions, 273
Consent to treatment, 259–60
    adolescents, 395
Constipation, 408–9
    infant, 106
    physical handicap and, 500
    preschool child, 109
Constitutional delay in growth and puberty, 142
Constitutional short stature, 142
Consultants
    outreach clinics and, 196
    secondary/tertiary care, 184
Consultations
    emotional demands of, 31
    GP, morbidity statistics from, 20
    GP, rates, 190–1
        factors affecting, 197–8
Consulting with children, school nurses, 213
Continence problems
    in cerebral palsy, 505
    faecal, see Soiling
    learning-disabled child, 581
    support organisation, 593
    urinary, see Enuresis
Continuing (ongoing) professional development, 35, 186
Contracts for Health (government's), 7, 9
Control, feelings of lack, 31
Convulsions (fits/seizures), 416–18, see also Epilepsy
    febrile, 14–15
Cope Street Centre, 333
Copper deficiency, 359
Coronary heart disease, see Heart disease
Cortical visual impairment, 530–1
Corticosteroids, asthma, 405
Cortisol, 138
Corynebacterium diphtheriae, 305–6, see also DTP vaccine
Cost(s) (financial and other in health economics), 155, 173, see also Economics; Finance; Socioeconomic factors
    and consequences, 157
    in injury prevention, 312
        Nottingham Safe at Home Project, 160–5
    screening tests, 24–6
    sharing, 172
Cost–benefit analysis, 159–60
Cost–effectiveness analysis, 158

Nottingham Safe at Home Project, 160, 163
Cost–utility analysis, 158–9
Cot death (sudden unexpected infant death), 361
    reduction programme, 210
    support organisation, 592
Cough in asthma, 403
Council Tax Benefit, 251
Council for Voluntary Service, 268
Counselling, 469–77
    child, 469–77
        effective, basic requirements, 469–71
        first session, 471–3
        how to conduct sessions, 473–7
        longer-term, 469
    by school nurse/doctors, 132
    genetic, see Genetic counselling
Counsellor, characteristics, 470
Counter-transference, 33
Court of Appeal, 261–2
Court Report (1976), 5, 395
Court witness, see Witness
Cover test, 537, 538
Cows' milk
    infant, 103
    preschool child, 108
    protein intolerance, 118, 407
Craniosynostosis, 416
Crime and Disorder Act (1998), 253, 259, 260
Criminal behaviour, 391–2
Crisis Loan, 250
Cruelty to children (older term for child abuse), 197, see also Child abuse
Crying, 431
Cryptorchidism (undescended testes), 415
CTFR (cystic fibrosis gene), 68, 69, 72, 88
    testing for, 88
Cues and changes in behaviour, 125–8
Cultural issues (impacting on health), 329, see also Ethnic groups
    child abuse and, 378
    schooling and, 517–18
Cycle accidents, 312
Cystic fibrosis, 68, 69, 72, see also CTFR
    diagnosis, 403
    genetic tests, 88
    support organisation, 592
Cytogenetics
    nomenclature, 67–8
    techniques (laboratory tests), 82–3
        interpretation, 87
        learning disability and, 577

D
DARE, 281
Data
    essential core data set in health
        promotion, 277
    numerical, sources, 17–20
Day assessment units, 183
Day care, 235
Day centres, 232
Day nurseries, *see* Nurseries
Day wetting, 414, 447
Deafness, *see* Hearing loss
Death, *see* Bereaved children;
        Mortality; Terminally ill
Decision-making (choice) in health
        economics, 155, 156
Decision-making as stressor, 30
Defences
    collective, 33–4
    individual defence mechanisms,
        33
Deformities (and their
        management)
    cerebral palsy, 505
    equipment preventing
        deformities, 501
Deletion, *see also* Microdeletions
    chromosomal, 68
    gene, 69
Demand and resources, balancing,
        174
Denial, 33
Dentition (teeth)
    caries and sugars, 107
    physically-disabled child, care,
        496
Denver II, 64
Department of Education and
        Employment (DfEE), 217, 222
    special educational needs and,
        219, 219–21
Department of Health, *see*
        Government
Department of Public Health in
        health promotion, 275
Depression
    child, 433, 460–2, 517
    maternal, 278, 430
Deprivation, *see* Poverty
Dermatology, *see* Skin conditions
Descriptive epidemiological studies,
        12–14
Desmopressin, 448
Developing countries, visual
        impairment, 527–9
Development, 49–65, *see also* Child
        Development Programme;
        Child development team;
        Growth
    assessment (incl. screening tests),
        63–5
        pitfalls, 271, 272
    delay/impairment in, 445–6
        child abuse and, 362, 363

enuresis as, 445–6
    handicapped child, 497
    investigation, 491
    language and speech, *see*
        Language; Speech
    language and speech delay
        associated with other, 563–5
    learning disability vs other
        disabilities, 574
    nutrition and, 330, 515
    syndromes of delayed global
        development, 564
equipment (disabled child's)
    . allowing, 501
    visual, 531–3, 537
    visual loss and its impact on,
        533–5
Diabetes, 411–12
    diet in, 117–18
    support organisation, 591
Diagnosis, clinical, community
        paediatrician in, 1
Dialect, 515
Diaphyseal fractures, 358
Diarrhoea, infant and toddler, 106,
        109, 407–8
    nursery outbreak, 109
Diary, 170
Diet, 330, *see also* Eating problems;
        Feeding; Food; Nutrition
    in disease, 117–20
    growth and, 136–7, 330
    in iron-deficiency anaemia,
        modification, 410
    preschool child, 106–8, 279
        poor habits, 109–10
    recommended daily amounts, 95
    reference values, 95–6
    school-age child, 113
Difficult and/or disobedient child
        (difficult child syndrome;
        conduct disorders), 425,
        453–4
    parenting, 425, 453, 454–5
    schooling, 516–17
Digestive tract problems, *see*
        Gastrointestinal problems
Diphtheria, 305–6
Disability (handicap), 377–8, *see also*
        Special needs *and specific
        disability*
    acquired, 573
    adolescents, 397
    benefits system, *see* Benefits
    care/services, 169, 178
    causes, 481
    child abuse and, 377–8
    concept/models, 42–3
    education, 224–6, *see also* Special
        educational needs
        compared with medical
            perspectives, 224–6, 227
        Education (Handicapped
            Children) Act, 218

legislation, 218, 256, 479, 486,
        488
    equipment, *see* Equipment
    international classification of
        functioning and, 479–80
        definition of disability, 480
    management, 483–6
    mental, *see* Learning difficulty
    physical, *see* Physical disability
    prevalence, 480, 481
    recognition/news of, 480–1
        family reaction after, 481–3
    school-leaver with, 488
Disability Adjusted Life Years
        (DALY), 14
Disability centres, equipment from,
        503
Disability Discrimination Act (1995),
        488
Disability Income Guarantee, 241
Disability Living Allowance, 243–8
    components, 243–6
    decision-making process, 246–7
    how to claim, 246
    learning disability and, 584
    other benefits and, 247–8, 249,
        250–1
    payment method, 247
    revisions and appeals, 247
Disability Living Foundation, 488
Disabled Persons Act (1986), 488
Disabled Persons Act (1995), 479
Disabled Person's Tax Credit, 251
Discipline, helping with, 454–5
Discourse analysis, 41–2
Discretionary Social Fund, 250
Disease/medical
        conditions/physical illness
        (in general), 401–22, *see also*
        Syndromes *and specific (types
        of) disease*
    adolescents, 383–4
    chronic/long-standing, *see*
        Chronic disease
    counselling in, 469
    dietary management in, 117–20
    distribution, describing, 14
    explaining cause, 14
    in general practice, spectrum, 191,
        192
        example from one GP, 193
        referral reasons and, 196
    injury causing, 309–11
    in learning-disabled children, *see*
        Learning difficulty
    overall burden of, 14
    parental, 430
    psychiatric morbidity, 426
    stress causing, 32
Disobedience, *see* Difficult and/or
        disobedient child
Distraction test (for hearing)
    diagnostic, 550
    screening (health visitor), 546–7

Distribution of disease, describing, 14, *see also* Geography
DMK, 74
DNA bases/kilobases/megabases, 67
DNA tests (diagnosis of genetic disorders), 82, 83
  interpretation, 87–8
Doctors, school, health promotion, 131–2
Domestic violence, 377
Dominant mutations causing disease, autosomal, 70
'Don't Forget Us', 581–2
Down's syndrome (trisomy 21), 70, 586, 587, 588
  medical problems, 586, 587
    cardiac lesions, 413, 587
    specialist care, 585
  screening, 158
  support organisations, 592
Down's syndrome Medical Interest group, 584, 587, 592
Drink(s)
  infants, 104
  preschool child, excessive use, 109–10
  school-age children, 114–15
Drinking (alcohol), 385
Drug abuse, 386–90, 517
  classification of illegal drugs, 386
  clinical conditions arising, 287
  commonly used drugs and their effects, 387, 388–9
  education about, 390
    Drug Abuse Resistance Education, 281
  education and effects of, 517
  recreational use, 386
  serious, 387
  services, 390
  support organisations, 592, 593
Drug therapy
  asthma, 404, 405
  emotional and behavioural problems, 464
    attention deficit and hyperactivity disorder, 450–1
    enuresis, 448
    learning-disabled child, 583
    tics, 440
Dry powder inhalers, 406
DTP vaccine, 302
Duchenne muscular dystrophy, 506, 588
  support organisation, 593
Duplication
  chromosome, 68, 74–6
  gene, 69–70
Dyslexia, 522, 523
  support organisation, 591
Dysmorphic child
  genetic assessment, 85–6
  tall stature, 146

Dyspraxia
  developmental verbal, 562
  support organisation, 592

E
Ear, glue, *see* Glue ear
Ear, nose and throat problems, learning-disabled child, 580
  Down's syndrome, 587
EAR (estimated average requirement), 95, 96
Early growth response 2 gene, 87
Early years, *see* Preschool children
Eating problems, 440–2, *see also* Diet; Feeding; Nutrition
'Ecological' epidemiological studies, 12–13
Economics (health), 155–65, 173, *see also* Cost; Income; Socioeconomic factors
  definitions/terminology, 155
  economic evaluation (of health care), 156–65
    injury prevention, 160–5, 312
    types, 157–60
  immunisation programmes, 295–6
Ecstasy, 389
Education, 217–39, *see also* Education services; Health education; Learning; School
  asthma, 404–6
  deprived children, preschool, 7–8, 331
  disabled persons, *see* Special educational needs
  drugs, *see* Drug abuse
  peer, in local authority care, 345–6
  phases, 220
  sex, 280–1, 397
  special needs in, *see* Special educational needs
  visually-impaired child, 224, 536
Education Action Zones, 274
Education Acts, 218
  1893/1899 Acts, 4
  1907 (Administrative Provisions) Act, 4
  1944 Act, 4, 218
  1970 Act (Handicapped Children), 218
  1971 Act, 568
  1974 Act, 486
  1981 Act, 218, 486, 568
  1982 Act, 218
  1992 (Schools Act), 218
  1993 Act, 486
  1996 Act, 218, 256, 479, 487
  1997/1998 Acts, 218
Education services, 185, 217–39
  interface with community paediatrics, 6, 185
  key principles, 218–22
  people in, roles/responsibilities, 222–4

  structure, 217, 218
Education welfare service, 224
Educational psychology services, 224
Edward's syndrome, 70
Effectiveness (of intervention), 15, *see also* Cost–effectiveness
  accidental injury prevention, 315
    Nottingham Safe at Home Project, 161–2
  health visiting, 209
Efficacy (of intervention), 15
EGR2, 87
'Eight Guidelines for a Healthy Diet', 115
Elastin gene, 75
ELN, 75
Emergency referral clinics, 183
Emotion(s), child's, 426–7
  development (and maturity), 59, 279, 431–4, 434
    delayed/slow (immature emotions), 426–7, 434
    promoting, 434–5
    visual loss and, 534–5
  growth and, 137
  negative/unpleasant, 431
  positive/pleasant, 431, 432
  psychiatric disorders and emotional state, 426–7
Emotion(s), community paediatrician's (and demand of families/children), 30–1, 32–3, 35
  emotional self-care, 36
Emotional abuse, 352–3, 356, 362–3
Emotional and behavioural difficulties, 437–67, *see also* Difficult and/or disobedient child
  4–15 y/olds, data, 19
  charity providing help, 267
  education/learning and, 516–17
    specialist support teaching staff, 224
  learning disability and, 581–3
  neglect leading to, 362
  prognosis, 464
  symptoms indicating serious disturbance, 437–8
  treatment failure, reasons, 464
  treatment principles, 462–5
  visual loss and, 535
Emotional congruence as motivation for abuse, 355
Employment agencies, equipment provision, 503
Empowerment, school nursing, 212
Encopresis (soiling), 408–9, 445, 448
  treatment, 448, 449
Endocrinology, 411–12
  Down's syndrome-related problems, 587

growth
  normal, 137–9
  short stature, 144
  tall stature, 147–8
Energy intake/requirements
  preschool child, 107
  school-age child, 113
Enforcement interventions, accident
    prevention, 315, 317
Engineering interventions, accident
    prevention, 315, 316
English as second language, 514–15
Enuresis (urinary incontinence;
    wetting), 413–14, 445–8, see
    also Continence problems
  learning-disabled child, 581
  physically-disabled child, 500
    neuropathic bladder, 414, 506
  support organisation, 592
Environmental factors, 327–8
  child abuse, 354
  infection spread, 290
Epidemiological studies, 12–17
  interpretation, 15–17
  types, 12–14
  uses, 14–15
Epilepsy, 417–18, 507
  juvenile myoclonus, 74
  learning-disabled child and, 581
    and behavioural problems, 582
  support organisation, 591, 593
EQ-5D (EuroQol), 158
Equipment and devices
  learning-disabled child, 584
  physically-disabled child, 488,
    501–3
    communication, 499–500
  primary care health promotion,
    275
Equity, school nursing, 212
Erikson's psychoanalytical theory,
    60–2
Error, 15–16
Erythema, perianal, 363–5
Essential core data set, 277
Estimated average requirement
    (EAR), 95, 96
Ethics, genetic tests, 86–7
Ethnic groups/minorities/
    communities (incl. Blacks
    and Asians), see also Cultural
    issues
  asthma, 402
  child abuse
    Asian communities, 378
    bruising in black children, 358
  English language and, 514–15
  obesity, 150
  voluntary organisations, 266
EuroQol, 158
Evidence-based practice, health
    promotion, 132–3
Evoked potential, steady state,
    549–50

Examination, see Physical
    examination
'Excellence in Schools', 214
Experimental epidemiological
    studies, 13, 14
Eye, see also Vision
  Down's syndrome-related
    problems, 587
  motor system, examination, 537
Eye/hand co-ordination, learning
    disability vs other
    disabilities, 574

F
Facial features, learning disability,
    576
Facilitator, school nurse as, 212–13
'Facipulation' (facilitation and
    manipulation), 130
Factitious disorder by proxy, 360
Factory Act (1833), 3
Faecal incontinence, see Soiling
Failure to thrive, 148–50, 361–2
  cause, 149
  definitions, 148
  dietary causes, 109–10
  interventions/management,
    149–50
  neglect and, 361–2
  significance, 148
Fainting, 418
Familial short stature, 142
Familial tall stature, 146
Family/families, 328–9, see also
    Carers; Parents; Single-parent
    families
  in accident prevention, working
    with, 315–16
  asthma impact, 404
  at-risk, health visitors and, 208
  benefits, 250–2
  birth and its impact in, 430–1
  breakdown, 428
  care in general practice, 197–8
  in child abuse
    abusing and neglecting
      families, 354
    meetings/conversations
      involving family members,
      371, 374
  children as carers in, see Carers
  concept, 42
  counselling covering, 472
  of disabled children
    benefits, 241
    equipment provision by, 503
    learning-disabled child,
      support, 583
    visual-impaired child, 534–5
  impact on community
    paediatrician of working
    with, 30–1, 32–3
  needs, see Needs
  psychiatric disorders and, 427–31

structure/size, and impacting on
    health, 328–9, 429–30
  support organisations, 592
Family centres, 235, 331
  Radford, 331–2
Family Fund Trust, 244, 251–2, 503,
    592
Family therapy, 462–3
Family tree, recording, 83–5
Fat, dietary, 116
  preschool child, 107, 108
  school-age child, 113
FBN1 (fibrillin-1 gene), 68, 69, 70
  tests for, 88
Fear, 432
Febrile convulsions, 14–15
Fecal incontinence, see Soiling
Feed(s)
  formula, see Formula feeds
  thickeners, 105
Feeding (eating and drinking), see
    also Diet; Eating problems;
    Food; Nutrition; Tube-
    feeding
  disabled child
    cerebral palsy, 504
    equipment, 502
  infant, 18, 96–106
    problems, 105–6
    weanling, 101–4
  preschool child, 108
    problems, 109–12
Feet, deprivation hands and, 362
Feingold diet, 112
Females, see Girls; Mothers; Women;
    Women's movement
Fetus, see Foetus
Fibre, dietary, preschool child,
    107–8
Fibrillin gene, see FBN1
Field social work, 232–3
Finance, 168, see also Benefits;
    Costs
Finger sucking, 439
Finished consultant episode, 20, 21
First aid training for parents, 160
FISH (fluorescent in situ
    hybridisation), 82, 83
Fits, see Convulsions; Epilepsy
Fluorescent in situ hybridisation,
    82, 83
Fluoride, 104
FMR-1, 73
Foetal alcohol syndrome, 588
Foetus (= antenatal/prenatal
    period), see also Birth
  disability acquired, 481
    hearing loss, 553
    learning disability, 571
  disability recognition, 480, 572
  growth and nutrition (and
    malnutrition), 136, see also
    Intrauterine growth
    retardation

chronic adult disease and, 14, 116–17, 136
screening and health promotion, 281
Folic acid and neural tube defects, 81–2
Follow-on milks, 101, 103
low birthweight babies, 104
Food, *see also* Diet; Eating problems; Feeding; Meals on wheels; Nutrition
additives, 112, 442
allergy, *see* Allergy
behaviour and, 112, 442
fads, 441
intolerance, 111, 112, 407
cows' milk protein, 118
learning problems and, 515
Foreign travel, child, 307
Formal operations, 63
Formula feeds/milks (bottle feeding), 98–101
cows' milk intolerance and, 118
gastroenteritis/diarrhoea and, 106
reasons for planning to use, 98
switching from breast feeding to, reasons, 98, 99
thickened, 106
tube-feeding, 119
Fostered children
psychiatric disorders, 431
support organisations, 591, 593
Fractures, non-accidental (= physical abuse), 358
infants, conditions mimicking/mistaken diagnosis, 358–9
Fragile X chromosome, 73, 74, 588, 592
'Framework for the assessment of children and need and their families', 369, 371, 372
Frataxin, 74
FRDA, 74
Friedreich's ataxia, 74
Frozen watchfulness, 361
Funny turns, 416
differential diagnosis, 417
Future (epidemiological studies in prediction of)
child's future, 15
service planning, 15

G
Galant's reflex, 50
Gastroenteritis, infant, 106
Gastrointestinal problems, 406–11
Down's syndrome, 587
Gastro-oesophageal reflux, 409–10
Gender (sex)
asthma and, 402
psychiatric disorders and, 425
Gene(s), 68, *see also* Mutations
sensorineural deafness-related, 78

General Household Survey, 20
General Medical Council's Revalidation Steering Group (1999), 201
General practice, 189–207, *see also* Primary care
accidental injury treatment in (in Nottingham Safe at Home Project), 161
care of child and family in, 197–8
current status/organisation, 189–90
history of child health care, 189–90
links with other services/organisations, 196
morbidity statistics from, 20
organisation of child health care in, 198
referrals from, *see* Referrals
workload, 190–3
General practitioners (GPs), 194
Contract (1990), 190
example of child health care by one GP, 192–3
learning-disabled child and, 585
payments for services, 201
training (in child health care), 190
Genetic counselling, 89
physically-disabled child, 500–1
Genetic databases, 85, 90
Genetic disorders and diseases (affecting children), 70–4, *see also* Syndromes
assessment/diagnosis, *see* Genetic tests/assessment
common, 80–2
growth effects, 136
short stature, 143–4
tall stature, 146–7
hearing loss, 68, 552
learning disability, 571
visual impairment, 531
Genetic factors, susceptibility to infection, 289–90
Genetic heterogeneity, 71, 76–80
Genetic tests/assessment, 82–8
dysmorphic child, 85–6
ethical dimensions, 86–7
interpretation of tests, 87–8
Genetics, 67–93, 327
asthma, 401–2
glossary, 90–1
language acquisition and, 559
nomenclature, 67–8
principles, 67–80
resources, 90
Genetics services, 89–90
Genital(s) (genitalia)
anomalies, boys, 415, 415–16
mutilation, female, 378
pubertal development, boys, 383
signs of sexual abuse, 365, 366
Genital herpes, 367–8

Genital warts, 367
Genomic imprinting, 69, 76
Geography, *see also* Distribution
infection and, 290
voluntary organisations and, 266–7
German measles (rubella), 300–1, *see also* MMR
Gesell's observations on child development, 59
Girls, puberty, 381–2, *see also* Gender; Siblings
pubic hair growth, 383
GJB1, 76
GJB2, 68, 78
Glasses, acceptance, 538
Glue ear (otitis media with effusion), 419–21, 564
learning-disabled child, 580
Gluten-sensitive enteropathy, *see* Coeliac disease
Goats' milk, 103
Gonadal mosaicism, 70
Gonorrhoea, 367
Governance, clinical, 186
Government/national health policies and advice (predominantly UK incl. Department of Health), 7, 44, 187–8, *see also* Legislation; Political aspects
child abuse, enquiries ordered, 351
Contracts for Health, 7, 9
diet/nutrition, 95, 115–17
disabled children's equipment, 503
education services, 217
health promotion and surveillance, 125, 187, 272–4, 275
accident (and accidental death) prevention, 273, 314, 318–19, 319
National Framework for Assessing Performance, 186
safeguard issues (away from home/in local authority care), 234–5
school nursing, 214
social services white paper, 237–8
Grammar, infant, 558
Grasp reflex, 50
Graves' disease, 411
Grief, 433–4
Griffiths Report (1988), 230
Griffiths Scales of Mental Development, 64–5
Grommets, 421
Group support, community paediatrician, 35
Growth, 135–53, *see also* Development; Height; Weight

failure, 142–5
   suspected, evaluation, 140–1
infant, *see* Infants
influences on, 136–9
   diet/nutrition, 136–7, 330
   intrauterine, retardation (IUGR),
      136, 142–3
learning disability and disorders
   of, 576
measurement/assessment, 139–
   40
   physically-disabled, 496–7
   reliability/timing, 140
normal patterns, 135–6
support organisations for growth
   problems, 591, 593
Growth charts, 135–6
Growth hormone (GH), 137–8
   administration
      GH deficiency, 145
      skeletal dysplasia, 144
      Turner's syndrome, 144
   deficiency, 142, 145
Guthrie test, 281

H
Habits, 438–9
   good habit training, 438
      sleep, 443
   pervasive habit-training disorder,
      438–9
   unwanted, 439
Haematological problems, Down's
   syndrome, 587
Haemophilus influenzae type B, 306
Hamartin, 71
Hand(s), *see also* Eye/hand co-
      ordination
   deprivation hands and feet, 362
   features, learning disability and,
      576
   functional assessment, 496
   X-ray (growth assessment), 141
Handicap, *see* Disability
Haplotype, determination, 83
Harm, *see also* Injury
   avoiding, *see* Protection
   significant (concept), 352
Head
   injury, non-accidental, 360
   shape/size abnormalities, 416
      learning disability and, 576
Headaches, 418–19
Heaf test, 304
Health/well-being (physical health
      and health in general), *see
      also* Disease; Mental health
   assessment, looked-after children,
      344
   behaviour impacting on, *see*
      Behaviour, health-related
   determinants, 124
   economics of, *see* Economics
   factors affecting, 326–34

inequalities, *see* Health
      inequalities
   learning and, 511
   monitoring and evaluation of
      plans to improve, 11
   poverty/deprivation effects on, 7,
      11, 325, 326
   public, *see* Public health
   strategic planning for, 11
Health Action Zones, 273
Health authorities
   child public health and, 10, 133
   in health promotion, 275
Health care, *see also* Medical
      treatment; Secondary care;
      Specialist care; Tertiary care
   economics, *see* Economics
   history, *see* History
   need inversely related to
      availability, 325–6
   new/changing styles and
      patterns of practice, 178, 182
   preventive, *see* Prevention
   primary/secondary/tertiary, *see*
      Primary care; Secondary
      care; Tertiary care
   pyramid of, 178
   services, *see* Services
   well-run programmes of, 172–3
Health clinics, *see* Clinics
Health education, *see also* Sex
      education
   accident prevention, 314, 315
      Nottingham Safe at Home
         Project, 160
   health visitor role, 208, 209
   infection prevention, 293
Health Education Authority, 133
'Health for all Children', 269
Health improvement, *see* Health
      promotion
Health Improvement Programmes
      (HIMPs), 319
Health inequalities, 43–5, 187,
      323–48, *see also* Poverty
   determinants/factors, 124, 323,
      326–34
   intervention schemes
      early, 7–8, 331–4
      young carers, 339–41
Health needs, *see* Needs
'Health of the Nation', 7, 115
Health professionals/personnel, *see*
      Professionals
Health Promoting School
      Programme, 279–80
Health promotion/improvement,
      123–34, 169, 180, 187, 269–
      87
   community in, *see* Community
   definitions and historical
      perspective, 123
   essential core data set, 277
   evidence-based practice, 132–3

government policies, *see*
      Government/national health
      policies and advice
   health professionals involved in,
      130, 274–7
      community paediatrician, 1–2,
         274
      health visitors, *see subheading
         below*
      school nurses, 131–2, 274
   health surveillance vs, 272
   health visitors, 208, 209, 274
      mental health promotion, 210
   looked-after children, 345–6
   opportunistic, 272
   programme, 278–86
   schools/school-age children,
      113–14, 131–2, 133, 279–80
   theory-driven practice, 125–8
Health record, child's personal, *see*
      Records
Health services, information on use
   of, 18–20
Health surveillance, 269–87
   age-specific advice at, in accident
      prevention, 318
   Down's syndrome (as model of
      conditions in learning-
      disabled children), 586
   government policies, *see*
      Government/national health
      policies and advice
   health promotion vs, 272
   principles, 270
   problems with surveillance
      checks, 271
   professional/agencies involved,
      274
      general practice/GPs and, 190,
         199–200
      health visitors and, 208
   screening and, distinction, 23
Health Survey for England, 18–20
Health visitor(s), and visiting, 184,
      194, 205–11
   assessment by health visitors, 208
   case management, 207–8
   core elements underpinning
      activities, 207
   future directions, 210–11
   GPs and visitors, working
      together, 195–6
   history, 205–6
   interventions based on
      programmes of care, 208
   learning-disabled child and, 585
   models of service delivery, 207
   principles, 206
   role and responsibilities of health
      visitor, 206–7, 208–10, 270
      new births, 281–2
      priority areas of work, 207
   skills and knowledge, 207
   success/effectiveness, 209

Index

Health visitor distraction test, 546–7
Hearing aids, 545
Hearing loss (deafness), 283–4, 497, 543–55, 578–9
  causes, 68, 551–3
  in cerebral palsy, 505
  conductive, *see* Conductive hearing loss
  congenital (prenatal), 548, 553
    genetic causes, 68, 552
  epidemiology, 551–2
  in glue ear, 420, 421, 564
  high-tone, 545
  investigations recommended, 554
  learning difficulties and, 578–9
    assessment of hearing loss, 578–9
    learning difficulty associated with (but not caused by) hearing loss, 514
    learning difficulty due to loss, 514
  sensorineural, *see* Sensorineural hearing loss
  sensory teachers (school), 224
  services, 554
  sign language, 499
  speech and language delay associated with, 563–4
  support organisations, 592, 593
  tests for, 283–4, 420, 546–8
    diagnostic, 548–51
    learning-disabled child, 578–9
    physically-disabled child, 497
    screening, 283–4, 546–8
  types/classification/degrees, 543–6, 552–3
Heart disease, 412–13
  adult (coronary)
    childhood diet and, 117
    government strategy of reducing death rate, 273
  congenital, 80, 412–13
    Down's syndrome, 413, 587
  support organisations, 592
  syncope in, 418
Heart murmurs, 412
Height (stature)
  on growth charts, 135–6
  measurement, 139
    parents' height, 141
    timing, 140
  shortness, 142–5
  tallness, 145–50
Hepatitis A/B/C, 306–7
Heredity, *see entries under* Genetic *and specific hereditary conditions*
Hernia
  inguinal, 415
  umbilical, 415
Heroin, 387, 389
Herpes, genital, 367–8
Highscope, 7, 10, 332

Hip, developmental dysplasia (congenital dislocation), 419
  screening, 285–6
Hirschsprung's disease, 408, 409
History (of child health/health care), 7, *see also* Legislation
  child abuse, 349
  health promotion, 123
  health visitors, 205–6
  services, 3–6
    general practice, 189–90
  social, 229–30
History, patient (child)
  dysmorphic child, 85
  learning difficulties and, 518
HIV, sexual abuse and, 368
Home, *see also* Housing; Housing Benefit; Residential care
  clinical care at, 183
  failure to thrive managed at, 149–50
  injuries at, 311–12
    prevention, 160–5
  learning and problems at, 516
  learning-disabled child, adaptations and equipment, 584
  nurse visits, pre-/postnatal, 332–3
  school and, agreements, 221
  social services' help at, 232
Home-Start, 265
Homelessness, 328, 390–1
Homocysteine and neural tube defects, 81–2
Homocystinuria, 146–7
Hormones, *see* Endocrinology
Hospital(s)
  admission
    adolescents, 384
    avoidance, 178–9, 182–4
  benefits and going into
    Disability Living Allowance, 248
    Income Support, 249–50
    Invalid Care Allowance, 249
  data on child use of, 20
  failure to thrive managed in, 149–50
  in health promotion, 274–5
  health visitors based in, 206–7
  at-home service, 183
  visits and travel to, help, 252
Housing, *see also* Home
  conditions, 327–8
  costs, Income Support and, 249
Housing Benefit, 251
HPV, genital warts, 367
Hub and spoke model, 183
Human immunodeficiency virus, sexual abuse and, 368
Human papillomavirus, genital warts, 367
Human rights, *see* Rights
Humour and anxiety, 458

Hydrocephalus, 506–7
  support organisation, 591
Hydrocoele, 415–16
Hygiene (personal), 293
  oral, physically-disabled child, 496
Hyperactivity and attention deficit disorder, *see* Attention deficit and hyperactivity disorder
Hypermetropia, 537, 538
Hyperphenylalaninaemia, 72
Hypertension, 413
Hyperthyroidism, 411
Hypospadias, 415
Hypothyroidism, 411
  acquired, 411
  congenital, 23, 411
  short stature, 144

I
ICD-10, learning disability in, 567, 568
ICIDH-2, 479–80
Ill-health, physical, *see* Disease
Imaging, brain, learning disability, 578
Immunisation (vaccination), 192, 200, 293, 293–307, *see also specific diseases*
  effectiveness/safety, 294
  history, infection susceptibility and, 290
  medical impact, 296
  passive, *see* Immunoglobulins
  physically-disabled child, 500
  programmes/schedules, 279, 295–6, 296
  theory of immunity, 293
  uptake, 296–7
    and herd immunity, 294–5
Immunoglobulins (passive immunisation), 293
  hepatitis A, 306
  measles, 300
Immunological problems, Down's syndrome, 587
Imprinting, genomic, 69, 76
Incidence, 12
Income, 328
Income Support, 244, 249–50
Incontinence, *see* Continence problems; Enuresis; Soiling
'Independent Enquiry into Inequalities in Health', 187
Infant(s) (up to 1 year), *see also* Age; Postnatal period
  death, 17
    rates, 18
    sudden unexpected, *see* Cot death
  diarrhoea, *see* Diarrhoea
  disability recognition, 481, 573
  emotions, 432
  feeding, 18

fractures, spontaneous, 358–9
growth, 135
    and chronic adult disease, 14,
        116
    health review, 282
    hearing tests, 283–4
    hip, developmental dysplasia,
        screening, 286
    immunisation programme, 295
    motor development
        fine skills, 54–5
        gross, 52
    newborn, see Neonates
    nutrition, see Nutrition
    premature, see Premature infants
    social and behavioural
        development, 56–7
        Erikson's theories, 60
    speech/sounds, 556–7
    visual assessment, 532
Infantile realism, 63
Infections, 289–308, see also specific
        diseases/pathogens
    blindness due to, 528–9
    data on, 20
    diagnosis and management,
        290–3
    immunisation, see Immunisation
    notifiable diseases, 289, 290
    recording, 289
    respiratory, and asthma, 402
    sexually transmitted, see Sexually
        transmitted diseases
    susceptibility to, 290–1
    urinary tract, 414–15
Influenza vaccine, 307
Information, 17–22
    community paediatrician role, 2
    in health services, 168, 173–4
    health-promoting, 127
    learning disability (for family),
        583–4
    literature reviews as sources, 20–2
    numerical data sources, 17–20
    school nurses and giving of, 212
Information bias, 16
Inguinal, hernia, 415
Inhalers, 404–6
Inheritance, see entries under Genetic
        and specific hereditary
        conditions
Injury, see also Fractures; Harm
    accidental, see Accidents
    brain, see Brain damage
    non-accidental (historical use of
        term), 349–50, see also
        Physical abuse; Self-harm
Inner city areas, disadvantages, 329
Intelligence (incl. IQ), see also Bright
        children
    language disorders and, 559
    learning disability, measurement
        in classification of disability,
        567–8

psychiatric disorders and, 425–6
Interdepartmental Enquiry on
        Physical Deterioration (1904
        report), 4
International Classification of
        Diseases (ICD-10), learning
        disability in, 567, 568
International Classification of
        Impairments, Disabilities and
        Handicap (ICIDH-2), 479–80
Internet (incl. websites)
    benefits system, 252
    genetic disease information, 90
    health promotion, 281
    literature reviews, 22
    support organisations, 591–4
Intrauterine causes of disability, see
        Foetus
Intrauterine growth retardation
        (IUGR), 136, 142–3
Invalid Care Allowance, 244, 248–9
    other benefits and, 247, 248
Inversely care law, 325–6
Inversion, chromosomal, 68
Iron
    breast feeding and, 97
    deficiency, 110, 334, 410
        anaemia, 110, 410
        correction, 334
        other effects, 110
    dietary sources, 110, 111
    supplements, 410
    vegetarianism and, 114

J
Jamaican Study (nutrition and
        development), 330
Jarman index, 324
Jobseekers' Allowance, 250
Joint, tuberculosis, 303
Juvenile myoclonus epilepsy, 74

K
Karyotype, 68
    abnormal, see Chromosomes,
        abnormalities
Klinefelter's syndrome, 147

L
Labelling of child with psychiatric
        disorder, 424
Lactose intolerance, 407
Landau–Kleffner syndrome, 562–3
Language, 514–15, 557–66
    assessment methods, 65
    development/acquisition, 557–9
        in hearing-impaired children,
            563–4
    developmental delay in acquiring
        (language difficulties), 498,
        514–15, 557–66
    causes (and classification by
        cause), 559, 561
    classification schemes, 561, 562

learning disability vs other
        disabilities, 574
    other developmental delays
        associated with, 563–5
    physically-disabled child with,
        497
    prevalence, 559
    prognosis, 565
    schemes/programmes
        preventing or helping with
        (incl. language therapy),
        333–4, 498, 565
    specific disorders, 562
    linguistic elements, 560–2
    power of (in social context), 40–1
    visual loss impacting on, 534
Laughter, 432
Law, see Legal issues; Legislation
Laxatives, 409
Leaflets, health-promoting, 127
Learning, 509–21, see also Education;
        School
    factors affecting, 509–11
Learning difficulty/disability
        (mental handicap), 567–90
    assessment and management,
        569–86
        people involved, 570–2
    behavioural difficulties and,
        581–3
    causes, 509–18, 568–9
        classification, 571
        investigation/diagnosis of, 575
    conditions confused with, 574
    education with severe disability,
        see also Special educational
        needs
        arrangements, 221
        past educational experience,
            221
    identification, 572–3
    investigations, 577–8
    medical problems and conditions
        associated with
        health surveillance, 586
        management, 579–81
        specialist health care, 585
    moderate (MLD) vs severe (SLD),
        567, 568, 570
        differences in characteristics,
            570
    physical examination, 575–7
    services, 585–6
    support for child and family, 264,
        583–5, 593
    terminology, 567–8
Learning theory, 59–60
Legal issues, 253–62, see also
        Legislation
    adolescent services, 394–5
    child abuse cases, 376
    sex education, 280
Legislation, 3–5, 253–6, see also
        specific Acts

education, 217, 218, 479
health visiting, 205–6
social services, 229, 230, 231
special needs, 479
special educational needs, 218,
256, 476, 479, 488
young carers, 337–8
Leisure/recreational activities (incl.
sports), *see also* Play
injuries, 312
physical disability and, 401
young carers, 339
Leiter International Performance
Scale Battery, 65
Leukotriene antagonists, asthma,
405
Lichen sclerosis and atrophicus, 366
Life events, impact, 331
Lifelong learning (continuing
professional development),
35, 186
Lifestyle choices, 7
Linguistic elements of speech and
language, 560–2
Linkage analysis, 83
Listening, school nurses, 212
Literacy (reading/writing)
problems, 522–4
prognosis, 565
Literature reviews, information
from, 20–2
Local authorities, 234–5
looking after/committed to care
of child, 234–5, 257–8, *see also*
Children's homes;
Residential care; Social
services
needs of child, 341–6
recommendations for change,
344
parenting role, 237
partnerships with NHS,
education and, 222
social services, *see* Social services
Local education
authorities/departments
(LEAs), 217, 219, 222
health promotion, 275
parent partnership schemes
(pupils with special
educational needs), 221, 222
special educational needs and,
486, 487
equipment provision, 503
hearing loss, 554
support services, 223–4
Local Government Act (1888), 4
Local service agreements, 172
Long-sightedness (hypermetropia),
537, 538
Low birthweight babies, *see also*
Small-for-gestational age
chronic adults disease and, 14,
136

follow-on milks, 104
Lower reference nutrient intake
(LRNI), 95, 96
LRNI (lower reference nutrient
intake), 95, 96
LSD, 389
Lung disease, chronic, infants, 402
Luteinising hormone (LH), 138, 139
Lymphadenopathy, cervical
tuberculous, 304

M
McCormick Toy Discrimination
Test, 551
Macrocephaly, 416
Magic mushrooms, 389
Makaton vocabulary, 499, 564
Development Project, 593
'Making a Difference', 214
Malnutrition, prenatal, *see* Foetus
Management
clinical, community paediatrician
in, 1
service, 167–76
community paediatrician in, 2
definitions/terminology, 167–9
Mantoux test, 304
Marfan's syndrome, 68, 69, 70–1,
146
genetic tests, 88
Masturbation, 439
Maternal issues, *see* Mothers
Maternity and Child Welfare Report
(1916) and Act (1918), 4–5
Meals on wheels, 232
Measles, 298–300, *see also* MMR
Meckel–Gruber syndrome, 82
Media, mass, health promotion, 127,
275
Medical conditions, *see* Disease
Medical history, *see* History, patient
Medical literature reviews,
information from, 20–2
Medical services, school, *see* School;
School nurses
Medical staff, 184
Medical treatment, *see also* Health
care
consent, *see* Consent
learning difficulties associated
with, 512
specialist, *see* Secondary care;
Specialist care; Tertiary care
Medication, *see* Drug therapy
Meetings, 173
Menarche, 381–2
Mencap website, 252
Meningitis
H. influenzae type B, 306
hearing loss, 552
meningococcal, 306
support organisation, 593
tuberculous, 303
Meningococcal disease, 306

Mental age, scoring in Griffiths
Scales of Mental
Development, 64–5
Mental handicap, *see* Learning
difficulty
Mental health, 423–67
adolescents, 385
government strategy in (reducing
death rate from mental
illness), 273
ill-health/dysfunction
(psychological difficulties),
423–67, *see also* Emotional
and behavioural difficulties;
Psychiatric disorders
counselling appropriate to, 469
in local authority care, 342–3
promotion, health visitors, 210
Mental Health Foundation's 'Don't
Forget Us', 581–2
Mental health needs (psychological
needs)
child, 11–12
local authority care and, 342–3,
343, 345
community paediatrician, 29–37
parental, 278
Mental health staff, 185
Mental retardation syndromes, 70,
73
Metaphase spread, 82
Metaphyseal fractures, 358
Metered dose inhalers, 404–6
5,10-α-Methylenetetrahydrofolate
reductase gene, 81
Methylphenidate (in ADHD), 450–1
Microcephaly, 416
Microdeletions and microdeletion
syndromes, 70, 74–6
congenital heart malformations,
81
Microduplication, chromosomal,
74–6
Midwives, 184, 194–5
in health promotion, 275
Migraine, 418
Miliary tuberculosis, 303
Milk, *see* Breast milk; Cows' milk;
Follow-on milk; Formula
feeds/milks
MMR (measles/mumps/rubella)
measles vaccine in, 299
mumps vaccine in, 300
rubella vaccine in, 300
Mobility, *see also* Movement
problems
assessment, 496
equipment, 502
Mobility Component of Disability
Living Allowance, 245–6
learning disability and, 584
'Modernising social services', 237–8
Molecular DNA tests, *see* DNA tests
Mongolian blue spots, 360

Morbidity statistics, 18–20
Moro reflex, 50
Mortality/death (and death rates),
    7, 17, see also Bereaved
    children; Suicidal children;
    Terminally ill
  adolescents, 384
    causes (other than drugs), 384
    drugs, 387, 387–90
  infant, see Infants
  information on death rates, 17, 18
  from injury (unintentional
    injuries), 309
    mechanisms/types of injury,
      309, 310
    reduction, 273, 314, 319
    reduction (incl. government
      strategies), 273
    accidents, 273, 314, 319
Mosaicism, 87
  gonadal, 70
Mothers, see also Parents; Pregnancy
  attachment problems, 428–9
  depression (postnatal), 278, 430
  nurse home visits (pre-
    /postnatal), 332–3
  teenage, 393–4
Motor and sensory neuropathy,
    hereditary, 76
Motor skills
  development, 50–6, see also
    Sensorimotor stage
    fine skills, 53–6
    gross skills, 51–3
    visual loss and, 533–4, 534
  problems
    in cerebral palsy, 504–5
    clumsiness, 519–22
    learning disability vs other
      disabilities, 574
Motor system, ocular, examination,
    537
Mouth co-ordination, 521, see also
    Oral hygiene
Movement Assessment Battery for
    Children, 65
Movement problems, cerebral palsy,
    504–5, see also Mobility
MTHFR, 81
Mucopolysaccharidoses, 588–9, 589
Multidisciplinary team, see Team
Multifactorial inheritance,
    disorders, 80
Mumps, 300, see also MMR
Munchausen syndrome by proxy,
    360
Murmurs, heart, 412
Muscular dystrophy, 506, 588
  support organisations, 592, 593
Musculoskeletal problems, see
    Orthopaedic problems
Mutations, 68, 69–70, see also Genes
  disease-causing, 70–4
  mechanisms, 69–70

Mutism, elective, 564
Myoclonus epilepsy, juvenile, 74
Myopia, 538
Myotonic dystrophy, 74

N
Nail biting, 439
National Child Development Study,
    323
  education and social inequality,
    510
National Children's Bureau (NCB),
    593
  looked-after children and, 345,
    346
National Framework for Assessing
    Performance, 186
National Health Service, see NHS
National Institute for Clinical
    Excellence (NICE), 185–6
National Insurance-based benefits
    and Invalid Care Allowance,
    248
National Service Frameworks,
    181
National Society for the Prevention
    of Cruelty to Children, 349,
    593
National Specialist Commissioning
    Advisory Group, 181
National Survey of Patient and User
    Experience, 186–7
NDN, 76
Neale Reading Test, 522
Necdin, 76
Neck reflex, asymmetrical tonic,
    50–1
Need, children in, 180, 352, 369–70,
    see also Special needs
  Children Act (1989) section 17
    definition, 325–6, 337, 352,
      371
  services for, 169, 180
  social, 236
Needs, health and other
    (child/family), 179–81, see
    also Special needs and specific
    needs
  adolescents, 383–4
    primary care and, 200–1
  assessment, 238, see also
    Framework for the
    assessment of children and
    need and their families
    developing new framework,
      238
    local authority, 233
    population-based, 10–11
    school nurses, 213
  general practice/primary care
    and consideration of, 198–9
    adolescents and, 200–1
  health care, inversely related to
    availability, 325–6

in local authority care (of child),
    341–6
  meeting, 180–1
  young carers', 337, 338
Neglect, 353, 361–2
  models/causation theory, 356
Neighbourhood, 328
Neisseria gonorrhoeae, 367
Neisseria meningitidis, 306
Neonates, 281–2, see also Age;
    Perinatal period; Postnatal
    period
  developmental dysplasia of hip,
    285
    undetected, 419
  health surveillance (e.g.
    screening), 281–2
    hearing, 548
    thyroid-stimulating hormone,
      raised, 22–3, 138
    vision, 284
  mortality, 17
    rates, 18
  new birth review, 281–2
  nutrition, see Nutrition
  reflexes, assessment, 50–1
  speech sounds, 557
  visual assessment, 531–2
Networks, sorting, 171–2
Neural tube defects, 80–2
Neurofibromatosis, 589
Neuroimaging (brain scan),
    learning disability, 578
Neurological problems, 416–18
Neuropathic bladder, 414, 506–7
Neuropathic bowel, 506–7
Neuropathy, hereditary motor and
    sensory, 76
Neuropsychiatric disorders, Down's
    syndrome, 587, see also
    Psychiatric disorders
Newborns, see Neonates
NHS
  1990s reforms, 180–1
  child public health and, 10
  local authority partnerships with,
    education and, 222
  quality in, see Quality
NHS Act (1946), 5
NHS Direct, 178
NHS Reorganisation Act (1973), 5
NHS trusts, 181
NICE (National Institute for
    Clinical Excellence), 185–6
Night-time enuresis, 414, 445, see
    also Enuresis
Nitrites, 389
Nocturnal enuresis, 414, 445, see also
    Enuresis
Non-accidental injury (historical use
    of term), 349–50, see also
    Physical abuse; Self-harm
Noonan's syndrome, 144, 588
Notifiable diseases, 289, 290

Nottingham
  Cope Street centre, 333
  general practice
    child health clinics, 198–9
    health surveillance, 199–200
  looked-after children, specialist
    health services, 345
  Self-Help Nottingham, 265
Nottingham and Nottinghamshire
  parent partnership scheme,
  222
Nottingham Safe at Home Project,
  160–5
Nottingham Young Disabled
  People, 266
NSPCC, 349, 593
Numerical data, sources, 17–20
Nurse(s) and nursing staff, 184–5,
  205–15
  general practice, 194
  home visits, pre-/postnatal, 332–3
  school, see School nurses
  specialist community paediatric,
    183–4, 184–5
Nursery, day, 235
  in infection prevention, 291–2
Nursery schools (infant schools),
  220
  in infection prevention, 291–2
Nurture and affection and forming
  of attachments, 330
Nut allergy, 111–12, 411
Nutrition, 95–121, 330, 406–11, see
  also Diet; Eating problems;
  Feeding; Food; Obesity
  adolescents, 115–18, 384
  development and, 330, 515
  growth and, 136–7, 330
  infant (incl. neonatal), 96–101
    chronic adult disease (and
      prenatal nutrition), 14,
      116–17, 136
    health visitors and, 209
    weanling, 101–4
  infection susceptibility and, 290
  learning-disabled child, 579–80
  national surveys and advice, 95,
    96, 115–17
  physically-disabled child, 496–7
  preschool child, 106–12, 279
  problems, 406–11
  school-age child/adolescent,
    112–15
  support (in medical conditions),
    118–19

O
Obesity, 137, 146, 150–1, 440–1
  aetiology, 151
  definitions, 150–1
  interventions, 151–2
  learning disability and, 579
  physically-disabled child, 497
  preschool child, 111

tall stature and, 146
Observational epidemiological
  studies, 13, 14
Obsessional compulsive disorders,
  458–9
Ocular problems, see Eye
Oestrogens, 139
Offending behaviour, 391–2
Office for National Statistics (ONS)
  censuses for, 17
  hospital episodes, 20
  infectious disease, 20, 21
  longitudinal study, 18
Omneo Comfort I and 2, 100–1
One-parent families, see Single-
  parent families
Ophthalmology, see Eye
Oral hygiene, physically-disabled
  child, 496
Organic solvents and congenital
  malformations, 16
Organisations
  collective defences, 33–4
  stressors in, 29–30
Orthopaedic (musculoskeletal)
  problems, 419
  Down's syndrome, 587
Osteogenesis imperfecta, 359
Otitis media with effusion, see Glue
  ear
Otoacoustic emissions, 548
Otology, see Ear
'Our Healthier Nation', see 'Saving
  Lives: Our Healthier Nation'
Out-of-hours care, 196–7
Outcomes
  in health service, 168, 175
  for young carers, 336–7
Outreach clinics, consultants
  running, 196
Outreach teacher, 224
Overwork, see Workload

P
P value, 15
Paedophile (child sex) rings, 353
Paget–Gorman sign system, 499
  in Landau–Kleffner syndrome,
    563
PAH, 72
Palmar grasp reflex, 50
Parachute reaction, 51
Parent(s), 257–8, see also Carers;
    Child abuse; Family;
    Mothers; Neglect;
    Parenthood; Positive
    Parenting Programme;
    Single-parent families
  benefits, 250–2
  bonding/attachments with, 330,
    428–9
  in child abuse
    failure to use services, 362
    talking to, 371

communication problems and,
  499
conflict/separation/divorce, 428
deafness suspected by, 548
death of, 429
difficult children,
  coping/interventions, 425,
  453, 454–5
disability recognition and
  reaction of, 481–3
failure to thrive related to, 149
genetic counselling, see Genetic
  counselling
health visitors and health
  promotion through, 208
height measurement, 141
in injury prevention, 315
  at home, 160
learning-disabled child
  information for, 583–4
  talking to, 583
mental health
  disorders, 278, 430
  needs, 278
in nutritional support, 119–20
role/responsibilities, 257–8
  consent and, 258
  sex education, 280–1
school agreements with, 221
in sleep problems, 442
  interventions, 443–5
visual loss and impact on, 534–5
Parenthood
  concept, 41–2
  individual's awareness of, 62
Parenting role, local authorities, 237
Parotitis (mumps), 300, see also
  MMR
Partnerships
  in education, 221–2
  school nursing, 212
Patau's syndrome, 70
'Patch', 2, 3
  patch directory for community
    paediatrician, 2–3
Payments for services in primary
  care, 201, see also Benefits
Peanut allergy, 111–12, 411
Pedestrian injuries, 312
Peer education in local authority
  care, 345–6
Peer support, community
  paediatrician, 35
Pendred's syndrome, 78
Perceptual problems, 515, see also
    Auditory–perceptual
    pathway
  cerebral palsy, 505
Performance tests
  hearing, 550–1
  learning disability vs other
    disabilities, 574
Perianal region and sexual abuse,
  363–5

Perinatal period, *see also* Birth
  disability acquisition, 481
    hearing loss, 553
    learning disability, 571
  disability identification, 572
  mortality, 17
    rates, 18
Peripheral myelin protein 22
  (*PMP22*), 76
Perry Preschool Program, 332
Personal Allowance (Income
  Support), 249
Personal child health record, *see*
  Records
Personal life, professional life and
  its impact on, 35
Personnel, *see* Professionals
Pertussis, *see* Whooping cough
Pharmacotherapy, *see* Drug therapy
Phenylketonuria, 72
Phobias, 458
Phones, 170
Phonological problems, 561, 562
Physical abuse, 352, *see also* Non-
  accidental injury
  clinical features, 357–60
  sexual abuse and, 363
Physical disability, 493–508
  assessment and management,
    494–6
  education, *see* Education
  epidemiology, 493–4
  medical review, 496–501
  support organisation, 593
Physical examination
  asthma, 403
  dysmorphic child, 85
  learning disability, 575–7
Physical features, learning
  disability, 575–6
Physical health, *see* Health
Physical illness, *see* Disease
Physiotherapy, cerebral palsy, 504–5
Piaget, Jean, 62–3
Picture pointing, 499
Place to Call Our Own, A
  (APTCOO), 267
Places of work, 3
Plagiocephaly, 416
Planning, services, 168, 172, *see also*
  Annual business plan
  epidemiological studies aiding, 15
  role of community paediatrician,
    2
Play, 56–9, *see also*
    Leisure/recreational
    activities
  autism and, 451
  physical disability and, 501
Playgroups, 235
PMP22, 76
Pneumatic otoscopy, glue ear, 420
Pneumococcal vaccine, 307
Point mutations, 69

Poisoning, 318, 360
Polio, 297–8
Political aspects, *see also*
    Government
  child abuse, 351
  immunisation programmes, 295
Pollution, air, and asthma, 402
Polygenic disorders, 80
Polyglutamine tracts, 73
Polymerase chain reaction, 83
Polymorphisms, 69, 87
  cystic fibrosis, 72
Polysaccharides, non-starch,
    preschool child, 108
Population, Census information, 17
Population-based needs assessment,
    10–11
Portable auditory response cradle,
    548
Portage Scheme, 334
Posetting, 105–6
Positive Parenting Programme, 209
Positive predictive value, 23–4
Posters, health-promoting, 127
Postnatal period
  disability acquisition, 481
    hearing loss, 553
    learning disability, 571
  disability identification, 573
Post-traumatic stress disorder, 459
Postural development, 51–3
Poverty/deprivation, 7–8, 43, 45, *see
    also* Health inequalities;
    Social class; Social factors
  in Acheson Report, 323–4
  adolescents, 390–1
  Child Poverty Action Group
    website, 252, 591
  definitions and measures, 43,
    324–5
  effects, 7–8
  health, 7, 11, 325, 326
Powder devices, asthma, 406
Power, health professionals, 45–6,
    see also Empowerment
Prader–Willi syndrome, 76, 77, 588
  support organisation, 593
Precocious puberty, 147, 382
Predictive genetic testing, 86
Predictive value, positive, 23–4
Pregnancy, *see also* Birth; Mothers
  teenage, 393–4
  termination, *see* Abortion
Premature adrenarche, 148
Premature infants (preterms)
  asthma, 402
  formula feeds after discharge,
    104
  fractures, spontaneous, 358
  retinopathy, 531
Premature puberty, 147, 382
Premature thelarche, 148, 382
Prenatal period, *see* Foetus
Preschool children/early years (1–5

years incl. toddlers), *see also*
    Age
  diarrhoea, *see* Diarrhoea
  diet and nutrition, 106–12, 279
  disability recognition, 481, 573
  education, 220, 222
    deprived children, and its
      effects, 7–8, 331
    early years worker, 224
    health promotion/surveillance
      programme, 278–9, 282–3
    hearing tests, 284
    vision tests, 284–5
  immunisation programme, 295
  motor development
    fine skills, 55–6
    gross, 52–3
  Perry Preschool Program, 332
  social and behavioural
    development, 57–9
    Erikson's theories, 60–1
Prescriptions in general practice,
    191–2, 193
Preterm infants, *see* Premature
    infants
Prevalence, 12
Prevention (preventive health care),
    22–3
  accident, *see* Accidents
  importance, 6
  infection
    environmental and personal
      measures, 291–3
    vaccines in, *see* Immunisation
  primary, *see* Primary prevention
  secondary, *see* Secondary
    prevention
  tertiary, *see* Tertiary prevention
Primary care, 177, 189–207, *see also*
    General practice
  accidental injury treatment in (in
    Nottingham Safe at Home
    Project), 162
  future directions, 201
  health promotion and, 274
    facilities and equipment
      required, 275
  health visitors and, 206, 207
  learning disability and, 585
  links with other
    services/organisations, 196
  medical staff, 184
  payments for services in, 201
  people involved, 193–6
  referrals from, *see* Referrals
Primary care trusts, 181, 189,
    201
Primary prevention/interventions,
    23, 269, 270
  child abuse, 376
  injuries (unintentional), 314
Primary school-age children, 220,
    see also School
  education, 220

Index

special educational needs
    coordinator, 223
    support assistant, 223
obesity interventions, 61
social/behavioural development,
    61
tests on starting school, 283
    sensory, 284, 285
Private medicine, 187
Process (in health service), 168
Professionals/personnel/staff
    (predominantly health
    professionals), see also Carers;
    Services and specific posts;
    Team
    allied to medicine, 185
    child protection and, see
        Protection
    court appearance, see Witness
    expectations of others, 29
    in health promotion, see Health
        promotion
    learning disability assessment
        and management, 570–2
    in local authority care
        concerns of, 343
        consultation to, 345
        training, 346
    physically-disabled child, 495–6
    power, 45–6
    in primary care, 193–6
    psychological needs, 29–37
    roles (in general), see Roles
    self-regulation, 186
    visually-impaired child, 535
Prognosis, epidemiological studies
    impacting on, 14–15
Projective identification, 33
Protection/safeguarding of child,
    349–80
    agencies involved, 368–9
        interagency working, 368–9
        social services, see Social
            services
    history-taking in protection cases,
        256
    legal aspects, 253–6
    professional/health professional
        involvement, 370–3
        health visitors, 208
        school nurses and, 212
        supervision and support, 379
    protection registers, 233–4
        numbers of children on, 351
Protein intolerance, cows' milk, 118,
    407
Psychiatric disorders, 423–35, see
    also Neuropsychiatric
    disorders
    child, 423–35
        assessment and aetiology,
            423–4
        family and, 427–31
        definition, 424

parent, 430
Psychiatry service, referral to, 464–5
Psychoanalytical theory, Erikson's,
    60–2
Psychological factors, GP
    consultation rates, 197–8
Psychological treatments, 462–4
Psychological well-being and
    difficulties, see Mental health
Psychology services, educational,
    224
Psychopathic states and child
    abuse, 353–4, 356
Psychosocial factors, child abuse,
    354–5
Psychotic disorder
    drug-induced, 387
    schoolwork and, 517
Psychotropic medication, learning-
    disabled child with
    behavioural problems, 583
Puberty, 381–2, see also Adolescents
    delay, 382
        constitutional, 142
    growth, 135
    hydrocephalus and, 507
    precocious, 147, 382
    recording, 140
Pubic hair development, 381, 382,
    383
Public attitudes, immunisation, 296
Public health (child), 7–27, see also
    Department of Public Health
    broad vs narrow approaches, 7, 8
    health visitors and, 208–9
    interface with community
        paediatrics, 6
    long time-scales, 7–8
    observations about, 11–12
    people/organisations involved,
        8–10
    specialists, functions, 10–11
Pulmonary disease, chronic, infants,
    402
Pulmonary tuberculosis, 303
Punishment fitting crime
    (undisciplined child), 454–5

Q
Quality, services
    in NHS, 167–8, 175, 185–7
        primary care, 201
        standards of, see Standards
    voluntary organisations, 264
Quality-adjusted life years (in
    cost–utility analysis), 159
Quality Protects, 236–7, 255, 344
Questions in counselling, open vs
    closed, 473–4

R
Race, see Cultural issues; Ethnic
    groups
Radford Family Centres, 331–2

Radiograph, see X-ray
Random error, 16
Rates (in epidemiology), 12
RDAs (recommended daily
    amounts), 95
Reading problems, see Literacy
Realism, infantile, 63
Recessive mutations causing disease
    autosomal, 71–2
    X-linked, 72–3
Recommended daily amounts
    (RDAs), 95
Records and record-keeping
    birth, 17
    child abuse, 378–9
    child's personal health record (=
        Red Book), 2, 275–7
        health visitors and GPs writing
            in, 195–6
    learning-disabled child, 583–4
    family tree, 83–5
    infection, 289
    puberty, 140
Recreational activities, see Leisure
    activities; Play
Recreational drug use, 386
Red book, see Records
Reference nutrient intake (RNI), 95,
    96
Referencing (language acquisition),
    558
Referrals
    to child and adolescent
        psychiatry service, 464–5
    schoolchildren making poor
        progress, 518–22
    to social services (in child abuse),
        370–1, 371
    to specialist care (from
        primary/GP care), 192, 196
        emergency (in A&E
            departments), 183
Reflection in counselling, 474–5
Reflex(es)
    neonatal, assessment, 50–1
    persistent primitive, in cerebral
        palsy, 505
    Piaget's ideas, 62
Reflux, gastro-oesophageal, 409–10
Refractive error, 538–9
    learning-disabled child, 581
    measurement, 539
Registers of individual diseases, 20
Relaxation (coping with anxiety),
    458
Remedial help, see Special
    educational needs
Renal tract problems, 413–15
Residential care (incl. children's
    homes), 231–2, 235
Resources
    allocative efficiency, 156
    demand and, balancing, 174
Respiratory disorders, 401–6

Respite care, learning-disabled
    child, 584
Retinitis pigmentosa, 78–80
Retinopathy of prematurity, 531
Reye's syndrome, case-control
    study, 13–14
Reynell Developmental Language
    Scale, 65
Reynell–Zinkin scales, 65
Rib fractures, 358
Rights (legal/human), 261–2
    adolescents, 395
    young carers, 337
Risk factors
    adolescent mental health
        problems, 385
    learning difficulties (moderate
        difficulties), 511
    retrospective ascertainments of
        exposure to, 16
    unintentional injury, high-risk
        children, 313–14
Risk management (in health
    service), 168
Risk-taking
    by child/adolescent, 279, 385–90
        altering risk-related behaviour,
            128
    by health professional, as stressor,
        30
Ritualistic abuse, 353
RNI (reference nutrient intake), 95,
    96
Road traffic accidents, 312
    deaths, 310
Roles (in child health), 6
    community paediatrician, see
        Community paediatrician
Rolls, 502
Rubella, 300–1, see also MMR
Russell–Silver syndrome, 143

S
Sadness, 433
Safeguarding, see Protection
Safety advice (accident prevention),
    314, 315–16
    home (Nottingham Safe at Home
        Project), 160
Sanfilippo's syndrome, 589
'Saving Lives: Our Healthier
    Nation', 7, 125, 187, 214, 219,
    272–3, 314
    accident prevention, 273, 314,
        319
Scalds, non-accidental, 359
Scar(s), non-accidental, 359–60
Scarcity (in health economics), 155,
    156
Schedule of Growing Skills, 64
Schema/schemata, Piaget's, 62
Schonell Test, 522
School(s), 509–21, see also Education;
    Learning

behavioural problems, 455–7
    counselling covering, 472
    disabled school-leaver, 488
    exclusion from (preventing
        infection spread), 291–2
    learning in, 509–21
        chronic illness affecting, 511–
            14
        influence of school, 509–10
        referral for poor progress,
            assessment, 518–22
    medical/health services, 256–7,
        see also School nurses
        adolescents, 396–7
        health promotion, 131–2
    non-attendance, 391–2, 456–7, 511,
        516–17
        in long-standing illness,
            511–12
    roles/responsibilities, 222–3
    sex education, 280–1, 397
    special needs pupils in
        communication problems,
            499
        specialist vs mainstream
            schools, 487, 494
School-age children, 279–80
    development
        (social/behavioural), 61
    health behaviour, 18
    health promotion/surveillance
        (incl. screening), 113–14,
        131–2, 133, 279–80
        obesity interventions, 152
        tests on starting school, 283,
            284, 285
    nutrition, 112–15
School effectiveness and
    improvement services, 224
School meals, 113–14
School nurses (and nursing), 184,
    211–15
    future directions, 213–14
    health promotion, 131–2, 274
    philosophy of nursing, 212
    process of nursing, 212–13
    range of activity, 211–12
Screening (and screening
    programmes), 22–6, 270–1,
    281–5
    advantage of early detection by,
        271
    antenatal, 281
    criteria for appraising screening
        programmes, 25, 26
    criteria for 'good' screening test,
        271
    developmental, 64
    Down's syndrome, 158
    hearing, 283–4, 546–8
    information required about
        screening programme, 172
    neonates/infants, see Infants;
        Neonates

opportunistic, 272
    pitfalls, 271
    preschool, 278–9, 284, 284–5
    sensitivity and specificity, 23–4
    sensory impairment, 283–5
    vision, 284–5, 539–41
    yield, 24
Seating, disabled child, 501–2
Seckel's syndrome, 589
Secondary care (specialist care),
    177
    medical staff, 184
Secondary
    prevention/interventions,
    22–3, 269, 270
    child abuse, 376
    injuries (unintentional), 314
Secondary school, 220, see also
    School
Segregation analysis, 83
Seizures, see Convulsions; Epilepsy
Selection bias, 16
Self-esteem, 427
Self-harm, deliberate, 462
Self-help groups, 264–5
    child protection and, 376
Self-regulation, professional, 186
Senior house office level, paediatric
    training at, 3
Sensitivity, screening test, 23–4
Sensitivity analysis (in economic
    evaluation), 157
    Nottingham Safe at Home
        Project, 163–4
Sensorimotor neuropathy,
    hereditary, 76
Sensorimotor stage of development,
    Piaget's, 62–3
Sensorineural hearing
    loss/deafness, 283, 497,
    545–6
    causes, 553
    investigation of, 551
    hereditary, 76–8
Sensory skills, see also Hearing;
    Vision
    impairment, 283–5
        learning difficulties with, 514
        sensory teachers (school), 224
    visual loss impacting on, 533–4
Separation (loss of
    parent/pet/friend etc.),
    phases, 433
Services (in/related to child health),
    177–268, see also
    Professionals; Team
    adolescents, 394–8
    community paediatrician in
        service management and
        frameworks, 2
    directories of, 172
    drug abuse, 390
    hearing-impaired, 554
    history, see History

information on use of, 18–20
integration, 181
learning-disabled child, 585–6
local, agreements, 172
looked-after children, new
    developments, 344–6
management, see Management
neglect and failure to use, 362
planning, see Planning
primary care, see Primary care
providers, 181, see also specific
    services
secondary care, see Secondary
    care
special needs children, 489
    audit, 489
tertiary care, see Tertiary care
unequal access to, 331
visually-impaired, 535–6
for young carers, 340
young carers projects, 339
Sex, see Gender
Sex chromosomes, see also Fragile X
    chromosome
aneuploidy, 70
recessive mutations causing
    disease, 72–3
Sex education, 280–1, 397
Sex steroids
female, 138–9
male (testosterone), 138–9
Sexual abuse, 353, 363–6, see also
    Child sex rings
clinical features, 363–6
homeless young women, 391
Sexual arousal as motivation for
    abuse, 355
Sexual health, 392–4
Sexual intercourse, age and law
    and, 395
Sexually transmitted diseases
adolescents, 392–3
sexual abuse and, 366–8
Sheeps' milk, 103
Sheldon Report (1967), 5
Shock (parents) with news of
    disability, 482
Short-sightedness (myopia), 538
Short stature, 142–5
Shunt (in hydrocephalus), 506–7
Siblings, learning-disabled child,
    support, 584
Sickle cell disease, 15
Sickle Cell Society, 266
Sign languages, 499
in globally delayed development,
    564
in Landau–Kleffner syndrome,
    563
Single-/one-parent families, 429–
    30
support organisations, 592, 593
Sites of work, 3
Skeletal dysplasia, 144

Skills, see also Schedule of Growing
    Skills
equipment helping disabled child
    with, 503–4
for reading, skills required, 523
sensorimotor, see Motor skills;
    Sensory skills
Skin conditions/problems, 419
learning disability and, 576
    Down's syndrome children, 587
Skin tests, asthma, 403
Skinfold measurements, 140, 150
Sleep problems, 442–5
learning affected by, 515
Small-for-gestational age, 136
Small nuclear ribonucleoprotein N,
    76
Smile, infant, 432
Smith–Lemli–Opitz syndrome, 589
Smith–Magenis syndrome, 75–6
Smoking, see also Cigarette burns
prenatal exposure, and asthma,
    402
teenagers, 7, 12, 385–6
Social class, see also Poverty; Social
    factors
consultation rates and, 197
health related to, 323
unintentional injuries, 313
Social development, 56–9
Erikson's theories and their
    impact on, 60–2
learning disability vs other
    disabilities, 574
visual loss and, 534–5
Social Exclusion Unit, 392
Social factors (incl. social
    deprivation), see also Poverty;
    Psychosocial factors; Social
    class
child abuse, 354, 356
learning/education affected by,
    510
psychiatric disorders, 430
Social Fund, 244, 250
Social index, 325
Social issues, adolescents, 385
Social misbehaviour, see Antisocial
    behaviour
Social paediatrics, community
    paediatrician in, 1
Social reforms and child abuse, 351
Social science, 39–47
definitions of sociology, 39–40
everyday life and, 46–7
history and current structure,
    229–30
Social security benefits, see Benefits
Social services (local authority etc.),
    169, 185, 229–39, see also
    Social workers
future changes, 237–8
interface with community
    paediatrics, 6, 185

protection/safeguarding of child,
    233–4, 237, 253–4, 254–5, 369
initial assessment, 371–2
initial child protection
    conference, 372–3
outcome of section 47
    enquiries, 372–3
paediatrician's contribution to
    case conferences, 376
referral to social services,
    370–1, 371
review conference, 374–5
special needs/disabled children
    and, 487–8
equipment provision, 503
leaving school, 488
types of service provided, 230,
    231–7
child-specific, 233
young carers and, 340
Social support, see Support
Social workers, looked-after
    children and training of, 346
Socioeconomic factors, asthma, 402
Sodium cromoglycate, asthma, 405
Soiling (faecal incontinence), see also
    Continence problems
non-organic cause, see Encopresis
physically-disabled child, 500
Solid foods, moving to, 101–4
Solvents
misuse, 386–7
deaths, 390
education and, 517
congenital malformations and, 16
Sotos' syndrome, 147, 589
Soya formulas, 103–4
in cows' milk protein intolerance,
    118, 407
Special educational needs (SEN)
    and remedial help, 219–21,
    486–8
definition, 479
legislation, 218, 256, 479
parents and, 221
physical disability, 494
hydrocephalus, 507
muscular dystrophy, 506
reading/writing problems, 522
special educational needs
    coordinator in primary
    school, role, 223
special needs teacher, 224
Special needs (children with),
    479–92, see also Disability
audit of services, 492
education, see Special educational
    needs
health visitors and, 209–10
multidisciplinary team, see Team
registers, 489–92
specialist health care, 585
support organisations, 593
Specialist care, special needs

children, 585, *see also*
   Secondary care; Tertiary care
Specialist community paediatric
   nurses, 183–4, 184–5
Specialist looked-after health teams,
   344–5
Specialist registrar level, paediatric
   training at, 3
Specialist role, health visitors, 206
Specialist support teaching staff, 224
Specialist young carers projects, 339
Specificity, screening test, 23–4
Speech, 557–66, *see also*
   Communication
   acquisition, 557–8
   discrimination (hearing test), 551
   linguistic elements, 560–2
   problems, 557–66
      classification schemes, 561
      interventions, 498, 565
      other developmental delays
         associated with, 563–5
      physically-handicapped child,
         497
      prevalence, 556
      prognosis, 565
Speech therapy, 498, 565
Spelling/writing problems, 522–4
Splints, 502
Sports injuries, 312
SPRPN, 76
Squint (strabismus), 536, 537
   cover test, 537, 538
   management, 537–8
Staff, *see* Professionals
Standards
   of quality (of care), 175, *see also*
      Clinical Standards Advisory
      Group
      delivering, 186
      monitoring, 186
   of school education, raising,
      218–19
Stature, *see* Height
Statutory Social Fund, 250
Steady state evoked potential,
   549–50
Stepping reflex, 50
Steroids, *see* Androgens;
   Corticosteroids; Sex steroids
Stickler's syndrome, 78
Stillbirth, 17
   rates, 18
Stimulation, inadequate, 329
Strabismus, *see* Squint
Strategic Heath Authorities, 181
Stress (and stressors), *see also* Post-
   traumatic stress disorder
   child
      emotional stress, 427
      enuresis and, 445
   professionals (incl.
      paediatricians), 29–30, 31–4,
      176

organisational stress, 29–30
   responses to stress, 31–4
Structure (in health service), 168
Sturge–Weber syndrome, 589
Substance abuse, *see* Drug abuse
Sugars, non-milk intrinsic,
   preschool child, 107
Suicidal children, 462
Sun safe educational intervention,
   209
Supervision, professional, child
   protection/children in need,
   379
Supine length, measurement, 139
Supplies, 168
Support
   of children, *see also* Support
      groups
      by counsellor, 471
      learning disability (and support
         of family), 583–5
      by school nurses, 212
   of professionals
      child protection/children in
         need and, 379
      social support of community
         paediatrician, 35–6
Support assistant, primary school,
   223
Support groups/organisations, 264,
   591–4, *see also* Voluntary and
   charitable organisations
   learning disability, 264, 585, 593
Support services, education, 223–4
Supports (for disabled child), 502
Sure Start, 273
'Surestart', 210–11
Surgical problems, 415–16
Surveillance, *see* Health surveillance
Syncope, 418
Syndromes, *see also* Genetic
   disorders *and specific*
   syndromes
   with global delay in
      development, 564
   with hearing loss, 552
   with learning difficulties, 518,
      587–9
   physical features, 576
Syntactic problems, 561, 562
Syphilis, 368
Systematic error, 15, 16

T
Talking, *see* Communication; Speech
Tall stature, 145–50
Tax credits/benefits
   Council Tax Benefit, 251
   Disabled Person's Tax Credit, 251
   Working Families Tax Credit,
      250–1
TCOF1, 68
Teachers, school
   health promotion and, 131–2

special needs/disability and, 225
   specialist support staff, 224
Teaching and training
   by community paediatrician, 2
   of community paediatrician (and
      other health professionals), 3,
      34–5, 184, *see also* Continuing
      professional development
   of GPs (in child health care), 190
   of local authority care staff, 346
   of school nurses, 214
Team/workforce
   (multidisciplinary), 2–3, 171,
   184–5, *see also* Professionals;
   Services *and specific posts*
   framework for, 171
   health visitors and, 206
   in primary care, 193–6
   skills mix and staffing, 168
   special needs children, 489
      assessment (by child
         development team), 483–6
      physical disability, 495–6
Teasing (school), 456
Technical efficiency, 156
Teenagers, *see* Adolescents
Teeth, *see* Dentition
Telephone, 170
Temper, bad (and temper tantrums),
   459–60, *see also* Anger
Temperament, 331, 425
Tension headache, 418–19
Teratogens and congenital heart
   malformations, 81, 82
Terminally ill, Disability Living
   Allowance, 245
Tertiary (specialist) care, 177
   medical staff, 184
Tertiary prevention/intervention,
   23, 269, 270
   child abuse, 376
   injuries (unintentional), 314
Testes, undescended, 415
Testosterone, 138–9
Tetanus, 305, *see also* DTP vaccine
Thelarche (breast development), 383
   premature, 148, 382
Therapists in health promotion,
   275
Think Children, 267
Thinking and anxiety, 458
Thoughts and anxiety, 458
Threshold criteria (care
   proceedings), 260
Thumb sucking, 439
Thyroid hormone (thyroxine), 138
   deficiency/excess, *see*
      Hyperthyroidism;
      Hypothyroidism
   treatment with, 411
Thyroid-stimulating hormone,
   raised, neonatal, 22–3, 138
Thyroxine, *see* Thyroid hormone
Tics, 439–50

Time
  management, 170
  stress due to pressures of, 30
Toddler, *see* Preschool child
Toilet (and toiletting)
  learning-disabled child, 581
  physically-disabled child,
    equipment helping, 502–3
  training, 447–8
Tonsillar infection, tuberculosis, 304
Tooth, *see* Dentition
Total communication system, 499
Townesend index, 325
Trachoma, 528
Training, *see* Teaching and training
Transference, 33
Translocation, chromosomal, 68, 70
Transport injuries, 310, 312
Travel
  carer/parent, to hospital, help
    with costs, 252
  child, abroad, 307
  paediatrician, 169–70
Treacher Collins syndrome, 68, 78
Trichomonas vaginalis, 367
Triplet repeat expansion disorders,
  69, 73–4
Trisomies, 70
  chromosome 21, *see* Down's
    syndrome
Truancy, 391–2, 456–7, 516–17
Tube-feeding, 119
Tuberculosis, 302–5
  diagnosis, 304
  presentation, 303–4
  prevention, 304–5
Tuberin, 71
Tuberose/tuberose sclerosis, 71, 589
  support organisation, 594
Tumours, CNS/brain, 507
Turner's syndrome, 143–4, 589
  classical (45,X), 70, 87
  mosaicism, 87
  short stature, 143–4
Tympanometry, 549
  glue ear, 420

U
UBE3A, 76
Ubiquitin-protein ligase E3A gene,
  76
Umbilical hernia, 415
Universal Neonatal Hearing
  Screening, 548
Urinary incontinence, *see* Enuresis
Urinary tract infections, 414–15
Usher's syndrome, 78, 553–4
Utility (in cost–utility analysis),
  158–9
Utting report, 234–5

V
Vaccination, *see* Immunisation
Vagina and sexual abuse, 365, 366

Vaginosis, bacterial, 368
Varicella/zoster immunisation
  active (= vaccine), 307
  passive (= immunoglobulin), 293
Vegetarianism, 114, 115
Ventricular septal defect, 413
Violence, domestic, 377
Viral respiratory infections and
  asthma, 402
Vision (and visual impairment),
  527–41, 578–9
  aetiology
    developing countries, 527–9
    UK, 529–31
  clinical signs of impairment,
    532–3
  colour, *see* Colour vision
  definitions of impairment, 527,
    528
  development, normal, 531–3, 537
  education, 224, 536
  epidemiology of impairment,
    527–9
  hearing loss accompanying visual
    problem, 553–4
  inherited impairment, 78–80
  learning difficulties and, 578–9,
    580–1
    assessment of vision, 578–9
    learning difficulty due to visual
      loss, 514, 578
  learning difficulties associated
    with (but not caused by)
    visual loss, 578–9
  physically-disabled child
    cerebral palsy, 505
    tests, 497
  screening, 284–5, 539–41
  services with impairment, 535–6
  severe/profound loss, *see*
    Blindness
  support organisations, 594
Visual acuity, 531
Visual reinforcement audiometry,
  550
Vitamin(s)
  requirements
    infants, 104
    school-age child, 113
  supplements
    infants, 104
    preschool child, 108
Vitamin A, 527–8
  breast feeding and, 97
  deficiency, 527–8
Vitamin B$_{12}$ and vegetarianism, 114
Vitamin D, breast feeding and, 97
Vocabulary
  infant, 558
  Makaton, *see* Makaton vocabulary
Voluntary and charitable
  organisations, 263–8, 591–4,
    see also Support groups
  activities, 264–7

child protection, 376
  special need children, 489
  contacting/working with, 267–8
  defining, 263–4
  geography and, 266–7
  primary care links with, 196
  quality issues, 264
  value, 267
Vulva and sexual abuse, 365, 366

W
Waardenburg's syndrome, 78, 82
War and child abuse, 350
Ward Infant Language Screening
  Test Assessment Acceleration
  Remediation, 334
Warts, genital, 367
Watch, 170
Water, drinking, infants, 104
Weanling, food, 101–4
Websites, *see* Internet
Wedges, 502
Weight
  excess, *see* Obesity
  on growth charts, 135–6
  low, at birth, *see* Low birthweight
    babies
  measurement, 139–40
  reduction programmes, 151
Welfare rights services, 232
Well-being, *see* Health
Weschler Intelligence Scale for
  Children, 65
Weschler Preschool and Primary
  Scale of Development, 65
Wetting, *see* Enuresis
Wheelchairs, 502
Wheezing, 403
Whey-dominant formulas, 98–9,
  100
WHO (World Health Organization)
  health promotion, 123–5
  health status monitoring, 133
  International Classification of
    Functioning and Disability,
    479–80
Whooping cough (pertussis), 301–2
  notification, 21
  vaccination, 302
    coverage figures, 21
Williams syndrome, 75, 589
WILSTAAR programme, 334
Wind, 105
Witness, professional, 260–1
  child abuse, 376
Women, *see also* Gender; Girls;
  Mothers
  child abuse by, 357
  domestic violence and, 377
  genital mutilation, 378
  homeless young, sexual abuse,
    391
Women's movement and child
  abuse, 351

Word(s), infant use, 558
Word boards, 499
Work place/work setting, pressures
    in, 29–32, 176
  managing, 34
Workforce, *see* Professionals; Team
Working Families Tax Credit,
    250–1
Workload
  excess (overwork)
    children, 516
    professionals, 30
  in general practice, 190–3

World Health Organization, *see*
    WHO
Wrist X-ray (growth assessment),
    141
Writing problems, *see* Literacy

X
X (chromosome), 72–3
  fragile site (= fragile X
    syndrome), 73, 74, 588, 592
  inactivation, 72, 73
  recessive disease mutations, 72–3
45,X, *see* Turner's syndrome

X-ray
  chest, asthma, 403
  hand/wrist (growth assessment),
    141
XXY (Klinefelter's syndrome), 147
XYY, 147

Y
York Centre for Reviews and
    Dissemination, website, 22
'Young Carers in the UK: a profile',
    335
Youth Offending Teams, 274